Prevention in Clinical Practice

Prevention in Clinical Practice

Edited by

Daniel M. Becker, M.D., M.P.H.

University of Virginia School of Medicine
Charlottesville, Virginia

and

Laurence B. Gardner, M.D.

University of Miami School of Medicine
Miami, Florida

Plenum Medical Book Company • New York and London

Library of Congress Cataloging in Publication Data

Prevention in clinical practice / edited by Daniel M. Becker and Laurence B. Gardner.
p. cm.
Includes bibliographies and index.

ISBN-13: 978-1-4684-5358-4 e-ISBN-13: 978-1-4684-5356-0
DOI: 10.1007/978-1-4684-5356-0

1. Medicine, Preventive. I. Becker, Daniel M. II. Gardner, Laurence B., 1941–
[DNLM: 1. Preventive Medicine. WA 108 P9422]
RA425.P718 1988 88-12568
614.4′4–dc19 CIP

233 Spring Street, New York, N.Y. 10013

Softcover reprint of the hardcover 1st edition 1988

Plenum Medical Book Company is an imprint of Plenum Publishing Corporation

For our wives,
Madaline and Behna
and to our late friend and mentor,
Eric Reiss, M.D.,
physician, scientist, teacher, pianist,
whose love of medicine and music enhanced all our lives

Contributors

Daniel M. Becker, M.D., M.P.H. • Department of Internal Medicine, University of Virginia School of Medicine, Charlottesville, Virginia 22908

Joseph R. Berger, M.D. • Departments of Neurology and Internal Medicine, University of Miami School of Medicine, Miami, Florida 33101

Randolph J. Canterbury, M.D. • Departments of Behavioral Medicine and Psychiatry and Internal Medicine, University of Virginia School of Medicine, Charlottesville, Virginia 22908

Joseph C. Chan, M.D. • Department of Medicine, University of Miami School of Medicine, Miami, Florida 33101

Julia E. Connelly, M.D. • Department of Internal Medicine, University of Virginia School of Medicine, Charlottesville, Virginia 22908

Eugene C. Corbett, Jr., M.D. • Department of Internal Medicine, University of Virginia School of Medicine, Charlottesville, Virginia 22908

Mark R. Cullen, M.D. • Occupational Medicine Program, Yale University School of Medicine, New Haven, Connecticut 06510

David C. Deitz, M.D., Ph.D. • Division of General Medicine and Primary Care, Department of Medicine, Beth Israel Hospital, Harvard Medical School, Boston, Massachusetts 02215

Gordon M. Dickinson, M.D. • Department of Medicine, University of Miami School of Medicine, Miami Veterans Administration Medical Center, Miami, Florida 33101

David S. Fedson, M.D. • Department of Internal Medicine, University of Virginia School of Medicine, Charlottesville, Virginia 22908

Arthur M. Fournier, M.D. • Department of Medicine, University of Miami School of Medicine, Miami, Florida 33101

Laurence B. Gardner, M.D. • Department of Medicine, University of Miami School of Medicine, Miami, Florida 33101

Richard L. Greenman, M.D. • Department of Medicine, Division of Infectious Diseases, University of Miami School of Medicine, Miami Veterans Administration Medical Center, Miami, Florida 33101

Mary P. Harward, M.D. • Department of Internal Medicine, Northwestern University School of Medicine, Chicago, Illinois 60611

Elizabeth Hodapp, M.D. • Department of Ophthalmology, University of Miami School of Medicine, Miami, Florida 33101

Roger E. Kelley, M.D. • Department of Neurology, University of Miami School of Medicine, Miami, Florida 33101

Mark Multach, M.D. • Department of Medicine, University of Miami School of Medicine, Miami, Florida 33101

Mark T. O'Connell, M.D. • Department of Medicine, University of Miami School of Medicine, Miami, Florida 33101

John T. Philbrick, M.D. • Department of Internal Medicine, University of Virginia School of Medicine, Charlottesville, Virginia 22908

Eric Reiss, M.D.† • Department of Medicine, University of Miami School of Medicine, Miami, Florida 33101

David V. Schapira, M.B., Ch.B. • H. Lee Moffitt Cancer Center, University of South Florida School of Medicine, Tampa, Florida 33612

Robert P. Smith, Jr., M.D., M.P.H. • Department of Medicine, Dartmouth–Hitchcock Medical Center, Hanover, New Hampshire 03756

Jay M. Sosenko, M.D., M.S. • Department of Medicine, University of Miami School of Medicine, Miami, Florida 33101

J. Donald Temple, M.D. • Department of Medicine, University of Miami School of Medicine, Miami, Florida 33101

Edward J. Trapido, M.D., Sc.D. • Department of Oncology, University of Miami School of Medicine, Miami, Florida 33101

James A. Wolff, Jr., M.D., M.P.H. • Management Services for Health, Boston, Massachusetts 02130

†Deceased.

Foreword

Prevention of disease and injury, including early identification of risks and disease and optimal control of potentially debilitating or fatal complications of chronic conditions, is the area of clinical medicine that holds the greatest promise for improving human health. Each year a long list of major, but potentially preventable health problems exacts a terrible human and financial toll. These problems urgently need our attention, especially as major advances in curative medicine become more complex and costly. Prevention of disease and injury may well be the central health issue of our time, an issue of vital concern to every quarter of our society.

Now is a very good time to promote prevention. Citizens and some social groups are increasingly aware of and interested in health and fitness issues. There is great enthusiasm about—even obsession with—health, and we are seeing an astonishing proliferation of health publications and media presentations for laymen, fitness and weight control centers, exercise programs, health food stores, disease support groups, health education programs, and do-it-yourself diagnostic kits. All of this betokens an increased health consciousness on the part of public and perhaps signals greater individual accountability for health.

Despite the indisputable value of prevention in general, there is a great deal of uncertainty, even confusion, on the part of the public and health professionals about specific preventive practices. What are the most important practices? What about their relative value and costs? What about this recommendation, or that?

We need accurate information about preventive interventions. Each measure must be assessed individually and analyzed in all its dimensions—benefits, risks, and costs. Although many preventive measures do improve health, they are not without risks and costs and, in fact, they seldom reduce medical expenditures. Only with documentation in hand will we be able to speak with conviction and authority about specific interventions and justify the allocation of resources to implement the most efficacious preventive practices.

People everywhere are showing greater willingness to take responsibility for their own good health. Physicians can foster this attitude by helping patients manage their health, by assisting them in making the daily choices that influence health and well-being, and by providing them with the facts and figures for informed decision making. But, like the public, physicians need accurate, authoritative information on the benefits, risks, and costs of practices that promote health and prevent disease and injury. *Prevention in Clinical Practice* will play an important role by providing much-needed information and by bringing into focus for health professionals those preventive practices and interventions of the greatest import and value.

Edward W. Hook

Introduction

It is a difficult time to practice medicine in the United States. Biomedical advances have led to increased precision and efficacy in the study and treatment of disease, yet physicians are increasingly hampered by the difficult ethical and economic issues raised in the wake of rapid technological and sociological change. It now seems clear that medical resources are limited even in the United States. Moreover, it is not clear how to get the most from what is available. From both clinical and financial perspectives rational practice would require an understanding of the harm done from either too little or too much medical care. Yet standards of minimal care have not been defined, and even if the ill effects of excessive care were easy to describe, decisions to limit care for the individual patient are extremely difficult. Despite the complexity and uncertainty inherent in evaluating the efficacy and fairness of health care, time for these analyses is short, and it appears inevitable that physicians will alter their practices before such data are available. Federal authorities are setting financial limits in the form of DRG reimbursement schedules; private third parties are planning prospective payment as well; and a more consumer-conscious public expects efficient as well as quality care. Somehow physicians must learn to achieve both cost restraint and a high standard of practice. To make this task even harder, growing medicolegal pressures can lead to defensive practices that undermine cost containment. Finally, amid these rising economic, governmental, consumer, ethical, and legal pressures, physicians also have to contend with increased competition. The public now has a greater choice of physicians, and in a freer market it is possible that physicians who are noncompetitive in terms of cost, quality, and efficiency will lose patients. Ironically, this competition might lead to excessive use of some expensive practices that appeal to the public conception of "good" care (e.g., executive physicals).

In response to the social and economic forces now helping to shape clinical practice, biomedical education and clinical training are changing. To guide health policy and to illuminate clinical thinking, methods for integrating social and clinical values into medical decision making are being developed and taught. To develop critical thinking and to broaden perspectives on health and disease, epidemiological principles are being applied in clinical settings. To reduce costs and to emphasize continuity of care, both patient care and clinical teaching are being shifted from the hospital to the clinic. To address health manpower issues, primary-care training is being encouraged as subspecialization is discouraged. With this emphasis on costs and benefits, rational clinical decision making, clinical epidemiology, and primary care, one would expect that the concept of prevention would be a rallying point for those learning how to apply medical technology fairly, effectively, and humanely.

Certainly preventive medicine is an important aspect of the new primary-care curriculum. However, limited studies suggest that preventive care is practiced poorly and erratically. Traditional and orthodox health care in this country has tried to cure disease. Medical schools and teaching hospitals teach their students and house staff to look for disease and then treat it. Traditional health insurance pays physicians to do this. In fact, preventive services may not be paid for while procedures of almost any sort are generously covered. Most of the time patients seek medical help when they are sick, not preventively. Taking into account the tradition of curative medicine and what its participants (physicians, patients, third parties) expect, it is still not clear why we do such a poor job of practicing preventive medicine. That we do a poor job of teaching preventive medicine no doubt contributes to this failure.

There are many ways to improve how we teach prevention. As previously mentioned, curricula and practice sites are changing. Disciplines such as epidemiology, biostatistics, management science, decision analysis, and economics are being taught at medical schools and in house staff programs. In teaching situations it is now possible to highlight a clinical problem, present a preventive intervention in epidemiological as well as biomedical terms, guide use of this preventive strategy in a practice site where continuous care is possible, and eventually measure the success or failure of such efforts.

To encourage preventive medicine and hopefully to make its practice easier, this book offers guidelines and rationales for disease prevention. It is written for physicians in primary-care settings, postgraduate trainees, medical students, and physician extenders, such as nurse practitioners and physician assistants. The book demonstrates how a public health perspective and epidemiological thinking can be used in daily practice. The book focuses on what can be done for the individual patient. Preventive care issues as they relate to public health policy are not specifically reviewed. Thus, for example, the argument for seat-belt use is not presented. The clinical situations are not limited to those where primary prevention (aimed at the disease) is possible. In a sense all medical care is preventive (aimed at complications). However, some chronic diseases with relatively long incubation periods for complications offer great opportunities for secondary preventive care. Diabetes mellitus, hypertension, and atherosclerosis were selected for discussion as common diseases whose complications can often be prevented. For the purposes of this book, the preventive aspects of the management of these diseases will emphasize early and accurate diagnosis, risk factor recognition and modification, and early nonpharmacological treatments. Tertiary prevention, as commonly practiced in hospitals and rehabilitation centers, will not be discussed.

As well as specific recommendations for preventive practice, the pertinent epidemiological principles, facts, and controversies are discussed. General chapters that review the major causes of morbidity and mortality in the United States and the interpretation of diagnostic tests are included. Although the book is a clinical guide written for practitioners, the epidemiological and socioeconomic justifications for recommended practices are stressed.

Implicit in this approach is the premise that clinical decisions and habits cannot rely solely on biomedical science. To deliver quality care at a reduced cost, it is now up to physicians to develop rational practices that integrate biomedical knowledge with the particular needs of society. Prevention as well as cure must be a major goal of those trusted with caring for patients.

Daniel M. Becker
Laurence B. Gardner

Contents

5. *Antimicrobial Prophylaxis*

Gordon M. Dickinson

6. *Hepatitis*

Richard L. Greenman

7. Streptococcal Pharyngitis

Mark Multach

8. Tuberculosis

David C. Deitz

9. Sexually Transmitted Diseases

Joseph C. Chan

14. Thromboembolism

Daniel M. Becker

15. Nephrolithiasis

Laurence B. Gardner

16. *Cancer*

David V. Schapira and J. Donald Temple

17. *Stroke*

Joseph R. Berger and Roger E. Kelley

20. *Health Advice for International Travelers*

Robert P. Smith, Jr., and James A. Wolff, Jr.

21. *Occupational Medicine*

Mark R. Cullen

25. Alcoholism and Drug Abuse

Randolph J. Canterbury

26. Periodic Health Examination

Julia E. Connelly

1

Patterns of Illness and Medical Practice in the United States

Daniel M. Becker

1. INTRODUCTION

Before discussing specific diseases and how they can be prevented or mitigated, it is useful to review in general terms both the health of the American people and why people visit physicians. There are abundant data describing the causes of morbidity and mortality in the United States. There are also studies that describe what kinds of problems are treated in primary-care practice. Comparing national statistics with patterns of office care should highlight where preventive efforts can be made and how the practitioner can participate in preventing early death and disability. In reviewing these data the health problems of adults will be emphasized.

2. MORBIDITY AND MORTALITY IN THE UNITED STATES

In 1979 the Surgeon General reported on the health of the American people.[1] Impressive health gains are described. The overall crude death rate from 1900 to 1979 has fallen from 17 per 1000 persons per year to less than nine per 1000. However, these gains vary according to the population studied (Fig. 1). The following sections describe the major health problems of adolescents and young adults, adults, and the elderly. The data are from the National Center for Health Statistics, as summarized in the Surgeon General's report.[1]

2.1. Adolescents and Young Adults

Since 1960 the death rate for adolescents and young adults (aged 15–24 years) has been increasing. Most deaths in this group are violent, related to motor vehicle accidents,

Daniel M. Becker • Department of Internal Medicine, University of Virginia School of Medicine, Charlottesville, Virginia 22908.

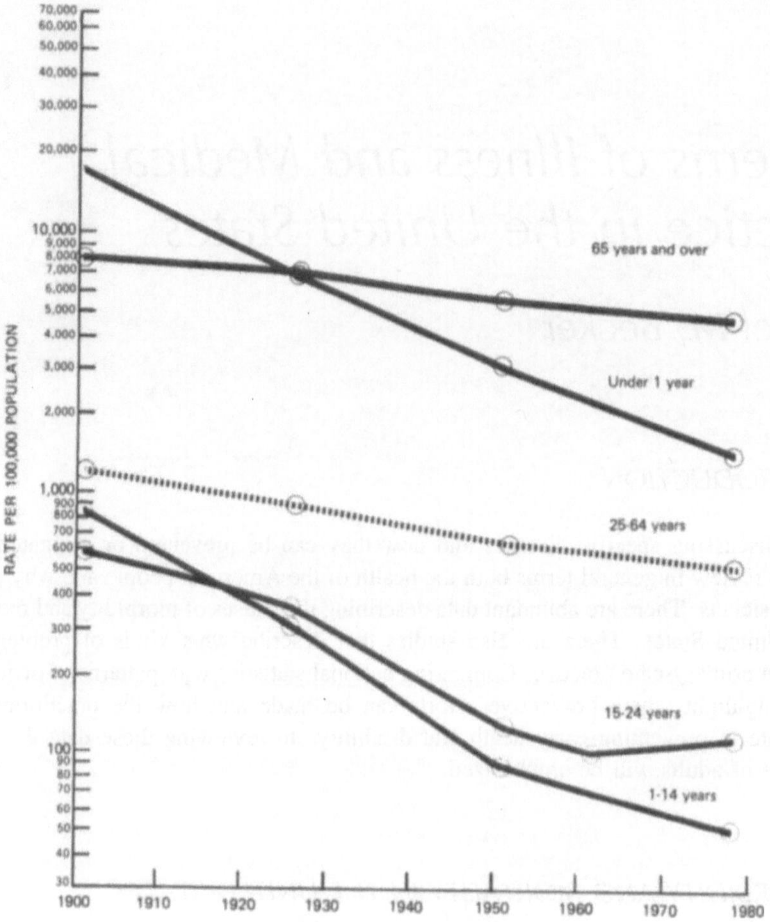

Figure 1. Death rates by age: United States, 1900–1977. Graphs based on data from 1906, 1950, 1960, and 1977. (Source: Ref. 1.)

industrial accidents, and homicides (Fig. 2). Young men are more likely than women to die violently, and black men are at particularly high risk to become homicide victims.

Alcohol and substance abuse underlie much of this violence. Half of the highway fatalities have blood alcohol levels that imply intoxication (greater than 100 mg/dl). Homicide is also associated with alcohol use. Substance abuse other than alcohol is becoming increasingly prevalent. It seems likely that illicit drugs such as cocaine, hallucinogens, sedatives, and amphetamines are contributing to the various categories of accidental and violent deaths in this age group.

Suicide is the third leading cause of death in this category. Since 1950 the suicide rate in young people has increased approximately five times. The United States is not alone with this problem. Other industrialized nations (Japan, Sweden, Germany) have even higher rates of suicide.

Childbearing during adolescence is hazardous for the mother and for the child. By

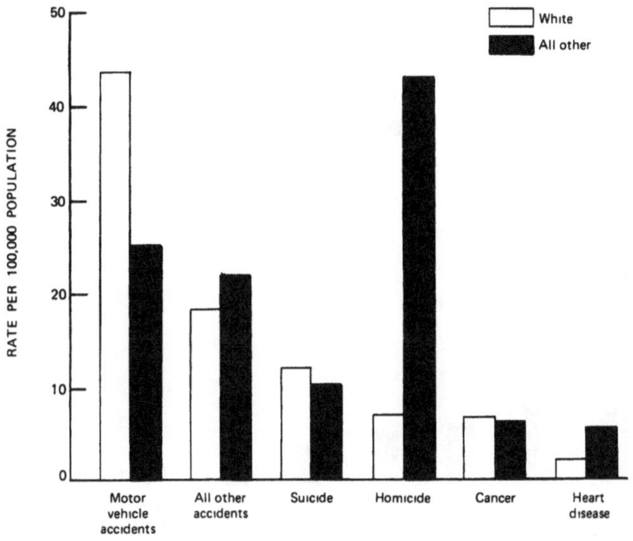

Figure 2. Major causes of death for ages 15–24 years: United States, 1976. (Source: Ref. 1.)

age 19 approximately 25% of American teenage girls have been pregnant at least once. Infants of teenage mothers are twice as likely to be of low birth weight and thus at risk for a host of neonatal and developmental problems. Young mothers are less likely to have received perinatal care and more likely to experience complications during pregnancy and at term.

More than 80% of reported sexually transmitted diseases occur among 15- to 29-year-olds. Although the incidence of syphilis and gonorrhea seems to be decreasing overall, both diseases are increasing in teenagers. Other "newer" venereal diseases such as herpes and nonspecific urethritis are most prevalent in this age category. Aside from the acute illness, these infections can cause permanent morbidity. Pelvic inflammatory disease leads to sterility in an estimated 75,000 women of childbearing age per year.

2.2. Adults

Within the age range of 25–64 years, the death rate since 1900 has fallen from 1200 per 100,000 population per year to less than 540. However, the overall gains in life expectancy during this century tail off with advancing age. For an infant, life expectancy has increased more than 26 years since 1900. For a 45-year-old man, further life expectancy has increased only 5 years compared to a 45-year-old at the turn of the century. Although preventive measures have dramatically changed infant mortality rates, the chronic diseases that afflict adults remain difficult to treat.

Heart disease, cancer, stroke, and cirrhosis are the leading causes of death in adults aged 25–64 years (Fig. 3). Together heart disease and stroke account for approximately one-third of these deaths. Reductions in mortality for these diseases have been occurring, and in large part these changes explain the overall decline in mortality.

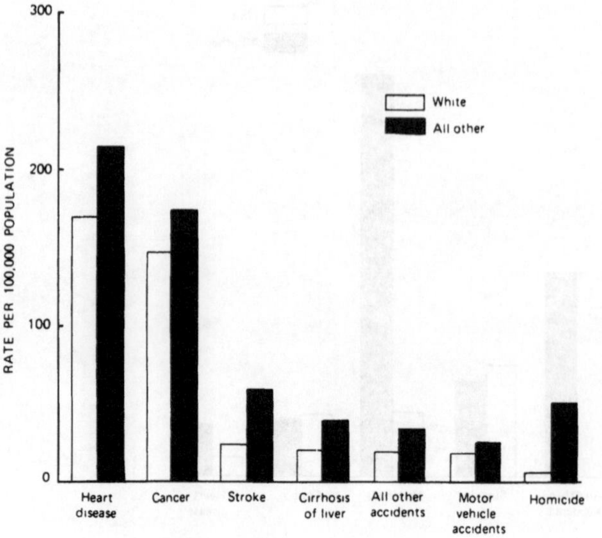

Figure 3. Major causes of death for ages 25–64 years: United States, 1976. (Source: Ref. 1.)

Preventive efforts have probably been important in reducing cardiovascular mortality.[2,3] Hypertension and smoking are major risk factors for the development of coronary artery disease and cerebrovascular disease. Control of hypertension can now be achieved for the vast majority of patients, and fewer adults in this age group are continuing to smoke. Elevated cholesterol is the third major risk factor for early cardiovascular mortality. More specific laboratory testing (e.g., high-density lipoprotein and apoproteins, as well as total cholesterol) allows more specific assessment of this risk. Dietary habits seem to be changing in the United States, and indirect evidence that such changes reduce or retard atherosclerotic heart disease is available.[2,3] Similarly, more Americans are exercising regularly, and it is possible to relate this behavioral change to the decline in cardiovascular mortality.

More than one-third of cancer deaths occur between the ages of 35 and 64 years. Because the population is aging, the crude cancer rate is increasing. After age adjustment the cancer rate for men since 1937 has increased slightly, while for women it has decreased slightly. Cigarette smoking is a major risk factor for many cancers and leads to more cancer deaths than any other known exposure. Compared to nonsmokers, smokers have 10 times as much lung cancer, more than three times as much oral and laryngeal cancer, and at least twice as much bladder cancer. Other important and modifiable exposures include alcohol, radiation, occupation, and environmental pollution. Geographical differences in cancer rates may in part be explained by dietary differences. If food additives and lack of dietary fiber prove to be important as cancer risks, opportunities for prevention will be obvious.

Alcohol use is a major contributor to morbidity and mortality in the United States. Alcohol is a factor in approximately 10% of all United States deaths. In 1977 there were an estimated 10 million alcoholics in the country and 30,000 deaths from cirrhosis. Alcohol use is also an important factor in deaths from accidents, homicides, and suicides. Alcohol is associated with cancer at several sites, including head and neck, liver, and esophagus. Excess alcohol use is socially disruptive, interfering with employment and family life. Domestic violence such as spouse and child abuse can often be related to alcohol.

The acquired immunodeficiency syndrome (AIDS) has become a major contributor to mortality in certain risk groups.[4] Male homosexuals are the largest risk group for AIDS. Presently in Manhattan and San Francisco, for single males aged 25–44 years, AIDS is the most important cause of mortality. Intravenous drug abuse and repeated exposure to blood products are also important risk factors for AIDS. Changes in blood banking will reduce the latter risk. Drug abuse is a risk that is theoretically preventable. Male homosexuals can alter their sexual behavior to reduce their risk, and there is evidence that this is occurring.[4]

2.3. Elderly

The population of the United States is growing older as the death rate for the elderly falls. In 1900 only 4% of the population was older than 65 years. By 2030 that figure will be 17% and will include 50 million people. In 1900 the death rate for those over 65 years was 8300 per 100,000, and by 1977 the death rate for these ages was 5400. The major decline in this rate has been for the ages 65–74. In fact mortality curves for those older than 85 years have declined only slightly in the last 30 years.

The major categories of mortality are slightly different for the ages 65 years and older compared to adults aged 24–64 years. Cardiovascular disease and cancer are important for both groups. Influenza, pneumonia, atherosclerosis, and diabetes mellitus become more important with aging, while accidents and liver disease are less common causes of mortality (Fig. 4). Many of the elderly have multiple chronic problems. Eighty percent have one or more chronic conditions, and these illnesses require more than 30% of

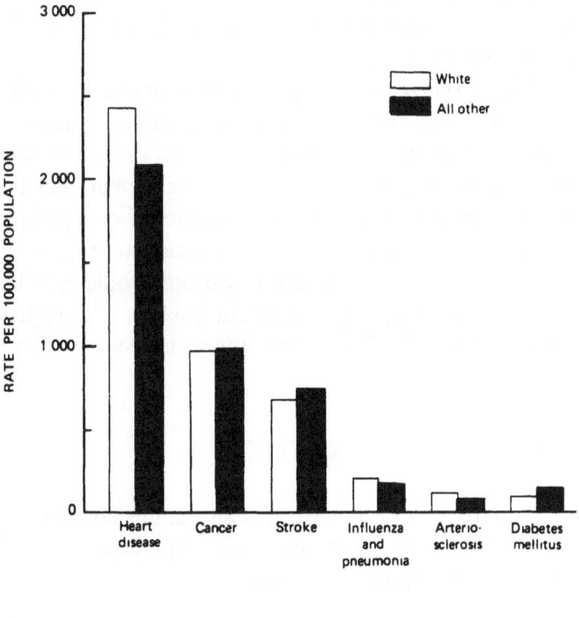

Figure 4. Major causes of death for ages 65 years and over: United States, 1976. (Source: Ref. 1.)

Table I. Death Rates by Race and Sex, 1983[a]

		Ratio of age-adjusted rate	
Rank	Cause of death	Male : female	Black : white
	All causes	1.76	1.47
1	Heart disease	1.96	1.31
2	Malignancy	1.49	1.33
3	Cerebrovascular disease	1.18	1.82
4	Accidents	2.82	1.21
	Motor vehicle	2.74	0.85
	Other	2.93	1.64
5	Chronic lung disease	2.47	0.76
6	Pneumonia and influenza	1.84	1.43
7	Diabetes mellitus	1.01	2.21
8	Suicide	3.50	0.49
9	Chronic liver disease	2.16	1.70
10	Atherosclerosis	1.29	1.02
11	Homicide and legal intervention	3.57	5.51
12	Perinatal disease	1.26	2.35
13	Renal disease	1.46	2.70
14	Septicemia	1.46	2.79
15	Congenital anomalies	1.11	1.01

[a]Source: Ref. 5.

national health care expenditures. Mortality statistics fail to portray the impact of these problems. More than 40% of the elderly have functional limitations due to chronic illness. These physiological limitations include mental impairment, visual and auditory difficulty, and arthritis. Accidents, although less important as a cause of mortality, remain significant. Orthopedic injuries, particularly hip fractures, can be severely disabling. The day-to-day difficulty of chronic disease is compounded by social and economic problems. These factors together with physical problems often lead to complete dependency and a need for institutional care.

Health statistics can say something about the social and economic factors related to fatal or disabling diseases and events. Table I summarizes in demographic terms recent data on leading causes of death.[5] Some of the differences in sex- and race-related risk are due to socioeconomic differences. Black men are much more likely than white men to be murdered or executed. Perhaps because of occupational differences, women are three times less likely than men to die in accidents. Figure 5 represents years of potential life lost between age 1 and 65 due to various problems.[6] These data need to be compared to the list of leading causes of death in Table I. Although cardiovascular disease and cancer cause more overall deaths, their impact is lessened compared to accidental injury because they occur later in life.

3. *PATTERNS OF PRACTICE*

Another way of looking at health in this country is to review the reasons why people visit physicians. Descriptions of office practice are available from individual physicians and also from national surveys.

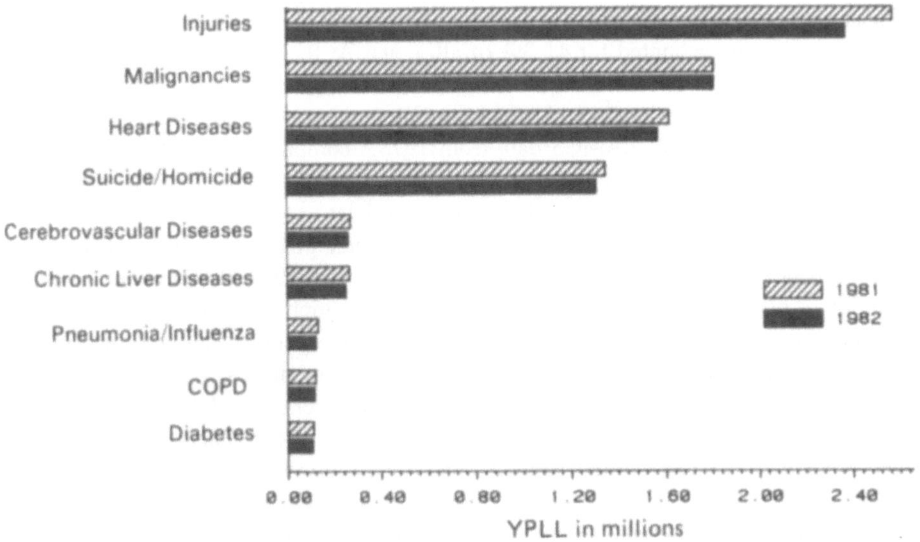

Figure 5. Years of potential life lost (YPLL) in millions, from age 1 until the 65th birthday, United States, 1981–1982. COPD, chronic obstructive pulmonary disease. (Reprinted with permission from Ref. 6.)

The National Ambulatory Medical Care Survey (NAMCS) is a study of 50,000 visits to a sample of 3000 physicians in office-based private practice. It has been conducted annually from 1974 to 1981, and since 1984 it is scheduled for every 3 years. The most recent available data are from 1981.[7] In that year, there were approximately 585,177,000 visits to physicians, with an average of 2.6 visits per person per year. For those persons over 65 years old, there were 4.3 visits per year. The annual visit rate for women was higher than for men (3.1 visits versus 2.1 visits). Whites, comprising 85.7% of the overall population, accounted for 89% of all visits.

These data allow comparisons between specialties. Table II presents the distribution

Table II. Visits according to Selected Physician Specialties, 1981[a]

Specialty	Number of visits (in thousands)	(Percent)
All visits	585,177	100[b]
General and family practice	189,966	32.5
Internal medicine	74,539	12.8
Pediatrics	64,539	11.0
General surgery	32,769	5.6
Obstetrics and gynecology	53,912	9.2
Psychiatry	15,954	2.7

[a]Source: Ref. 7.
[b]Subspecialty data are not included. Therefore, the overall percentage is less than 100%.

of visits by specialty. The contribution from family–general practice has declined steadily since 1975, when it accounted for 41.3% of all visits. At the same time internists have increased their share from 10.9% to 12.8%.

The basis for these visits can be listed according to the patient's reason for seeing the doctor. Table III, based on NAMCS data from 1975,[8] compares internists and family–general practitioners for the 18 most common problems or symptoms. In addition to data from national sources, descriptions by individual physicians of their private practices are useful. The categorical results of surveys are particularly difficult to interpret in areas related to patient education and psychosocial support. In 1973 Burnum published a description of his general internal medicine practice. He emphasized the idea of care for the "total person."[9] Patients with disabling emotional problems accounted for 11% of Burnum's practice. Many of these patients had coexisting organic disease. Burnum found that "human behavior . . . was largely inseparable from internal medicine" and that for most patients "functional" and "organic" problems were combined. NAMCS data suggest that internists and family–general practitioners provide support for emotional problems in less than 4% of patient visits.[8] This figure underestimates the supportive care given as more concrete complaints are explained, investigated, and treated.

Table III. Common Symptoms and Problems: Comparison of Internists and Family–General Practitioners[a]

Reason	Rank: Family or general practitioner[b]	Rank: Internist[c]
Back pain	1	8
Lower-extremity pain	2	4
Abdominal pain	3	5
General examination	4	1
Required examination	5	14
Fatigue	6	3
Upper-extremity pain	7	10
Headache	8	13
Chest pain	9	2
Sore throat	10	17
Cough	11	12
High blood pressure	12	6
Cold	13	16
Vertigo/dizziness	14	11
Shortness of breath	15	7
Medication	16	18
Diabetes mellitus	17	15
No complaint	18	9

[a]Source: Ref. 8.
[b]Forty-seven percent total practice time.
[c]Fifty-two percent total practice time.

4. PREVENTION

Patients visit physicians for treatment, prevention, or explication of findings. Table IV displays NAMCS data from 1977 and 1978 in these terms. Diseases, symptoms, treatments, and injuries explain 78% of visits. During this period preventive care was the major reason for 17% of visits. Table V compares various specialties in terms of their preventive practices.[10] The 10 items compared account for almost all of the preventive care noted by this survey. Eye visits are not included, but eye examination accounts for 19% of visits to ophthalmologists. The data in Table V do not represent all the preventive care provided during the survey period. In addition, the preventive items listed were mentioned as secondary reasons for 19.6 million visits to physicians.

Although a significant proportion of ambulatory practice can be considered preventive, there is some evidence that preventive efforts by physicians are inadequate and erratic. Expert panels have published recommendations for periodic health examinations, and physicians have been surveyed to see how they compared to idealized standards of preventive care.[11–13] It should be noted that there is substantial disagreement between experts. The Canadian Task Force on the Periodic Health Examination offers the most conservative advice based only on properly evaluated practices.[11]

Romm and others showed that practicing internists followed expert opinion in terms of periodic health examinations for about 60% of items.[14] Surprisingly, physicians in this survey agreed least often with the most carefully established guidelines (Canadian Task Force). Furthermore, there was substantial disagreement between the practitioners and the experts on what should be included in a periodic examination. This study revealed both a lack of consensus regarding specific preventive measures and a failure to implement those measures which were acceptable.

A group of Massachusetts primary-care physicians were surveyed by mail to examine their role in health promotion.[15] Although they agreed that stopping smoking, eating a balanced diet, and wearing seat belts were "very important," less than half felt that moderating alcohol use, decreasing salt consumption, avoiding saturated fats and choles-

Table IV. Reasons for Visits to Physicians[a]

Reason for visit[b]	Percent distribution of visits
Symptom	56.2
Disease	8.7
Treatment	9.0
Injuries and adverse effects	4.2
Diagnostic, prevention, screening	18.3
Test results	0.5
Administrative	1.7
Other	1.3

[a]Source: Ref. 10.
[b]National Ambulatory Medical Care Survey 1977–78: 1,154,550,000 office visits.

Table V. Preventive Care by Specialty[a]

Preventive practice	Physician specialty (% of visits) General and family practice	Internal medicine	Pediatrics	Obstetrics–gynecology
1. General examination	4.3	7.7	16.0	5.5
2. Well baby examination	0.9	—	8.5	—
3. Routine prenatal care	2.2	0.0	0.1	29.1
4. Postpartum examination	0.2	—	—	3.0
5. Breast examination	0.0	0.1	—	0.2
6. Gynecological examination	0.3	0.1	0.1	11.1
7. Blood pressure test	3.2	5.5	0.0	0.1
8. Pap smear	1.0	0.4	0.0	2.2
9. Prophylactic inoculations	0.9	0.5	1.2	0.2
10. Family planning	0.4	0.1	0.0	1.7

[a]Source: Ref. 10.

terol, and exercising regularly were "very important." Regardless of what the physician believed was important, only 3–8% thought they were "very successful" in helping their patients change harmful behaviors.

Another mailed survey asked members of a California county medical society if they preached what they practiced in their health-counseling habits.[16] Physicians with better personal health habits were more likely to try to help patients break unhealthy habits. Again, as in the Massachusetts survey, a low percentage of respondents (12%) thought they were effective in counseling against pernicious behaviors such as smoking. Internists and family practitioners in this survey counseled more frequently than surgical specialists.

Assuming that too little preventive care is provided, what are the reasons? There are barriers to preventive practice for both physicians and patients. Just as physicians disagree about the benefits and applicability of some preventive methods, patients can easily underestimate the value of early diagnosis or intervention. Most practice settings and schedules make little allowance for the extra time and effort needed for counseling, education, and testing. Furthermore, the majority of health insurers exclude reimbursement for health maintenance or prevention. Some physicians resort to using creative diagnoses to shift payment for screening tests to the insurance company. A comprehensive review of the problems of implementing preventive care has recently been published.[17,18]

Although it seems that prevention is the exception rather than the rule in ambulatory practice, there is some evidence that physician education does improve adherence to preventive standards. A randomized trial at Cleveland Metropolitan Hospital showed that house officers routinely taught preventive guidelines actually increased their preventive practices.[19] The experimentally educated groups of residents ordered significantly more screening mammograms and immunizations than the control groups. Long-term data from similar experimental interventions are not available. Systems changes in clinical practice have also been shown to improve preventive efforts. Computers can monitor the ongoing physician–patient relationship and provide reminders when preventive measures are indicated. In Indianapolis computer reminders were tested in a 2-year randomized trial.[20]

Occult blood testing, mammographic screening, weight reduction diet, and vaccination for influenza or pneumococcus were increased in the experimental group. A nurse reminder system was used in a similar way in a North Carolina study.[21] Significant changes in stool occult blood testing, breast examination, and influenza vaccination were documented.

Preventive strategies can be part of the hospital routine as well as the office. Fedson argues persuasively that previous hospitalization is a common risk factor for serious pneumococcal infection. It follows, therefore, that the hospital could be an important site for vaccination.[22]

In the present economically austere health care climate, preventive medicine must prove to be a sound investment. Although cost–benefit analyses are promising, data that demonstrate savings from actual preventive programs are lacking.[18] The potential savings from preventive medicine are enormous. For example, in 1976 the direct costs of alcohol-use and smoking-related disease were estimated at $20.5 billion. If indirect costs such as lost earnings are also considered, the total cost of these two personal habits would amount to $59.6 billion, or one-quarter of the total cost of illness in the U.S. population for that year.[23] Scheffler and Daringer describe a program for stopping smoking that costs $125 per person and is 25% successful.[23] Treating 22 million smokers would "cure" 5.5 million. This many fewer smokers would reduce annual health costs by $2.35 billion. There are other dramatic examples of potential savings: rubella vaccination programs; fluoridation of community water; screening for hypothyroidism in newborns; and work site hypertension screening and treatment. Kristein points out the favorable cost–benefit ratio of early diagnosis and treatment of hypertension, breast and colon cancer screening, and treatment for tobacco and alcohol addiction.[24]

These brief descriptions of national health statistics and patterns of ambulatory practice reveal the potential for prevention within a health care system that mainly treats diseases and symptoms. Theoretically and practically, preventive medicine offers many solutions that would ease the national burden of largely avoidable injury and chronic disease. Physicians in their offices can prevent illness as well as diagnose and treat it. Primary-care physicians should be leaders in the national effort to reduce mortality and morbidity by avoiding sickness.

REFERENCES

1. *Healthy People: The Surgeon General's Report on Health Promotion and Disease Prevention.* U.S. Dept. of Health, Education, and Welfare. US Govt. Printing Office, Washington, DC, 1979, pp. 43–80.
2. Stern, M. P.: The recent decline in ischemic heart disease mortality. *Ann. Intern. Med.* **91**:630–640, 1979.
3. Goldman, L., and Cook, E. F.: The decline in ischemic heart disease mortality rates: An analysis of the comparative effects of medical interventions and changes in lifestyle. *Ann. Intern. Med.* **101**:825–836, 1984.
4. Curran, J. W., Morgan, W. M., Hardy, A. M., *et al.*: The epidemiology of AIDS: Current status and future prospects. *Science* **229**:1352–1357, 1985.
5. Advance report of final mortality statistics 1983. *National Center for Health Statistics Monthly Vital Statistics Report.* **34**(6, suppl. 2):1–44, 1985.
6. Centers for Disease Control: Annual summary 1983: Reported morbidity and mortality in the United States. *Morbid. Mortal. Wkly. Rep.* **32**(54):108, 1984.
7. Lawrence, L., and McLemore, T.: *1981 Summary: National Ambulatory Medical Care Survey.* Advance Data 1983, No. 88. National Center for Health Statistics, US Dept. of Health and Human Services.

8. Noren, J., Frazier, T., Altman, I., *et al.:* Ambulatory medical care: A comparison of internists and family-general practitioners. *N. Engl. J. Med.* **302**:11–16, 1980.
9. Burnum, J. F.: What one internist does in his practice: Implications for the internist's disputed role and advocation. *Ann. Intern. Med.* **78**:437–444, 1973.
10. Cypress, B. K.: *Office Visits for Preventive Care, National Ambulatory Medical Care Survey: United States, 1977–78.* Advance Data 1981, No. 69. National Center for Health Statistics, US Dept. of Health and Human Services.
11. Canadian Task Force on the Periodic Health Examination: The Periodic Health Examination. *Can. Med. Assoc. J.* **121**:1–46, 1979.
12. Medical Practice Committee, American College of Physicians: Periodic health examination: A guide for designing individualized preventive health care in the asymptomatic patient. *Ann. Intern. Med.* **95**:729–732, 1981.
13. Breslow, L., and Somers, A. R.: The lifetime health monitoring program: A practical approach to preventive medicine. *N. Engl. J. Med.* **296**:601–608, 1977.
14. Romm, F. J., Fletcher, S. W., and Rulka, B. S.: The periodic health examination: Comparison of recommendations and internists' performance. *South. Med. J.* **74**:265–271, 1981.
15. Wechsler, H., Levine, S., Idelson, R., *et al.:* The physician's role in health promotion—A survey of primary care practitioners. *N. Engl. J. Med.* **308**:97–100, 1983.
16. Wells, K., Lewis, C. E., Leake, B., *et al.:* Do physicians preach what they practice? A study of physician's health habits and counseling practices. *JAMA* **252**:2846–2848, 1984.
17. Inus, T. S., Belcher, D. W., and Carter, W. B.: Implementing preventive care in clinical practice. I. Organizational issues and strategies. *Med. Care Res.* **38**:129–153, 1981.
18. Carter, W. B., Belcher, D. W., and Inus, T. S.: Implementing preventive care in clinic practice. II. Problems for managers, clinicians, and patients. *Med. Care Res.* **38**:195–215, 1981.
19. Cohen, D. I., Littenberg, B., Wetzel, C., *et al.:* Improving physician compliance with preventive medicine guidelines. *Med. Care* **20**:1040–1045, 1982.
20. McDonald, C., Hui, S. L., Smith, D. M., *et al.:* Reminders to physicians from an introspective computer medical record: A two year randomized trial. *Ann. Intern. Med.* **100**:130–138, 1984.
21. Davidson, R. A., Fletcher, S. W., Retchin, S., *et al.:* A nurse initiated reminder system for the periodic health examination: Implementation and evaluation. *Arch. Intern. Med.* **144**:2167–2170, 1984.
22. Fedson, D. S.: Improving the use of pneumococcal vaccine through a strategy of hospital based immunization: A review of its rationale and implications. *J. Am. Geriatr. Soc.* **33**:142–50, 1985.
23. Scheffler, R. M., and Daringer, L.: A review of the economic evidence on prevention. *Med. Care* **18**:473–484, 1980.
24. Kristein, M. M.: Economic issues in prevention. *Prev. Med.* **6**:252–264, 1977.

2

History of Preventive Medicine

Daniel M. Becker

1. INTRODUCTION

The concept of preventive health care is not modern. Before the 20th-century biomedical revolution, important advances had been made in the understanding and prevention of infectious diseases and nutritional deficiency. Long before the advent of scientific investigation into disease processes, men were explaining disease and attempting to avoid illness. In surveying historical efforts to prevent communicable diseases and nutritional deficiency diseases three categories of prevention are apparent; (1) individual control over personal health through adherence to dietary and hygiene codes; (2) social control over health by means of isolating diseased individuals or protecting large groups of people from environmental dangers; (3) application of increased scientific understanding of disease.

2. PERSONAL HEALTH

The dietary and personal hygiene code of the ancient Hebrews, described in Leviticus, Numbers, and Deuteronomy of the Old Testament, provided protection from food-borne and person-to-person spread of disease by calling for personal cleanliness, dietary restrictions, and proper sexual conduct. Greek and Roman medicine, exemplified in the writings of Hippocrates and Galen, considered disease to be a disturbed equilibrium between "natural" (innate) forces and "nonnatural" (external) forces. The ideal healthy life was one in which nutrition and excretion, exercise and rest were properly balanced according to age, sex, and season. Theoretically, diet and exercise could regulate health. This view has remained throughout history.

Although one does not usually associate the Middle Ages with an interest in healthy lifestyles, this was indeed an important concern. During the Crusades the medical school at Salerno developed as a center for recuperation from the religious wars. Its faculty successfully promoted personal health by publishing what was to be one of the most popular secular books of the era, *Regimen Sanitalis Salernitum.* Written originally in

Daniel M. Becker • Department of Internal Medicine, University of Virginia School of Medicine, Charlottesville, Virginia 22908.

Latin verse but soon translated into common European languages, it gave simple, common-sense advice on sleep, diet, drink, and sex. For example[1,2]:

> Joy, temperance, and repose
> Slam the door in the doctors' nose

and

> Wine, women, baths by art or nature warme,
> used or abused do men much good or harme

Similar advice regarding proper lifestyle appears in the 18th century in Jeremiah Wainewright's *Mechanical Account of the Non Naturals.*[1] Finally, in our own times, there is a continuing fascination with diet and exercise as routes to spiritual as well as physical health.

3. SOCIETY

There is archeological evidence of sanitary engineering in the earliest Mesopotamian civilizations. The Hebraic codes mentioned previously mandated both protection of the water supply from fecal contamination and sanitary disposal of excreta. Sanskrit writings from 2000 B.C. recommend use of copper plumbing and charcoal filtration of water. Among the Roman engineering accomplishments were aquaducts to deliver relatively clean water to cities, indoor plumbing, and sewer systems. Specific deities overlooked these sanitary works: Cloacina (hence *cloaca* or *sewer*), the Goddess of Drains, and Stercutius, the Dung-God.[2]

With the Renaissance and rebirth of civilization came the invention of the water closet in 1596 by Sir John Harrington, a nephew of Queen Elizabeth. However, widespread use of toilets did not occur until the 19th century. In Europe and the United States the mid-19th century brought the "great sanitary awakening." In 1850 in Massachusetts, Lemmuel Shattuck, inspired by English sanitary reformers, published *A Report of the Sanitary Commission of Massachusetts,* which called for wide-scale public health improvements, including a clean water supply and proper sewage.[3] During the 19th century urban water systems were progressively purified, with the introduction of filtration, chlorination, and bacterial oxidation techniques. Most of these sanitary reforms were established before their microbiological rationale was formulated.

The recommendation that diseased individuals should be separated from society originates from the Old Testament (Leviticus), which linked spiritual and physical uncleaness. Leprosy, urethral discharge, and menstruation required separation from the community as well as a purification rite. In the Middle Ages the church policy of isolating lepers was based on biblical admonitions. Later, plague victims were dealt with similarly. Not only were the diseased isolated, but their homes and social contacts were also restricted. Quarantine policies, which required visitors to communities to be isolated and observed to ensure they were not plague carriers, developed in the 14th century. The efficacy of these quarantine efforts was dubious since knowledge of disease spread was limited. In the 18th century James Lind recommended that newly impressed seamen in the

British Navy be bathed and held in "slop ships" before joining their regular ships for prolonged tours of duty.[1]

Even before general acceptance of germ theories of contagion, quarantine methods were extended in large-scale efforts at controlling disease spread. Rather than removing the sick individual from his environment, the environment itself was changed. Sanitary and social reformers in the late 19th century, assuming that a clean city is a healthy city, attempted to improve living conditions. Slum clearance, provision of bathing facilities, and improved personal hygiene reduced the incidence of urban typhus by affecting louse transmission, even though this mode of typhus spread was not understood.[1]

In large cities in the 19th century, infants were increasingly fed raw cow's milk rather than breast milk, and diseases such as typhoid fever, scarlet fever, tuberculosis, and infant diarrhea became rampant. Concern about milk as a vehicle for disease grew.[2] Abraham Jacobi, a crusading pediatrician in New York City, began advocating boiling milk in 1873. In the 1890s milk stations appeared in large cities, and large quantities of treated (pasteurized) milk were distributed. Condensed and evaporated milk also provided a disease-free milk source. Along with other social improvements, the provision of a safe milk supply contributed to the dramatic decline in infant mortality from typhoid fever and diarrhea in the early 20th century. Such efforts to "decontaminate" milk preceded the microbiological understanding of milk-borne disease.

There are several important modern examples of how society gropes toward solutions of public health problems despite limited scientific insight. At present there is great public concern and controversy over poorly understood environmental health threats. Ground water is threatened by industrial and agricultural pollutants. Safe storage and transport of hazardous materials such as nuclear waste and toxic chemicals are not guaranteed. The risks of nuclear accidents at power plants are real. Most frightening is the potential for nuclear war, the ultimate public health concern. Society is trying to contend with these dangers, but effective technological solutions are not yet available.

Society is also trying to deal with a modern plague, acquired immunodeficiency syndrome (AIDS). As in the Middle Ages, there is social pressure to quarantine AIDS victims, even without scientific evidence that this would prevent disease spread. With increased understanding of the epidemiology, immunology, and virology of AIDS, effective means of interrupting transmission will be available.

4. APPLIED SCIENCE

By the second half of the 19th century and the early 20th century, public health improvements were informed by tremendous advances in microbiology and nutrition. The application of scientific discoveries and specific preventive strategies is relatively recent, but the evolution of modern disease concepts has occurred over hundreds of years.

As mentioned, Greek and Roman physicians recognized that disease was caused by environmental factors. Occupational health risks were noted as early as the 1st century A.D. when Pliny observed that palsy followed lead dust exposure.[4]

In the Middle Ages Arabian physicians preserved and elaborated Greco–Roman medical traditions. Rhazes' vivid descriptions of measles and smallpox were the first to group clinical signs and symptoms into distinct diseases with unique natural histories.[5,p.129] He thus made it conceptually possible to separate causes, treatments, and preventive methods for various diseases.

Among the new ideas of the Renaissance were theories of disease spread and a concern for work-related illness.[2] In the 16th century, hundreds of years before Pasteur and the new science of microbiology, Fracastoro theorized the contagious nature of diseases such as syphilis, smallpox, measles, tuberculosis, and rabies. Also in the early 16th century, Paracelsus, best known for his investigations of the toxic and pharmacological affects of various chemicals, recognized occupational diseases in miners and smelters and suggested means of protecting workers. Neurological disease following occupational mercurial poisoning was described by Jean Fennel in 1557.[4]

In the 17th century in England, Sydenham, an astute bedside observer, classified disease according to specific historical and clinical features and then for the first time applied treatments specific to the illness.[5] Although he incorrectly attributed epidemics to atmospheric phenomena (''miasmas''), his clear descriptions of epidemic disease and his inference that transient environmental factors underlie changes in disease frequency are fundamental contributions in the history of epidemiology and preventive medicine.

In the 18th and early 19th centuries clinical and epidemiological experimentation was used to test theories of disease.[1] In experiments with British sailors, Lind showed that citrus fruit prevents scurvy. Jenner used cowpox to vaccinate against smallpox (although this was the first use of vaccination to prevent disease, for thousands of years previously in China and the Middle East, inoculums of infected material from smallpox victims were used to transmit what was incorrectly understood to be milder disease). Epidemiological evidence was used by Snow in 1854 to explain outbreaks of cholera in London. Although the discoveries of Lind, Jenner, and Snow utilized scientific methodology, they were made without an accurate understanding of the pathophysiology of the disease in question.

Even though the contagious nature of many diseases was long suspected, it was not until the 19th and early 20th centuries that microbiological and clinical evidence finally changed medical and public health practices.[2,6] The simple exigency of hand washing was urged by Oliver Wendell Holmes (1843) and Semmelweis (1848) to reduce obstetrical infection (puerperal fever). Lister encouraged aseptic methods in the operating room to prevent surgical wound infection. Basic discoveries in microbiology by Pasteur and Koch in the late 19th century created opportunities for controlling rabies, anthrax, cholera, and tuberculosis. In the tropics work by Manson, Ross, and Findlay established the vector role of mosquitoes in transmitting filariasis, malaria, and yellow fever. Mosquito control projects were then used with marked efficacy (e.g., the Panama Canal project). The gonococcus was described and implicated in ophthalmia neonatorum in 1879, and soon thereafter silver nitrate prophylaxis was available. The causative agent of syphilis was identified in 1905, and serological testing (Wassermann test) as well as chemotherapy (Salvarsan) were available a few years later. By 1900 acute as well as chronic diphtheria (carrier state) could be diagnosed by specific microbiological means, immunity could be assessed (Schick test), and antitoxin could be provided for treatment. Active immunization using diphtheria toxoid was employed in large scale by 1920.

Parallel to the rapid advances in microbiology, the science of nutrition developed quickly in the late 19th and early 20th centuries.[1,6] Although Lind was able to prevent scurvy using citrus, it was not until 1932 that the antiscorbutic factor was identified as vitamin C. In an early clinical trial (1905), Fletcher showed that people fed uncured rice (thiamine depleted) developed beriberi. Later, cured rice corrected the symptoms. In the 1920s in the rural south, Goldberger used epidemiological methods to show that pellagra is a dietary disease. Xerophthalmia, described by Roman physicians, was associated with vitamin A deficiency in 1917 by McCollum and Simmonds. Rickets was shown to be experimentally inducible (in dogs) and then correctable with cod liver oil in 1919 by Mellanby. In 1922 the antirachitic factor in cod liver oil was isolated by McCollum.

Progress in preventing disease was particularly rapid in the early part of this century. Discoveries in microbiology, immunology, and nutrition led quickly to preventive interventions which markedly reduced childhood mortality from communicable disease. Advances in preventive care have continued since World War II. New vaccines have brought control over many childhood infections, in particular polio, and have reduced adult complications from influenza and pneumococcal infections. Prevention of congenital birth defects and reduction of neonatal morbidity and mortality have become possible with *in utero* screening techniques, genetic counseling, improved control of diabetes during pregnancy, increased awareness of fetal risks from certain maternal infections (e.g., rubella, herpes simplex), and screening for Rh compatibility. Occupational health risks have been reduced with the promotion and institution of wide-scale industrial hygiene programs. Fluoridization of water has markedly reduced the incidence of dental caries in children. Many other examples of improvements in preventive care as they pertain to adult medical practice are the subject of later sections of this book.

5. UNITED STATES

Despite advances in preventive care, diagnostic testing, and therapeutics, as well as huge investments in medical care, the nation's health in the 20th century is only slowly improving. Early mortality from communicable diseases has been replaced by delayed mortality from vascular and malignant disease. At present, the life expectancy of a 45-year-old American man is just 5 years longer than it would have been in 1900.[7] This small change highlights the limitations of medical technology in curing today's important diseases. The chronic diseases that afflict Americans as they age should be easier to prevent than to cure. The current potential for preventive care depends more than ever on physicians in practice. To clarify the physician's position vis-à-vis preventive care, it will be useful to trace the evolution of public health in the United States during the 19th and 20th centuries. During this time, social changes and scientific discoveries led to a public health movement concerned with individual health care as well as community sanitation and hygiene. With these changes it became necessary for physicians to be concerned with more than diagnosing and treating patients.

The late 19th century brought industrialization, urbanization, and immigration to the United States.[6] From 1860 to 1910, the urban portion of the U.S. population grew from 19% to 45%. By the late 19th century, the black migration from the rural south to the urban north had begun also. Most of the European immigrants and American blacks arriving in northern cities had poorly paid jobs (not infrequently in unsafe factories) and crowded housing. Their children were particularly prone to nutritional deficiency states, such as rickets, and communicable diseases, including tuberculosis, scarlet fever, diphtheria, whooping cough, smallpox, typhoid fever, infant diarrhea, and malaria.

The plight of the urban poor did not go unrecognized. At the turn of the century, a broad reform movement attempted to deal with housing, child labor, prostitution, sweat shops, and the health consequences of poverty. This movement represented several distinct ideological concerns and social developments. In the early 20th century, conservation of natural resources became popular, and some social observers saw unnecessary disease as a waste of human resources. The National Conservation Commission stated in 1910 that "natural resources are of no avail without men and women to develop them, and only a sturdy and sound citizenship can make a nation permanently great."[6] This sentiment became prophetic a few years later when an alarming number of young men were deemed physically unfit for the armed services during the World War I draft. Also early in the century, there was increased attention to occupational health. The Prudential Life Insurance Company estimated that in 1913 there were 25,000 fatal accidents, 300,000 serious injuries, and two million other injuries in U.S. workers. Although following the Civil War state labor bureaus began to investigate worker health, it was not until the first decade of the 20th century that this became a national issue involving a broad coalition of concerned physicians, lawyers, labor leaders, politicians, and social scientists. Another important element of this reform spirit was the feeling that newly arrived immigrants, in addition to their basic needs for food, shelter, work, and health, needed to be "Americanized." Concern over maternal and child health reflected the push to Americanization. Thus milk stations, orange juice and cod liver oil distribution, immunization campaigns, and lessons in infant feeding were programs aimed directly at health problems and indirectly at the necessity of assimilating newly arrived immigrants into American life.

With the recognition that ill health accompanies poverty (the New York Charity Organization in 1909 estimated that there was serious physical disability in three-quarters of its families), reforms arose from three directions: (1) government, (2) local health agencies with professional staffs, and (3) volunteer agencies. The scale of the problems required government action at local, state, and national levels. Initially, government action came only after prodding by private citizens who, galvanized by social conscience, formed groups that promoted community health. The National Tuberculosis Association, founded in 1904 is the oldest such group. The Society of Social and Medical Prophylaxis was formed in 1905 to combat venereal disease. Present organizations such as the March of Dimes, the American Heart Association, and the National Cancer Society reflect both the changes in major illnesses that have occurred in the past 70 years and the continued spirited involvement of concerned citizens in disease control. These organizations educate people about their health and raise funds for research and treatment. In similar roles in the present era major philanthropic foundations are important participants in health care delivery and research. To conceive and administer the reforms called for by governments and citizens groups, local health agencies were required. In 1866 New York City created the Metropolitan Board of Health, which served as a model for other cities. Public health laboratories were integral components of these local health agencies. New York City set the standard with the laboratory organized in 1893 and directed by William H. Park. The first diphtheria antitoxin used in the United States came from this laboratory. One of the oldest bacteriological laboratories in the United States was part of the Marine Hospital Service on Staten Island. This laboratory later moved to Washington as the hygienic laboratory of the Public Health Service, eventually becoming the nucleus of the National Institutes of Health.

Despite increasing preventive activities within communities, most physicians were committed exclusively to diagnosing and treating disease. Lack of physician interest and involvement in community health contributed to the development of a new profession of nonphysician public health workers. The American Public Health Association (APHA) was founded in 1872. In 1897 80% of the 568 APHA members were physicians.[8] In 1900 physicians represented 63% of professional health workers. In 1960 physicians accounted for 21% of American professional health workers. By 1969 physicians accounted for only 29% of APHA membership. The School of Hygiene and Public Health was established at Johns Hopkins University in 1916. By 1974 there were 18 accredited schools of public health in the United States.

With the appearance of a cadre of public health professionals, the boundary between clinical practice and public health required clarification.[9] The new sciences of bacteriology and nutrition allowed public health workers to deal with individual health problems (e.g., immunization) as well as the general problems of community health such as sanitation. Inevitably, conflicts with practicing physicians arose. At issue was the conviction among physicians that they should be free from competition or control in their dealings with patients. Several examples illustrate this emphasis on physician autonomy. Controversies developed when public health laboratories began to compete with physicians and pharmacists in the performance of diagnostic tests (e.g., serological testing for syphilis, Schick test for diphtheria immunity) or the production of serum. Physicians objected vociferously to mandatory reporting of tuberculosis and syphilis instituted near the turn of the century by the New York City Health Department. School examination programs, tuberculosis clinics, and maternal and child health centers intruded on the physician domain of patient examination.

Physicians did not want to do public health work any more than they wanted public health workers to provide individual patient care. One reason for this has been that preventive care and public health receive relatively little attention at schools of medicine. When the APHA was founded (1872), its first president called for the addition of "sanitary science" to the medical school curriculum in order to encourage the profession to be "as much devoted to the practice of the art of preventing as it is in curing disease."[8] In response to the "lack of due emphasis of the practitioner's role as an apostle of hygiene no less than therapy," the Rockefeller Foundation helped found the nation's first public health school at Johns Hopkins University in 1916.[6] In 1913 William Osler lectured on preventive medicine at Yale University.[10] He referred only to community measures of hygiene and sanitation and did not mention the relevance of preventive medicine to clinical training or individual practice. With the rapid growth of medical science following World War II the increasingly crowded medical school curriculum left little room for public health topics. In fact, students wanted to deemphasize instruction in this area.

The meager public health content of medical school curricula reflected the lack of status and economic reward of public health work compared to private practice.[11,12] In

1886 an article in the *Journal of the American Medical Association* ascribed the limited opportunity for preventive practice to a system that "makes the physician's income dependent on the amount of sickness"; in other words, "millions for care and not one cent for prevention."[13] Traditionally, the tangible rewards of medicine, both financially and personally, are found at the bedside. Surveys of medical students, house staff, and practicing physicians bear this out.[14,15] Few students are interested in public health careers, and the perceived importance of public health topics in medical education falls steadily during medical school, residency training, and practice.

Encouragingly, the situation in medical schools has changed in the past 25 years, and most medical schools now have separate departments responsible for teaching and promoting the various tenets of public health.[16,17] As the public health profession became more oriented to individual care in the early part of this century, the medical profession gained a public health perspective while attempting to deal with chronic disease and skyrocketing health care costs. The increasing government role in health care research, planning, and financing has helped to shape this outlook. Topics such as preventive care, clinical epidemiology, cost–benefit analysis, and biostatistics have been linked to primary-care clinical specialties, and thus in a sense validated.[16] In the 1950s the specific specialty of preventive medicine emerged, embracing occupational health and preventive care. Growing numbers of primary-care specialists in academic settings help to bridge schools of medicine and public health.

At present the turn-of-the-century distinction between individual and community health is blurred. Preventive care has been popularized, and despite organizational as well as fiscal constraints, physicians are attempting to practice prevention.[12] The epidemiological and clinical rationale of this type of health care is the major subject of this book.

REFERENCES

1. Rosen, G.: Historical evaluation of primary prevention. *Bull. NY Acad. Med.* **51**:9–26, 1975.
2. Wain, H.: *A History of Preventive Medicine*. Charles C Thomas, Springfield, IL, 1970.
3. Winslow, C. E. A.: Foreword, in Shattuck, L., *A Report of the Sanitary Commission of Massachusetts*, 1850 (facsimile edition). Harvard University Press, Cambridge, Massachusetts, 1948, pp. v–ix.
4. Neurotoxic disorders. *Morbid. Mortal. Wkly. Rep.* **35**:113–116, 1986.
5. Garrison, F. H.: *An Introduction to the History of Medicine*. Saunders, Philadelphia, 1929.
6. Rosen, G.: Preventive medicine in the United States 1900–1975: Trends and interpretation, in *Preventive Medicine USA*, Prodist, New York, 1976, pp. 715–808.
7. *Health People: The Surgeon General's Report on Health Promotion and Disease Prevention*. DHEW Pub. No. 79-55071, US Government Printing Office, Washington, DC, 1979, p. 53.
8. Terry, M.: Evolution of public health and preventive medicine in the United States. *Am. J. Public Health* **65**:161–168, 1975.
9. Starr, P.: *The Social Transformation of American Medicine*. Basic Books, New York, 1982, pp. 180–197.
10. Osler, W.: *The Evolution of Modern Medicine*. Gryphon Editions, Birmingham, Alabama, 1982, pp. 218–233.
11. Neuhauser, D.: Don't teach preventive medicine: A contrary view. *Public Health Rep.* **97**:220–222, 1982.
12. Relman, A. S.: Encouraging the practice of preventive medicine and health promotion. *Public Health Rep.* **97**:216–219, 1982.
13. Hutchinson, W.: Health insurance, or our financial relation to the public. *JAMA* **7**:477–481, 1886.
14. Coker, R. E., Back, K. W., Donnelly, T. G., *et al.*: Public health as viewed by the medical student. *Am. J. Public Health* **49**:601–609, 1959.

15. Task Force Report—John E. Fogarty International Center for Advanced Study in the Health Sciences and The American College of Preventative Medicine: Education and training of health manpower for prevention: An assessment of physician's attitudes toward prevention, in *Preventive Medicine USA*. Prodist, New York, 1976, pp. 458–464.
16. Berg, R. L.: Prevention: Current status in undergraduate medical education. *Public Health Rep.* **97**:205–209, 1982.
17. Lewis, C.: Teaching medical students about disease prevention and health promotion. *Public Health Rep.* **97**:210–215, 1982.

3

Screening for Early Disease
Interpretation of Diagnostic Tests

John T. Philbrick and Daniel M. Becker

1. INTRODUCTION

Diagnostic tests play an important role in the clinical strategies of preventive medicine. Some aspects of disease prevention are applicable to all and can be recommended unselectively. Examples include wearing seat belts and avoiding excessive use of alcohol. Other aspects of prevention require the selection of certain higher-risk groups in whom intervention would be beneficial. This selection is often done clinically, as with the use of pneumococcal and influenza vaccines in the elderly or in patients with pulmonary disease. However, many areas of preventive medicine rely on diagnostic tests in the implementation of a clinical strategy. Diagnostic tests are used in prevention in three ways.

1.1. Diagnosis of Asymptomatic Disease

Patients may be afflicted with a disease at an early stage, before they note symptoms that lead them to seek medical attention. Use of tests to diagnose these asymptomatic diseases is usually referred to as "screening." Examples of screening are the blood pressure testing performed by rescue squads or other groups in shopping malls and the legal requirement for premarital syphilis serology. Use of tests to diagnose asymptomatic disease in the doctor's office is sometimes referred to as "case finding," because the tests are performed on patients who have already presented themselves to providers of medical care for other reasons. Examples of case finding are the yearly performance of testing for blood in bowel movements and yearly mammograms ordered by a physician. In recent years, little distinction is made between screening and case finding. Most authorities consider them both screening activities.

1.2. Identification of Risk Factors for the Development of Disease

Some screening tests do not directly uncover an asymptomatic disease, but rather identify risk factors for the development of a disease. For example, hypercholesterolemia

John T. Philbrick and Daniel M. Becker • Department of Internal Medicine, University of Virginia School of Medicine, Charlottesville, VA 22908.

usually is clinically relevant only insofar as high cholesterol is a risk factor for atherosclerosis.

1.3. Monitoring the Result of an Intervention Aiding in Disease Prevention

Tests can be used to monitor the effect of an intervention aimed at prevention. There is, perhaps, a fine line between what is "preventive" activity and what is treatment of a disease. However, to the extent that hypercholesterolemia is a risk factor and not a disease, monitoring serum cholesterol to assess the effect of diet and drug therapy can be included in this category.

The interpretation of results of tests used in preventive health care involves more than knowing the magnitude of the result or whether it is positive or negative. The interpretation of screening tests is fraught with difficulty. The following sections provide the background necessary to understanding the role of diagnostic tests in preventive health care.

2. TERMINOLOGY

The purpose of this section is to define terminology useful in discussing diagnostic tests. See Table I for help in understanding this section.

2.1. Two-by-Two Table

Most test results are classified as either positive or negative (or normal or abnormal). Patients can usually be divided into two groups, those with the disease for which the

Table I. Definitions Used with Diagnostic Tests[a]

	Confirmed disease	
Result of diagnostic test	Present	Absent
Positive	*a* (true positives)	*b* (false positives)
Negative	*c* (false negatives)	*d* (true negatives)

[a]Sensitivity $= \dfrac{a}{a + c}$

Specificity $= \dfrac{d}{b + d}$

Accuracy of positive prediction $= \dfrac{a}{a + b}$

Accuracy of negative prediction $= \dfrac{d}{c + d}$

Prevalence $= \dfrac{a + c}{a + b + c + d}$

patient is being tested, and those without the disease. The results of tests performed on a group of patients in which disease state (presence or absence) has been determined can be organized in a two-by-two table, as in Table I. Once the data are arranged in this fashion, the important indices of test efficacy can be calculated.

2.2. Gold Standard

It is essential in dealing with diagnostic tests to have some definitive way of determining whether the patient actually has the disease in question. Only after a patient has been accurately classified as "diseased" or "nondiseased" can we make a two-by-two table to calculate the indices of test efficacy. The definitive test used to establish the disease state is known as the "gold standard." With some diseases, such as cancer of the colon, this is a simple task. A pathology report is all that is needed. Establishing the disease state is less clear-cut with coronary disease. A coronary angiogram is usually accepted as the gold standard of coronary disease, but what constitutes a positive angiogram? Is it 50% luminal diameter narrowing? Or should it be 75%? Or should it be some other criterion? An even more difficult situation is chronic pancreatitis. What is the gold standard for presence of disease, especially if the amylase is normal? Fortunately, for most diseases, a reasonable gold standard is available.

2.3. Sensitivity and Specificity

These are the two indices of test efficacy most commonly used to describe how good a test is. Values for sensitivity and specificity are obtained by performing the test on groups of patients who have the disease in question and on other groups who are free of the disease. Sensitivity is calculated by dividing the number of patients with both a positive test and the disease by the total number of patients with the disease. An ideal test would be positive in all diseased patients and thus would have a sensitivity of 1.0. Specificity is calculated by dividing the number of patients with a negative test and who are free of the disease by the total number of patients tested who do not have the disease. An ideal test would have no false negatives and would have a specificity of 1.0. Both these indices are calculated "vertically" on the two-by-two table (Table I). That is, sensitivity is calculated using only the information in the first column on the table, and specificity is calculated using only the information in the second column. This fact has major implications for the usefulness of these two indices. These indices can be defined in probabilistic terms: sensitivity is the likelihood, given a patient is diseased, that the test will be positive; specificity is the likelihood, given the patient is disease free, that the test will be negative. Unfortunately, this information is not what the clinician needs to know. The clinician performs a test on patients in whom the disease state is unknown and wishes to use the test result to predict the likelihood of the disease being present. This information is supplied by the indices discussed in the next section.

2.4. Accuracy of Positive Prediction and Accuracy of Negative Prediction

Accuracy of positive prediction is calculated by dividing the number of those with both a positive test and the disease in question by the total number of patients with a positive test. Accuracy of negative prediction is calculated by dividing the number of patients with both a negative test and no disease by the total number of those with a negative test. These are the "horizontal" indices because each one deals with only one row of the two-by-two table. These indices provide just the information that clinicians need to know to interpret the results of the test. They provide the likelihood, given the test result, of whether the patient has the disease or is free of the disease. Unfortunately, as will be discussed in the next section, these indices are not constant, but rather vary widely depending on the ratio of diseased to nondiseased patients in the population in which the test is being performed.

These indices have been referred to by many other terms, including predictive value of a positive (or negative) test, positive (or negative) predictive accuracy, and even diagnostic sensitivity (or specificity).

2.5. Prevalence

Prevalence is defined as the number of patients with the disease in question divided by the total number of patients in the population being studied. Prevalence varies from population to population. For example, the prevalence of coronary disease (defined by a "significant" narrowing on coronary angiogram) in a group of patients with typical anginal pain is probably about 90%. Of course, the prevalence of coronary disease in a group of patients with no symptoms will be much lower, perhaps 5%.

2.6. Reliability

A test is sometimes repeated in the same patient. Reliability, or reproductibility, is the likelihood that the same test result will be obtained each time the test is performed.

3. EFFECT OF PREVALENCE ON PREDICTIVE VALUES

In the best of worlds, a positive test would prove beyond doubt the presence of disease, and a negative test would likewise exclude disease. The next best would be for the test, if it could not absolutely rule in or rule out disease, to at least give the same accuracy of positive prediction and accuracy of negative prediction in all persons to whom the test is applied. Unfortunately, unless the test is "perfect" (i.e., has a sensitivity of 1.0 and a specificity of 1.0), the predictive accuracies are not constant, but vary depending on the prevalence of disease in each group of patients tested. This variation is often great. Table II shows the theoretical variation of accuracy of positive prediction of an imaginary test with both sensitivity and specificity of 0.95. Note how low the accuracy of positive prediction is for the lower prevalence values.

This principle is best made clear using a real example. The treadmill exercise test is frequently used to determine the presence or absence of significant coronary artery disease. It is often used in three different clinical situations: (1) in asymptomatic patients to screen for coronary disease; (2) in patients with chest pains "atypical" for angina to determine the etiology of the pain; (3) in patients with typical angina to "rule in"

Table II. Variation of Accuracy of Positive Prediction with Prevalence[a]

Prevalence (%)	Accuracy of positive prediction
0.01	0.002
0.1	0.02
1	0.16
10.0	0.68
50.0	0.95
90.0	0.99

[a]Sensitivity = 0.95; specificity = 0.95.

coronary disease. Table III gives an estimate for the prevalence of coronary disease (determined by coronary angiography) in each of these three situations.[1]

A pooling of the results of 33 exercise testing studies provides a rough estimate for the sensitivity (0.65) and specificity (0.88).[2] Using these values along with the prevalence estimates, it is simple to calculate the expected distribution of test results among the cells of the two-by-two table for any size patient group.

Tables IV through VI show the expected results of three theoretical studies of 100 patients each: Table IV gives the results for a group of asymptomatic men, Table V the results for a group with atypical chest pain, and Table VI the results for a group of patients with typical angina. Once the cell numbers for each of the tables are calculated, it is easy to determine the indices of predictive accuracy. The accuracy of positive prediction varies from 0.22 to 0.98 over the three clinical groups. The accuracy of negative prediction varies from 0.98 to 0.22. This variation occurs because the indices of predictive accuracy are calculated "horizontally." As the prevalence of disease changes in each of the theoretical studies, the ratios from which the "horizontal" indices are calculated [$a/(a + b)$; $(d/c + d)$] necessarily change. The only exception to this rule would be the case of the perfect test, where if sensitivity and specificity were both 1.0, there would be no false positive tests (b would be zero) and no false negative tests (c would be zero).

Clinicians who have never heard of diagnostic test theory often intuitively come to the same conclusions concerning predictive accuracy. For example, a clinician who obtains a negative sputum cytology in a patient with a lung mass usually concludes that

Table III. Approximate Angiographic Prevalence of Coronary Disease in Men

Clinical subset	%
Asymptomatic	5
Typical angina	90
Atypical angina	50

Table IV. Calculation of Predictive Accuracies of the Exercise Test for Coronary Disease: Asymptomatic Men[a]

	Angiogram		
Stress test	Positive	Negative	Row total
Positive	3.25	11.4	14.65
Negative	1.75	83.6	85.35
Column total	5	95	100

[a]Accuracy of positive prediction $= \frac{3.25}{3.25 + 11.4} = 0.22$

Accuracy of negative prediction $= \frac{83.6}{1.75 + 83.6} = 0.98$

Prevalence = 5%; N = 100; sensitivity = 0.65; specificity = 0.88.

the test is falsely negative and continues to pursue the diagnosis. A clinician who obtains a very high potassium level in a healthy person who is not on potassium supplementation or does not have renal disease usually assumes that the test is a false positive owing to hemolysis of the blood sample and arranges for the test to be repeated.

4. CHARACTERISTICS OF A GOOD SCREENING TEST

A number of factors must be taken into consideration in selecting a screening test. These factors are discussed in the sections that follow.

4.1. High Sensitivity

The purpose of a screening test is to detect the presence of disease whenever it is present. This requires that there be few false negative tests. Since this means that c in

Table V. Calculation of Predictive Accuracies of the Exercise Test for Coronary Disease: Atypical Angina[a]

	Angiogram		
Stress test	Positive	Negative	Row total
Positive	32.5	6	38.5
Negative	17.5	44	61.5
Column total	50	50	100

[a]Accuracy of positive prediction $= \frac{32.5}{32.5 + 6} = 0.84$

Accuracy of negative prediction $= \frac{44}{17.5 + 44} = 0.72$

Prevalence = 50%; N = 100; sensitivity = 0.65; specificity = 0.88.

Table VI. Calculation of Predictive Accuracies of the Exercise Test for Coronary Disease: Typical Angina[a]

	Angiogram		
Stress test	Positive	Negative	Row total
Positive	58.5	1.2	59.7
Negative	31.5	8.8	40.3
Column total	90	10	100

[a]Accuracy of positive prediction $= \frac{58.5}{58.5 + 1.2} = 0.98$

Accuracy of negative prediction $= \frac{8.8}{31.5 + 8.8} = 0.22$

Prevalence = 90%; N = 100; sensitivity = 0.65; specificity = 0.88.

Table I must be relatively small and sensitivity must be high [remember, sensitivity is defined as $a/(a + c)$].

4.2. Relatively High Specificity

Even though sensitivity is quite high in a good screening test, if the specificity is low an excessive number of false positive tests would result (b in Table I). This would create a low accuracy of positive prediction [$a/(a + b)$, Table I], especially in populations in which the disease for which the test is performed is uncommon. This type of test might still be satisfactory if a reasonable confirmatory test were available that was highly specific. (See Section 8.1 for an example.)

4.3. Simplicity

A screening test is intended to be applied to large numbers of people on a regular basis. The simpler the test procedure, the more likely that it will be widely used. It should not require lengthy training for those performing the test, it should not require complicated patient preparation, and it should be relatively easy to perform. For example, colonoscopy is a highly sensitive and specific test for colon carcinoma, but would be unwieldy as a screening test because it is not simple enough to be applied on a large scale. On the other hand, blood pressure screening is simple and therefore is commonly performed.

4.4. Safety

Since the majority of people on whom screening is performed are healthy, or at least have no complaints referrable to the disease for which they are being screened, the test must be very safe. It would be unacceptable to cause injury by the screening activity itself, or by the workup of many false positive tests created by screening, unless the possible injury is heavily outweighed by the benefits of the screening activity.

4.5. Acceptability

A screening test must not be so difficult, uncomfortable, or unpalatable as to be unacceptable to the patient. Screening tests are performed on people who have no symptoms, so an uncomfortable test could easily dissuade patients from undergoing them. A rigid sigmoidoscopy is one such test that is often refused on that basis. A flexible sigmoidoscopy, because of its greater comfort, is more readily accepted.

4.6. Low Cost

The benefits of screening must justify the cost. As far as society is concerned, limited health dollars should be used where the greatest benefit to health can be obtained. If a screening program is so expensive that the cost of finding one case is too high, then it is discouraged even if effective. On the other hand, the patient's out-of-pocket costs for screening can limit wide application. An individual may refuse an effective screening test just because it is not covered by his insurance policy.

5. FACTORS THAT AFFECT SENSITIVITY AND SPECIFICITY

Although in theory the sensitivity and specificity of diagnostic tests are independent of disease prevalence, these characteristics are nevertheless affected by aspects of the population that is tested. Thus, the defined sensitivity and specificity of a particular test should not be taken for granted. As diagnostic aids are developed and promoted, their sensitivity, specificity, and ultimate efficacy vary considerably among different investigators over time. This variation arises from differences in the spectrum of disease within the tested population and from various types of bias incorporated into the evaluation process.[3]

5.1. Spectrum of Patients

In defining a test's sensitivity it is important that the diseased population represents a wide spectrum of pathological and clinical features. For example, although carcinoembryonic antigen (CEA) is often elevated in cancer patients, it may be negative early in disease but easily measured in the later stages.[4] Sensitivity of this test among patients with widely metastatic disease is fairly high. However, if the spectrum of disease were broad, there would be more false negative tests and CEA measurement would be an insensitive disease marker.

Similarly, the nondiseased or control population used for estimating specificity should include patients with different diseases that would challenge the test's specificity. Thus angiotensin converting enzyme (ACE) as a marker for sarcoidosis seems specific only if patients with other granulomatous diseases are excluded from the control groups.[5] It turns out that other granulomatous and pulmonary diseases, many of which are important to distinguish from sarcoidosis, have elevated (false positive) ACE levels.

5.2. Bias

In addition to an adequate spectrum of disease, accurate and nonbiased determination of both disease state (present or not present) and test results (positive or negative) is important for the proper evaluation of test efficacy. Unless these determinations are made independently, the test may seem better than it really is.

Thus a positive or negative test result, if known to the investigator, may change the disease workup. Positive results may lead to further efforts to find disease, whereas negative results may inhibit such diagnostic enthusiasm. False positive tests would be discovered if the subsequent workup were negative. On the other hand, false negative results may not be pursued. If disease is thus underdiagnosed, the test's sensitivity (positive test in diseased patients) is exaggerated. Ransohoff and Feinstein offer as an example the evaluation of a new gallbladder scan in which only positive scans had further tests to document cholecystitis.[3]

Another type of bias applies if the investigator knows the diagnosis before the test result is interpreted. It would be hard to ignore the pulmonary angiogram result when reading a lung scan. ''Monday morning quarterbacking'' should not be used in judging a study positive or negative.

5.3. Exercise Testing as an Example

Problems of both spectrum and bias have been noted in the literature that discusses exercise testing for coronary artery disease. In a review of 33 studies of exercise testing, sensitivity varied from 35% to 88%, and specificity varied from 41% to 100%.[2] This wide range of test efficacy was noted amid equally variable research methodology. Many of the studies did not take steps to limit biased interpretations of the stress test results. A group of biased studies would be expected to have variable results. An important aspect of this variation also was related to the limited spectrum of patients available for the research.[6] Of 205 consecutive exercise tests from two hospitals, only 3% of the studied patients would have been eligible for a study of the exercise test's efficacy. Reasons for exclusion included coexisting diseases or medications that make electrocardiogram interpretation difficult, technical problems in performing the tests, and physician unwillingness to subject the patients to angiography. The patients ultimately eligible represented the tip of the clinical iceberg. It would be hazardous to generalize their results to the total heterogeneous population receiving exercise tests.

6. CHARACTERISTICS OF DISEASES FOR WHICH SCREENING IS WORTHWHILE

Assuming that a screening test is sensitive, specific, practical, and reliable, and therefore potentially beneficial if applied to large populations, there remain important issues regarding the efficacy of large-scale testing.[7] These issues involve characteristics of the disease for which screening is performed.

6.1. Relatively High Prevalence

To justify the cost of screening, the disease in question must be relatively prevalent in the overall population. The prevalence of the disease (i.e., the number of people with the disease at any point in time) depends on its frequency and duration. Screening for rare diseases is generally not feasible because the cost per case detected is high. Furthermore, with rare diseases the accuracy of positive prediction of even a very specific test is low. Screening for phenylketonuria (PKU) illustrates these problems.[8] In most states screening neonates for PKU is mandated by the legislature. At a cutoff of blood phenylalanine levels where no PKU cases would be missed, the test has a sensitivity of 100% and a specificity of 99.95%. However, if the incidence of PKU is one case per 10,000 live births, then the accuracy of positive prediction is only 17%. It is estimated that $10 million is spent annually to screen three million neonates to find 300 cases. Despite the very high sensitivity and specificity of the test, the screening program is very inefficient and the cost per case detected is quite high.

6.2. Long Duration

Among more common diseases, those with long durations are more likely to benefit from screening. Diseases with long natural histories have higher proportions of preclinical, detectable cases. For example, breast and cervical carcinoma develop relatively slowly, and there is ample opportunity to search for early disease. Hematological malignancies are relatively common, but because they often develop and progress quickly, it is harder to detect an early, treatable phase of the illness.

6.3. Serious Consequences

The screened disease should have serious consequences. Diseases that are morbid and ultimately fatal are suitable for screening. In these terms most cancers are eligible.

6.4. Treatable Disease

Early detection of an untreatable disease does not change the ultimate outcome. For example, biochemical markers of genetic diseases can be measured. Huntington's chorea can now be diagnosed years before symptoms, yet there is no treatment that then alters the natural history. Most diseases, however, have some mode of therapy, and even if cure is not possible early treatment often improves the outcome. Detection and treatment of moderate or severe hypertension prevents morbid outcomes such as stroke even though the hypertension is not cured. Very few cancers can be cured, but in some instances treatment offers prolonged survival and improved quality of life. The hope for a surgical cure of cancer is based on early detection. Screening programs can be aimed at diseases treatable in some sense, but the benefits of early detection can be difficult to measure properly.[9]

7. DISTORTIONS CREATED BY SCREENING

An important problem in determining the efficacy of large-scale screening is the potential distortion of the natural history of diseases by screening.

7.1. Pseudodisease

Screening might uncover lesions that would never have caused clinical disease (see Fig. 1b), hence the term *pseudodisease*. Some cases of pseudodisease would remain

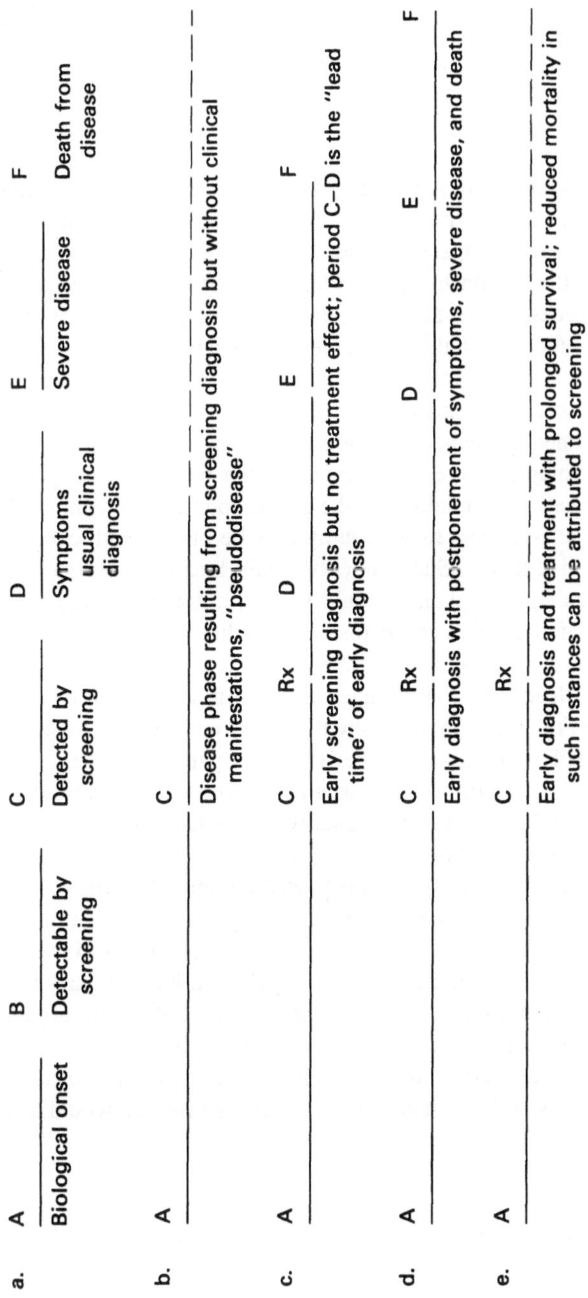

Figure 1. Natural history of disease: effects of screening. (Modified from Ref. 7.)

asymptomatic or even regress to pathologically normal states. Other cases might get worse, but coexisting and severe diseases would interrupt the natural history of the pseudodisease. The presence of cases of pseudodisease in the screened population accounts for some of the reports of successful screening programs. For example, some of the colonic polyps found by screening undoubtedly are pseudodisease.

7.2. Bias

Experimental evaluations of screening programs are expensive and impractical. Nevertheless, randomized clinical trials in which the mortality rates of the screened and unscreened populations are compared provide the most valid means of evaluating screening results. In the 1960s the Health Insurance Plan (HIP) of Greater New York completed a randomized trial of breast cancer screening using mammography.[10] Over 60,000 women were enrolled, and reduced mortality for screened women between the ages of 50 and 59 was demonstrated. This study is unique in its size and detail. There are only a few such randomized trials of screening interventions. Most screening programs have been evaluated using nonexperimental methods and are thus prone to several types of bias.

The effects of voluntary screening programs can be estimated by comparing mortality between the screened population and the general population within the area. However, patients who are self-selected for screening may be more health conscious or may be aware of a personal risk factor. Such patients would bias the results of screening since neither their risk nor their compliance would vary in a random fashion.

Another means of evaluation compares the mortality of screening-diagnosed patients with symptom-diagnosed patients. The time between screening diagnosis and clinical diagnosis is termed "lead time." Prolonged survival in a screened patient may only be due to lead time (see Fig. 1a,c). In the figure the time from C to F is longer than from D to F, but the time of death is the same. In the HIP study patients with a diagnosis made by screening had an average lead time of 1 year, and to avoid lead time bias their survival at 6 years was compared to the survival of clinically diagnosed patients at 5 years.

"Length bias" is another problem that complicates comparisons between screening-diagnosed cancer patients and symptom-diagnosed patients. Slowly growing tumors are easier to detect and have a better prognosis than rapidly growing tumors. The slowly growing tumors would also be more prevalent. Length bias refers to the overrepresentation of slowly growing tumors in the screened population. Even if early treatment has no effect, the screened patients would survive longer because their tumors are biologically different. It is difficult to measure or correct for length bias. If screening is repeated, patients diagnosed by later screening (i.e., initially negative) would have fast-growing tumors, and comparisons at these stages of the screening program would be relatively free of length bias.

8. APPLICATION OF DIAGNOSTIC TEST THEORY TO SCREENING TESTS

This section discusses several examples of diagnostic tests that have been used or considered for use as screening tests to illustrate the principles outlined.

8.1. Syphilis Screening

Serological testing for syphilis has been widely used for screening purposes. The relevant tests illustrate several principles of screening. Following infection by *Treponema pallidum* two general classes of antibodies can be measured: nonspecific (nontreponemal) reagins directed against a host–parasite-derived lipoidal antigen and specific anti-treponemal antibodies. The sensitivity of these tests during various states of syphilis is shown in Table VII.[11–13] The specificity (Table VII) varies somewhat with the population surveyed.

The FTA–ABS test seems superior to the VDRL since it is clearly the more sensitive and specific test. However, the FTA–ABS is more expensive and more difficult to perform than the VDRL. Although in general the most sensitive test is used for screening, in this example the practicality of testing determines policy. Since the VDRL test is cheap, simple to perform, and reliable, it is recommended by the Centers for Disease Control for screening asymptomatic populations.[14] If the VDRL is positive and there are no associated clinical findings, the diagnosis of syphilis can be confirmed by a treponemal antibody test. Figure 2 illustrates how sequential testing works. This example is modified from Griner *et al.*[15]

8.2. Screening for Coronary Artery Disease

Screening for coronary artery disease is often advocated, especially in certain occupation groups such as airline pilots and firefighters and also in middle-aged persons desiring to embark on an exercise program. The standard treadmill test is often used in this situation. Table IV shows the results of a screening program of this type applied to a group of 100 men with 5% prevalence of coronary disease. The 85 men with a negative stress test would be quite relieved. However, two of these tests are false negatives. Fifteen men would have positive tests, but only three would be true positives. Since coronary disease is such a worrisome problem and since it has no simple treatment, further testing is usually obligatory to eliminate the false positives. This is done with a stress thallium test or the more risky coronary arteriography. Thus, the relatively low sensitivity of the exercise test

Table VII. Sensitivity and Specificity of Serological Tests for Syphilis

Stage	VDRL[a]	FTA–ABS[b]
	Sensitivity	
Primary	0.78	0.85
Secondary	0.97	0.99
Late	0.77	0.95
Latent	0.74	0.95
	Specificity	
Noninfected patients	0.80–1.0	>0.99

[a]Venereal Disease Research Laboratory.
[b]Fluorescent treponemal antibody absorption.

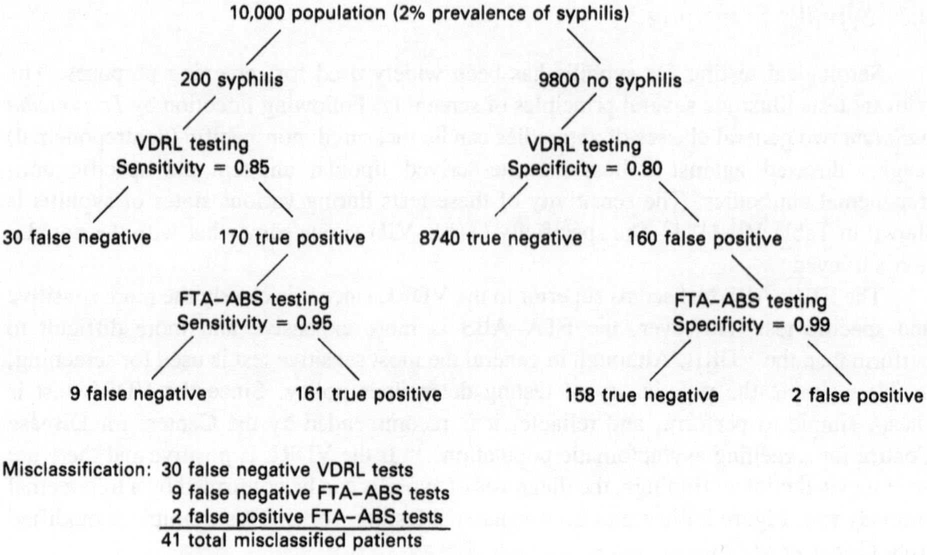

Figure 2. Sequential testing for syphilis. (Modified from Ref. 15.)

results in close to four false positives for every true positive found. This low accuracy of positive prediction, along with the high cost of the test, makes exercise testing for coronary disease a poor screening activity.

Another factor to consider in screening for asymptomatic coronary disease is the lack of proven treatment for the asymptomatic patient. Many physicians would not change or initiate therapy for those patients.

8.3. Screening for Breast Cancer

Cancer of the breast is the most common cause of cancer death in women.[16] Because evidence exists that early detection and treatment result in decreased mortality, screening for breast cancer has been a high priority for those interested in prevention.[17] There are two widely advocated screening modalities for breast cancer: breast self-examination and mammography.

Breast self-examination is clearly inexpensive and simple to perform. However, it has several drawbacks. Few women actually do breast examination regularly.[18] The

Table VIII. Sensitivity and Specificity of Breast Cancer Screening Modalities

Modality	Sensitivity	Specificity
Self-examination	0.35	—
Physical examination	0.38	0.90
Mammogram	0.75	0.90

technique is so insensitive (Table VIII), that most cancers are missed.[19] Because of the low prevalence of breast cancer in the general population compared to fibrocystic disease, the accuracy of positive prediction of a lump found by breast self-examination is only about 20%.[20] Although several studies have shown benefit of self-examination measured by earlier disease detection, no reduction of mortality has been demonstrated.[21]

Mammography is recommended as a preferable screening tool. Despite the higher cost and increased complexity of the test over breast self-examination or even physical examination by a physician, the mammogram has a great advantage in its higher sensitivity (Table VIII).[19] Also, mammography screening has been shown to reduce mortality from breast cancer by 30% in women between ages 50 and 59.[10] For these reasons, policy makers have concluded that mammograms are a necessary ingredient of breast cancer screening.

REFERENCES

1. Diamond, G. A., and Forrester, J. S.: Analysis of probability as an aid in the clinical diagnosis of coronary artery disease. *N. Engl. J. Med.* **300:**1350–1358, 1979.
2. Philbrick, J. T., Horwitz, R. I., and Feinstein, A. R.: Methodologic problems of exercise testing for coronary artery disease: Groups, analysis and bias. *Am. J. Cardiol.* **46:**807–812, 1980.
3. Ransohoff, D. F., and Feinstein, A. R.: Problems of spectrum and bias in evaluating the efficacy of diagnostic tests. *N. Engl. J. Med.* **299:**926–930, 1978.
4. Fletcher, R. H.: Carcinoembryonic antigen. *Ann. Intern. Med.* **104:**66–73, 1986.
5. Shultz, T., Miller, W. C., and Bedrossian, C. W. M.: Clinical application of measurement of angiotensin-converting enzyme level. *JAMA* **242:**439–441, 1979.
6. Philbrick, J. T., Horwitz, R. I., Feinstein, A. R., *et al.*: The limited spectrum of patients studied in exercise test research: Analyzing the tip of the iceberg. *JAMA* **248:**2467–2470, 1982.
7. Morrison, A. S.: *Screening in Chronic Disease.* Oxford University Press, New York, 1985, pp. 3–40.
8. Galen, R. S., and Gambino, S. R.: *Beyond Normality: The Predictive Value and Efficiency of Medical Diagnosis.* Wiley, New York, 1975, pp. 53–60.
9. Cole, P., and Morrison, A. S.: Basic issues in population screening for cancer. *J. Natl. Cancer Inst.* **64:**1263–1272, 1980.
10. Shapiro, S.: Evidence on screening for breast cancer from a randomized trial. *Cancer* **39:**2772–2782, 1977.
11. Sparling, P. F.: Diagnosis and treatment of syphilis. *N. Engl. J. Med.* **284:**642–653, 1971.
12. Goldman, J. N.: FTA–ABS and VDRL slide test reactivity in a population of nuns. *JAMA* **217:**453–455, 1974.
13. Duncan, W. C., Know, J. M., and Reuben, D. W.: The FTA–ABS test in dark-field-positive primary syphilis. *JAMA* **228:**859–860, 1974.
14. Jatte, H. W.: The laboratory diagnosis of syphilis. *Ann. Intern. Med.* **83:**846–850, 1975.
15. Griner, P. F., Mayeski, R. J., Mushlin, A. I., *et al.*: Selection and interpretation of diagnostic tests and procedures: Principles and applications. *Ann. Intern. Med.* **94**(4 pt 2)**:**553–600, 1981.
16. *Facts and Figures.* American Cancer Society, New York, 1984.
17. Health and Public Policy Committee, American College of Physicians: The use of diagnostic tests for screening and evaluating breast lesions. *Ann. Intern. Med.* **103:**143–146, 1985.
18. Mahoney, L. J., Bird, B. L., and Cooke, G. M.: Annual clinical examination: The best available screening test for breast cancer. *N. Engl. J. Med.* **301:**315–316, 1979.
19. Mushlin, A. I.: Diagnostic tests in breast cancer. *Ann. Intern. Med.* **103:**79–85, 1985.
20. Baker, L. H.: The Breast Cancer Detection Demonstration Project: Five year summary report. *CA* **32:**194–225, 1982.
21. Shapiro, S., Venet, W., Strax, W., and Roose, R.: 10–14 year effect of screening on breast cancer mortality. *J. Natl. Cancer Inst.* **69:**349–355, 1982.

4

Adult Immunization

David S. Fedson

1. INTRODUCTION

Among all of the challenges of clinical preventive medicine, immunization offers the most clear-cut benefits and greatest likelihood for success. Nonetheless, vaccines often are not regarded as examples of high-technology medical care (which they are),[1] and their use among adults has not been widespread. In contrast, almost all children in the United States receive their required childhood immunizations by the time of school entry. So successful has this been that a substantial proportion of the remaining morbidity and mortality from these vaccine-preventable diseases of childhood now occurs in older adolescents and adults. Thus successful implementation of adult immunization programs is still one of the major challenges in prevention facing physicians.

Current programs for promoting adult immunization focus on the major diseases for which vaccines are given in childhood—tetanus, diphtheria, measles, mumps, rubella, and poliomyelitis—together with two diseases—influenza and pneumococcal infections—to which selected groups of adults may be at increased risk. The vaccines for these diseases are reviewed in this chapter. Hepatitis B vaccine, bacille Calmette Guérin (BCG) vaccines, and vaccines for foreign travel are discussed elsewhere in this book.

The vaccines and toxoids recommended for all adults are summarized in Table I. In addition, some of these vaccines are indicated for selected groups of adults whose medical conditions, occupations, or living circumstances place them at increased risk of infection. Detailed information on each of the vaccines can be found in the statements issued by the Immunization Practices Advisory Committee (ACIP), which are published in *Morbidity and Mortality Weekly Report,* in the American College of Physicians' *Guide for Adult Immunization,*[2] and in other texts.[3,4] Physicians must be thoroughly familiar with each product, and patients must be fully informed about the potential risks associated with immunization as well as the important benefits of preventing disease in both the individual and in the community.

David S. Fedson • Department of Internal Medicine, University of Virginia School of Medicine, Charlottesville, Virginia 22908.

Table I. Vaccines and Toxoids Recommended for All Adults

Vaccine or toxoid	Age group (years)		
	18–24	25–64	65+
Influenza[a]	—	—	+
Pneumococcal[b]	—	—	+
Tetanus/diphtheria (Td) toxoids[c]	+	+	+
Measles[d], mumps[e], rubella[f] (MMR)	+	+	—
Poliovirus[g]	—	—	—

[a]Influenza vaccine should be given annually to younger persons with high-risk conditions and can also be given to any healthy adult who wishes to avoid influenza virus infection.

[b]Pneumococcal vaccine is indicated for younger persons with high-risk conditions, particularly surgical or functional asplenia.

[c]Booster doses of combined tetanus and diphtheria (Td) toxoids should be given every 10 years.

[d]Measles vaccine is indicated for persons born after 1956 and for those who received inactivated measles vaccine from 1963–1967.

[e]Mumps vaccine itself is indicated primarily for susceptible men, but can be given safely to all adults.

[f]Rubella vaccine is recommended for women of childbearing age (≤45 years). Rubella vaccine and MMR vaccine are contraindicated during pregnancy, and adequate contraception should be ensured for 3 months following immunization.

[g]Poliovirus vaccine is not routinely recommended for adults, but inactivated poliovirus vaccine (IPV) can be given to nonimmune parents of children who are to be immunized with live oral poliovirus vaccine (OPV).

2. INFLUENZA VACCINE

Epidemics of influenza are among the most significant causes of acute respiratory disease in the United States. They occur in most communities every year and are marked by increased rates of school and work absenteeism, physician visits, and hospitalization.[5,6] Influenza remains a significant cause of excess mortality, and of 10,000–40,000 or more deaths associated with each epidemic, 80–90% occur in persons 65 years of age and older.[7] The overall economic cost of each epidemic exceeds several billion dollars.

Influenza type A viruses that infect man are classified into subtypes on the basis of their two surface antigens—hemagglutinin (H1, H2, H3) and neuraminidase (N1, N2). Since 1977 variants of H3N2 and H1N1 have cocirculated. Although each subtype has been responsible for epidemic disease, excess mortality has been associated primarily with H3N2 outbreaks. The antigenic "drift" characteristic of type A influenza viruses occurs less frequently with type B viruses. Infections with these viruses generally have been less widespread, although in some years type B viruses have been the predominant cause of severe disease and death.

Current influenza vaccines are trivalent preparations containing 15 μg of each hemagglutinin antigen from the type A (H3N2 and H1N1) and type B variants that are expected to cause outbreaks of disease. Antigenic drift necessitates periodic reformulation of the vaccine. Occasionally antigenic change is not recognized in time to meet the production schedule of the manufacturers, and a supplemental vaccine must be prepared, as occurred with the monovalent A/Taiwan/86 (H1N1) vaccine in 1986–1987. Influenza vaccine is administered intramuscularly (0.5 ml/dose) and generally leads to the development of serum and secretory antibodies to both surface antigens. Protection against clinical illness is best correlated with a serum antihemagglutinin titer of 1 : 40 or greater. This antibody level is achieved in 90% or more of immunocompetent adults, including the elderly. Clinical protection is dependent on the closeness of the "match" between the vaccine and epidemic strains. When there is a good match, influenza vaccine is usually 60–80% protective against clinical illness in younger adults. Among the elderly protection may be less than 50%, although protection against pneumonia, hospitalization, and death is much greater.

Influenza vaccine is extremely safe. It contains inactivated virus and thus cannot cause influenza itself. Side effects attributable to the vaccine have virtually disappeared since modern methods of vaccine production were introduced 15–20 years ago. In adults local reactions are uncommon, and serious systemic reaction are very rare. Importantly, no increased risk of adverse neurological reactions, including Guillain-Barré syndrome, has been observed over the past decade. The only contraindication to receipt of influenza vaccine is known anaphylactic hypersensitivity to eggs. Although immunization may alter the hepatic clearance of several drugs, including warfarin, theophylline, and phenytoin, none of these changes has been shown to be clinically significant.

Annual influenza immunization is recommended for all persons who are at increased risk of lower respiratory complications and death following influenza virus infection. Highest priority is given to (1) persons with chronic conditions, especially cardiopulmonary disorders, who have required regular medical followup or hospitalization within the past year, and (2) residents of nursing homes and other chronic-care institutions. Others who should be immunized include persons 65 years of age and older and persons with diabetes mellitus or other metabolic conditions, chronic renal disease, severe anemia, asthma, or immunosuppression, regardless of cause. In addition, physicians, nurses, and other health care personnel who have contact with high-risk persons, particularly those who work in intensive-care units, should be immunized to reduce the risk of nosocomial influenza. The same rule applies to home health care workers and family members of high-risk patients.

The ACIP has strongly recommended annual influenza immunization for over 20 years. Nonetheless, vaccination rates have not improved in persons aged 65 years and older; they have remained steady at 21–23% for several years.[8] For younger persons with high-risk conditions the rates have declined to approximately 10%. By any measure, the failure of influenza vaccine to prevent infection in high-risk patients is largely the result of the failure to use the vaccine, rather than a lack of vaccine efficacy. This reflects the general absence of organized approaches to vaccine delivery. Well-organized immunization programs in the office-practice setting and in hospitals can immunize 50–70% or more of high-risk patients who are offered the vaccine. In addition, once patients are immunized, they are likely to expect or even ask for the vaccine in subsequent years. Programs for influenza immunization should be organized at least 1 year in advance. Orders for the vaccine are generally taken in late fall, and these orders let the manufacturers know how much vaccine should be produced the next year. Vaccine is usually available the following September, and immunization programs should be conducted from then through the end of February, or until the end of an outbreak should it occur.

For persons who have not received (or cannot receive) influenza vaccine, the antiviral agent amantadine can be given prophylactically. It is effective against type A but not type B infections, and must be taken daily throughout the epidemic period. Alternatively, for persons who can be vaccinated, amantadine can be given for 2 weeks following immunization to ensure both immediate and longer-lasting protection. Amantadine also is useful therapeutically when given early in the course of disease. This drug can be especially helpful in persons who by virtue of their underlying medical conditions might be expected to respond poorly to the vaccine. Nonetheless, the problem of daily compliance with a prophylactic or therapeutic regimen, together with the occurrence of drug side effects in the presence of reduced renal function, emphasizes the overwhelming importance of immunization as the mainstay of efforts to control influenza and prevent its complications in high-risk patients. If such a program were widely implemented, the resulting health benefits and the cost-effectiveness of influenza immunization would be substantial.[9]

3. *PNEUMOCOCCAL VACCINE*

The annual incidence of serious pneumococcal infections is not known, although estimates for the United States suggest 70–260 cases per 100,000 population for pneumococcal pneumonia and 7–25 cases per 100,000 population for pneumococcal bacteremia. Pneumococcal infections remain the most common cause of hospitalization for community-acquired pneumonia, accounting for 34% of all diagnosed cases in a recent multicenter prospective study conducted in England.[10] More important, appropriate antimicrobial therapy and intensive-care support have not had an appreciable effect on mortality from pneumococcal bacteremia; it remains 20–30% overall and can exceed 40% or more among the elderly and in those with nosocomial infection.[8,11]

Pneumococcal vaccine contains purified capsular polysaccharides representing types that account for most cases of serious bacteremic pneumococcal pneumonia and meningitis. The initial 14-valent vaccine which came into use in 1978 contained 50 μg of each capsular polysaccharide from types accounting for approximately 80% of serious illnesses. In 1983 a second-generation, 23-valent vaccine took its place. This vaccine contains only 25μg of each capsular polysaccharide. Antigenic subtypes of improved antigenicity and new types have been added to increase vaccine coverage to almost 90% of serious pneumococcal infections.

Protection against pneumococcal infection is dependent on a number of factors, including adequate numbers of normally functioning polymorphonuclear leukocytes, intact complement function, and type-specific antibody directed at the capsular polysaccharide. Of these, specific antibody generally is the most important. Most immunocompetent adults develop a twofold rise in type-specific antibody following a single 0.5-ml dose of vaccine given intramuscularly. There are few data to indicate the specific titers of antibody that are protective for each serotype, although some evidence suggests that levels of 200–400 ng of antibody nitrogen per milliliter, as measured by radioimmunoassay, are protective. Serial observations indicate that adequate levels of antibody generally persist for 5 years in most vaccine recipients, although in some persons antibody titers may decline after 8–10 years.

Pneumococcal vaccine is extremely safe. Although mild local side effects are not unusual, fever and other constitutional symptoms occur in fewer than 1% of recipients, and severe reactions are extremely rare. Reimmunization with pneumococcal vaccine has not been recommended, although the frequency of adverse reactions following reimmunization probably is less than what was reported in earlier studies and is likely to be even lower in persons whose initial vaccination occurred many years ago. Pneumococcal vaccine can be given at the same time as influenza vaccine, provided each vaccine is administered at separate sites.

Recommendations for pneumococcal immunization have evolved since the vaccine was first licensed, as reflected in the three statements issued by the ACIP. From the beginning there has been no doubt the vaccine should be given to all persons who have surgical or functional asplenia, including sickle cell disease. This is to protect against the syndrome of overwhelming pneumococcal sepsis that occurs in such patients. Also, there has been general acceptance of the recommendation to give pneumococcal vaccine to patients with Hodgkin's disease, lymphoma, and multiple myeloma, recognizing that these patients are at increased risk of infection primarily because they have a poor antibody response to pneumococcal capsular polysaccharide antigens. However, there has been continued controversy over whether pneumococcal vaccine should be given to immunocompetent adults with underlying high-risk conditions such as cardiopulmonary diseases and diabetes mellitus, and to healthy persons 65 years of age and older. It should be remembered that the efficacy of pneumococcal vaccine was unequivocally demonstrated in randomized controlled trials among novice gold miners in South Africa who, because of their working and living conditions, were at greatly increased risk of acquiring pneumococcal infection. It has been difficult to obtain similar evidence in randomized controlled trials in open populations of elderly persons; the low incidence of nasopharyngeal carriage of pneumococcal organisms and the often high titers of naturally acquired type-specific antibodies result in a low incidence of infection. Consequently, other methods have been used to assess the efficacy of pneumococcal vaccine in the elderly, including case-control and retrospective studies.[12,13] In these studies the efficacy of pneumococcal vaccine in preventing pneumococcal bacteremia has been estimated to be 60–80%, although the confidence intervals have been broad, and in subgroups of patients with immunocompromise the vaccine has not been effective.

The results of the Veterans Administration Cooperative Study were reported recently.[14] This multicenter, randomized controlled trial attempted to assess the efficacy of the vaccine in preventing pneumococcal infections in older high-risk patients. The study failed to demonstrate protection against pneumococcal bacteremia, pneumonia, or bronchitis in vaccinated subjects. Interpretation of the study results is hampered by a lower-than-expected incidence of vaccine-type infection in control as well as vaccinated subjects, and a significantly higher frequency of previous pneumococcal infection among vaccinated subjects. Also, the sample size was too small to preclude the likely occurrence of a type II (beta) error (i.e., a false-negative result). The VA study results emphasize once again the importance of adequate levels of antibody as indicators of protection; only two of seven vaccinated patients with probable pneumonia caused by vaccine-type organisms had antibody levels greater than 600 ng/ml antibody nitrogen by radioimmunoassay. The VA Cooperative Study does not provide a basis for modifying current 1984 ACIP recommendations for pneumococcal immunization. The results demonstrate the difficulty of conducting a clinical trial of a disease of low frequency, while emphasizing the need to improve the antigenicity of the vaccine, perhaps by using protein-conjugated polysaccharides.

The target populations for pneumococcal and influenza immunization are quite similar, the major exception being persons with splenic disorders, as mentioned earlier. During the period 1978–1985, approximately 13.5 million doses of pneumococcal vaccine were distributed in the United States.[8] It is not known with any certainty the proportion of elderly and high-risk persons who have been immunized; certainly it is no greater than 20–25%, and it probably is lower. Also, there is no convincing evidence that the Medicare policy authorizing reimbursement for pneumococcal (but not influenza) immunization has had any effect on vaccine use. As with influenza vaccine, it is likely that improvements in the use of pneumococcal vaccine will come about only as a result of organized programs for vaccine delivery. In this respect, programs that target patients at the time of hospital discharge would be particularly useful.[11] Approximately two-thirds of patients hospitalized with serious pneumococcal infections have been discharged at least once in the previous 5 years. With organized programs almost 80% can be immunized.[8]

4. MEASLES, MUMPS, AND RUBELLA VACCINES

It might be argued that childhood immunization has been the most important preventive health success of the past decade. As a result of the Childhood Immunization Initiative launched in 1977 more than 95% of all children are fully immunized at the time of school entry. In 1984 the Centers for Disease Control (CDC) received reports of only 2587 cases of measles, 3021 cases of mumps, and 752 cases of rubella.[15] At least 93% of U.S. counties were free of measles and rubella, and 78% of counties were free of mumps. Although congenital rubella syndrome is thought to be underreported, only five cases were brought to the attention of the CDC.

The decline in the incidence of these three diseases has brought about a shift in the age distribution of the cases reported. In 1984 approximately 33% of cases of measles, 25% of cases of mumps, and 48% of cases of rubella occurred in persons 15 years of age or older.[15] Serological surveys show that by 20 years of age most persons are immune to mumps, but 20% of young adults may be susceptible to measles,[16] and 10–15% remain susceptible to rubella.[17] In the last few years the incidence of measles has actually risen. Whether this is due to faltering immunization programs or to epidemiological variation in the natural history of the disease is not known. Many recent outbreaks of measles have occurred on college campuses, and outbreaks of rubella have affected both colleges and hospitals. Both infections are more serious in young adults; measles virus infection can cause encephalitis, and rubella virus infection during the first trimester of infection leads to fetal wastage or congenital rubella syndrome in 80% of fetuses carried to term. Mumps virus infection, though generally mild, can cause meningeal reactions, orchitis, and rarely deafness or sterility. Thus current ACIP recommendations stress the need to address the ''bulge of susceptibility'' among young adults to these three diseases.

Measles, mumps, and rubella (MMR) vaccines contains live, attenuated viruses. A single dose induces protective levels of antibodies against measles and rubella in 95% of recipients and against mumps in 90% of recipients. Because adults who are susceptible to one of the viruses are often at risk of infection by the others, it has become common practice to give combined MMR vaccine. Measles vaccine is indicated for persons (1) who were born after 1956 who lack documented immunity, (2) who were vaccinated before 12 months of age, (3) who received only killed measles vaccine, (4) who received live measles vaccine within 3 months of killed vaccine, or (5) who received vaccine of unknown type between 1963 and 1967. Rubella vaccine is indicated for all young adults, particularly nonpregnant women of childbearing age, who lack documented immunity (an immunization record or positive serology, not simply physician-diagnosed disease). Susceptibility should be assessed at the time of all visits for medical care, premarital screening, and hospital discharge. Serological testing is unnecessary for nonpregnant women with no known history of rubella immunization; MMR can be given without fear of adverse reactions. Although most younger adults have natural immunity to mumps, the vaccine may benefit those who received only killed mumps vaccine, which was available from 1950 to 1978.

MMR vaccines produce mild infections that generally are short-lived and well tolerated. In addition, rubella vaccine is frequently associated with transient arthralgias in smaller peripheral joints. Allergic reactions are uncommon, although persons with a history of anaphylactic reaction to eggs should be given measles and mumps vaccines with caution because these vaccines (but not rubella vaccine) are prepared in chick embryo cell cultures. The major contraindication to giving MMR vaccine is pregnancy or the likelihood of pregnancy occurring within 3 months. However, inadvertent rubella immunization during pregnancy has not been associated with congenital rubella syndrome, nor has measles vaccine, unlike measles virus infection itself, been associated with subacute sclerosing panencephalitis. The three vaccines also should not be given to persons with immunocompromise and should be delayed for at least 3 months after administration of immune globulin.

The benefits associated with MMR immunization have been striking; estimates suggest that without vaccine the cost of the three diseases in 1983 would have been $1.4 billion, whereas the cost of immunization, together with the costs of disease in the smaller number of cases, was so reduced that immunization had a benefit–cost ratio of 14 to 1.[18] Rigorous immunization programs have virtually eliminated these diseases among military recruits. Nonetheless, outbreaks of measles and rubella have continued to occur on college campuses. They often have been costly to control, and for measles they have been associated with fatalities. For these reasons the American College Health Association has commited itself to organizing effective immunization programs. Continued success with childhood immunization programs should bring about the eventual elimination of these three diseases among young adults.

5. POLIOMYELITIS VACCINES

Universal immunization with live oral poliovirus vaccine (OPV) has virtually eradicated wild strains of polioviruses from the United States.[19] Protection against poliomyelitis can be ensured only by maintaining high levels of immunization. Either OPV or inactivated poliovirus vaccine (IPV) is protective against all three strains of poliovirus infection in more than 95% of cases. However, because most persons older than 18 years of age are already immune, widespread immunization of adults is not regarded as necessary.

There are certain situations in which immunization with polio vaccine may be advisable. Adults who have not been immunized as children and who might be at greater risk of exposure to wild polioviruses (e.g., foreign travelers or certain laboratory workers) should be given a primary series of IPV—three doses each 4–8 weeks apart, followed by a fourth dose 6–12 months later. OPV should be avoided because the risk of OPV-associated paralytic disease is slightly greater in adults than it is in children. When children are given OPV, adults in the household who are not fully immunized have a very small risk of OPV-associated paralytic disease; they may be given IPV if they wish, but full immunization of children should never be delayed unless there is no doubt that waiting for the adult to be immunized will not unduly delay the subsequent full immunization of the child.

Adverse reactions to poliomyelitis vaccines are extremely rare. IPV causes almost no reactions, although it should be avoided by persons with anaphylactic hypersensitivity to streptomycin and neomycin, which may be present in the vaccine in trace amounts. In immunocompetent recipients of OPV the risk of vaccine-associated paralysis is one case per nine million doses of vaccine distributed. Of the eight cases of paralytic poliomyelitis reported to the CDC in 1984, seven were OPV-associated.[15] Neither OPV nor IPV has been shown to adversely affect the pregnant woman or the fetus; the choice of which vaccine should be given is determined by the urgency of the need for immediate protection.

6. COMBINED TETANUS AND DIPHTHERIA TOXOID

The occurrence of tetanus and diphtheria in the United States has declined dramatically. In 1984 only one case of diphtheria was reported.[15] There were 74 cases of tetanus, only two of which occurred in persons with histories of complete immunization. Most cases of tetanus and many of diphtheria now occur in elderly persons—53% of the cases of tetanus in 1984 occurred in persons aged 60 years and older. These findings parallel those from serological surveys indicating that 40–80% of older persons lack protective levels of antitoxin to the two diseases.[20] Because immunization is virtually 100% protective, all adults should be assured immunization.

Once a primary series of combined tetanus and diphtheria (Td) toxoid has been given (two doses 4 weeks apart, followed by a third dose 6–12 months later), immunity should be maintained with booster doses every 10 years. A mid-decade birthday serves as a convenient reminder. Local adverse reactions can occur but are well tolerated; systemic reactions are far less common. A more severe Arthus-type local hypersensitivity reaction can occur in persons who previously have received multiple doses of tetanus toxoid. Booster doses should be given cautiously and no more frequently than once in 10 years. Severe hypersensitivity reactions are extremely rare and are the only contraindication to combined Td toxoid.

The use of combined Td toxoid and tetanus immune globulin in routine wound

Table II. Tetanus Prophylaxis in Routine Wound Management

	Clean, minor wounds		All other wounds	
History of tetanus immunization	Td[a]	TIG[b]	Td	TIG
Unknown, uncertain, 0–2 doses	Yes	No	Yes	Yes[c]
Three or more doses[d]	No[e]	No	No[f]	No

[a]Combined tetanus–diphtheria (Td) toxoid. For children less than 7 years of age, DTP (DT if pertussis vaccine is contraindicated) is preferred to tetanus toxoid alone. For persons 7 years of age or older, Td is preferred to tetanus toxoid alone.
[b]Tetanus immune globulin.
[c]When Td and TIG are given simultaneously, adsorbed and not fluid tetanus toxoid should be used.
[d]If only three doses of fluid toxoid have been received, a fourth dose of adsorbed toxoid should be given.
[e]Td should be given if more than 10 years since the last dose.
[f]Td should be given if more than 5 years since the last dose. More frequent boosters may increase side effects and are unnecessary.

management is outlined in Table II. Tetanus prophylaxis in hospital emergency rooms is widespread, but often it is given incorrectly.[21] One recent study has shown that overtreatment was more common than undertreatment, but only 27% of persons with the most serious wounds were correctly treated with both tetanus toxoid and tetanus immune globulin.

7. CONCLUSION

In the next few years the vaccines and toxoids currently available for adult immunization will be supplemented by modified preparations (e.g., live attenuated influenza vaccine, protein conjugated pneumococcal vaccine) and entirely new vaccines (e.g., live attenuated varicella vaccine). However, the future success of adult immunization will depend even more on the development of new approaches to vaccine delivery. Relatively little research has been conducted on the microepidemiology of immunization practices—who gives and who receives vaccines. The determinants of effective immunization practice need to be defined more precisely. In all likelihood, expanded educational programs that focus only on the characteristics of the diseases and the vaccines will not be sufficient.[3,4,8] Administrative and organizational interventions will probably be needed. They have dramatically improved immunization practices in a variety of settings and should be aggressively pursued and extended to all sites where physicians care for adults.

REFERENCES

1. Thomas, L.: The technology of medicine. *N. Engl. J. Med.* **285:**1365–1368, 1971.
2. Committee on Immunization: *Guide for Adult Immunization.* American College of Physicians, Philadelphia, 1985.

3. Fedson, D. S.: Immunizations for health care workers and patients in hospitals, in Wenzel, R. P. (ed.): *Prevention and Control of Nosocomial Infections*. Williams & Wilkins, Baltimore, 1986, pp. 116–174.
4. Fedson D. S.: Adult Immunization, in Noble J. (ed.): *Textbook of General Medicine and Primary Care*. Little, Brown, Boston, 1987, pp. 1681–1695.
5. Perrotta, D. M., Decker, M., and Glezen, W. P.: Acute respiratory disease hospitalization as a measure of impact of epidemic influenza. *Am. J. Epidemiol.* **122**:468–476, 1985.
6. Barker, W. H.: Excess pneumonia and influenza associated hospitalization during influenza epidemics in the United States, 1970–78. *Am. J. Public Health* **76**:761–765, 1986.
7. Lui, K. J., and Kendal, A. P.: Impact of influenza epidemics on mortality in the United States from October 1972 to May 1985. *Am. J. Public Health,* **77**:712–716, 1987.
8. Fedson, D. S.: Influenza and pneumococcal immunization strategies for physicians. *Chest* **91**:436–443, 1987.
9. Riddiough, M. A., Sisk, J. E., and Bell, J. C.: Influenza vaccination. Cost effectiveness and public policy. *JAMA* **249**:3189–3195, 1983.
10. Research Committee of the British Thoracic Society and the Public Health Laboratory Service: Community-acquired pneumonia in adults in British hopsitals in 1982–1983: A survey of aetiology, mortality, prognostic factors and outcome. *Q. J. Med.* **62**:195–220, 1987.
11. Fedson, D. S.: Improving the use of pneumococcal vaccine through a strategy of hospital-based immunization: A review of its rationale and implications. *J. Am. Geriatr. Soc.* **33**:142–150, 1985.
12. Shapiro, E. D., and Clemens, J. D.: A controlled evaluation of the protective efficacy of pneumococcal vaccine for patients at high risk of serious pneumococcal infections. *Ann. Intern. Med.* **101**:325–330, 1984.
13. Bolan, G., Broome, C. V., Facklam, R. R., *et al.:* Pneumococcal vaccine efficacy in selected populations in the United States. *Ann. Intern. Med.* **104**:1–6, 1986.
14. Simberkoff, M. S., Cross, A. P., Al-Ibrahim, M., *et al.:* Efficacy of pneumococcal vaccine: Results of a Veterans Administration cooperative study. *N. Engl. J. Med.* **315**:1318–1327, 1986.
15. Centers for Disease Control: Annual Summary 1984: Reported morbidity and mortality in the United States. *Morbid. Mortal. Wkly. Rep.* **33**(54):3, 1986.
16. Hinman, A. R., Eddins, D. L., Kirby, C. D., *et al.:* Progress in measles elimination. *JAMA* **247**:1592–1595, 1982.
17. Orenstein, W. A., Bart, K. J., Hinman, A. R., *et al.:* The opportunity and obligation to eliminate rubella from the United States. *JAMA* **251**:1988–1994, 1984.
18. White, C. C., Koplan, J. P., and Orenstein, W. A.: Benefits, risks and costs of immunization for measles, mumps and rubella. *Am. J. Public Health* **75**:739–744, 1985.
19. Kim-Farley, R. J., Bart, K. J., Schonberger, L. B., *et al.:* Poliomyelitis in the USA: Virtual elimination of disease caused by wild virus. *Lancet* **2**:1315–1317, 1984.
20. Weiss, B. P., Strassburg, M. A., and Feeny, J. C.: Tetanus and diphtheria immunity in an elderly population in Los Angeles County. *Am. J. Public Health* **73**:802–804, 1983.
21. Brand, D. A., Acampora, D., Gottlieb, L. D., *et al.:* Adequacy of antitetanus prophylaxis in six hospital emergency rooms. *N. Engl. J. Med.* **309**:636–640, 1983.

5

Antimicrobial Prophylaxis

Gordon M. Dickinson

1. INTRODUCTION

The proverb "An ounce of prevention is worth a pound of cure" is particularly appropriate to infections. Infections account for a majority of illnesses that cause patients to seek medical care.[1] Although many of these infections are self-limited upper-respiratory-tract infections, serious infections with much greater morbidity and economic impact are also common. A study of community-acquired infections in hospitalized patients conducted over a 3½-year period in the early 1970s, led the authors to estimate that there were more than three million infections per year in hospitalized patients in the United States.[2] A contemporary study of nosocomial infections estimated that more than two million hospital-acquired infections occurred yearly.[2] It is clear that infections will continue to account for a large proportion of illnesses that require medical care.

On the other hand, tremendous strides have been made in the control of infections, and once-important infections have been eradicated from many parts of the world. The programs responsible for these dramatic successes are often forgotten or taken for granted. Control of mosquito breeding through drainage projects and widespread use of insecticides eliminated endogenous malaria from the United States more than 40 years ago. Widespread vaccination programs have completely eradicated smallpox. Polio, diphtheria, and pertussis are infrequently encountered in the United States because of universal vaccination. The establishment of safe water supplies and construction of adequate sewage systems are two public health measures that have made epidemics of hepatitis A, salmonellosis, and shigellosis rare events. These public health measures may be applied to other diseases, or refined further, but are unlikely to lead to equally great progress in the future.

A chemoprophylactic approach to the prevention of infections began soon after the introduction of antimicrobials. The extent of prophylactic antibiotic use today is unknown, although studies suggest that prophylaxis for surgical infections accounts for a significant proportion of antibiotic use in hospitals.[3,4] It is likely that prophylaxis accounts for a significant proportion of antibiotic use in ambulatory patients, too. Prophylaxis is a controversial subject, however. Though the goals of prophylaxis are clear,

---

Gordon M. Dickinson • Department of Medicine, University of Miami School of Medicine, Veterans Administration Medical Center, Miami, Florida 33101.

the actual benefit of prophylaxis often remains unproven. Because infections typically occur in a minority of persons at risk, or only at infrequent intervals, large numbers of subjects are usually necessary to allow statistically significant inferences about the efficacy of a particular agent in prevention of an infection. It is often not possible to enroll sufficient numbers of subjects and follow them long enough to achieve statistical significance. Consequently, many studies suggest, but do not conclusively demonstrate, efficacy. Concern over toxicity, particularly when it occurs in an otherwise healthy person, tends to temper enthusiasm for prophylaxis. The emergence of antimicrobial resistance to agents used in prophylaxis is always a potential problem. The indications for antimicrobial prophylaxis are reviewed in this chapter.

2. INDICATIONS FOR USE

There are three basic indications for antimicrobial prophylaxis (Table I). Exposure to a specific pathogen is the major indication for patients outside the hospital setting. The person is typically healthy but has had or will have an exposure to a virulent pathogen, and thus is at risk for subsequent infection and disease. Antibiotics are usually given for a short time, though in cases where the exposure is prolonged the prophylaxis also may be long term. The second indication is a predisposition for infection due to an anatomical defect or to a deficiency in host defenses. Prophylaxis for these persons typically must be given for long periods of time because the abnormality is usually permanent. Prophylaxis may be directed against one specific pathogen, or several. The last indication is a surgical procedure that is known to be associated with significant risk for infection. Prophylaxis often must be directed against multiple pathogens. Specific pathogens are not precisely known, although from historical data the likely pathogens can be predicted and antibiotic agents selected accordingly.

Table I. Indications for Chemoprophylaxis of Infection

1. Exposure to a specific pathogen
   - A. *Neisseria meningitidis*
   - B. *Neisseria gonorrhoeae*
   - C. *Plasmodium* species
   - D. *Mycobacterium tuberculosis*
   - E. *Hemophilus influenzae*
   - F. Influenza
2. Predisposition to infection
   - A. Endocarditis
   - B. Rheumatic carditis
   - C. Recurrent urinary tract infections
3. Surgical procedures
   - A. Contaminated surgery
   - B. Clean–contaminated surgery
   - C. Clean surgery with potential for catastrophic consequences if infection occurs

2.1. Exposure to a Specific Pathogen

2.1.1. *Neisseria meningitidis*

Disease caused by *N. meningitidis* is typically fulminant and severe, and in spite of our ability to diagnose these infections and the availability of effective antibiotics, the mortality rate ranges up to 19%.[5] There are two epidemiological patterns of meningococcal disease: epidemic and endemic. There have been no serious epidemics of meningococcal disease for more than 40 years in the United States, although extensive outbreaks have occurred elsewhere in recent years. Endemic disease caused by *N. meningitidis* occurs at a rate of 1–3 per 100,000 persons per year in the United States, with the highest rates occurring in late winter and early spring.[6] Isolates of *N. meningitidis* can be serotyped. Type A, B, C, and Y account for most serious infections.

Epidemic meningococcal disease was once a serious problem in military training camps where young recruits from various parts of the United States were concentrated. One of the most dramatic uses of antimicrobial prophylaxis was the elimination of these epidemics by the administration of sulfonamides in the 1940s.[7] Several outbreaks caused by sulfonamide-resistant strains occurred in the 1960s, however, and the continued presence of resistant strains now precludes the use of sulfonamides unless the susceptibility of the strain to be targeted is known. Several vaccines have been developed and proven to be highly effective. Unfortunately, serotype B has eluded efforts to develop a vaccine effective against it. One polyvalent vaccine currently available induces protective antibodies against types A, C, Y, and W-135. Vaccination is primarily useful for preventing disease in large groups in whom increased risk of disease can be anticipated, such as military recruits. Vaccination may also be useful for terminating an epidemic caused by a serotype targeted by the vaccine. It is of limited usefulness for preventing secondary infections, however, because secondary cases often occur within an interval of time too brief for the development of individual immunity. Thus, there is still a need for chemoprophylaxis.

Infection is acquired in the nasopharynx, probably by droplet spread directly from a carrier and, in the susceptible individual, is followed by invasive disease. The purpose of chemoprophylaxis is eradication of nasopharyngeal carriage of *N. meningitidis,* which in turn eliminates the potential for invasive disease. Because sulfonamide resistance is widespread, other antimicrobials must be used. Rifampin and minocycline are both effective.[8,9] Minocycline is often associated with vertigo and is therefore not well tolerated. Rifampin is well tolerated and is currently the drug of choice for chemoprophylaxis.[10] Because the administration of rifampin has been associated with the emergence of rifampin-resistant strains of *N. meningitidis,*[11] it is not suitable for mass prophylaxis against epidemics. It is, however, considered satisfactory for prophylaxis for contacts of sporadic cases. The usual dose is 600 mg every 12 hr for 2 days for adults and 10 mg/kg every 12 hr for 2 days for children. Those persons for whom prophylaxis is recommended are shown in Table II. Often, the history of exposure is not convincing; close observation may be an appropriate alternative to chemoprophylaxis for such patients. Penicillin and a number of other agents active against *N. meningitidis* are not effective in eradicating *N. meningitidis* from the nasopharynx, presumably because bactericidal levels are not achieved in saliva.[12]

Table II. Persons at Risk for Meningococcal Disease

Household contacts
Day-care center contacts
Medical personnel with intimate contact (resuscitating or suctioning a patient)
Persons in contact with a patient's secretions

2.1.2. *Neisseria gonorrhoeae*

Sexual partners of persons who have gonorrhea are at high risk for infection: one study found that 78% of male sexual contacts and 86% of female sexual contacts of persons with gonorrhea were infected, many of whom had no symptoms.[13] Because *N. gonorrhoeae* is readily passed from one individual to another, chemoprophylaxis of contacts of persons with gonorrhea will not only prevent the complications of infections in the contact but will also interrupt the chain of transmission. Treatment is recommended for all identified partners.[14] Persons who have had sexual intercourse with the diagnosed patient within the past 30 days should be considered at risk. The choice and dosage of chemoprophylaxis are identical to those used in the treatment of gonorrhea.[14] The emergence of penicillinase-producing *N. gonorrhoeae* strains has limited the effectiveness of benzylpenicillin in many parts of the world, including parts of the United States, and alternative agents are now supplementing benzylpenicillin in the treatment of gonorrhea. Ceftriaxone, 250 mg administered intramuscularly one time, is currently recommended for penicillinase-producing *N. gonorrhoeae.*[14] Other agents such as tetracycline or spectinomycin can also be used. The choice of treatment should be based on the current prevalence of penicillinase-producing *N. gonorrhoeae* in the patient's community. If pharyngeal infection is suspected, only benzylpenicillin or ceftriaxone should be used, since oral ampicillin, amoxicillin, or spectinomycin are not effective in the eradication of pharyngeal gonorrhea. Administration of antimicrobial agents before or after sexual activity has been attempted to prevent infection and can decrease the incidence of infection. Because of uncontrolled variables associated with sexual activity, the need for prolonged prophylaxis of many individuals, problems with compliance, and the emergence of resistance, this approach should be discouraged.

2.1.3. *Chlamydia trachomatis*

The epidemiology of sexually transmitted *C. trachomatis* is similar to that of *N. gonorrhoeae,* and contacts of infected persons should also be treated regardless of symptoms. The current recommended treatment is tetracycline, 500 mg by mouth four times a day for 7 days. Current recommendations for treatment of gonorrhea include administration of tetracycline to persons with gonorrhea because the frequency of concurrent infection with *C. trachomatis* approaches 50%. Recent sexual partners of persons with syphilis and chancroid should also be treated with a regimen appropriate to the treatment of these infections.

2.1.4. *Hemophilus influenzae*

The leading cause of meningitis in children between the ages of 6 months and 6 years is *H. influenzae,* type B. Humans are the natural host for *Hemophilus* species, and disease is thought to occur in a susceptible person after colonization is acquired from another infected person in a manner similar to the pathogenesis of *N. meningitidis* disease. Epidemics of *H. influenzae* disease do not occur, but it is known that family contacts of a person with systemic *H. influenzae* disease have a significantly higher risk of infection than the general population.[15] Outbreaks of systemic infection have occurred in day care centers.[16] The secondary cases are found chiefly among children less than 6 years of age, the age group at risk for invasive *H. influenzae* infection. Most persons over the age of 6 are not susceptible to *H. influenzae* disease, though they can develop pharyngeal colonization and pass the organism to other susceptible persons.

Efforts to develop a vaccine have had limited success because the age group at greatest risk, children less than 12 months of age, do not reliably develop protective antibodies. Because antibiotic prophylaxis may prevent secondary cases, the American Academy of Pediatrics recommends that all household, nursery, and day care center contacts of a person with systemic *H. influenzae* disease, both children and adults, receive antibiotic prophylaxis.[17] The recommended regimen is rifampin, 20 mg/kg per day (up to 600 mg/day) given once a day by mouth for 4 days. Granoff and War have reviewed the status of prophylaxis for *H. influenzae* infections.[18] They stressed that data defining the risk of secondary infection are incomplete, that the logistical difficulties of administering prophylaxis to all contacts are great, and that problems with compliance all contribute to a great deal of uncertainty in this area.

2.1.5. *Mycobacterium tuberculosis*

Tuberculosis has steadily decreased in the United States, but it remains a serious problem in some communities, particularly in poor inner-city neighborhoods. A total of 20,000 cases were reported to the Public Health Department in 1985, In spite of the availability of potent drugs for treatment, tuberculosis remains a potentially lethal disease with significant morbidity. Since bovine tuberculosis has been essentially eradicated from the United States, tuberculosis is now a disease limited to humans. The infection is readily transmitted by the airborne route, and virtually all infections are acquired by inhalation of the tubercle bacillus. The risk for contacts developing active tuberculosis undoubtedly varies with the extent of their exposure, but for persons who become tuberculin reactive, it is considered to be approximately 5%. Isoniazid has been advocated for many years for prophylaxis for tuberculosis in persons exposed to a patient with disease. It was considered both an effective and safe prophylactic agent. Treatment of contacts is 60–80% effective in the prevention of active tuberculosis.[19] Failure of chemoprophylaxis is probably related to poor compliance. Recognition that isoniazid could cause severe hepatotoxicity has led to the reevaluation of prophylaxis. The incidence of hepatitis ranges from a rate of 1 per 100,000 in persons under age 20, 300 per 100,000 between ages 20 and 34, 1200 per 100,000 between ages 35 and 49, 2300 per 100,000 between ages 50 and 64, to 800 per 100,000 over age 64.[20] Most cases of isoniazid-associated hepatitis are insidious in onset and are characterized by asymptomatic elevations of serum transaminases. Continued administration of isoniazid can lead to hepatic failure; therefore, periodic monitoring of liver enzyme levels is necessary.

There is considerable controversy over the question of who should be given chemoprophylaxis. Persons of any age who develop a positive skin reaction to tuberculin after exposure to an active case of tuberculosis and children with a positive skin reaction of unknown duration have a sufficiently high risk of developing active disease that most authorities would recommend prophylaxis. Persons exposed to an active case, but who are initially tuberculin negative should be closely followed and retested in 3 months. Children with significant exposure, i.e., living in a home with an active case, should be given isoniazid during the 3 months pending the repeat tuberculin test. In virtually all other situations, it is unclear as to what is the most advantagous course. Adults over the age of 35 who are tuberculin positive at initial testing may have recently acquired infection and thus be at relatively high risk for developing active disease, or they may have acquired their infection many years earlier and have very little risk of disease. Adults with a positive skin reaction and a chest film suggestive of inactive disease are at increased risk for developing active disease if they have never been treated for tuberculosis and may benefit from prophylaxis. The risk, however, of active disease developing decreases over several years of observation. Persons with a positive tuberculin reaction who receive chronic corticosteroids, or who are immunosuppressed by malignancy or other debilitating conditions, have an increased, but poorly defined risk of developing active tuberculosis, and the benefit of prophylaxis has not been established. The benefit from prophylactically treating all tuberculin-positive members of population groups with high rates of tuberculosis is also undefined. The picture is clouded by the fact that these groups may harbor isoniazid-resistant *M. tuberculosis* (Indochinese refugees, Haitians) and have shown difficulty achieving adequate compliance with the prophylactic regimen. Table III lists persons recommended for chemoprophylaxis by the Committee on Isoniazid Preventive Treatment of the National Consensus Conference on Tuberculosis.[21]

The standard regimen for prophylaxis is isoniazid, 300 mg/day for 12 months. Pyridoxine, 50 mg/day, should be given to prevent the neurotoxicity that may be seen with isoniazid. Patients should be monitored clinically every 2–3 months, and serum transaminase levels should be checked periodically (especially for persons over the age of 35). If mild elevations occur, isoniazid can be continued; however, if progressive in-

Table III. Candidates for Chemoprophylaxis of Tuberculosis[a]

1. Contacts of newly diagnosed cases
2. Newly infected persons
3. Persons with radiographic abnormalities suggestive of tuberculous parenchymal scarring and positive tuberculin reaction
4. Tuberculin reactors in special situations
   - A. Hematological or reticuloendothelial malignant neoplasm
   - B. Long-term systemic high-dose corticosteroid therapy
   - C. Silicosis
   - D. Diabetes mellitus
   - F. Conditions associated with nutritional deficiency
   - G. Heroin addicts
5. Tuberculin reactors aged 35 years or less

[a]Adapted from the recommendation of the Committee on Isoniazid Preventive Treatment, National Consensus Conference on Tuberculosis.[21]

creases are seen or if the patient develops symptoms, the drug should be discontinued. Patients at high risk for severe disease, after infection with known isoniazid-resistant organisms, should be considered for chemoprophylaxis with rifampin for 1 year, with the standard dose used in treatment.

2.1.6. Malaria

Malaria is endemic in many parts of the world and it represents a hazard to visiting American tourists and businessmen, especially if their travels take them out of large urban areas. Chemoprophylaxis has been used for many years and should be considered for all persons traveling to potentially infested areas. Information is available from the Public Health Service about the current status of malaria throughout the world, and the service publishes a pamphlet, *Health Information for International Travel,* that updates malaria prophylaxis recommendations annually. The standard agent for prophylaxis has been chloroquine, one table of 500 mg/week, given 1 week before the traveler enters an endemic area and continued weekly until 6 weeks after the endemic area is vacated. The emergence of chloroquine-resistant strains of *Plasmodium falciparum* in many parts of the world has limited the efficacy of chloroquine. Fansidar (pyrimethamine and sulfadoxine) is active against most chloroquine-resistant strains of *P. falciparum.* It is administered as one tablet per week, for the same duration as chloroquine. One disadvantage of Fansidar is its limited activity against non-*falciparum* species; thus it must be given in addition to chloroquine. Serious reactions to Fansidar, including agranulocytosis and Stevens–Johnson syndrome, have been reported and are another disadvantage.[22] Patients should take Fansidar only if they will have extended significant exposure to mosquitoes in an area known to have chloroquine-resistant *P. falciparum.* Strains of *P. falciparum* resistant to chloroquine, Fansidar, and quinine have emerged in Indochina and pose further difficulties.[23] Often overlooked are measures that travelers can take to avoid being bitten by mosquitoes. Avoidance of mosquito-infected areas, remaining indoors at dusk when mosquitoes are most active, wearing clothing that minimizes exposed skin, sleeping under mosquito nets, and liberal use of insect repellant will do much to prevent infection. The importance of these measures should be emphasized to all persons visiting endemic areas.

2.1.7. Influenza

Influenza can be a serious infection for patients with chronic pulmonary disease or other chronic debilitating diseases, and even in healthy adults it can cause considerable morbidity and loss of time from work. Influenza spreads rapidly by the respiratory route, and epidemics occur every few years. Since the 1940s, vaccines have been in use that are effective in reducing both the frequency and the severity of influenza infection.[24] Antigenic drift, caused by minor changes in the proteins of a particular strain of influenza, occur with relative frequency and limit the efficacy of the influenza vaccines; therefore, vaccines are updated from year to year. Amantadine has been used for many years for prophylaxis against influenza. It is effective against influenza type A, but not against type B. The need for patient compliance with a twice-daily regimen for weeks to months during an influenza outbreak and the risk of adverse neurological effects have limited the acceptance and efficacy of amantadine in the United States. When taken regularly, it is reported to be 75% or more effective in preventing illness due to influenza A.[25] Prophylaxis with amantadine should be considered an adjunct to vaccine administration. Persons who should be considered for prophylaxis are those with chronic illness, the elderly, persons holding critical jobs who have not yet received vaccination, and household contacts of a person with influenza. A drug not yet available, rimantidine, appears to be equal in efficacy to amantadine when it is approved for clinical use.

2.2. Predisposition to Infection

Some patients are at increased risk for infections because of a physical problem unique to themselves and may therefore benefit from specific preventive action, including antimicrobial prophylaxis (Table I). It should be noted that the recommendations for prophylaxis of infection in these patients are based on theoretical reasons that are not always supported by conclusive studies. It is possible that our understanding of the prevention of infection in these patients will change, and so physicians need to keep abreast of current literature. Rheumatic fever is discussed in Chapter 7 and will not be considered here.

2.2.1. Endocarditis

Endocarditis is a serious infection associated with significant morbidity, crippling complications, and residual effects that may lead to congestive heart failure many years after the acute infection has resolved. Fatal outcomes are not rare. Endocarditis can occur in persons without an identifiable predisposition, but the population at greatest risk includes patients with structural abnormalities of cardiac valves. Most episodes of endocarditis can be bacteriologically cured, but residual damage may be associated with significant future morbidity. Because the infection is located in the relatively avascular tissue of cardiac valves where white blood cells cannot readily penetrate, antibiotics must be administered parenterally in high doses for 2–6 weeks. Thus, the costs of treating endocarditis are extremely high.

Bacteremia is a necessary step in the pathogenesis of all cases of endocarditis except those acquired at the time a prosthetic valve is implanted. Prevention of bacteremia is the immediate goal of prophylaxis for endocarditis. Most endocarditis is caused by streptococci that arise from the oral cavity or genitourinary tract, and a smaller proportion of cases is caused by other bacteria originating from the oral cavity. Dental or surgical procedures of the oral, gastrointestinal, and genitourinary tract are often associated with bacteremia, and consequently these procedures are the focus of most efforts to prevent endocarditis.[27] Controversy about the details of prophylaxis exists. First, the risk of any particular procedure is known only indirectly and is undoubtedly very low. The fact that most endocarditis is caused by organisms commonly found in the oral, gastrointestinal, or genitourinary tracts, coupled with the anecdotally noted temporal association of endocarditis caused by these organisms with surgical or dental procedures, is the basis for prophylaxis. However, endocarditis after such a procedure is a distinctly uncommon event,[28] and many patients who do develop endocarditis in association with a procedure do not have cardiac lesions identified at the time of the procedure.[29] Also, many episodes of endocarditis occur in persons who have not had recent procedures. Thus, it has been estimated that only about 10% of all cases of endocarditis are preventable.[28] Another controversy centers on the relative risk for endocarditis that is associated with any particular defect. Prosthetic valves as well as congenital and acquired abnormalities of mitral and aortic valves are accepted as high-risk factors for infection, whereas with idiopathic hypertrophic subaortic stenosis and mitral valve prolapse the risk is far less clear. Other conditions, such as secundum atrial defects or previous coronary artery bypass graft surgery, carry no recognizable risk. Cardiac abnormalities for which endocarditis prophylaxis is recommended are shown in Table IV. Less controversy surrounds the question of what constitutes appropriate duration of prophylaxis. Experimental studies in animals have demonstrated that the critical period occurs at the time of the bacteremia and that prolonging the administration beyond that time is of no demonstrable benefit.[30] Administration of prophylaxis earlier than is needed to achieve high levels at the time of surgery is also thought to be of no benefit and to possibly predispose the patient to colonization with resistant bacteria.

The optimal antimicrobial regimen must be based on probabilities and empiricism. While virtually any organism can occasionally cause endocarditis, most endocarditis is caused by streptococci or by one of a handful of other organisms thought to originate in the mouth. *Staphylococcus aureus,* which accounts for a certain proportion of cases of endocarditis, often involves normal valves and is typically associated with intravenous drug use or soft tissue infections and is therefore not an infection subject to prophylaxis. If a procedure will involve the oral cavity, penicillin-susceptible streptococci or other penicillin-susceptible bacteria are to be expected, whereas surgery of the genitourinary tract is more likely to give rise to enterococci. The current recommendations of the American Heart Association committee on endocarditis prophylaxis, shown in Table V, represent a consensus view (not accepted by all authorities) of what constitutes appropriate regimens for various procedures.[31] Oral antimicrobials have been used for prophylaxis because of the convenience of this route of administration. In 1977, however, the American Heart Association committee on endocarditis prophylaxis recommended that antibiotics be given parenterally to achieve high serum levels. The recommendation was made because of occasional reports of apparent failure of oral regimens to prevent infection and because of data from animal experiments that showed lack of efficacy with low serum antibiotic levels.[30,32] Unfortunately, the parenteral mode of administration poses logistic problems, and a survey of practicing dentists found that only 15% actually follow the recommendations.[33] The most recent recommendations from this committee, therefore, once again include oral antibiotics.[31] It is probable that these recommendations will continue to evolve over time.

Table IV. Indications for Endocarditis Prophylaxis

Prosthetic cardiac valves
Congenital cardiac malformations
Surgically constructed systemic–pulmonary shunts
Rheumatic and other acquired valvular dysfunction
Idiopathic hypertrophic subaortic stenosis
Previous history of bacterial endocarditis
Mitral valve prolapse with valvular insufficiency

Table V. Recommendations for Prophylaxis of Endocarditis[a]

Standard regimen	For dental procedures and oral or upper-respiratory-tract surgery	Penicillin V, 2 g orally 1 hr before, plus 1 g 6 hr later
Special regimen	For GI or GU tract procedures	Ampicillin, 2 g i.m. or i.v., plus gentamicin, 1.5 mg/kg or i.v. 1/2 hr before surgery
	Penicillin-allergic patients	Erythromycin, 1 g orally 1 hr before, plus 0.5 g 6 hr later
		Vancomycin, 1 g over 1 hr, starting 1 hr before, or plus gentamicin, 1.5 mg/kg i.m. or i.v., for GI or GU tract procedures

[a]Source: Shulman *et al.* [31]

2.2.2. *Urinary Tract Infections*

Recurrent urinary tract infections may constitute a reason for antimicrobial prophylaxis in certain patients. Symptomatic urinary tract infections in otherwise healthy persons are primarily a problem in sexually active women, occur sporadically, and are easily managed. For reasons that are not entirely clear, some women have recurrent infections in the absence of stones, structural abnormalities, or other plausible explanations. Most recurrent infections in these women represent reinfections rather than relapses. Reinfections are identified by isolation of a different causative organism with each episode, whereas relapses are caused by the same strain each time. Relapses usually are associated with renal stones, obstructions of urine flow, or foci of infection in kidney. Since each relapse represents an exacerbation of a chronic infection, treatment is surgical correction of any structural abnormality, physical removal of stones, or eradication of parenchymal disease with a high-dose, prolonged course of antibiotics. Reinfections, on the other hand, are relatively easy to treat. Though they usually do not represent a serious threat to the health of the afflicted individual, each episode may cause marked discomfort and disruption of daily activities. Successful prophylaxis of reinfections can be achieved by several antibiotic regimens[34–36] (Table VI). The decision about when to give prophylaxis must be individualized, but it is usually based on the frequency of infections, the severity of symptoms, and the willingness and ability of the individual to comply with long-term medication. Generally, a history of three or four infections per year is an indication for prophylaxis, while infections occurring only once a year or less can easily be managed by treatment as they arise.

Table VI. Regimens for Prophylaxis of Symptomatic Urinary Tract Infections

Antibiotic	Dosage
Trimethoprim–sulfamethoxazole	1/2 tablet/day
Trimethoprim	40 mg/day
Nitrofurantoin	50 mg/day

2.3. Surgical Infections

Infections that complicate surgery range from simple subcutaneous abscesses to fatal sepsis. All contribute unnecessary morbidity to the postoperative convalescence. The impact of postoperative infections is reflected in the prolongation of hospitalization and increased cost of medical care.[37] Rates of surgical infections varied from less than 2% for "clean operations" to 10–20% for some "clean contaminated" operations in a multicenter study published in the early 1960s.[38] Enthusiasm for preventive measures has now led to widespread use of antimicrobial prophylaxis that is often clearly inappropriate.[4,39] Minimizing the potential for infection includes not only appropriate antimicrobial prophylaxis but also attention to other factors.

Factors that influence infection rates include the type of surgery, the duration of operation, operative technique, and underlying diseases.[38,40–42] Prolonged hospitalization before surgery is associated with an increase in the rate of infection compared to the rate in patients operated on shortly after admission.[38] This is presumably related to colonization of the hospitalized patient with virulent organisms acquired in the hospital. Efforts to reduce the incidence of infections also have an effect, though not always a favorable one. Antiseptic washes the night before surgery are associated with a lower rate of infection.[40] Razor shave of the operative site the day before surgery increases the infection rate, apparently because shaving traumatizes skin and increases the local bacterial flora.[41] Placement of surgical wound drains is an established practice, but drains can also provide a route of infection, and unnecessary drains increase the risk of infection. Mechanical cleansing of the bowel before bowel surgery decreases the chance for gross contamination without significantly reducing the intestinal flora.[43] Bowel preparation with oral nonabsorbable antibiotics diminishes the bowel flora and has been thought to decrease the rate of infection,[43] although some authorities challenge this opinion.

For many years, the use of prophylactic antibiotics was controversial, and reports in the medical literature did not support their use.[44] More recent work has demonstrated that antibiotics, when appropriately administered, do diminish the incidence of infection.[42,45–47] The successful use of prophylactic antibiotics at the time of surgery is based on recognition of the levels of risk for infection associated with a particular operation and the use of prophylaxis only for those with higher risk. Surgical operations can be classified as clean, clean–contaminated, or contaminated (Table VII). Clean surgery involves cutting of normal skin and sterile tissues only. Herniorrhaphy, open heart surgery, transcutaneous neurosurgery, and hip arthroplasty are examples of clean surgery. Clean–contaminated surgery is defined as surgery that requires cutting through tissue surfaces that are heavily colonized with bacteria. Colorectal surgery, vaginal hysterectomy, prostatic resection, and appendectomy are examples of clean–contaminated surgery. Contaminated surgery is defined as surgery in an area where bacterial contamination or infection of normally sterile tissue has already occurred. Examples of contaminated surgery include abdominal laparotomy for a ruptured appendix or perforated bowel, prostatic surgery in a man with chronic bacteriuria, and open reduction of a contaminated compound fracture. The risk of infection after clean surgery is negligible, and except for operations in which an infection would be catastrophic, prophylactic antibiotics are not indicated. For cases of clean–contaminated surgery, prophylactic antibiotics can lower the rate of infection, and it is for this classification of surgery that the indications for prophylaxis are the most

Table VII. Classification of Selected Surgical Operations

Clean surgery
Craniotomy
Coronary artery bypass
Mastectomy
Elective plastic surgery
Herniorrhaphy
Clean–contaminated surgery
Appendectomy
Laryngectomy
Cholicystectomy
Gastric reaction
Colon resection
Prostatectomy
Hysterectomy
Contaminated surgery
Exploratory laparotomy for perforated colon, ruptured appendix
Internal fixation of compound fracture
Burn wound debridement

firmly established. Antibiotics are also indicated for contaminated surgery, although their role is probably treatment rather than prophylaxis, since an infection is already present.

Thus, there are two indications for the use of prophylactic antimicrobial agents: if the complicating infection would be catastrophic, or if the procedure is associated with a high risk of infection. Infections that involve joint prostheses, artificial heart valves, or central nervous system shunts occur at a very low rate but with catastrophic effects. Procedures that require cutting through heavily colonized mucosal surfaces (clean–contaminated surgery) carry a high risk of infection, and prophylactic antimicrobials can significantly lower the rate of infection.

Several principles of prophylaxis are applicable to all cases. First, the antimicrobial should be administered only shortly before surgery. Antimicrobials administered in advance of surgery tend to alter the host flora in favor of resistant bacteria.[43] Antimicrobials are initiated within minutes to 1 hr of surgery. Second, the dosage should be sufficient to achieve high tissue levels at the time of surgery. In practice, this means that the antimicrobial is given parenterally. Experimentally, it has been shown that prophylactic antibiotics are the most effective if present in tissue before contamination occurs,[50] which suggests that they should be given shortly before surgery commences. Third, the duration of prophylaxis should be no longer than is needed to achieve maximum benefit. Studies have demonstrated that regimens of 24–48 hr are as effective as longer regimens in the prevention of infection, with less complications, less adverse reactions, fewer problems with resistant bacteria, and less expense.[45–48] Fourth, the choice of an antimicrobial should be based on the recognition of which pathogens are likely to cause infection. The safest, most convenient, and least expensive drug that will be effective should be used. Because their spectrum of activity includes most gram-positive cocci and gram-negative bacilli, cephalosporins have been used in many of the studies of prophylaxis; they are active against most gram-positive cocci and gram-negative bacilli. Because anaerobic bacteria are not uniformly susceptible to the first generation of cephalosporins, agents with better anaerobic activity have also been used for bowel surgery. There is a tendency for physicians to reach for the newer, more potent agents that have a wider spectrum of activity than some of the older agents. However, with very few exceptions, there is no need to use these newer antibiotics. Their potency and spectrum do not offset their greater expense, and they have potential for induction of resistance that may eventually curtail their efficacy for treatment of serious infections. An exception to this principle exists if the patient is known or suspected to be colonized with bacteria resistant to the standard agents that would normally be given for a particular operation. As patterns of resistance change, so will our choices of antimicrobial agents, but for the present the older agents are preferred.

REFERENCES

1. Moffett, H. L.: Common infections in ambulatory patients. *Ann. Intern. Med.* **89**(Part 2):743–745, 1978.
2. Dixon, R. E.: Effect of infections on hospital care. *Ann. Intern. Med.* **89**(Part 2):749–753, 1978.
3. Kass, E.: Antimicrobial drug usage in general hospitals in Pennsylvania. *Ann. Intern. Med.* **19**(Part 2):800–801, 1978.
4. Shapiro, M., Townsend, T. R., Rosner, B., and Kass, E. H.: Use of antimicrobial drugs in general hospitals: Patterns of prophylaxis. *N. Engl. J. Med.* **301**:351–355, 1979.
5. Anderson, B. M.: Mortality in meningococcal infections. *Scand. J. Infect. Dis.* **10**:271–282, 1978.
6. Centers for Disease Control: Annual summary 1979: Reported morbidity and mortality in the United States. *Morbid. Mortal. Wkly. Rep.* **28**:14–7,53, 1980.
7. Kuhns, D. M., Nelson, T., Feldman, H. A., and Kuhn, L. R.: The prophylactic value of sulfadiazine in the control of meningococcic meningitis. *JAMA* **123**:335–339, 1943.
8. Guttler, R. B., Counts, G. W., Avent, C. K., and Beaty, H. N.: Effect of rifampin and minocycline onmeningogoccal carrier rates. *J. Infect. Dis.* **124**:199–205, 1971.
9. Devine, L. F., Johnson, D. R., Rhode, S. L., *et al.*: Rifampin: Effect of two-day treatment on the meningococcal carrier state and the relationship to the levels of drug in sera and saliva. *Am. J. Med. Sci.* **2661**:79–83, 1971.
10. Apicella, M. A.: Neisseria meningitidis, in Mandell, G. L., Douglas, R. G., Jr., and Bennett, J. E. (eds.): *Principles and Practice of Infectious Diseases,* 2nd ed. Wiley, New York, 1985, pp. 1186–1195.
11. Weidmen, C. E., Dunkel, T. B., Pettyjohn, F. S., *et al.*: Effectiveness of rifampin in eradicating the meningococcal carrier state in a relatively closed population: Emergency of resistant strains. *J. Infect. Dis.* **124**:171–178, 1971.
12. Hoperich, P. D.: Prediction of antimeningococci chemoprophylactic efficacy. *J. Infect. Dis.* **123**:125, 1971.
13. Thelm, I., Wnnstrom, A. M., and Mardh, P. A.: Contact tracing in patients with genital chlamydial infections. *Br. J. Vener. Dis.* **56**:259, 1980.
14. Centers for Disease Control: 1985 STD treatment guidelines. *Morbid. Mortal. Wkly. Rep.* **34**(suppl 4):75s–108s, 1985.
15. Ward, J. I., Fraser, D. W., Baraff, L. J., and Plikaytis, B. D.: *Haemophilus influenzae* meningitis: A national study of secondary spread in household contacts. *N. Engl. J. Med.* **301**:122, 1979.
16. Granoff, D. M., and Daum, R. S.: Spread of *Haemophilus influenzae* type B: Recent epidemiologic and therapeutic considerations. *J. Pediatr.* **97**:854, 1980.
17. Centers for Disease Control: Prevention of secondary cases of *Haemophilus influenzae* type b disease. *Morbid. Mortal. Wkly. Rep.* **31**:672–680, 1982.
18. Granoff, D. M., and Ward, J. I.: Current status of prophylaxis for *Haemophilus influenzae* infections, in Remington, J. S., and Swartz, M. N. (eds.): *Current Clinical Topics in Infectious Diseases.* McGraw-Hill, New York, 1984.
19. Des Prez, R. M., and Goodwin, R. A., Jr.: Mycobacterium tuberculosis, in Mandell, G. L., Douglas, R.

G., Jr., and Bennett, J. E. (eds.): *Principles and Practice of Infectious Diseases,* 2nd ed. Wiley, New York, 1985, pp. 1383–1406.
20. Kopanoff, D. E., Snider, D. E., Jr., and Caras, G. J.: Isoniazid-related hepatitis. A U.S. Public Health Service cooperative surveillance study. *Am. Rev. Respir. Dis.* **117**:991, 1978.
21. Bailey, W. C., Byrd, R. B., Glassroth, J. L., *et al.:* Preventive treatment of tuberculosis. *Chest* **87**(suppl):128–132, 1985.
22. Centers for Disease Control: Adverse reactions to Fansidar and updated recommendations for its use in the prevention of malaria. *Morbid. Mortal. Wkly. Rep.* **33**:713–714, 1986.
23. Wyler, D. J.: Malaria—Resurgence, resistance and research. *N. Engl. J. Med.* **308**:875–878, 1983.
24. Centers for Disease Control: Recommendations of the Immunization Practices Advisory Committee (ACIP): Prevention and control of influenza. *Morbid. Mortal. Wkly. Rep.* **35**:317–325, 1986.
25. Monto, A. S., Gunn, R. A., Bandyk, M. G., and King, C. L.: Prevention of Russian influenzae by amantadine. *JAMA* **241**:1003–1007, 1979.
26. Dolin, R., Reichman, R. C., Madore, H. P., *et al.:* A controlled trial of amantadine and rimantadine in the prophylaxis of influenza A infection. *N. Engl. J. Med.* **307**:580–584, 1982.
27. Hook, E. W., and Kaye, D.: Prophylaxis of bacterial endocarditis. *J. Chronic Dis.* **15**:635–646, 1962.
28. Durach, D. T.: Prophylaxis of infective endocarditis, in Mandell, G. L., Douglas, R. G., Jr., and Bennett, J. E. (eds.): *Principles and Practice of Infectious Diseases,* 2nd ed. Wiley, New York, 1985, pp. 539–544.
29. Kaye, D.: Prophylaxis against bacterial endocarditis: A dilemma, in Kaplan, E. L., and Taranta, A. V. (eds.): *Infective Endocarditis.* AHA Monograph No. 52. American Heart Association, Dallas, 1977, pp. 67–69.
30. Durock, D. T., Petersdorf, R. G.: Chemotherapy of experimental streptococcal endocarditis: Comparison of commonly recommended prophylactic regimens. *J. Clin. Invest.* **52**:592–599, 1973.
31. Shulman, S. T., Amren, D. P., Bisno, A. L., *et al.:* Prevention of bacterial endocarditis: A statement for health professionals by the Committee on Rheumatic Fever and Infective Endocarditis of the Council on Cardiovascular Disease in the Young. *Circulation* **70**:1123A–1127A, 1984.
32. Durack, D. T., Bisno, A. L., and Kaplan, E. L.: Apparent failures of endocarditis: Analysis of 52 cases submitted to a national registry. *JAMA* **250**:2318–2322, 1983.
33. Brooks, S. L.: Survey of compliance with American Heart Association guidelines for prevention of bacterial endocarditis. *J. Am. Dent. Assoc.* **101**:41–43, 1980.
34. Harding, G. K. M., and Ronald, A. R.: A controlled study of antimicrobial prophylaxis of recurrent urinary infection in women. *N. Engl. J. Med.* **291**:597–601, 1974.
35. Stamey, T. A., Condy, M., and Mihara, G.: Prophylactic efficacy of nitrofurantoin macrocrystals and trimethoprim–sulfamethoxazole in urinary infections: Biological effects on the vaginal and rectal flora. *N. Engl. J. Med.* **296**:780–783, 1977.
36. Stamm, W. E., Counts, G. W., Wagner, K. F., *et al.:* Antimicrobial prophylaxis of recurrent urinary tract infections: A double-blind, placebo-controlled trial. *Ann. Intern. Med.* **92**:770–775, 1980.
37. Green, J. W., and Wenzel, R. P.: Postoperative wound infection: A controlled study of the increased duration of hospital stay and direct cost of hospitalization. *Ann. Surg.* **185**:264–268, 1977.
38. Post-operative wound infections: The influence of ultraviolet irradiation of the operating room and of various other factors, National Academy of Sciences–National Research Council, Division of Medical Sciences, Ad Hoc Committee of the Committee on Trauma. *Ann. Surg.* **160**(suppl. 2):1–192, 1964.
39. Crossley, K., and Gardner, L. C.: Antimicrobial prophylaxis in surgical patients. *JAMA* **245**:722–726, 1981.
40. Cruse, P. J. E., and Ford, R.: A five-year prospective study of 23,649 surgical wounds. *Arch. Surg.* **107**:206–209, 1973.
41. Cruse, P. J. E., and Ford, R.: The epidemiology of wound infection—A ten year prospective study of 62,939 wounds. *Surg. Clin. North Am.* **80**:27–40, 1979.
42. Shapiro, M., Munoz, A. Tager, J. B., *et al.:* Risk factors for infection at the operative site after abdominal or vaginal hysterectomy. *N. Engl. J. Med.* **307**:1661–1666, 1982.
43. Nichols, R. L., Condon, R. E., Gorback, S. L., and Nylus, L. M.: Efficacy of preoperative antimicrobial preparation of the bowel. *Ann. Surg.* **176**:227–323, 1972.
44. Sanford, J. P.: Prophylactic use of antibiotics: Basic considerations. *South. Med. J.* **70**(suppl. 2):2–3, 1977.

45. Stone, H. H., Haney, B. B., Kob, L. D., *et al.:* Prophylactic and preventive antibiotic therapy-timing, duration and economics. *Ann. Surg.* **189:**691–699, 1979.
46. D'Angelo, L. J., and Sokol, R. J.: Short-versus long-course prophylactic antibiotic treatment in cesarean section patients. *Obstet. Gynecol.* **55:**583–586, 1980.
47. Conti, J. E., Jr., Cohen, S. N., Roe, B. B., *et al.:* Antibiotic prophylaxis and cardiac surgery. A prospective double-blind comparison of single-dose versus multiple-dose regimens. *Ann. Intern. Med.* **76:**943–949, 1972.
48. Higgins, A. F., Lewis, A., Noone, P., *et al.:* Single and multiple dose cotrimoxazole and metronidazole in colorectal surgery. *Br. J. Surg.* **67:**90–92, 1980.
49. Hemsell, D. L., Reisch, J., Nobles, B., *et al.:* Prevention of major infection following elective abdominal hysterectomy: Individual determination required. *Am. J. Obstet. Gynecol.* **147:**520–528, 1983.
50. Burke, J. F.: The effective period of preventive antibiotic action in experimental incisions and dermal lesions. *Surgery* **50:**161–168, 1961.

6

Hepatitis

Richard L. Greenman

1. INTRODUCTION

In addition to a number of viruses, toxins and drugs can cause injury to the liver. Ethanol is perhaps the most common example of a toxin/drug etiology of hepatitis. This chapter will, however, deal exclusively with the viral etiologies of hepatitis, the epidemiology of these agents, and clinical strategies for prevention of disease.

At least four viruses are known to be causes of hepatitis. These are: (1) hepatitis A virus, (2) hepatitis B virus, (3) the non-A–non-B viral agents, which probably represent more than one virus, and (4) the delta agent. In addition, two ubiquitous herpes viruses commonly causes hepatitis as part of the syndrome of clinical infection. These agents, cytomegalovirus and Epstein–Barr virus, are not classified as hepatitis viruses because the spectrum of disease they cause is broad and hepatitis is not the major clinical manifestation in most infections. Other unusual viruses, such as yellow fever virus, also cause hepatitis but are rare in the practice of medicine outside the tropics. Thus, four types of viral hepatitis important in the clinician's understanding of this disease will be discussed in this chapter.

2. HEPATITIS A

2.1. The Virus

The causative agent of type A hepatitis is a small, nonenveloped single-stranded RNA virus of the picornavirus family. Hepatitis A virus (HAV) is similar in size, structure, and nucleic acid content to members of the enterovirus genus and has been classified as enterovirus 71. HAV infectivity in humans has been shown to survive at 60°C for 1 hr, but is destroyed by boiling (100°C) for as little as 1 min. Infectivity can also be destroyed by chlorination.

Hepatitis A virus was first detected in the stool of infected patients by immunoelec-

Richard L. Greenman • Department of Medicine, Division of Infectious Diseases, University of Miami School of Medicine, and Miami Veterans Administration Medical Center, Miami, Florida 33101.

tron microscopy.[1] Provost and Hilleman have reported propagation of HAV in fetal rhesus-monkey kidney cells.[2] An efficient animal model of infection exists in the marmoset.

2.2. Epidemiology

Hepatitis A virus appears to have a worldwide distribution. Infection occurs primarily by the oral route, with infectious virus subsequently being shed in the feces. A chronic carrier state does not appear to exist for HAV. Because there is no persistent infection with viremia, parenteral transmission by blood is not important in HAV infection. With no form of chronic infection and with no known natural nonhuman reservoir of HAV, the virus is maintained by transmission from acutely infected patients to susceptible hosts.

2.3. Mode of Transmission

The most frequent mode of transmission of HAV is by the fecal–oral route, thus requiring close person-to-person contact.[3] This mode of transmission is probably also important in the spread of disease among homosexual males by direct oral–anal contact. Contamination of food by a food handler with acute hepatitis A infection may lead to sporadic cases or moderate-size point source epidemics.

In addition to personal contact, well-documented outbreaks of hepatitis A have occurred through sewage contamination of water supplies.[4] Sewage contamination of shellfish harvested from effluent fouled waters has also led to epidemics when these mollusks have been consumed raw.[5]

Rare reports of transmission of HAV by percutaneous transmission from a viremic patient late in the incubation period of hepatitis A exist. However, this route is infrequent and not of major importance. Intrauterine infection of the fetus when the mother has developed HAV infection has not been proven.

2.4. Incidence

Approximately 30,000 cases of hepatitis A are reported yearly to the Centers for Disease Control (CDC), but it is estimated that the true number of HAV infections is greater than one million per year. Many cases are subclinical and reporting is incomplete. Seroprevalence studies show that one-fourth to one-half of all adults in the United States have antibody of HAV.[6] The incidence of HAV infection is highest in low socioeconomic groups, presumably because of increased crowding and poor sanitation.

Prisons, day care centers, and schools are all areas of increased transmission. Young children whose hygiene is less fastidious are particularly efficient spreaders of infection. Worldwide differences in prevalence of antibody to HAV exist. In developing countries over 90% of the population has evidence of infection by early adulthood.

2.5. Incubation Period and Period of Communicability

The incubation period from exposure to development of clinical disease is from 15 to 50 days, with a mean incubation of approximately 28 days.[3]

Infectious HAV has been found in the feces as early as 3 weeks prior to the onset of clinical disease. Stool appears infectious for at least 1 week after onset of jaundice. However, peak infectivity (stool shedding) appears to occur just before or at the time of onset of symptoms.[7]

2.6. Strategies for Prevention of Infection

Prevention of infection with HAV or modification of the disease in hepatitis A depends on interrupting the transmission of the virus or immunologically rendering susceptibles immune or partially immune to the virus. At present there is no available vaccine for HAV, so that immunization takes the form of passive immunization with immune serum globulin (ISG).

2.7. Prevention of Viral Spread

2.7.1. Isolation

Isolation of patients with clinical hepatitis A in the home situation is unnecessary and probably not useful. Exposure to HAV, if it is to occur, has probably already occurred because infectivity is maximal in the period shortly before clinical disease occurs. Reasonable measures to decrease the chances of transmission if it has not yet occurred include the following: (1) infected patients should not prepare food for other family members, (2) infected patients should have their own utensils of personal hygiene (e.g., toothbrushes, eating utensils, and, for young children, toys), and (3) surfaces soiled with contaminated material from infected patients or other inanimate objects such as toys should be disinfected with a 0.2% hypochlorite solution (household bleach diluted 1 part to 25 parts water). Most important is fastidious hand washing by the patient and by susceptibles after contact with the patient or with potentially contaminated materials.

Isolation in the hospital should revolve around good personal hygiene and hand washing, as mentioned. Infectivity decreases dramatically after onset of jaundice, but infectious HAV may remain in feces for up to 1 week. Eating utensils, objects of personal hygiene, and medical instruments should be decontaminated for this same time period if they are to be used for other susceptible patients. Patients with fecal incontinence or diarrhea should be placed in single rooms. Other patients who are cooperative about their personal hygiene do not need to be placed in single rooms or confined to their rooms.

2.7.2. Prevention of Transmission through Food

Prevention of spread of HAV by food handlers is best effected by removing any infected patients from food-handling duties. If this cannot be done, food handlers need to be well instructed and able to carry out scrupulous hand washing.

Shellfish-associated hepatitis A can be reduced if only shellfish from waters known to be free of sewage effluent are ingested.

2.7.3. Prevention of Transmission through Water

Potable water standards in the United States and most developed countries provide for water that is free from HAV. In instances where transient decreases of potable water pressure occur owing to pump failure or fracturing of water mains, "boil water" advisories should be issued until it can be shown that the water has not become contaminated by fecal material (assay for coliforms and chlorine residual). Boiling of water for 3 min at a "rolling boil" will inactivate HAV along with other potential viral or bacterial pathogens.

2.8. Passive Immunoprophylaxis

The efficacy of normal pooled human gamma globulin (ISG) administered intramuscularly in preventing or modifying HAV infection has been demonstrated on numerous occasions.[8] ISG is prophylactically useful in both preexposure and postexposure situations. Preexposure prophylaxis is limited to persons traveling to areas of HAV endemicity. Several studies suggest that while the incidence of icteric clinical hepatitis A is reduced by 80–90%, the incidence of HAV infection is little changed. Thus this mode of prophylaxis confers a form of "passive–active immunity." Recipients are largely protected from clinical disease but subclinical infection leads to active immunity. Significantly higher doses of ISG may block HAV infection entirely so that only passive immunity is conferred and the recipient is once more susceptible after passively transferred antibody is cleared. Thus ISG prophylaxis should comply with dosage guidelines listed in Table I. Low-dose ISG is given for trips where exposure will be for less than 2 months. For exposure times of 2–6 months the higher dose (0.06 ml/kg) of ISG is utilized. For prophylaxis for periods of time greater than 6 months, repetition of the ISG dosage is necessary. For postexposure prophylaxis ISG should be given as early as possible. No protection is demonstrable if administration is delayed beyond 2 weeks after exposure. Table II lists indications for the use of ISG in postexposure situations.

3. HEPATITIS B

3.1. The Virus

The causative agent of type B hepatitis is a small DNA virus with unique properties that distinguish it from previously described viruses. This agent, along with three similar animal viruses, recently described in woodchucks, ground squirrels, and Peking ducks is classified in a new viral family termed the Hepadnaviridae.[9] They have a unique small, circular DNA that is partially single stranded, a unique viral DNA polymerase, and a marked tropism for hepatocytes. The complete virus in human hepatitis B (HBV) is identical to the previously described "full Dane particle" and consists of a virion core

Table I. Immune Serum Globulin Prophylaxis of Hepatitis A

Type of exposure	ISG dose	Duration of protection
Postexposure	0.02 ml/kg	—
Preexposure	0.02 ml/kg	2 months
	0.06 ml/kg	6 months

Table II. Indications for Postexposure ISG for Hepatitis A

1. Close personal contacts, including household and sexual (homosexual or heterosexual), of hepatitis A cases
2. Residents and staff of institutions (e.g., mental health facilities, prisons), during documented hepatitis A outbreaks
3. Members of the household of staff working at, or children attending, day care facilities during documented hepatitis A outbreaks
4. Medical care personnel after mucous membrane or percutaneous exposure to feces, blood, or body fluids of known hepatitis A patients

containing DNA, DNA polymerase, and protein kinase. The core has on its surface the core antigen, termed HBcAg. The core is surrounded by a complex surface antigen (HBsAg) made up of at least seven polypeptides. The hepatitis B e antigen (HBeAg) determinant appears to be made up of a complex of antigens associated with the virion core.[10]

High levels of surface antigen particles (22-nm HBsAg particles) circulate in the blood of the chronic carrier as well as the patient with acute hepatitis B. These particles, which are found in concentrations of 10^{11}–10^{14} particles/ml, outnumber complete viral particles by a factor of 10^4–10^6. Thus large numbers of infective virions circulate in the serum of patients with acute infection or chronic carriage. HBV infectivity is destroyed by boiling at 100°C for 10 min, autoclaving at 121°C for 15 min, or by dry heat at 160°C for 2 hr. Chemical methods that destroy HBsAg antigencity include 0.5% sodium hypochlorite for 10 min and 40% aqueous formalin for 12 hr.[10]

3.2. Spectrum of Disease

Hepatitis B virus infection may lead to acute hepatitis B or clinically inapparent infection. Approximately 1% of acute hepatitis B cases may progress to fulminant hepatitis. Approximately 10% of those infected go on to chronic HBV carriage usually lifelong and frequently with chronic liver disease. Chronic HBV infection is clearly associated with hepatocellular carcinoma. In some parts of the world where HBV infection is very common, hepatocellular carcinoma is the most common cancer. Several lines of evidence support an etiological role of HBV infection in hepatocellular carcinoma.[11]

Several interesting extrahepatic syndromes are associated with HBV infection. These include a serum sickness–like syndrome with fever, rash, and arthritis; polyarteritis nodosa; membranous glomerulonephritis; aplastic anemia; and essential mixed cryoglobulinemia.

3.3. Epidemiology

Hepatitis B virus appears to have a worldwide distribution. In the United States it has been estimated that there are approximately 200,000 new HBV infections each year. For the population at large the lifetime risk of HBV infection is estimated at 5–10%. However, within certain high-risk groups individuals may reach a nearly 90% chance of infection over their lifetime. Table III lists some of the important high-risk groups.[12]

Table III. Prevalence of HBV Markers in Relation to Population Group[a]

Population group	Prevalence of serological markers of HBV infection (%)
High risk	
Immigrants from HBV highly endemic areas	70–85
Parental drug abusers	60–80
Homosexual males	35–80
Institutionalized mentally retarded patients	35–80
Intermediate risk	
Staff of institutions for the retarded	10–25
Health care workers with frequent blood contact	15–30
Low risk	
Health care workers with infrequent blood contact	3–10
Healthy adult blood donors	3–5

[a]Adapted from Ref. 12.

Socioeconomic status is associated with risk of infection. Cherubin *et al.* found the prevalence of anti-HBs in adults to be 44% in Harlem, 18% in Staten Island, and 10% in upper-middle-class Manhattan residents.[13]

HBV infections occur at markedly increased rates in areas of Asia, Africa, and Oceania. In these areas maternal–child transmission appears to be the major route of infection.

3.4. Modes of Transmission

Hepatitis B virus infection appears to be exclusively a human–human disease without any known, important animal reservoirs of the virus. Blood and blood products are the most efficient transmitters of HBV infection. Semen has also been shown to contain infectious HBV.[14] Other body secretions may be infectious but their infectivity appears significantly lower than that of blood or semen.

There is no evidence for fecal–oral transmission as in HAV infection. Consequently food and water do not appear to be important in the spread of HBV infection. Infection through the oral route probably occurs by blood, saliva, or semen passing small breaks in the oral mucosa.

Thus the most important routes of infection appear to be blood or blood product transfusion, sharing of parenteral needles or medical instruments, homosexual and heterosexual intercourse, and minor trauma allowing small blood exchanges (shaving, tatooing, ear piercing). The presence of a relatively large pool of chronic HBV carriers accounts for much more frequent possibilities of exposure than in HAV infection, where a carrier state does not exist.

Another important mode of transmission is from the mother, either a chronic carrier or who acute hepatitis B in the third trimester, infecting the fetus or, more commonly, the newborn infant. This route of transmission does occur in the United States but is of much less importance than in areas such as China or Taiwan, where almost half of all HBV infection is acquired perinatally.[15]

3.5. Incubation Period and Period of Communicability

The incubation period for symptomatic HBV infection ranges from 1 to 6 months, with the usual period being 60–100 days. HBsAg and infectious HBV appear in the blood 1–7 weeks before the onset of clinical hepatitis. HBsAg and infectious HBV remain in the blood for an average of approximately 6 weeks. However, they may persist for as long as 4–6 months even in patients who are not becoming chronic carriers. Patients who remain antigen positive for longer than 6 months appear to fall into the 10% of patients who become chronic carriers. Chronic carriage of HBV may be a lifelong event, though it appears there is a spontaneous cure rate of approximately 2% per year.[10] Patients who remain positive for HBsAg should be considered to be infectious, although there are rare examples of patients with HBsAg carriage who apparently produce no infectious HBV. Patients who are positive for HBeAg or viral DNA polymerase are generally more highly infectious than those in whom these markers cannot be demonstrated.

3.6. Strategies for Prevention of Infection

Prevention of HBV infection and hepatitis B depends on several approaches. These include (1) interruption of the transmission of HBV, (2) passive immunoprophylaxis of infection with immune globulin, and (3) active immunoprophylaxis against HBV with an effective vaccine.

3.6.1. Interruption of HBV Transmission

The most important steps taken to date to interrupt HBV transmission have occurred in the field of blood banking. Before 1972 hepatitis B was a common sequela of transfusion of blood or blood products. Since then, two milestone changes in policy have occurred. Since 1972 all blood banks have been required to test all units of blood for HBsAg. Current testing utilizing a sensitive radioimmunoassay identifies over 90% of potentially infectious units.[16] Such units are disposed of and the donors are precluded from further blood donation. A second important policy has been an attempt to convert all blood donations to a true volunteer donor population. Eliminating paid donors has had an effect almost equal to the HBsAg screening.[17] Between the two, posttransfusion hepatitis B has been reduced by over 90%. A small number of HBV infectious units still exist, undetected by HBsAg testing. Other measures for detecting such blood including anti-HBc testing and transaminase screening (primarily useful for non-A–non-B hepatitis) are being evaluated. Elimination of unnecessary transfusions along with use of autotransfusion of precollected blood for elective surgical procedures is also useful to ensure that infective blood is not transfused.

Special problem populations regarding the transmission of HBV virus include parenteral drug abusers and promiscuous sexually active persons, particularly male homosexuals. Interruption of transmission in drug abusers is theoretically possible if only sterile needles and syringes are used or if no needle sharing were to occur. However, the "social" aspects of parenteral drug abuse make this quite difficult. Needle sharing and injection in communal "shooting galleries" is apparently important to many addicts. This makes interruption of HBV transmission nearly impossible. Similarly, changes in sexual practice to discourage promiscuity would be helpful in decreasing HBV transmission. Again, social patterns are such that this is unlikely to occur to a great enough extent to significantly decrease transmission. Thus, immuprophylaxis becomes the most important strategy in these populations.[18]

Interruption of viral transmission is an important adjunctive means of preventing HBV transmission in families, in the hospital care setting, and in situations such as dentistry. For example, in the household setting, family members without sexual contact with an infected patient should be educated to wash hands after contact with blood or body secretions or excretions. Razors, toothbrushes, and other personal hygiene items should not be shared. Routine immunization of all household members is a financial problem and will remain such until less expensive vaccines are developed. However, susceptible sexual contacts of HBsAg carriers or patients with acute hepatitis B should receive immunoprophylaxis as the risk of acquiring infection is much higher unless the additional risk factor (sexual contact) is eliminated.

Similarly in the hospital setting, patient care and laboratory personnel should be instructed in appropriate hygiene to decrease the risk of infection, but the cost–benefit ratio of immunization appears to favor this mode of protection for most patient care and laboratory personnel. The same conclusions can be drawn for practicing dentists, whose risk of acquiring HBV infection is among the highest of all health care personnel.

Education, hand washing, appropriate decontamination, barriers, and avoidance of mucosal contact with blood or secretions has assumed new importance in this era of the acquired immune deficiency syndrome (AIDS). HTLV-III/LAV transmission, though apparently significantly less efficient than HBV transmission by routes other than blood transfusion or intercourse, makes attention to hygiene of continued importance even in the HBV immune person. Considerations relating to non-A–non-B (NANB) hepatitis also support a continued role for good hygiene in prevention of virus transmission.

3.6.2. Isolation

The patient with either HBsAg carriage or acute hepatitis B does not need to be isolated in the hospital unless unable to adhere to a reasonable degree of hygiene. However, "hepatitis precautions," which include appropriate disposal or decontamination of potentially contaminated objects, special labeling of patient blood sent to the laboratory, and appropriate protection (gloves, masks, eyeglasses) to prevent inoculation of open cuts or mucous membranes with potentially infectious blood or secretions, should be utilized.

HBsAg-positive hemodialysis patients should be segregated by placing them on separate dialysis machines along with geographical separation if possible. Such patients should be cared for only by immune nursing staff (natural or immunized). Such measures have been effective in limiting spread between patients and to dialysis unit staff.

3.6.3. Immunization

Immunoprophylaxis against HBV infection cannot be conveniently separated into passive (ISG) and active (vaccine) immunization. Most situations relating to postexposure prophylaxis utilize both types of immunization in a large proportion of exposures.

Preexposure active immunization with hepatitis B vaccine is a more straightforward situation. The current vaccine, derived from highly purified plasma of chronic HBsAg carriers, is 80–95% effective in most situations.[19] The vaccine has been free of serious adverse effects. Specifically any early concern about possible transmission of an AIDS agent has been shown to be without any basis. HTLV-III is inactivated by several of the steps in the preparation of the vaccine. No patient who has received hepatitis B vaccine who has not been in an HTLV-III risk group has become HTLV-III positive. The real concerns pertaining to hepatitis B vaccine center about cost–benefit ratios for this extremely expensive ($100/series) product. In addition, decreased efficacy after injection into adipose tissue rather than muscle has been demonstrated. Other interesting aspects of active immunization include the possibility of decreasing cost by intradermal injection where one-tenth the amount of vaccine appears equally effective as standard doses of intramuscular vaccine and, eventually, the production of less expensive second- and third-generation vaccines produced through recombinant genetic technology or chemical synthesis. Specifics of hepatitis B vaccine use are covered in Chapter 4 which discusses immunization in the adult.

Postexposure immunoprophylaxis for HBV exposure is useful in several settings. Frequently a combination of passive and active immunization has been shown to be superior to either modality alone.

In the adult after a single parenteral exposure to potentially infectious material (see Table IV), hepatitis B hyperimmune serum globulin (HBIG) is indicated. Prospective trials comparing HBIG to standard ISG have yielded conflicting results. Some series demonstrate a significant advantage of HBIG over ISG.[20] However, series in which the ISG had significant anti-HBs titers show no difference between HBIG and ISG limbs.[21] True placebo-controlled trials have not been carried out, but the trials where the ISG employed had no anti-HBs titer have shown significant protection of HBIG over these ISG lots. When used, HBIG should be given as soon as possible after exposure. A second dose, though frequently recommended, is of questionable value. If the interval since exposure is greater than 7 days, no benefit has been shown.

The recommended dose of HBIG is 0.06 ml/kg (5 cc maximum) given within 7 days after exposure. A second dose is repeated 1 month later. If the source of the exposure is unknown, of unknown status regarding HBsAg, or is known to be negative for HBsAg, then ISG 0.06 ml/kg (5 cc maximum) is given. This is given as prophylaxis against NANB hepatitis but would also offer some protection against HBV. If the exposed person is known anti-HBs positive naturally or from immunization or is a known HBsAg carrier, ISG should still be administered for prophylaxis against NANB agents.

While the regimens cited are appropriate for single-exposure situations, the presentation of a patient with a hepatitis B contact must raise the question of how likely are further exposures. For health care personnel, intravenous drug abusers, active homosexual males,

Table IV. Exposures for which Use of HBIG Is Recommended

1.	Needlestick from known HBsAg-contaminated needle
2.	Mucous membrane splashed with blood from HBsAg-positive patient
3.	Exposure of broken skin to HBsAg-positive blood or secretions
4.	Sexual intercourse with HBsAg-positive partner
5.	Sharing of razor, toothbrush, etc., with HBsAg-positive person

or spouses of chronic HBsAg carriers, repeated exposure is likely. In such situations both passive and active prophylaxis should be instituted and a series of hepatitis B vaccine immunizations begun. If a determination of anti-HBs status is performed to preclude wasting of vaccine in already immune individuals, this determination must be performed on blood obtained prior to the administration of ISG or HBIG. There has not been any evidence to suggest interference with the development of active immunity by coadministration of ISG or HBIG with the hepatitis B vaccine.

Prevention of HBV transmission is also extremely important in the newborn child. Infants born of mothers with acute hepatitis B infection in the third trimester or of mothers who are HBsAg carriers, particularly if they are also HBeAg positive, have a very high chance of becoming infected with HBV. In addition, up to 90% of these infants become chronic HBsAg carriers.[22] Studies have shown that when HBIG is administered to these infants within the first 48 hr of life, the rate of infection is reduced by approximately 70%.[23] The passive protection afforded by HBIG is rather short lived and many infants so protected are infected later in the first year of life. One recent study utilizing combined HBIG and hepatitis B vaccine demonstrated a 94% protection rate in infants receiving both modalities of prophylaxis.[24] The recommended regime is to administer 0.5 cc of HBIG intramuscularly immediately after delivery followed by a first dose of vaccine (0.5 ml) within the first week of life. The series of active immunizations is then completed with a second and third dose at 1 and 6 months, respectively. Elimination of neonatal transmission is an extremely important goal in the prevention of chronic hepatitis B infection and the potential sequelae of cirrhosis and primary hepatocellular carcinoma. Current CDC guidelines suggest that only high-risk mothers (previous history of hepatitis, intravenous drug abuser, immigrant from area of high risk) be screened, but recently acquired data suggest that such guidelines may miss as many as 50% of potentially infective mothers in the setting of a large municipal hospital (E. Schiff, personal communication, 1986). The impact of interruption of neonatal transmission in many developing countries is potentially enormous. Unfortunately these countries do not have the resources to implement the screening and combined passive and active regimen of prophylaxis. The observation that vaccine alone produces an antibody response in almost all neonates raises the possibility of a more affordable regimen, particularly with the development of less expensive vaccines with newer technologies.

4. DELTA AGENT

4.1. The Virus

The delta agent is a defective 35- to 37-nm RNA virus-like particle that requires coinfection with HBV for its replication and clinical expression. It consists of a coat of HBsAg with an internal structure that includes the delta antigen (HBdAg) and a linear single-stranded RNA.[25]

4.2. Spectrum of Disease

Delta infection does not appear to occur without coinfection with HBV. Initial coinfection with both HBV and the delta agent may lead to a higher incidence of fulminant hepatitis than does HBV infection alone.

The delta agent infection may also be superimposed on prior HBV infection with chronic HBsAg carriage. In this situation delta appears to be an important cause of severe exacerbations of hepatitis and an increased incidence of chronic liver disease.

4.3. Epidemiology

Delta agent infection appears to be more geographically limited than infection by the other agents of viral hepatitis. Serological surveys have shown a high prevalence of antibody to this agent in the Mediterranean basin, particularly in the south of Italy.[26] Africa, Oceania, and South America have also been sites of outbreaks of delta-related disease. The prevalence of delta agent infection appears quite low in the United States, although increasing rates of infection have been found in intravenous drug abusers and in patients who have received many transfusions. Recently an outbreak of delta agent hepatitis has been reported in drug addicts in Worcester, Massachusetts.

4.4. Modes of Transmission

The delta agent appears to be transmitted primarily by blood and blood products. The prevalence in intravenous drug abusers and multiply transfused persons supports this premise. The relative lack of disease in the homosexual, non-drug-abusing population suggests that transmission through intercourse is much less efficient than for HBV. The incubation period of experimental delta agent infection in chimpanzees ranges from 2 to 10 weeks. In humans the incubation period is not firmly established.

A chronic carrier state of delta infection coexisting with HBV infection clearly exists, and such blood appears to be infectious for the duration of delta agent infection. Not all delta infection becomes chronic, as demonstrated by the lack of infectivity, in the chimpanzee model, for a proportion of human blood that is antidelta positive.[27]

4.5. Strategies for Prevention of Infection

Studies relating to the prevention of delta agent infection are only now underway. It seems that many of the precautions relating to prevention of HBV infection should be useful in preventing delta agent infection. Blood that is negative for all HBV markers should be delta agent free because of the apparent requisite for coinfection. Similarly, prophylaxis of HBV infection should be important in reducing delta agent infection in that if an individual never becomes infected with HBV it appears he is immune to infection with delta agent.

Further understanding of the epidemiology and pathophysiology of delta agent infection is necessary to better formulate strategies for prevention of delta agent infection. Further, it will be important to know whether coinfection with HBV remains an obligate condition for delta agent infection or disease.

5. NON-A–NON-B HEPATITIS

5.1. The Virus

NANB remains a relatively poorly understood disease. One of the major roadblocks in understanding this disease is the lack of a clearly identified agent or agents that cause the disease. Similarly there are no serological antigen or antibody markers that are reproducibly associated with NANB infection. Preliminary data suggest that there is more than one agent of NANB hepatitis. Currently it appears that there may be one agent implicated in non-blood-borne disease and two agents that can cause transfusion or blood associated NANB hepatitis.[28] The candidate agent in the non-blood-borne form of NANB disease appears to be a small, 27-nm virus, probably with RNA as the nucleic acid. This virus would, at least superficially, resemble HAV. At least two blood-borne agents have been proposed based on differences in incubation periods and multiplicity of infections.[29] There is a suggestion that the blood-borne agents contain reverse transcriptase, which would place them in the family of retroviruses.[30]

5.2. Spectrum of Disease

The NANB agents appear divisible in their disease spectrum along the same lines as their mode of transmission. The non-blood-borne form of NANB hepatitis closely resembles hepatitis A in its clinical spectrum. It generally presents with fever and jaundice. There is little fulminant hepatitis, although this complication may be more common than with hepatitis A, especially in pregnant women. Chronic hepatitis does not appear to occur as a result of infection with this NANB agent.

In contrast, blood-borne NANB hepatitis appears to present in a more insidious fashion. Fulminant hepatitis occurs in a small, but significant proportion of cases, estimated at 0.5–2%. The most striking aspect of blood-borne NANB infection is the high rate of chronic liver disease seen after infection. A carrier state definitely occurs, and 20–40% of patients, generally those with less severe acute infections, progress to chronic liver disease, frequently with cirrhosis. Data relating NANB infection with primary hepatocellular carcinoma do not exist.

5.3. Epidemiology

The non-blood-borne type of NANB hepatitis appears to be transmitted by the fecal–oral route, with several water-borne epidemics described. The incubation period appears similar to HAV, with one epidemic demonstrating incubation periods of 10–40 days with a mean incubation of 2 weeks.

Blood-borne NANB agents now cause over 90% of cases of posttransfusion hepatitis. A significant proportion of hepatitis in parenteral drug abusers is also caused by this agent or agents. The incubation period in several posttransfusion studies has displayed a mean of approximately 8 weeks, although the range has been wide (2–26 weeks). A shorter incubation period, averaging 20 days, has been reported for NANB hepatitis following factor VIII concentrate administration in hemophiliacs. A lack of any marked increase of incidence of NANB hepatitis in active male homosexuals suggests that these agents are not frequently transmitted by sexual routes.

5.4. Strategies for Prevention of Infection

Strategies for prevention of NANB hepatitis logically fit into two patterns. For the non-blood-borne form, prevention of breakdown in sanitation systems along with fastidious personal hygiene should be helpful. The role of ISG in this form of NANB infection is not known. There are no prospects for a vaccine in the near future.

For blood-borne NANB agents, the hygienic measures discussed in Section 3.6.1 seem appropriate but are untested. Clearly, avoidance of shared needles by illicit parenteral drug abusers would be helpful in decreasing transmission. If passive immunoprophylaxis is to be utilized for accidental parenteral exposure, ISG should be used although its value is not proven.

The major question relating to blood-borne NANB hepatitis is how it can be eliminated as the major cause of posttransfusion hepatitis (PTH). Several approaches have been studied. Use of exclusively volunteer donor blood results in approximately a fourfold reduction of NANB PTH from 17 to 35% with paid donor units to 6–7% with all volunteer donor blood. A second approach has been to screen donor blood for elevated hepatic enzymes that would indicate chronic hepatitis in the donor. Aach *et al.* showed that 10 of 11 recipients of blood units with serum alanine aminotransferase (ALT) levels greater than 45 IU developed PTH.[31] Using a cutoff of ALT greater than 45 IU would have eliminated 45% of NANB PTH hepatitis while excluding approximately 3 of every 100 units of donor blood. Alter *et al.*, in a similar study, used an ALT level of 2 SD above the mean as a proposed cutoff for donor units.[32] This level excluded 1.6% of donor units while eliminating approximately one-third of infectious units of blood. Yet another strategy for eliminating NANB positive units is to exclude blood positive for hepatitis B markers other than HBsAg. The premise that donors with HBV experience probably have greater NANB agent experience is probably true. Elimination of as much as 10% of the donor pool based on anti-HBs or anti-HBc positivity would be a stress on the blood supply. Further study to demonstrate or estimate the protective effect of such measures is necessary.

Attempts at protection from NANB PTH by passive immunoprophylaxis with ISG have been carried out. Results have been conflicting, with several studies showing no protection while others demonstrated significant reduction in active NANB PTH. ISG is expensive and would be scarce if given after all transfusions. Possible suppression of icteric disease after transfusion, possibly without eliminating infection, raises the question of whether such prophylactic attempts would only increase the amount of chronic NANB carriage. One study concluded that ISG should be given to all recipients of more than two units of blood in a single transfusion.[33]

As with the non-blood-borne form of NANB hepatitis, there is no prospect in the near future for a vaccine for the agent or agents of blood-borne NANB hepatitis.

REFERENCES

1. Feinstone, S. M., Kapikian, A. Z., and Purcell, R. H.: Hepatitis A: Detection by immune electron microscopy of a viruslike antigen associated with acute illness. *Science* **182:**1026, 1973.

2. Provost, P. J., and Hilleman, M. R.: Propagation of human hepatitis A virus in cell culture *in vitro*. *Proc. Soc. Exp. Biol. Med.* **160:**213, 1979.
3. Krugman, S., Ward, R., and Giles, J. P.: The natural history of infectious hepatitis. *Am. J. Med.* **32:**717, 1962.
4. Rindge, M. E., Mason, J. O., and Elsea, W. R.: Infectious hepatitis: Report of an outbreak in a small Connecticut school due to water-borne transmission. *JAMA* **180:**33, 1962.
5. Portnoy, B. L., Mackowiak, P. A., Caraway, C. T., *et al.*: Oyster associated hepatitis: Failure of shellfish certification program to prevent outbreaks. *JAMA* **233:**1065, 1975.
6. Dienstag, J. L., Szmuness, W., Stevens, V. E., *et al.*: Hepatitis A virus infection: New insights from seroepidemiologic studies. *J. Infect. Dis.* **137:**328, 1978.
7. Dienstag, J. L., Feinstone, S. M., Kapikian, A. Z., *et al.*: Fecal shedding of hepatitis A antigen. *Lancet* **1:**765, 1975.
8. Mosley, J. W., Reiser, D. M., Braholl, D., *et al.*: Comparison of two lots of immune serum globulin for prophylaxis of infectious hepatitis. *Am. J. Epidemiol.* **85:**539, 1968.
9. Robinson, W. S.: Genetic variation among hepatitis B and related viruses. *Ann. NY Acad. Sci.* **354:**371, 1980.
10. Robinson, W. S.: Hepatitis B virus and the delta agent, in Mandell G. L., Douglas, R. G., Jr., and Bennet, J. E. (eds.): *Principles and Practice of Infectious Diseases*, 2nd ed. Wiley, New York, 1985, p. 1002.
11. Szmuness, W.: Hepatocellular carcinoma and the hepatitis B virus: Evidence for a causal association. *Prog. Med. Virol.* **24:**40, 1978.
12. Centers for Disease Control: Inactivated hepatitis B virus vaccine. *Morbid. Mortal. Wkly. Rep.* **31:**318, 1982.
13. Cherubin, C. E., Purcell, R. H., Landers, J. J., *et al.*: Acquisition of antibody to hepatitis B antigen in three socioeconomically different medical populations. *Lancet* **2:**149, 1972.
14. Alter, J. H., Purcell, R. H., and Gerin, J. L.: Transmission of hepatitis B to chimpanzees by hepatitis B surface antigen-positive saliva and semen. *Infect. Immun.* **16:**928, 1977.
15. Okada, K., Kainiyama, I., Inometa, M., *et al.*: e Antigen and anti-e in the serum of asymptomatic carrier mothers as indicators of positive and negative transmission of hepatitis B virus in their infants. *N. Engl. J. Med.* **294:**746, 1976.
16. Hoofnagle, J. H., Seef, L. B., Bales, Z. B., *et al.*: The Veterans Administration Hepatitis Cooperative Study Group. Type B hepatitis after transfusion with blood containing antibody to hepatitis B core antigen. *N. Engl. J. Med.* **298:**1379, 1978.
17. Alter, H. S., Holland, P. V., and Purcell, R. H.: The emerging pattern of post-transfusion hepatitis. *Am. J. Med. Sci.* **270:**329, 1975.
18. Perspectives on control of viral hepatitis type B. *Morbid. Mortal. Wkly. Rep.* **25**(suppl. 1, no. 17)**:**3, 1976.
19. Szmuness, W., Stevens, C. E., Harley, E. J., *et al.*: Hepatitis B vaccine: Demonstration of efficacy in a controlled clinical trial in a high risk population in the United States. *N. Engl. J. Med.* **303:**833, 1980.
20. Seef, L. B., Wright, E. C., Zimmerman, H. J., *et al.*: Type B hepatitis after needlestick exposure: Prevention with hepatitis B immunoglobulin. A final report of the Veterans Administration Cooperative Study. *Ann. Intern. Med.* **88:**285, 1978.
21. Grady, G. F., Lee, V. A., Prince, A. M., *et al.*: Hepatitis B immune globulin for accidental exposures among medical personnel. Final report of a multi-center controlled trial. *J. Infect. Dis.* **137:**131, 1978.
22. Beasley, R. P., Trepo, C., Stevens, C. E., *et al.*: The e antigen and vertical transmission of hepatitis B surface antigen. *Am. J. Epidemiol.* **105:**94, 1977.
23. Beasley, R. P., Hwang, L. Y., Lin, C. C., *et al.*: Hepatitis B immunoglobulin (HBIG) efficacy in the interruption of perinatal transmission of hepatitis B carrier state. *Lancet* **2:**388, 1981.
24. Beasley, R. P., Hwang, L. Y., Lin, C. C., *et al.*: Prevention of perinatally transmitted hepatitis B virus infections with hepatitis B immune globulin and hepatitis B vaccine. *Lancet* **2:**1099, 1983.
25. Rizetto, M., Hoyer, B., Canese, M. G., *et al.*: Delta agent: The association of delta antigen with hepatitis B surface antigen and ribonucleic acid in the serum of delta-infected chimpanzees. *Proc. Natl. Acad. Sci. USA* **77:**6124, 1980.
26. Rizetto, M., Purcell, R. H., and Gerin, J. L.: Epidemiology of HBV-associated delta agent: Geographical distribution of anti-delta and prevalence in polytransfused HBgAg carriers. *Lancet* **1:**1215, 1980.
27. Nicholson, K. G.: Hepatitis delta infections. *Br. Med. J.* **290:**1370, 1985.
28. Tabor, E.: The three viruses of non-A non-B hepatitis. *Lancet* **1:**743, 1985.

29. Brotman, B., Prince, A. M., and Huima, T.: Non-A, non-B hepatitis: Is there more than a single blood-borne strain? *J. Infect. Dis.* **151**:618, 1985.
30. Seto, B., Coleman, W. G., Iwarson, S., *et al.:* Detection of reverse transcriptase activity in association with the non-A, non-B hepatitis agent(s). *Lancet* **2**:941, 1984.
31. Aach, R. D., Szmuness, W., Mosley, J. W., *et al.:* Serum alanine aminotransferase of donors in relation to the risk of non-A, non-B hepatitis. *N. Engl. J. Med.* **204**:989, 1981.
32. Alter, J. H., Purcell, R. H., Holland, P. V., *et al.:* Donor transaminase and recipient hepatitis: Impact on blood transfusion service. *JAMA* **246**:630, 1981.
33. Seeff, C. B., and Hoofnagle, J. H.: Immunoprophylaxis of viral hepatitis. *Gastroenterology* **77**:161, 1979.

7

Streptococcal Pharyngitis

Mark Multach

1. INTRODUCTION

Two hundred years have passed since the recognition that rheumatic fever affects the heart.[1] Since that time, our understanding, diagnosis, and treatment of the disease have changed dramatically. The recognition that pharyngitis was related to acute rheumatic fever (ARF) came in the early 1930s. In the early 1950s Wannamaker and co-workers showed that ARF could be prevented by early treatment of group A β-hemolytic streptococcal (GABHS) pharyngitis with penicillin.[2,3] The association of a preceding GABHS pharyngitis, along with the discovery that early treatment of this infection could essentially eradicate the risk of rheumatic heart disease, has produced a remarkable change in the morbidity and mortality of this complication.

In 1979 pharyngitis accounted for more than 40 million visits to physicians' offices.[4] Inappropriate utilization of diagnostic examinations could represent a large economic burden, even with a test as inexpensive as a throat culture. On the other hand, empirical treatment of all patients with "sore throats" could lead to both an inordinate expense and considerable morbidity due to anaphylactic reactions. In spite of the frequency with which we are faced with pharyngitis, there is still much controversy surrounding its diagnosis and treatment. This chapter will review the current epidemiology, diagnosis, and treatment of this disease and its complications.

2. EPIDEMIOLOGY

2.1. Streptococcal Pharyngitis

Pharyngitis is one of the most common illnesses bringing adult patients into a physician's office, comprising as much as 15–20% of patient visits[2] in a general practice. Surveys of physician practices show that approximately 50% of these have throat cultures performed. Cultures are positive for GABHS in approximately 20–30% of these patients.

One must keep in mind which patients have a high risk of streptococcal pharyngitis. First, the relative contribution of GABHS in acute pharyngitis decreases above the age of

Mark Multach • Department of Medicine, University of Miami School of Medicine, Miami, Florida 33101.

18 years, as does the incidence of ARF in this population (ARF occurs most frequently in those with the most frequent and intense infections). Second, certain adults are at higher risk for GABHS-induced pharyngitis: (1) anyone with frequent contact with patients with a high incidence of GABHS pharyngitis (e.g., parents of young children—especially school-age children, school teachers, physicians, nurses, allied medical personnel); and (2) military personnel. Finally, the incidence and severity of streptococcal pharyngitis, and the immune response to it, are related to various epidemiological features of GABHS infections, including altitude, season, age, economic factors, and crowding (e.g., military barracks, closed institutions, large families in small quarters, residents of densely populated areas of major cities), which leads to increased person-to-person spread of the more virulent GABHS.

One difficulty in dealing with acute pharyngitis is determining the meaning of a positive throat culture. Throat cultures will grow GABHS in 5–15% of individuals tested from an asymptomatic population. In all patients with a positive culture for GABHS, only 50% develop serological evidence of infection.[5] It then becomes important to find some way to discriminate between acute pharyngitis secondary to GABHS and acute pharyngitis in a carrier of GABHS. Several criteria have been used, and criticized, in an attempt to differentiate between the carrier state and acute infection:

1. Degree of growth (number of colonies) on the throat culture: It has been proposed by several authors that patients with fewer than 10 growing colonies on culture are chronic carriers and not acutely infected by GABHS. Although this is an attractive theory, no data yet support it. In fact, in the Fort Warren study,[2] there was no difference in the risk of ARF in patients with light growth of organisms versus those with moderate or heavy growth. Komaroff *et al.*[6] showed no significant association between growth (heavy or light) and increases of antistreptococcal antibodies. The severity of the infection is correlated with the intensity of the resultant immune response, which is directly correlated with the incidence of ARF.
2. Extent of increase in antistreptococcal antibodies: First, this is not useful clinically, as the increase is seen up to several weeks after the time frame for effective prophylaxis; its utility is in studies testing the value of other parameters in estimating the risk of streptococcal pharyngitis. Even in patients treated with antibiotics within 24 hr, there is a measurable increase in antibodies, although the increase is much greater in untreated patients with positive cultures.[7] This brings up one difficulty in interpreting the literature since the advent of antibiotic therapy: studies use the serological response as the "gold standard" to diagnose GABHS pharyngitis. However, treated patients will often not show a significant serological response (in fact, treatment is aimed at decreasing the immune response, and thereby, the incidence of ARF). This leads to an underestimation of the disease in treated patients.

2.2. Rheumatic Fever

In epidemic outbreaks, approximately 3% of patients with cultures positive for GABHS will go on to develop ARF if left untreated.[2] In nonepidemic cases, 0.6–2.6% of

GABHS pharyngitis will lead to ARF if untreated. The attack rate for ARF is related to the rheumatogenicity of the streptococcal strains involved in the infection. In epidemics, there is an increased incidence of strains with high rheumatic potential, and there is a high degree of spread. In nonepidemic outbreaks, the tendency is toward isolated cases, with less spread of the high-risk strains.

In the last 70 years, there has been a dramatic decrease in the incidence of ARF in most parts of the United States and western Europe. Thirty years ago, the incidence of ARF ranged from 50 to ≥200 per 100,000; this has declined to as low as 0.5 per 100,000 in some populations. In the 1930s it was recognized that prophylaxis of patients having a history of ARF with various antibiotics (sulfanilamide, penicillin) reduced the occurrence of recurrent episodes. Furthermore, in 1951–1952 Wannamaker and co-workers, in a randomized clinical trial, showed that ARF could be prevented by early treatment of GABHS pharyngitis with penicillin.[2,3] Initiation of antibiotic therapy within 3–7 days brought the ARF rate from 3% to ≤0.6%. These discoveries were responsible, in part, for the decline in the attack rate of rheumatic fever.

The beginning of this decline, however, antedated the discoveries of these beneficial effects of antibiotics in the prevention of ARF. The rate of decline was due initially to improvements in living conditions. However, the rate of decline in the incidence of ARF accelerated in the 1950s and 1960s, decreasing from 25–50 per 100,000 in the 1950s to 0.5–2 per 100,000 in the late 1970s, coincident with initiation of antibiotic therapy of streptococcal pharyngitis. While the incidence of GABHS pharyngitis has remained essentially unchanged through the years, the recognition of GABHS as the etiological agent in ARF, along with early treatment and secondary prophylaxis, has had a significant impact. Recognition and treatment of populations at risk for ARF have played an important role also. The risk factors include the following:

1. Crowded living conditions—evidenced by a high incidence in military camps and cities with high population density.[2]
2. Indigent populations.
3. Genetic factors—some factors seems to limit susceptibility to ARF in less than 3% of those with GABHS pharyngitis. Along these lines, monozygotic twins have a higher incidence of ARF than dizygotic twins. However, the concordance (percentage of identical twin pairs in which both members exhibit a certain trait; in this case, the trait is development of ARF following GABHS pharyngitis) of ARF is only 20%,[8,9] indicating low penetrance of genetic predisposition to ARF. Monozygotic twins also show concordance in manifestations of ARF, whether living in close proximity or not.[8] Finally, one research group has shown a correlation between HLA-D4 and susceptibility to ARF in Caucasian populations.[10]
4. Past history of ARF, especially with rheumatic valvular disease or Sydenham's chorea. Chronic rheumatic valvular disease is a greater risk factor than acute disease which resolves.

Finally, change in the rheumatogenicity of various streptococcal strains has had a significant affect on the incidence of ARF. Epidemiological evidence suggests that certain group A serotypes have a greater ability to cause ARF.[11] It appears that there has been a shift in the GABHS strains involved in acute pharyngitis. This shift has been away from the more rheumatogenic strains seen in the Wannamaker studies (M-types 5, 14, 19, 24) to less rheumatogenic strains (especially M-type 12) found to be prevalent in more recent studies that involved typing of organisms isolated from patients with cultures positive for GABHS.

While the incidence of ARF has declined in the United States and western Europe as a whole, it has remained high within some populations. In this respect, incidence figures quoted earlier (0.5 cases of ARF per 100,000) are misleading, as seen in Table I.[12]

Very high rates are seen in Indian reservations, where recent attack rates for ARF approximate 9.5–13.5 per 100,000.[13] Of course, the classic example of the variability of ARF attack rates is Wannamaker's study of military recruits, in which the rates were up to 5 times higher than in similar studies in other populations.

Prior ARF increases the attack rate of subsequent ARF: the risk of recurrent ARF following GABHS-induced pharyngitis may reach 60–70% versus a risk in the general population of <3%. The recurrence rate decreases as the time from the initial episode of ARF becomes greater: during the first 5 years, the yearly incidence is 19%, decreasing to 11%, 6%, and 1.4% in the succeeding 5-year periods, respectively. Certain subpopulations are at particular risk[14]:

1. Patients with residual heart disease (by physical examination, echocardiogram).
2. Patients who had ARF that included carditis, with or without current evidence of rheumatic heart disease. Patients with recurrent ARF tend to have the same manifestations as in previous episodes, with the exception of chorea.
3. Patients who had a greater immune response during the episode of GABHS pharyngitis that led to the first episode of ARF—the underlying process in ARF appears to be an immune response against myocardial tissue. This immune response may be induced by reaction against streptococcal antigens, which are similar in structure to myocardial antigens. Immunological cross-reactivity has been noted between some streptococcal cell wall antigens and human myocardial antigens.

   In early studies of the association of GABHS pharyngitis and ARF,[2,7] it was noted that the greater the immune response to streptococcal antigens (rise in antibody titers to antigens such as antistreptolysin) following GABHS pharyngitis, the higher the subsequent risk of ARF. Following the treatment of GABHS with antibiotics, the immune response—and subsequent risk of ARF—were markedly diminished.

Table I. Incidence of Acute Rheumatic Fever

	Incidence (per 100,000)		
Age (years)	Total	Black	White
<5	0.32	0.63	0
5–17	1.73	2.69	0.76
18–64	0.43	0.79	0.07

3. RATIONALE FOR TREATMENT

Several arguments support the treatment of patients with acute pharyngitis:

1. For symptomatic relief: Several studies[15–17] have shown that early antibiotic therapy decreases the symptomatic period of pharyngitis by 12–24 hr; although this difference has been shown to be statistically significant, it is short lived, so that by 48–72 hr there is no difference in the extent of symptoms between treatment and control patients.[18] Penicillin for presumed GABHS pharyngitis may help the patient by treating another pharyngeal pathogen. Komaroff *et al.* note that organisms such as *Neisseria gonorrhoeae, Hemophilus influenzae,* and *Corynebacterium diphtheriae* respond to penicillin and cause pharyngitis.[19]
2. Prevention of supporative complications: Several early studies[20,21] showed a decreased incidence of supporative complications following GABHS pharyngitis in patients receiving treatment. These findings were especially true for local complications (peritonsillar abscess) compared to distant spread (metastatic foci, bacteremias).
3. For the prevention of ARF.

The latter reason remains the most compelling. Numerous studies have shown that early treatment of GABHS pharyngitis, with elimination of GABHS from the throat, shows a direct correlation with the reduction of consequent ARF. In addition, a relationship has been established between the timing of the treatment and the degree of reduction of consequent ARF[22]: treatment within 48–72 hr of onset of symptoms is 95% effective; within 1 week, 90%; 2 weeks, 67%; and 3 weeks, 42%.

4. DIAGNOSIS

4.1. Clinical Diagnosis of GABHS Pharyngitis

The clinical diagnosis of GABHS pharyngitis has been studied extensively, using both historical and physical findings. Various signs and symptoms show the frequencies listed in Table II compared to non-GABHS pharyngitis.[23,24] As can be seen, no set of signs or symptoms is unique to GABHS pharyngitis.

It is necessary to make the proper diagnosis with the greatest efficiency and the lowest rate of false-negative results. Several investigators have studied the ability of clinicians to make the diagnosis of GABHS pharyngitis based on their clinical skills. These studies use a positive culture as the "gold standard" of diagnosis. Clinicians are able to correctly predict the results of cultures in only 30–70% of cases.[23,25] Even under ideal conditions (e.g., experienced physicians treating pediatric cases, in which the clinical picture is, in general, more "typical" than that seen in adults), at least 30% of cases will be missed.[23,26] The conclusion of those authors and their successors has been that while "certain symptoms and signs were suggestive of streptococcal infection . . . none were diagnostic."[23]

Nevertheless, clinical findings can be quite helpful. For example, the presence of a

Table II. Signs and Symptoms of Pharyngitis

Signs/symptoms	GABHS (%)	Non-GABHS (%)
Sore throat	79	44
Odynophagia	65	32
Pharyngeal erythema	92	75
moderate/severe	~50	20–25
Exudate	54	27
moderate/large	~16	~1
Cervical adenopathy	80–90	≤60
Fever	15–30	—
Cough	10–15	25–35
Coryza	10–15	>25

moderate or severe pharyngeal exudate is seen 16 times as often in GABHS pharyngitis as in non-GABHS pharyngitis, while coryza is seen twice as commonly in non-GABHS pharyngitis. The presence of coryza and cough showed a strong negative correlation with GABHS pharyngitis, being present in fewer than 4% of cases. This has led to the development of diagnostic strategies or clinical decision rules to increase the diagnostic yield, decrease the false-negative rate, and obviate the need for throat cultures.[22,27–33] These strategies utilize signs and symptoms but give them relative weights according to the correlation with disease seen in other studies.

Walsh *et al.*[30] scored patients on five factors: oral temperature (3 points for each degree over 36.1°C/97°F), recent exposure to streptococcal infection (17 points), recent cough (−7 points—e.g., a negative predictor), pharyngeal exudate (6 points), and enlarged or tender cervical nodes (11 points). Breese[32] used 13 factors to separate patients into varying degrees of risk for GABHS pharyngitis: age, season, sore throat, fever, white-blood count, cough, headache, abnormal pharynx, abnormal cervical glands, coryza, diarrhea, abnormal lungs, and abnormal ears. The latter four criteria were deleted from the study as having no additional value. A summary of these decision strategies, as well as two others noted prominently in the literature, is shown in Table III.

Using these factors, it was possible to sort patients according to levels of probability of a culture positive for GABHS. Walsh *et al.*[30] found that patients with a score of less than 10 points (for example, a patient with enlarged/tender cervical nodes—but without exudate, or recent exposure to GABHS—cough, and no more than low-grade fever) had a 4% culture positivity rate. On the other hand, patients with a score greater than 10 had a 21% culture positivity rate. The results are shown in Table IV.

By way of example, Tables III and IV can be used to evaluate several sample patients:

1. Patient 1 presents with a sore throat, a scratchy sensation in her eyes, and a history of a slight cough; on examination, she has tender cervical adenopathy and marked tonsillar exudate.
2. Patient 2 presents with malaise and a ''dry'' throat without a sore throat; on examination, he has pharyngeal erythema.

Table III. Scores for Clinical Parameters in Four Diagnostic Strategies[a]

Symptom	Walsh[30]	Breese[32]	Komaroff[34]	Centor[27,31]
Tonsillar exudate	6	4	1 or 2[h]	1
Anterior cervical adenopathy	11	4	1	1
Temperature >100°F	9[b]	4	NA	1[j]
History of recent exposure to GABHS	17	NA	1[i]	NA
Headache	NA[c]	4	NA	NA
Cough	−7	2[d]	NA	1
No rhinorrhea	NA	NA	NA	NA
Myalgias	NA	NA	1	NA
Itchy eyes	NA	NA	−1	NA
Season	NA	Varies[e]	NA	NA
Age	NA	Varies[f]	NA	NA
WBC	NA	Varies[g]	NA	NA

[a]Ref. 27,30,31,32,34.
[b]3 points for each degree over 36.1°C (97°F).
[c]NA, not applicable.
[d]Presence of a cough adds 2 points, absence adds 4.
[e]Winter (Feb.–Apr.), 4; (Jan., May, Dec.), 3; (June, Oct., Nov.), 2; (July, Aug., Sept.), 1.
[f]5–10 yrs, 4; 4 or 11–14, 3; 3 or >15, 2; ≤2, 1.
[g]0–8.4, 1; 8.5–10.4, 2; 10.5–13.4, 3; 13.5–20.4, 5; ≥20.5, 6; not done, 3.
[h]Marked tonsillar exudate, 2; Pinpoint tonsillar exudate, 1.
[i]Positive throat culture for GABHS in the preceding year.
[j]For any history of fever 1 point.

Table IV. Probabilities of Positive Cultures for GABHS[a]

Study	Clinical score	Probability of culture + for GABHS (%)
Walsh[30]	≥17	28
	5–16	15
	<5	4
Breese[32]	18–25	6
	26–29	36
	30–38	78
Komaroff[34]	0	10
	>1	≥20
Centor[27,31]	0–1	11
	≥2	32

[a]These probabilities are calculated on populations with known overall frequency of GABHS-positive cultures among all adult patients presenting with sore throat at that particular center (~15% for Walsh,[30] ~54% for Breese,[32] ~20% for Komaroff,[34] ~17% for Centor,[31] and ~26% for Centor[27]).

Table V. Sample Patients: Clinical Prediction of Positive Culture

	Walsh[30]		Breese[32]		Komaroff[34]		Centor[27,31]	
	Score	Risk[a]	Score	Risk[a]	Score	Risk[a]	Score	Risk[a]
Patient 1	10	15%	17	<6%	2	>20%	0	32%
Patient 2	0	4%	4	<6%	0	10%	0	11%
Patient 3	22	28%	14	<6%	2	>20%	4	32%

[a]Risk = the probability of a culture positive for GABHS.

3. Patient 3 presents with sore throat, a recent cough, and fevers (undocumented) recently; on examination, cervical adenopathy, pinpoint tonsillar exudate, and a temperature of 101°F are found. (See Table V.)

It is clear that there is variability from strategy to strategy. Most notable is the low yield of the assessment using Breese's strategy. This is due in large part to the development of this strategy using children as the cohort. The presentation of GABHS pharyngitis in children is somewhat different than in adults. In addition, when comparing rules, one must take into account population characteristics of the original test population, as well as the population being tested. Certain characteristics of the populations, such as the prevalence of GABHS in acute pharyngitis in a geographical area, will change the relative values of individual components of the decision rule.[27,35]

4.2. Throat Culture

With the realization in the 1950s that the clinical diagnosis of streptococcal pharyngitis was misleadingly low, it has become popular to perform throat cultures. The proper technique for this culture is to take a sterile cotton swab and rub it on the tonsils and posterior pharynx. Swabs can sit in sterile conditions for several hours before inoculation of the culture plate. The swab should be used to inoculate a sheep blood agar plate, and this culture is allowed to grow at 35°C overnight. Efforts to increase the specificity of this test by adding Bacitracin discs lead to a higher false-negative rate (reduced sensitivity), apparently due to lack of uniformity in reading zones of hemolysis. Therefore, at this time it is not recommended to add the antibiotic disc for further grouping of the β-hemolytic streptococcus.[36,37]

The yield (i.e., sensitivity) of such a single swab throat culture is in the range of 75–85%. Use of a second swab and a second culture plate increases the yield to ≥90%.[38] The increased yield may represent patients with a light growth, the significance of which has been discussed.

Throat cultures performed and grown in the physician's office are estimated to cost approximately $3.00 (excluding the cost of the incubator). Additional cost must be added for staff time.

4.3. Rapid Tests Utilizing Group A Streptococcal Antigen

The most recent tool added to the physician's armamentarium is testing based on the presence of streptococcal antigen on pharyngeal swabs. These tests have been developed over the past decade and have appeared on the market recently. In part, their attraction can be attributed to the rapidity and ease with which a diagnosis can be made, usually within 1 hr. These tests extract the streptococcal antigen directly from the pharyngeal swabs, using either enzymatic (an enzyme is the active agent utilized to extract the antigen from the swab; this requires 1 hr) or chemical (a chemical, micronitrous acid, is utilized to extract the antigen from the swab; this requires 3–5 min) extraction. The antigen is then visualized either by agglutination or by enzyme-linked immunosorbent assay.

Studies to test the sensitivity and specificity of antigen tests have used throat cultures as the standard of comparison. A sensitivity of 90% for one of the antigen tests means that it has correctly detected antigen in 90% of the cases where a culture is positive.[39–42] These studies show sensitivities (true positives/true positives plus false negatives) of 90–95%. That is, if a culture is positive, there is a 90–95% probability that the antigen test will be positive. Combining these two sensitivities (antigen test plus throat culture) yields a combined sensitivity for the antigen tests of 87% (the antigen tests have 94% of the sensitivity of throat cultures, which themselves have a sensitivity of 95%). Specificities (true negatives/true negatives plus false positives) have been 90–97%. Thus, if a culture is negative, there is a 90–97% probability that the antigen tests will be negative. The combined specificity is 90%.

Most of the difference in results between these tests and cultures (e.g., the 5–10% of instances where cultures are positive and antigen tests are negative) is seen in cultures with low growth of organisms, e.g., less than 10 colonies. It is often mentioned in the literature that patients whose cultures grow fewer than 10 colonies probably represent pharyngeal colonization with GABHS, rather than GABHS pharyngitis. These patients are therefore assumed to be at low risk for ARF. This assumption has not been confirmed by prospective studies, as discussed previously. Although no such evidence exists now, should it be shown that patients with light growth have a lower risk of GABHS pharyngitis and ARF, then results with rapid antigen assays would be almost identical to those of culturing. In the same studies, physicians' clinical estimates showed sensitivity of approximately 70% and specificity of approximately 55%.

The cost of the test itself ranges from $1.34 to $2.75 per patient.[43] Additional cost must be added for staff time.

4.4. Use of Tests in Clinical Situations

An ideal test would be 100% sensitive and specific and give a result without delay so that therapy could be initiated immediately. Such a test does not exist as yet. Therefore, one has to choose tests to use according to the specific clinical situation. In the case of the throat culture, athough it is more sensitive, it requires 24–48 hr to complete. On the other hand, the antigen tests are slightly less sensitive, but are nearly equally specific, and a result can be obtained within 1–2 hr. These characteristics help determine which tests will be of advantage in different clinical settings.

In an emergency room or other settings where poor follow-up would be expected, the approach should be to maximize the number of patients with GABHS pharyngitis who will be treated. The use of streptococcal antigen tests would avoid treatment of a significant number of patients who are assessed clinically (and incorrectly) to have GABHS pharyngitis (e.g., false-positive clinical assessment), while treating a number of patients with a positive antigen test who would otherwise have been missed on clinical grounds (e.g., false-negative clinical assessment). In episodic settings such as emergency rooms, poor follow-up of throat culture results is the rule and would effectively nullify the high degree of specificity of that test. This would, in turn, lead to a number of patients with GABHS infection going untreated and potentially to an increased incidence of ARF.

For example, in a population of 100 patients with pharyngitis there will be 15 patients with GABHS pharyngitis (i.e., a prevalence of 15%). Using the specificities and sensitivities for antigen tests and clinical assessment noted in the previous section, 10 of 15 (i.e., sensitivity of 67%) patients with GABHS pharyngitis would be treated based on clinical assessment alone, while 13 of 15 would be treated based on antigen tests (sensitivity of 87%). Table VI summarizes this information. Tables VII and VIII show the breakdown of the treatment (Table VII) and no-treatment (Table VIII) data presented in Table VI.

The office is a setting where one would expect good follow-up and thus be better able to delay therapy for 24–48 hr while awaiting the results of the throat culture. This approach will yield the highest sensitivity and specificity, thus maximizing the number of patients with GABHS pharyngitis receiving treatment, while minimizing the number of patients with non-GABHS pharyngitis who are treated.

For example, in the same population of 100 patients with pharyngitis, there will be 15 who have GABHS pharyngitis (prevalence of 15%). Using the specificities and sensitivities for antigen tests and throat cultures noted in the previous sections, 10 of 15 (i.e., sensitivity of 67%) patients with GABHS pharyngitis would be treated based on clinical assessment alone, 13 of 15 (i.e., combined sensitivity of 87%) would be treated based on antigen tests, and 14 of 15 (i.e., sensitivity of 90%) would be treated based on throat cultures.

At the same time, clinical assessment would diagnose GABHS pharyngitis in 48 patients (sensitivity of 67%, specificity of 55%), so 38 patients without GABHS pharyngitis would be treated with antibiotics. Assessment based on throat cultures or antigen tests, with much higher specificities, would result in treatment of 19 and 22 patients, respectively; so that only five or nine patients without GABHS pharyngitis would be treated unnecessarily with antibiotics. Tables VI, VII, and VIII summarize this information.

In an office setting, there are further disadvantages to the antigen tests. Namely,

Table VI. Comparison of Antigen Test, Clinical Judgment, and Throat Culture in a Population of 100 Patients with Pharyngitis (Utilizing Sensitivities and Specificities from the Text)

GABHS	Treat	Do not treat
Clinical judgment	48	52
Antigen test	22	78
Throat culture	19	81

Table VII. Breakdown of Patients Treated in Table VI

GABHS	True positive	False positive
Clinical judgment	10	38
Antigen test	13	9
Throat culture	14	5

these results are obtained using specially trained laboratory technicians, a commodity rarely available in a private office, and although it is quick, the technique requires that a staff person be taken away from other responsibilities for 20–30 min for each test (not a good alternative in a private office). Alternatively, the tests could be run in a batch at the end of the day, but this would negate much of the benefit of a rapid diagnosis compared to the overnight culture technique.

5. PREVENTION OF RHEUMATIC FEVER

Before presenting a general strategy for preventing the complications of GABHS pharyngitis, several points should be emphasized. First, even if all patients with pharyngitis are found and treated, roughly 25–33% of patients with ARF have no history of pharyngitis. Second, no matter the strategy, some physicians continue antibiotics regardless of a negative culture. One study has shown that 42% of primary-care physicians start antibiotics before culture results are available, and 42% of primary-care physicians did not discontinue antibiotics in the light of negative cultures. To make any strategy effective, improved physician compliance is necessary. Finally, patient education must be an important part of developing cost-effective strategies. Many patients expect antibiotics for a sore throat. Explaining the risks and limited benefits of overzealous treatment may decrease the pressure on physicians to treat in situations in which therapy is not really necessary.

Strategies for the diagnosis and treatment of acute pharyngitis must address the morbidity and mortality of unrestrained penicillin usage. About 1 per 10,000 penicillin recipients will have a fatal allergic reaction to penicillin (see Table IX).

In 1977, Tompkins *et al.*[44] performed an extensive cost-effectiveness analysis of the management of pharyngitis. They compared three different diagnostic/treatment strategies and performed a threshold analysis to see what prevalence of GABHS pharyngitis

Table VIII. Breakdown of Patients Not Treated in Table VI

GABHS	True negative	False negative
Clinical judgment	47	5
Antigen test	76	2
Throat culture	80	1

Table IX. Incidence of Various Penicillin Reactions

	Intramuscular benzathine PCN[a]	Oral PCN G
Allergic reaction	2–4%	1%
Death	0.0094%	0.0055%
Serious allergy	0.64%	0.25%

[a]PCN = penicillin.

needed to be reached in order to make it more cost-effective to (1) treat only patients with group A streptococci-positive cultures; (2) treat all patients; or (3) treat none of the patients. Several criticisms of this analysis have been pointed out: namely, that in a litigious society, failure to treat or culture a patient is an unexceptable alternative, and estimates of costs of such factors as premature death are based on nonscientific value judgments. In spite of these criticisms, the study still stands as the cornerstone of the literature on the cost-effective approach to treatment. The conclusions of their analysis follow:

1. In epidemic streptococcal pharyngitis, as seen in the military camps in the 1950s when Wannamaker did his original study,[2] the most effective strategy, both economically and medically, is to treat all patients. In this way, a slightly higher rate of allergic reactions is expected. However, there would be a 40% reduction in cases of ARF and a 32–35% reduction in cost when compared to culturing and treating.
2. In endemic streptococcal pharyngitis, the cost per patient and the incidence of ARF depend on the prevalence of GABHS pharyngitis in the population studied. In populations in which the proportion of GABHS ranges between 0.05 and 0.20 (as mentioned previously, Walsh's clinical prediction rule[30] can separate out a group of patients with an expected culture rate less than 20%), it is more cost-effective to culture the throats of the patients and wait to treat those with positive cultures. For populations with an expected culture rate greater than 0.20, the cost-effective strategy is to treat. Their final conclusion was not to treat or culture patients with a culture rate of less than 0.05. However, from a medico-legal standpoint this is a difficult stand, and more sensibly one would put these in the "culture and treat if positive" group.

Using these strategies, one could decrease inappropriate antibiotic usage in the roughly 80–90% of patients with non-GABHS pharyngitis and reduce the cost per patient per episode of pharyngitis by as much as 25%.

In summary, the most cost-effective and medically sensible approach to acute GABHS pharyngitis is to utilize a clinical decision rule that assesses weights for the various clinical data.[30,34] In using this rule, heavier emphasis is placed on the presence of cervical adenopathy, pharyngeal exudate, and history of recent exposure to *Streptococcus*. Symptoms such as coryza, rhinorrhea, and cough reduce the likelihood of streptococcal infection. Using the positive culture rate predicted by this rule, one would either treat, or culture and treat, as outlined earlier.

6. PREVENTION OF RECURRENCES OF RHEUMATIC FEVER

Because of the high recurrence rate of ARF (see Section 2), it is recognized that patients with a history of ARF should be treated more aggressively for the prevention of streptococcal pharyngitis. Recommendations in the literature and in the clinics vary from author to author and from clinician to clinician.

It has been shown that monthly injections of benzathine penicillin G are more effective than oral prophylaxis with either penicillin or sulfonamides. The parenteral regimen is as much as 10 times as effective in preventing recurrences. In large part this is due to poor compliance with oral regimens. However, i.m. injections are also more effective in maintaining adequate systemic levels of antibiotic and eradicating the majority of streptococci from the oropharynx.

The question of the duration of prophylaxis is a controversial one. Keeping in mind the recurrence rates for the succeeding 5-year periods, it is recommended that patients receive i.m. prophylaxis for at least 5 years after their last episode of ARF. In assessing prophylaxis beyond these recommendations, the physician will need to take into account the individual patient's circumstances. For example, patients often do not want the inconvenience of monthly office visits for painful injections. In the case of an older person without evidence of cardiac sequelae and without a high exposure rate to GABHS, oral prophylaxis may be considered.

7. TREATMENT OF STREPTOCOCCAL PHARYNGITIS

The treatment of choice for streptococcal pharyngitis is penicillin, either i.m. benzathine penicillin, 600,000 units (patient weight less than 60 lb) or 1,200,000 units, or oral penicillin G, 250,000 units (equivalent to penicillin V 250–500 mg) every 6 hr for 10 days. The length of therapy is important, as adequate levels of antibiotic are necessary for a prolonged period of time to eradicate the organisms from the oropharynx.

The alternate therapy for patients with penicillin allergy is erythromycin, 250 mg every 6 hr for 10 days. Although tetracycline is used by some physicians, it is not an acceptable alternative. In Japan, where tetracyclines are more frequently prescribed, more than 50% of GABHS were resistant to tetracycline in 1977, and this resistance rate has continued to be high. Equally disturbing has been the increasing trend toward resistance to erythromycin, with resistance as high as 20–30% in the late 1970s in Japan. Sulfonamides, although effective for prophylaxis, are ineffective in clearing the organism from the oropharynx in acute pharyngitis and therefore are not an acceptable alternative.

8. ENDOCARDITIS PROPHYLAXIS

Patients undergo many invasive procedures during routine medical care. For a patient with prior history of ARF, these procedures, with their associated bacteremia, pose a particular threat for endocarditis. The incidence of transient bacteremia[45] is estimated to be 0% for cardiac catheterization or insertion of an intrauterine device, 10% for sigmoidoscopy and upper endoscopy and barium enema, 14–16% for liver biopsy and nasotracheal intubation, 12–47% for transurethral resection of the prostate, 35% for manipulation of septic foci, and 60.9–84.9% for tooth extraction.

The American Heart Association has set out recommendations for antibiotic usage for the prevention of bacterial endocarditis. These recommendations have recently been updated[46] and are reviewed in Chapter 5 of this book.

9. FUTURE DEVELOPMENTS

Finally, some words about future trends in the treatment of streptococcal pharyngitis. For several years investigators have been working on a vaccine against the M protein (the antigen against which the immune system develops immunity in endocarditis) of the more rheumatogenic strains of GABHS. The work thus far has been frought with technical difficulties. Concern about the consequences of injecting M proteins into patients has also slowed this project. After all, it is the immune response to the capsular proteins that eventually leads to cardiac damage in the case of ARF.

A second area of research has been to identify genetic risk factors for ARF. There is a 20% concordance of ARF in identical twins, indicating a genetic predisposition with low penetrance. Perhaps by better identifying these genetic factors health care providers will be more able to direct preventive strategies at a more select population.

REFERENCES

1. Comroe, J. H., Jr., and Dripps, R. D. (eds.): *The Top Ten Clinical Advances in Cardiovascular–Pulmonary Medicine and Surgery between 1945 and 1975*. Vol. I. *Data and Discussion. Final Report*. United States Department of Health, Education, and Welfare, Washington, DC, 1977.
2. Denny, F. W., Wannamaker, L. W., Brink, W. R., *et al.*: Prevention of rheumatic fever: Treatment of the preceding streptococcic infection. *JAMA* **143**:151–153, 1950.
3. Wannamaker, L. W., Rammelkamp, D. H., Jr., Denny, F. W., *et al.*: Prophylaxis of acute rheumatic fever by treatment of the preceding streptococcal infection with various amounts of depot penicillin. *Am. J. Med.* **10**:673–695, 1951.
4. Cypress, B. K.: Office visits for diseases of the respiratory system. U.S. Department of Health, Education, and Welfare, Washington, DC, 1979.
5. Wannamaker, L. W.: Perplexity and precision in the diagnosis of streptococcal pharyngitis. *Am. J. Dis. Child.* **124**:352–358, 1972.
6. Komaroff, A. L., Pass, T. M., Aronson, M. D., *et al.*: The prediction of streptococcal pharyngitis in adults. *J. Gen. Intern. Med.* **1**:1–7, 1986.
7. Brock, L. L., and Siegel, A. C.: Studies on the prevention of rheumatic fever: The effect of the time of initiation of treatment of streptococcal infections on the immune response of the host. *J. Clin. Invest.* **32**:630–632, 1953.
8. Spagnuolo, M., and Tarata, A.: Rheumatic fever in siblings. Similarity of its clinical manifestations. *N. Engl. J. Med.* **278**:183–188, 1968.
9. DiSciascio, G., and Taranta, A.: Rheumatic fever in children. *Am. Heart J.* **99**:635–658, 1980.
10. Ayoub, E. M.: The search for host determinants of susceptibility to rheumatic fever: The missing link. *Circulation* **69**:197–201, 1984.
11. Stollerman, G. H.: Nephritogenic and rheumatogenic group A streptococci. *J. Infect. Dis.* **120**:258–263, 1969.

12. Land, M. A., and Bisno, A. L.: Acute rheumatic fever. A vanishing disease in suburbia. *JAMA* **249**:895–898, 1983.
13. Coulehan, J. L., Baacke, G., Welty, T. K., and Goldtooth, N. L.: Cost-benefit of a streptococcal surveillance program among Navajo indians. *Public Health Rep.* **97**:73–77, 1982.
14. Catanzaro, F. J., Rammelkamp, C. H., Jr., and Chamovitz, R.: Prevention of rheumatic fever by treatment of streptococcal infections. II. Factors responsible for failures. *N. Engl. J. Med.* **259**:51–57, 1958.
15. Nelson, J. D.: The effect of penicillin therapy on the symptoms and signs of streptococcal pharyngitis. *Pediatr. Infect. Dis.* **3**:10–13, 1984.
16. Hutchison, B., and Yassi, A. L.: Resolving the sore throat dilemma. *Can. Fam. Physician* **27**:471–477, 1981.
17. Haight, T. H.: Erythromycin therapy of respiratory infections. I. Controlled studies on the comparative efficacy of erythromycin and penicillin in scarlet fever. *J. Lab. Clin. Med.* **10**:300–308, 1954.
18. Merenstein, J. H., and Rogers, K. D.: Streptococcal pharyngitis. Early treatment and management by nurse practitioners. *JAMA* **227**:1278–1282, 1974.
19. Komaroff, A. L., Aronson, M. D., Pass, T. M., *et al.*: Serologic evidence of chlamydial and mycoplasmal pharyngitis in adults. *Science* **222**:927–929, 1983.
20. Bennike, T., Bruchner-Mortenson, K., Kjaor, E., *et al.*: Penicillin therapy in acute tonsillitis, phlegmonous tonsillitis and ulcerative tonsillitis. *Acta Med. Scand.* **139**:253–274, 1951.
21. Chamovitz, R., Rammelkanp, C. H., Wannamaker, L. W., *et al.*: The effect of tonsillectomy on the incidence of streptococcal respiratory disease and its complications. *Pediatrics* **26**:355–367, 1960.
22. Lowe, R.: Early Treatment of streptococcal pharyngitis. *Ann. Emerg. Med.* **13**:440–448, 1984.
23. Breese, B. B., and Disney, F. A.: The accuracy of diagnosis of B streptococcal infections on clinical grounds. *J. Pediatr.* **44**:670–673, 1954.
24. Eggenberger, K., Christen, J-P., Delarue, C., *et al.*: Streptococcal pharyngitis-tonsillitis in Swiss children. Diagnosis and management. *Pediatrician* **9**:295–308, 1980.
25. Siegel, A. C., Johnson, E. C., and Stollerman, G. H.: Controlled studies of streptococcal pharyngitis in a pediatric population. *N. Engl. J. Med.* **265**:559–566, 1961.
26. Poses, R. M., Cebul, R. D., Collins, M., *et al.*: The accuracy of experienced physicians' probability estimates for patients with sore throats. *JAMA* **254**:925–929, 1985.
27. Wigton, R. S., Connor, J. L., and Centor, R. M.: Transportability of a decision rule for the diagnosis of streptococcal pharyngitis. *Arch. Intern. Med.* **146**:81–83, 1986.
28. Wood, R. W., Tompkins, R. K., and Wolcott, B. W.: An efficient strategy for managing acute respiratory illness in adults. *Ann. Intern. Med.* **93**:757–763, 1980.
29. Greenfield, S., Bragg, F. E., McCraith, D. L., *et al.*: Upper respiratory tract complaint protocol for physician–extenders. *Arch. Intern. Med.* **133**:294–299, 1974.
30. Walsh, B. T., Bookheim, W. W., Johnson, R. L., *et al.*: Recognition of streptococcal pharyngitis in adults. *Arch. Intern. Med.* **135**:1493–1497, 1975.
31. Centor, R. M., Witherspoon, J. M., Dalton, H. P., *et al.*: The diagnosis of strep throat in adults in the emergency room. *Med. Decis. Making* **1**:239–246, 1981.
32. Breese, B. B.: A simple scorecard for the tentative diagnosis of streptococcal pharyngitis. *Am. J. Dis. Child.* **131**:514–517, 1977.
33. Lowe, R.: Early treatment of streptococcal pharyngitis. *Ann. Emerg. Med.* **13**:440–448, 1984.
34. Komaroff, A. L., Pass, T. M., Aronson, M. D., *et al.*: The prediction of streptococcal pharyngitis in adults. *J. Gen. Intern. Med.* **1**:1–7, 1986.
35. Poses, R. M., Cebul, R. D., Collins, M., and Fager, S. S.: The importance of disease prevalence in transporting clinical prediction rules. *Ann. Intern. Med.* **105**:586–591, 1986.
36. Hoffman, S.: Lack of reliability of primary grouping of beta-hemolytic streptococci by culture of throat swabs with streptocult supplemented with bacitracin disks in general practice. *J. Clin. Microbiol.* **22**:497–500, 1985.
37. Larsson, P., and Lind, L.: The need for control of throat streptococcal cultures in general practice. *Scand. J. Infect. Dis.* **39**(suppl.):79–82, 1983.
38. Todd, J. K.: Throat cultures in the office laboratory. *Pediatr. Infect. Dis.* **1**:265–270, 1982.
39. DuBois, D., Ray, V. G., Nelson, B., *et al.*: Rapid diagnosis of group A strep pharyngitis in the emergency department. *Ann. Emerg. Med.* **15**:157–159, 1986.
40. Fischer, P. M., and Mentrup, P. L.: Comparison of throat culture and latex agglutination test for streptococcal pharyngitis. *J. Fam. Pract.* **22**:245–248, 1986.

41. Schwartz, R. H., Hayden, G. F., Mccoy, P., *et al.*: Rapid diagnosis pharyngitis in two pediatric offices using a latex agglutination kit. *Pediatr. Infect. Dis.* **4**:647–650, 1985.
42. Roddey, O. F., Clegg, H. W., Clardy, L. T., *et al.*: Comparison of a latex agglutination test and four culture methods for identification of group A streptococci in a pediatric office laboratory. *J. Pediatr.* **108**:347–351, 1986.
43. The Medical Letter: Rapid diagnostic tests for streptococcal pharyngitis. **27**:49–51, 1985.
44. Tompkins, R. K., Burnes, D. C., and Cable, W. E.: An analysis of the cost-effectiveness of pharyngitis management and acute rheumatic fever prevention. *Ann. Intern. Med.* **86**:481–492, 1977.
45. Lowy, F., and Steigbigel, N. H.: Infective endocarditis. Part III. Prevention of bacterial endocarditis. *Am. Heart J.* **96**:689–695, 1978.
46. Shulman, S. T., Amren, D. P., Bisno, A. L., *et al.*: Prevention of bacterial endocarditis: A statement for health professionals by the Committee on Rheumatic Fever and Infective Endocarditis of the Council on Cardiovascular Disease in the Young. *Circulation* **70**:1123A–1127A, 1984.

8

Tuberculosis

David C. Deitz

1. INTRODUCTION

For many primary-care physicians in Canada and the United States, tuberculosis has become a rare disease. The Centers for Disease Control (CDC) report 21,801 cases of tuberculosis in 1985, equivalent to a case rate of 9.1 per 100,000 population.[1] This is still a significant public health problem, but when compared with estimates of over 500,000 physicians in the United States by 1990, it becomes clear that many North American physicians will not encounter the disease in regular practice. Advances in our understanding of how to detect, cure, and prevent tuberculosis have greatly changed the course of the disease. As the prevalence of active cases declines, the role of preventive strategies as implemented by individual physicians requires continued emphasis. The challenge for primary-care physicians for the future will be to identify groups and individuals at risk for tuberculosis, screen for infection when appropriate, and prescribe prophylaxis when indicated—all without necessarily encountering an active case for long intervals.[2]

This chapter reviews these concepts with respect to disease caused by *Mycobacterium tuberculosis*. Basic principles of modern antituberculous chemotherapy are briefly reviewed, but readers are directed elsewhere for more comprehensive discussions of treatment and for information on disease caused by other mycobacteria. The discussions of screening and skin test interpretation are intended to be relevant to clinical practice in the United States and Canada. They are inapplicable to many parts of the world where the frequency and nature of tuberculous infections are quite different.

2. EPIDEMIOLOGY

An individual's risk of developing tuberculosis depends on many factors. The most important of these, of course, is the probability of exposure to the disease, which in the United States and many developed countries is considerably less than 0.1% per year. Acquisition of infection is not sufficient to produce active tuberculosis (tuberculosis disease). Between 5 and 10% of infected individuals will develop active tuberculosis over

---

David C. Deitz • Division of General Medicine and Primary Care, Department of Medicine, Beth Israel Hospital, Harvard Medical School, Boston, Massachusetts 02215.

the course of their lives[3,4]; most, therefore, will not. The risk of developing active tuberculosis following exposure is dependent on a variety of individual factors that have little to do with the probability of exposure. Epidemiological data on case and death rates for tuberculosis among various subgroups are not necessarily helpful in distinguishing between risks for exposure and infection and risks for development of active disease.[5]

In considering risk factors for tuberculosis, it is important that this distinction between risk of infection and risk of disease remains clear. For the primary-care physician, an individual patient's risk of infection will be important primarily in deciding whom and when to screen. Management decisions regarding prophylaxis and follow-up care of tuberculin-positive patients will depend on an assessment of the risk of disease, along with any possible risk associated with prophylaxis.

2.1. Risk of Infection

Geographical variation in the prevalence of tuberculosis has historically been an important determinant of an individual's risk of infection. Recent geographical trends in the United States (Fig. 1) reflect the historically higher prevalence of tuberculosis in more southern states as well as the recent influx of refugees to certain cities (e.g., Miami, San Francisco). In 1984, case rates ranged from a high of 21/100,000 in Hawaii to a low of 1/100,000 in Wyoming.[7] Regardless of regional prevalence, residence in urban areas is usually associated with increased risk (Table I).

The interpretation of most risk factors for tuberculous infection is simplified by

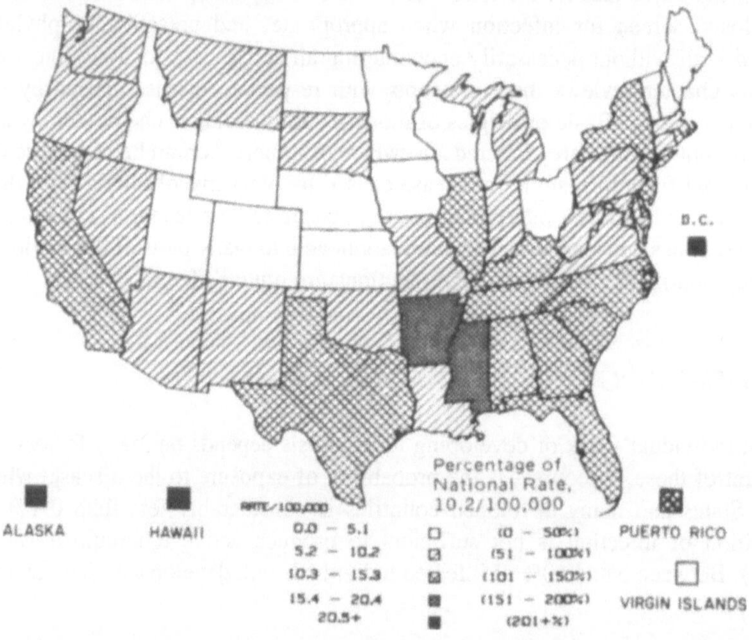

Figure 1. Reported tuberculosis cases per 100,000 population, by state, United States 1983. (Source: Ref. 6.)

Table I. 1984 Tuberculosis Case Rates for Selected Cities with Populations Greater than 250,000[a]

Highest		Lowest	
City	Case rate/100,000	City	Case rate/100,000
Miami, FL	49.9	Columbus, OH	6.5
Newark, NJ	44.2	Virginia Beach, VA	6.0
Atlanta, GA	40.2	Toledo, OH	5.1
San Francisco, CA	38.2	Albuquerque, NM	4.5
Tampa, FL	31.9	Omaha, NE	2.3

[a]Source: Ref. 7.

considering what they all seem to represent: the probability of contact with an individual with active tuberculosis.[5] In studies that have examined household contacts of persons with active tuberculosis, the severity of disease in the index case has the greatest influence on likelihood of infection in other household members.[8] Factors that affect aerosol spread (i.e., cavitary disease, degree of crowding, patterns of ventilation systems) will modify the probability of infection in these situations.[9] Most of the epidemiological risks listed in Table II are associated with a higher risk of exposure to tuberculosis disease. Many are clearly clustered—for example, recent immigrants are often urban residents with lower-than-average incomes, living in crowded conditions where the probability of contact with active disease is increased.

Institutional settings represent situations in which the potential for transmission of disease is great. Risks are probably multifactorial; crowding, increased prevalence of active cases in some groups, and increased susceptibility to disease in situations such as shelters and nursing homes are likely all important factors. Recognition of risks and periodic screening for tuberculosis in these settings is valuable.[10] Physicians and other health care workers, particularly house staff, are at markedly increased risk for infection and development of active tuberculosis in some institutions.[11,12]

In the United States, the incidence of tuberculosis is lowest in white females and

Table II. Risk Factors for Infection with M. tuberculosis

Contact with case of *M. tuberculosis*
Age—increased risk in infancy, late adolescence, and old age
Sex—M > F
Socioeconomic status (low > high)
Urban residents (especially inner-city)
Recent immigration from high-prevalence region (Southeast Asia, Central America, Haiti)
Institutional residence—prison, nursing home, shelter
Occupation
Health care workers
Institutional caretakers (e.g., nurses, prison guards)
Migrant workers
Miners (with silicosis)

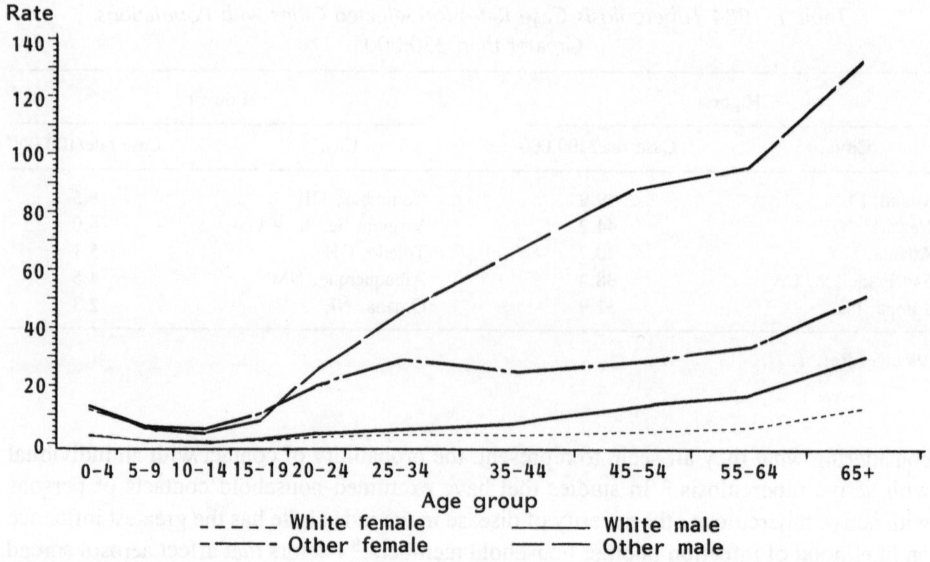

Figure 2. Reported tuberculosis cases per 100,000 population, by age group, race, and sex, United States 1983. (Source: Ref. 6.)

highest in nonwhite males (Fig. 2). Certain ethnic or racial groups are at increased risk, for a variety of reasons. Blacks, Hispanics, and Native Americans all represent identifiable groups at increased risk,[7,13] as do recent immigrants from Asia (especially Southeast Asian refugees), Central and South America, and the Caribbean (particularly Haiti).[14–16] In Canada, 32.3% of all new cases of tuberculosis from 1971 to 1976 has been attributed to immigrants.[17] It has not been possible to sort out the effects of race, socioeconomic class, nutrition, and other variables, such as substance abuse, on rates of infection. It seems likely that racial and cultural differences in case rates are largely artifacts of environmental factors that influence both probability of exposure and risk of active disease by those infected.[18,19]

2.2. Risk of Active Disease

Once infected, individuals may develop overt primary disease or, after a period of latency, develop reactivation tuberculosis, which classically presents with involvement of the pulmonary apices.[9,20] From studies of household contacts, it appears that the risk of developing active disease is greatest for the first few years after infection and declines rapidly thereafter.[21,22] Risk of active tuberculosis for the first year in tuberculin-positive young men may be greater than 4%[4]; a cumulative risk of approximately 6% for the first 5 years after infection has been reported for young men in the Netherlands, where overall prevalence of tuberculosis is less than in the United States.[22] Subsequent risk of reactivation is much lower after the first few years. Age is an important factor affecting risk of reactivation. After early childhood, case rates decline for several years before peaking again in late adolescence/early adulthood and then declining.[3] Risk of active disease increases again beginning about age 45–50, though reinfection may also be important in older age groups.[23–25]

The presence of abnormal findings on chest x-ray has long been recognized as a risk factor for the development of active pulmonary tuberculosis. The risk of activation for individuals with fibrotic lesions and a positive tuberculin test may be 20 times greater than that for those with a normal radiograph.[26] An additional important predictive factor is the size of the tuberculin reaction when initially tested.[4] Risk of active tuberculosis in individuals with a large tuberculin reaction ($\geq$12 mm) may be more than 3 times greater than in persons with smaller reactions (6–11 mm)[27] (see Section 3.2). It is not clear whether the influence of tuberculin reactivity on risk for subsequent disease is related to host factors (such as decreased resistance), virulence of the infecting organisms, or size of the initial inoculum.

An interesting and persistent association between leanness and increased risk for tuberculosis has been noted by several investigators.[4,28,29] Though this may be due in part to nutrition, a relationship to heritable differences in susceptibility has also been postulated.[5] Genetic differences in susceptibility probably do exist, and there is evidence linking certain HLA antigens with increased (HLA-Bw15, -DR5) or decreased (-DR6y) probability of active disease in blacks.[30,31]

A variety of pathological conditions are associated with increased risk for active tuberculosis (Table III), though the degree of increased risk is poorly documented for most of those listed.[32] Routine tuberculin testing is reasonable in all of these situations. Most are presumed to increase susceptibility by interfering with host defenses in some way. In future years, the acquired immunodeficiency syndrome (AIDS) may become one of the most significant illnesses associated with tuberculosis (see Section 5.3).

At present, alcoholism is probably the most prevalent illness associated with increased risk for tuberculosis. Alcoholics have multiple risks, which are summarized in Table IV.[33–37] Factors associated with alcoholism, such as low socioeconomic status, nutritional deficiencies, other pulmonary illnesses, and chronic liver disease, are likely in part to be responsible for increased rates of tuberculosis. Studies that have attempted to control for confounding suggest that alcoholism itself, possibly via impairment of cellular

Table III. Conditions Associated with Increased Risk for the Development of Active Tuberculosis[a]

Hematological or reticuloendothelial neoplasms
Corticosteroid therapy equivalent to 15 mg prednisone per day, or other prolonged immunosuppressive therapy
Silicosis
Chronic renal insufficiency
Diabetes mellitus, particularly if poorly regulated
Alcoholism
Conditions associated with nutritional deficiency and substantial weight loss, including gastrectomy and intestinal bypass
Heroin addiction
Acquired immunodeficiency syndrome

[a]Source: modified from Ref. 32.

Table IV. Factors Influencing Development of Tuberculosis in Alcoholics

Increased prevalence of tuberculous infection (+PPD)
Socioeconomic factors that affect exposure
Impaired cellular immunity
Increased probability of active disease
Nutrition, exposure, cellular immunity, intercurrent illness
More extensive disease at time of presentation
Increased probability of cavitary disease
Increased probability of peritoneal and possibly other extrapulmonary manifestations
Difficulties with treatment
More extensive disease at time of presentation
Longer duration of treatment necessary
Poor compliance
Increased incidence of complications from antituberculous chemotherapy
Increased probability of drug-resistant tuberculosis
Increased relapse rate
Secondary to factors cited above
Increased probability of reinfection even if adequately treated

immunity, is also important.[34,38–41] The success of supervised chemotherapy programs suggests that poor compliance with treatment is by far the most important reason for treatment failures and relapses in alcoholic patients.[38,39]

3. PREVENTIVE STRATEGIES

3.1. Primary Prevention—BCG vaccination

Despite the widespread use of bacille Calmette Guérin (BCG) vaccine in many countries for over 50 years, no consensus exists today on the degree of protection it provides against tuberculous infection. As has been pointed out elsewhere,[42] even a demonstrably effective vaccine would not be cost-effective for use in most of the United States and Canada, where the incidence of tuberculosis is low. BCG vaccination is an important element of tuberculosis control in many countries where incidence is higher.

Much of the controversy about BCG involves the interpretation of conflicting results obtained in large-scale trials of the vaccine, in which efficacies have ranged from 0 to 80% (summarized in Refs. 43, 44). One recent analysis has suggested that the vaccine trials that have shown the highest degree of protection for BCG are also methodologically superior.[45] Epidemiological evidence from Canada and the United Kingdom supporting the effectiveness of BCG has led to its continued use among Inuit populations in Canada, where the incidence of tuberculosis, particularly in children, remains high.[46,47] The duration of protective effect is unclear. Tuberculin reactivity gradually wanes after vaccination (see Section 3.2.1b); this may signal a return in susceptibility to exogenous infection. Other than questions of effectiveness, the principal disadvantage of BCG involves loss of the use of skin test conversion as a diagnostic test for tuberculous infection.

Serious side effects from the vaccine, such as osteomyelitis and disseminated BCG infection, are extremely rare.[48]

The strain of BCG currently available in the United States has not been objectively tested. It is recommended that BCG in the United States be used only where tuberculosis is epidemic, as defined by a new case rate of greater than 1% per year *and* where other control measures at present are ineffective.[49] Its use in travelers is suggested only if there are to be prolonged stays in endemic areas where the disease is poorly controlled and where the vaccinee will be out of reach of medical services.

3.2. Secondary Prevention

3.2.1. Detection of Tuberculosis Exposure

The decline in prevalence of tuberculosis in North America has made mass-screening strategies impractical for most of the population because of the low yield of active cases. In most of the Southeast and in some other regions, widespread exposure to nontuberculous mycobacteria (NTM) still accounts for considerable cross-reactivity to tuberculin (Fig. 3).[50,51] As the incidence of tuberculosis decreases, the probability that a given skin reaction is due to NTM ("false" positive) becomes progressively greater (see Section

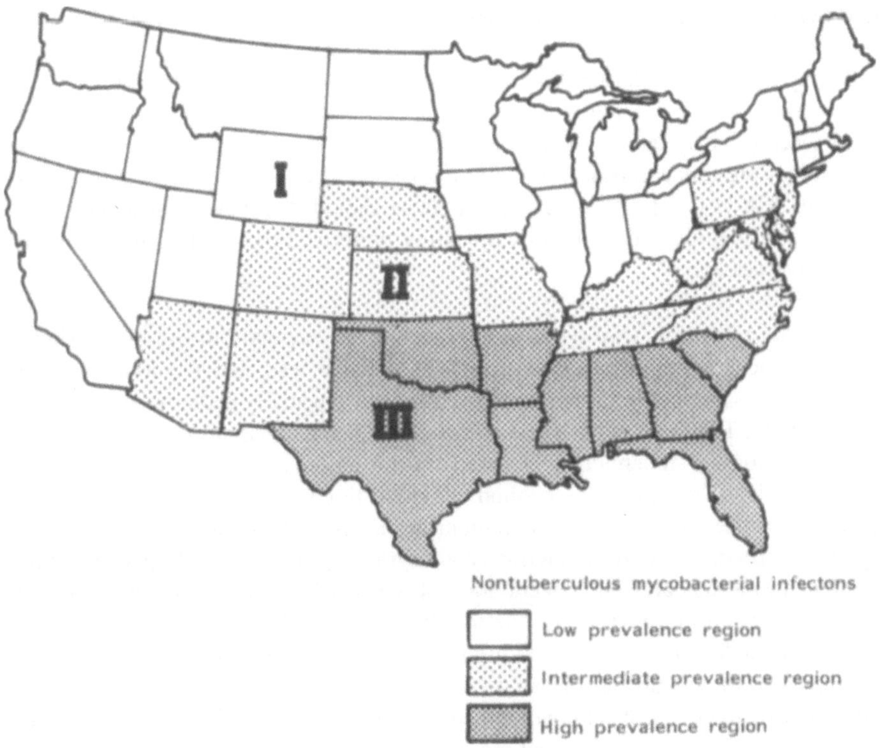

Figure 3. Prevalence of nontuberculous mycobacterial infection in the United States defined by level of prevalence. (Source: Ref. 50.)

3.2.1b). Chest radiographs are cost-ineffective for mass screening because of low sensitivity and specificity.[52,53] They also provide no information on the status of tuberculous infection in the absence of active pulmonary disease.

With the decline of mass screening, it has become more important for primary-care physicians to identify individuals and subgroups for whom screening *is* still necessary because they are at continued risk for tuberculosis. Tuberculin status of individuals in most of the epidemiological risk groups listed in Table II should be determined and recorded. This is particularly important for institutional residents and employees at the beginning of their residence or employment. A surprisingly high incidence of new tuberculin reactors and active tuberculosis has been documented in nursing homes in Arkansas.[54] Conversion rates (skin test newly reactive) of 5% for the first year of residence have been recorded.[55] There is reason to expect similar problems in other states and in other institutional settings such as prisons.[56–58]

Immigrants arrive with a risk for tuberculosis proportional to the prevalence of tuberculosis in their native country.[17] Risks in Haitian and Southeast Asian refugees have been well documented,[14–16] but almost all less-developed countries have a higher prevalence of tuberculosis than the United States or Canada. Some immigrants will have received BCG vaccination, but most will not recall the details. Since BCG vaccination programs in most countries do not approach complete coverage of the population,[43] Mantoux testing should be performed and the history of BCG vaccination recorded (if given). Interpretation of reactivity in persons who have received BCG is discussed in Section 3.2.1b.

It is important to emphasize that skin testing of contacts is *always* indicated regardless of risk, unless tuberculin reactivity has been previously documented. Since cutaneous reactivity may take up to 10 weeks to develop following infection, a negative test following a presumed exposure should be repeated after 10–12 weeks. All persons with positive skin tests regardless of contact status should then have a medical history taken and a physical examination and chest x-ray performed to identify any additional risks for active disease.

3.2.1a. Skin Testing. Two types of skin testing are currently in use in the United States and Canada: multipuncture tests, such as the tine test, and the Mantoux test. Multipuncture tests are preferred by many practitioners, especially pediatricians, because of their simplicity. They also provide less information. Much of our current understanding of the epidemiology of tuberculosis is based on the Mantoux test. It is still the gold standard and is the only appropriate method of skin testing for most clinical situations.[59]

The Mantoux test is performed by administering five tuberculin units (TU) of purified protein derivative (PPD) intradermally via syringe with a 26- or 27-gauge needle. PPD is diluted to a standardized concentration of 5 TU/0.1 ml, and a detergent (Tween 80) is added to retard loss of activity due to adsorption by glass. For convenience, the volar surface of the forearm is the site traditionally used. The site of administration should be reexamined in 48–72 hr and the amount of induration measured in millimeters. A transparent plastic ruler is probably one of the most convenient tools for this. Some prefer using a ballpoint pen to assess the exact margins of induration: with this method a pen is drawn slowly across the skin toward the center of induration and a mark made where resistance is first encountered at the edge.[60] Erythema or any reactivity occurring at less than 48 hr is not specific for tuberculosis and should be discounted, but indurations of 10 mm or more that persist for 96 hr or longer are still significant. Results should be recorded in the patient's medical record and should include the dates of administration and reading, site of administration, amount of tuberculin administered (5 TU in almost all situations), and the diameter of induration. Other antigens, such as mumps, *Candida,* or streptokinase–streptodornase, are often administered simultaneously at a separate site to provide evidence that the person being tested is not anergic. Results of these tests, if done, should also be recorded. Use of control antigens may be helpful if there is a suspicion of active tuberculosis or concomitant disorder that might suppress cutaneous hypersensitivity, but their interpretation has not been standardized.

3.2.1b. Interpretation of Mantoux Tests. Accurate interpretation of the results of Mantoux tests requires more than a measurement of the diameter of induration. Age, immunocompetence, exposure history, and geographical location of principal lifetime residence are all helpful and important factors. Much of this has been reviewed elsewhere[61] but will be summarized briefly here.

The greatest difficulty in interpretation of tuberculin tests occurs because persons exposed to NTM will have some degree of cutaneous hypersensitivity when tested with PPD, even if they have never been exposed to *M. tuberculosis.* With the exception of exposure to *M. bovis,* the amount of induration in such persons is usually less than 10 mm. Unfortunately, skin testing of populations with known active tuberculosis or from regions that are essentially free of NTM has established that many individuals infected with tuberculosis will also have Mantoux tests of less than 10 mm induration (Figs. 4 and 5).[50,61] The probability that an individual is infected with *M. tuberculosis* increases with the extent of induration, with almost all induration greater than 12 mm due to *M.*

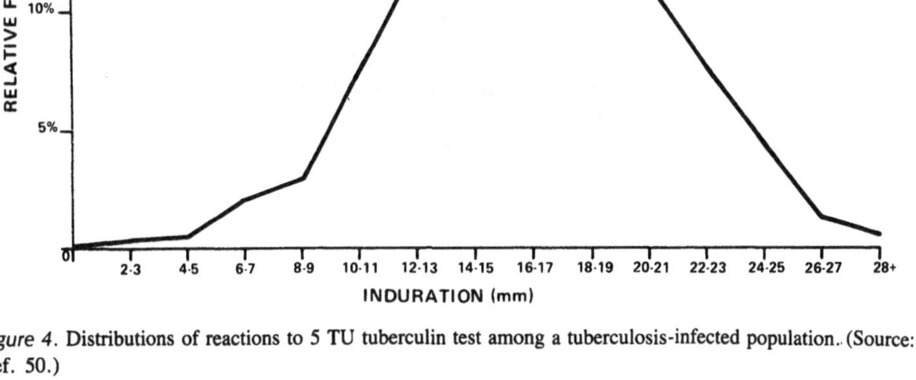

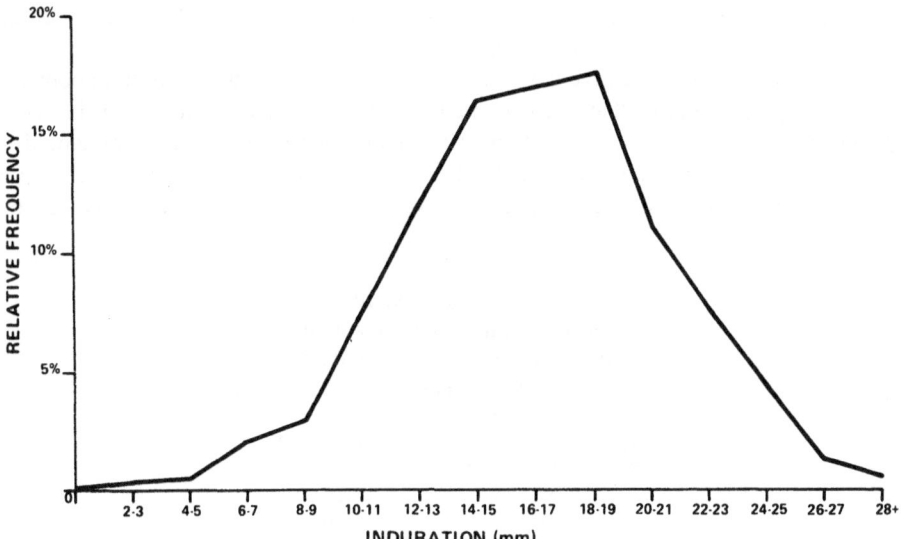

Figure 4. Distributions of reactions to 5 TU tuberculin test among a tuberculosis-infected population. (Source: Ref. 50.)

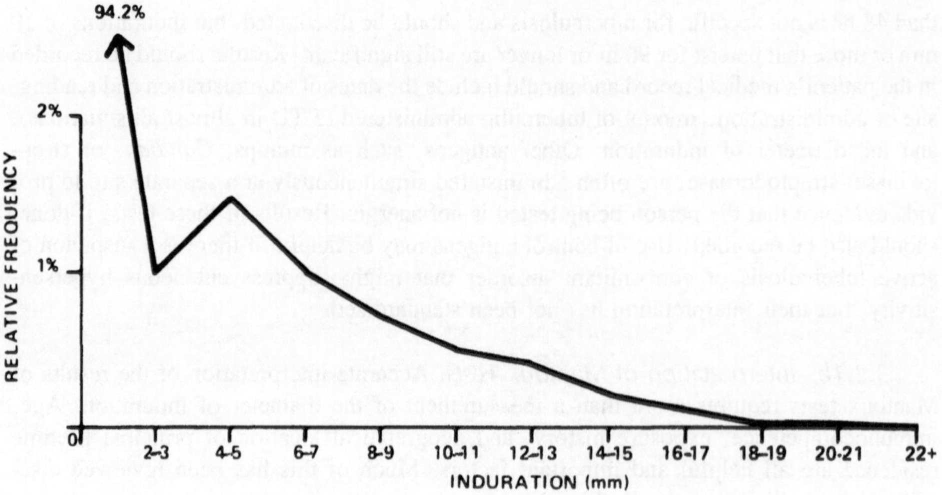

Figure 5. Distribution of reactions to 5 TU tuberculin test among a nontuberculosis-infected population. (Source: Ref. 50.)

tuberculosis.[50,61] The probability of subsequent active disease is also increased, as shown by data from a large study with a median follow-up of 35 months (Table V).[27,29]

In the United States, the traditional cutoff has been 10 mm of induration, with individuals whose reactions are 9 mm or less being considered tuberculin "negative." As reviewed by Snider[61] and summarized in Figs. 4–6, this cutoff point has provided the best compromise between misclassifying exposure to NTM as infection with *M. tuberculosis* and classifying small reactions due to *M. tuberculosis* as "negative."[50] While this is still a reasonable boundary between "positive" and "negative" tests for the general population, certain situations may dictate different cutoffs.

For recent contacts of active cases of tuberculosis, particularly household contacts, there is a high probability that even a small amount of tuberculin reactivity is due to exposure to *M. tuberculosis.*[4] In this situation, induration of 5 mm or more should be regarded as positive and managed accordingly. Similarly, persons who have lived most of their lives in areas where the prevalence of NTM infections is low will have a correspon-

Table V. Cases of Tuberculosis according to Size of Reaction to PPD among 1,124,883 White Navy Recruits[a]

Reaction size (mm)	Cases/100,000
0–5	36.3
6–11	110.3
> 11	378.2

[a]Source: Ref. 27.

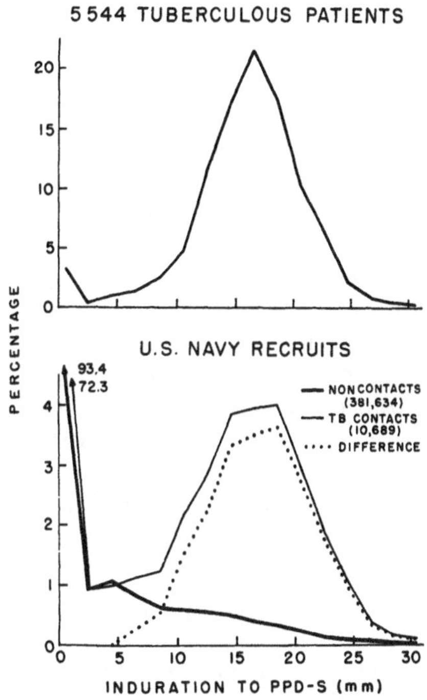

Figure 6. Reactions to PPD-S (0.0001 mg) in tuberculous patients and U.S. Navy recruits. (Source: Ref. 51.)

dingly low probability of prior skin sensitization. Any reaction to tuberculin in these areas is probably due to tuberculosis. This situation exists in Alaska, much of Canada, and some areas of the northern United States, where induration of 5 mm or more should be interpreted as positive (Fig. 3).

For individuals from regions where prior exposure to NTM is likely, selection of appropriate cutoffs depends on the prevalence of tuberculous infection. Individuals from many tropical regions such as Southeast Asia may be best managed by regarding 5 mm of induration as reactive. Though the probability of exposure to NTM is high, the risk of tuberculous infection is relatively high also, and a low cutoff may be advisable to minimize missed cases. A contrasting situation is seen in the southeastern United States, where the prevalence of tuberculosis relative to NTM infections has decreased. In such areas, some have advocated cutoffs as high as 15 mm of induration before considering a skin test positive.[61,62]

Persons with a history of known or possible BCG vaccination should be tested as appropriate to their clinical situation. Test interpretation in such individuals has recently been reviewed[63] and relies principally on knowledge of the time interval since vaccination and the probability of tuberculous infection or exposure. When tested 8–15 years after BCG vaccination, 44 of 63 individuals in one study had tuberculin reactions of 5 mm or less.[64] For individuals from high-prevalence areas, it is probably unwise to ascribe large reactions (10 mm) to prior BCG vaccination.

As is true for most tests, the Mantoux test may have false negative as well as false positive results. Some of these are dependent on interpretation, as discussed earlier; test performance will obviously vary as different cutoffs are chosen. It has long been known that skin tests may be negative in the presence of active tuberculosis.[65–67] Table VI summarizes other situations that must be considered in interpreting negative test results.[68] Reproducibility is also not ideal. In an attempt to quantify variability in Mantoux testing, Chaparas *et al.* administered duplicate tests to over 1000 individuals, some of whom had culture-proven *M. tuberculosis*. One test of each pair was arbitrarily chosen as the standard, and both standard and duplicate were read blindly by different experienced readers. Using a 10-mm cutoff after 48 hr, duplicate tests showed a "false negative" rate (1-sensitivity) of 14.5% and a "false positive" rate (1-specificity) of 2.5%; similar results were obtained using other cutoffs and other time intervals.[69]

Since the risk for development of active tuberculosis is highest in the first year of infection and declines with each succeeding year, identification of those recently infected is particularly important.[4,22] Individuals with a history of a previously nonreactive or insignificant skin test within the past 2 years who are found to be reactive on repeat testing are considered to be converters.[32] If the clinical history or records of prior skin tests suggest that this conversion is recent, a new infection is presumed. Because of the

Table VI. Potential Causes of Falsely Nonsignificant Tuberculin Test Reactions[a]

- Factors related to the person being tested
  - Infections
    - Viral (measles, mumps, chickenpox)
    - Bacterial (typhoid fever, brucellosis, typhus, leprosy, pertussis, overwhelming tuberculosis, tuberculous pleurisy)
    - Fungal (South American blastomycosis)
  - Live virus vaccinations (measles, mumps, polio)
  - Metabolic derangements (chronic renal failure)
  - Nutritional factors (severe protein depletion)
  - Disease affecting lymphoid organs (Hodgkin's disease, lymphoma, chronic lymphocytic leukemia, sarcoidosis, AIDS)
  - Drugs (corticosteroids and many other immunosuppressive agents)
  - Age (newborns, elderly patients with "waned" sensitivity)
  - Recent or overwhelming infection with *M. tuberculosis*
  - Stress (surgery, burns, mental illness, graft-versus-host reactions)
- Factors related to the tuberculin used
  - Improper storage (exposure to light and heat)
  - Improper dilutions
  - Chemical denaturation
  - Contamination
  - Adsorption (partially controlled by adding Tween 80)
- Factors related to the method of administration
  - Injection of too little antigen
  - Delayed administration after drawing into syringe
  - Injection too deep
- Factors related to reading the test and recording results
  - Inexperienced reader
  - Conscious or unconscious bias
  - Error in recording

[a]Source: Ref. 59.

variability with Mantoux testing, it has been recommended that in the absence of a contact history, an increase not be considered significant unless it is at least 6 mm larger than previously documented tests *and* at least 10 mm in size overall.[59]

A final confounding factor in interpreting tuberculin tests is the "booster" phenomenon. Up to 10% of individuals older than 50 with nonreactive tests initially will show significant reactions when retested 1 week to 1 year later.[70] Clinical and epidemiological investigations have determined that these "boosted" reactions do not represent recent infection.[70,71] Tuberculin reactivity declines with age and can apparently be recalled by exposure to the small amount of antigen present in the 5 TU Mantoux test. To avoid confusing these with conversions, it is now recommended that tuberculin testing of the elderly be done by a two-stage procedure.[59] Tests that are initially nonreactive are repeated in 1–2 weeks, with increases of 6 mm or more considered to be evidence for prior infection (boosted reactions).

While Mantoux tests require some training to be administered properly, multipuncture tests (tine, Heaf, Aplitest) can be given by inexperienced people after minimal instruction. These tests use a set of metal prongs to introduce antigen into the dermis. Their ease of administration and low cost has encouraged their use in situations such as mass screening of schoolchildren. They are also designed for self-interpretation with mail-in cards, which, it is hoped, improves compliance with test reading. Reactions from multipuncture tests cannot be quantified. Thus, Mantoux tests must be performed on patients with any amount of reactivity. Antigens used are not standardized; the tine test uses Old Tuberculin, a filtrate derived from cultures of *M. tuberculosis*, while others use PPD. Poor quality control in manufacture, particularly with respect to uneven coating of the tines with antigen, has been shown to affect test reliability.[72,73] Though some studies have reported high sensitivity and specificity of multipuncture tests when compared with Mantoux tests,[74,75] there are also several reports documenting lower sensitivities when the two are compared.[67,76–78] Paired multipuncture tests in known tuberculin reactors have shown an unacceptably high discordance rate in one other report.[79] For these reasons, multipuncture tests are not recommended for tuberculin testing of adults.[80,81]

3.2.1c. Serological Testing. Serological tests for *M. tuberculosis* infection are not at present clinically available. They are mentioned here because recent improvements in enzyme-linked immunosorbent assays (ELISA) suggest that they may soon be introduced. ELISAs using antibody to PPD and to antigen 5 (derived from *M. tuberculosis*) may potentially distinguish active from inactive tuberculosis without significant cross-reactivity to NTM. One ELISA using antigen 5 has been reported to have specificities as high as 98% in distinguishing active from inactive disease.[82] Other investigators have suggested the use of a combined sputum smear–ELISA strategy.[83] In clinical practice in North America, an ELISA with acceptable sensitivity and specificity would potentially be more useful than skin testing for high-risk groups, especially when some of the problems in the interpretation of Mantoux tests are considered.

3.2.2. Chemoprophylaxis

Chemoprophylaxis for tuberculosis involves identification of infected individuals, who are then treated to prevent the development of active disease. In a strict sense this is secondary rather than primary prophylaxis, since it actually represents treatment of a latent infection. However, it is clear from an epidemiological perspective that prevention of active disease in individuals already infected blocks transmission to others and decreases the incidence of tuberculosis in the population as a whole.[80,84]

The efficacy of isoniazid (INH) in decreasing the incidence of active disease is well established after several large trials,[4,85–87] and the subject of chemoprophylaxis in general has been reviewed.[21,88] Most commonly, INH is given to adults as a single daily dose of 300 mg for 12 months, but regimens using 600–900 mg taken twice weekly have also been effective. The twice-weekly regimens are especially attractive for supervised programs. Coadministration of pyridoxine (50 mg daily) to prevent peripheral neuropathy is recommended for patients with conditions in which neuropathy is common.[84] Benefits from INH are seen with as little as 3 months of treatment, but maximum efficacy seems to require 9–12 months of administration.[85,86] The efficacy of INH prophylaxis for 1 year is probably best estimated at 70–75% for the general population.[21,87] Compliance with therapy seems to be the most important variable influencing effectiveness. The protective effect is known to persist for at least 19 years after isoniazid administration.[89]

The principal adverse effect of INH is hepatitis. The risk of fatal hepatitis is almost nonexistent in individuals under 20 who are followed carefully, but increases with age.[90,91] The age-dependent risks of tuberculosis versus INH-induced hepatitis for adults have received much attention since their initial recognition.[92] The American Thoracic Society currently recommends treatment of all tuberculin reactors aged 35 or younger unless other contraindications exist.[59] Two decision analyses have been published, which, perhaps predictably, have reached different conclusions. The first of these has suggested that for adults aged 20–35 whose only risk factor for the development of active tuberculosis is a positive tuberculin reaction, potential benefits from treatment with INH do not clearly outweigh the risks.[93] A more recent model (which incorporates some newer data) suggests that INH prophylaxis reduces mortality at all ages.[94] As might be expected, disagreement over this recommendation hinges on the assessment of hepatitis mortality as determined in large trials, the lifetime risk that an infected individual will develop active disease, and the true efficacy of chemoprophylaxis in reducing that risk.[95,96] It is worth noting that the IUAT trial[86] documented a therapeutic efficacy for INH that is considerably higher than that cited by those questioning treatment for adults over 20 (75% versus 50%).

All analyses of the risks and benefits of INH chemoprophylaxis have dealt with asymptomatic, otherwise healthy adults who have a positive tuberculin test but no other risk factors for the development of active disease. It is important to emphasize that for those with a history of recent close contact with active tuberculosis, known recent skin test conversion, or other risk factors, treatment with INH is indicated regardless of age, though with appropriate supervision (Table VII).[88] INH has been well tolerated by most elderly patients in nursing-home settings when administered to recent converters or contacts at risk.[55] It is known to be particularly effective in preventing reactivation in groups with abnormal chest x-rays.[86,87]

Regardless of exact risk, clinical supervision of treatment with INH is essential in preventing fatalities from hepatitis. Most fatalities that have occurred have involved patients who continued to take INH despite jaundice or other clinical signs of hepatotoxicity.[86,95] The National Consensus Conference on Tuberculosis has recently recom-

Table VII. Preventive Therapy with Isoniazid[a]

Indications	Contraindications	Special attention
Household members, other close associates of newly diagnosed patients and newly infected persons	Progressive tuberculosis disease (more than one drug needed)	Concurrent use of other medications (possible drug interactions)
Positive tuberculin-skin-test reactors with abnormal chest roentgenogram	Adequate course of INH previously completed	Daily use of alcohol (possible higher incidence of INH-associated liver injury)
Positive tuberculin-skin-test reactors with special clinical situations	Severe adverse reaction to INH previously	Current chronic liver disease (difficulty in evaluating changes in hepatic function)
Other positive tuberculin-skin-test reactors up to age 35	Previous INH-associated hepatic injury Acute liver disease of any etiology	Pregnancy (prudent to defer until postpartum unless contact, new infection, or other urgent indication)

[a]Source: Ref. 88.

mended determinations of hepatic transaminases at 1, 3, 6, and 9 months during INH administration. Transaminase elevations up to four times normal are allowable, but call for closer monitoring. It is also suggested that patients receive no more than a 2-month supply of INH at one time.[32] Regardless of laboratory monitoring, it is important that patients be advised to stop taking INH at the onset of any symptoms suggestive of hepatotoxicity.

Despite the attention given to hepatitis, it should be recognized that the principal reason for failure of INH prophylaxis relates to incomplete courses of treatment. In clinical trials, INH has been discontinued for a variety of non-life-threatening side effects, such as nausea, rash, or dizziness.[86,90,97,98] A more significant problem is noncompliance. In the recent IUAT trial, INH prophylaxis for 1 year was 93% effective in those judged to be compliant with therapy, compared to 75% effectiveness for the entire study group. Similar results have been obtained in other trials,[21,85] along with similarly high rates of noncompliance with prophylaxis.[90] A recent cost–benefit analysis of the IUAT trial data suggests that from a public health perspective, 24 weeks rather than 1 year of INH may be the optimum duration for prophylactic therapy.[99] Because of noncompliance, only a small additional reduction in cases is obtained by continuing INH for 52 weeks, at a substantial incremental cost.[86,99] Patients who adhere to the regimen will, however, benefit more from a full 52 weeks of treatment.

4. ACTIVE TUBERCULOSIS

Management of active tuberculosis is no longer preventive medicine for the infected patient. However, early recognition and treatment of active disease is clearly instrumental in reducing spread to the community. In some instances large numbers of infections can be traced to contact with a single active case.[100,101]

Clinical, laboratory, and radiographic methods in diagnosis will not be reviewed here. It is important for primary-care physicians to consider the diagnosis in a variety of situations. Young adults may present with pulmonary illness consistent with either primary or reactivation tuberculosis,[102,103] and elderly patients, who have not been previously infected, may develop illnesses more consistent with primary disease than with typical reactivation tuberculosis.[54,55]

For reasons that are not clear, the incidence of extrapulmonary tuberculosis has remained constant while that of pulmonary disease has declined.[104–106] Thus, the ratio of extrapulmonary disease to pulmonary disease is actually increasing. Atypical presentations, confounding by other medical illnesses, and lack of familiarity with tuberculosis are all obstacles to diagnosis. Misdiagnosis of tuberculosis, especially as neoplastic disease, is not rare, and elderly patients are particularly likely to suffer from delay or confusion in diagnosis.[107–110]

Chemotherapy for active disease has steadily progressed toward shorter regimens with more drugs, in an effort to decrease costs and improve compliance.[111] In most instances, 9 months of INH (300 mg daily) and rifampin (600 mg daily) will be adequate; ethambutol should be added for the first month if drug resistance is suspected[84] (see Section 5.2). This may be given as a twice-weekly regimen (900 mg INH and 600 mg rifampin) after the first month and appears effective for pulmonary as well as extrapulmonary disease.[112] Special situations, alternative regimens, and the possible use of 6-month courses of treatment are discussed elsewhere.[39,84,112–115] Primary-care physicians need to be particularly involved with the issue of noncompliance, which one author has called "the most serious remaining problem in the control of tuberculosis in the United States."[116] Clinicians should not be reluctant to use supervised programs to ensure completion of therapy and monitor sputum conversion to negative. Not only are these more likely to be successful, they are also cost-effective when the costs of treatment of advanced disease and community spread are considered.[117–119]

5. SPECIAL SITUATIONS

5.1. Urban Tuberculosis and the Homeless

Many U.S. cities have considerably higher rates of tuberculosis than their surrounding communities; within cities, there may be clustering of risk groups within certain neighborhoods.[7,120] Inner-city residents may present with combinations of risks, including low socioeconomic status, poor nutrition, and increased rates of alcoholism and drug abuse. Crowded living conditions increase the probability of exposure to active cases and encourage aerosol spread. Immigrants from areas of high prevalence often constitute a portion of these inner-city residents. Homeless persons also combine multiple risks, and when these individuals are sheltered, they may transmit or acquire tuberculosis at rates comparable to those seen in developing nations.[10,121,122] Recent evidence suggests that homeless persons who have been successfully treated for tuberculosis may remain at high risk for reinfection.[123] Multiple host factors, such as stress, malnutrition, intercurrent illness, and alcoholism, combined with high exposure rates are presumed to explain this; by inference, other persons with multiple risks might likewise be at risk for reinfection.

Increased awareness of the epidemiology of tuberculosis by health care providers is essential in order to reduce disease transmission in these settings, and routine screening is recommended.[122] Though not usually cost-effective, chest x-ray screening in one study had an extremely high yield of 1 active case/240 radiographs among urban alcoholics and should be considered an important adjunct to other surveillance programs in high-risk settings.[10,53] As emphasized previously, aggressive screening and other case-finding programs will be of little value unless accompanied by effective supervision of treatment.

5.2. Drug-Resistant Tuberculosis

Though not common in American or Canadian citizens who acquire tuberculosis in North America, drug-resistant disease, especially INH resistance, is widespread among many immigrant groups.[14–16] The possibility of drug resistance should always be considered in evaluating exposure or active disease in such individuals. INH-resistant tuberculosis has recently become prevalent among the homeless in Boston and should probably be anticipated in other urban homeless groups.[121] Treatment failure, regardless of the degree of compliance with chemotherapy, increases the probability that drug-resistant tuberculosis is present. Susceptibility testing is essential in managing drug-resistant tuberculosis and should be performed routinely.

No controlled studies have been done to establish an effective prophylactic regimen for contacts of persons with INH-resistant organisms. The use of rifampin seems reasonable and is recommended if there is a significant probability of infection with an INH-resistant organism.[14,124] If INH resistance is not definitely known, INH should be given as well.[32]

5.3. Tuberculosis and Acquired Immunodeficiency Syndrome

Although the number of tuberculosis cases reported in the United States continued to decline in 1985, several individual states reported increases.[1] Preliminary data from 1986 suggest the decline may have stopped.[125] Several areas with increases in tuberculosis (New York City, California, Florida) are also among the leaders in reported AIDS cases.[1] Further analysis of data from Florida reveals that through December 31, 1985, 10% (109/1094) of all AIDS patients have also been diagnosed with tuberculosis.[126] Haitian AIDS patients appear to be at highest risk, with a reported 60% prevalence of tuberculosis.[127] The incidence of extrapulmonary tuberculosis, particularly lymphatic, is also increased in AIDS patients.[127,128]

The extent to which tuberculosis will increase among AIDS patients is unknown, but is surely a reason for concern. Patients with impaired cellular immunity such as occurs in AIDS are known to be at increased risk for tuberculosis, and some subgroups (Haitians, intravenous drug abusers) have been independently identified as being at risk for both diseases. As of 1986, there are an estimated 1.5 million individuals in the United States infected with human immunodeficiency virus (HIV) who are as yet without clinical AIDS.[129] Whether these individuals are also at increased risk for tuberculosis is unknown.

Current CDC guidelines for detection and management of tuberculosis in patients with known or suspected HIV infection include routine Mantoux testing as part of the initial evaluation. A positive tuberculin test in an HIV-infected patient is an indication for chemoprophylaxis at any age.[130] The efficacy of INH prophylaxis in these patients is unknown; clinicians should also assess the probability of drug-resistant tuberculosis and adjust management accordingly. Clinical suspicion of pulmonary and extrapulmonary tuberculosis should remain high in tuberculin-negative patients with appropriate symptoms. BCG vaccination of otherwise healthy HIV-positive individuals is contraindicated because of the risk of dissemination.[131]

Treatment of active tuberculosis in AIDS patients is beyond the scope of this chapter. Reports thus far suggest that the majority will respond, at least initially.[127,128]

6. SUMMARY

The emphasis on screening and prevention of tuberculosis in this chapter is possible only because of the large number of epidemiological studies that have been conducted to answer many of the questions clinicians face. The epidemiology of tuberculosis is better known than most other diseases physicians today will encounter. Decision analyses and other computer-assisted techniques are helpful, indeed almost essential, in distilling these data into clinically useful algorithms. They can also be misapplied, as a recent example illustrates.[12] Several medical house staff physicians who had recently become tuberculin reactors cited the analysis by Taylor *et al.*[93] as their rationale for rejecting INH prophylaxis (see Section 3.2.2)—not recognizing that recent converters were excluded from that analysis, and that prophylaxis was indicated for them regardless of age. Ironically, most of these physicians managed tuberculosis patients on an almost daily basis.

Tuberculosis has never been a disease that is evenly distributed throughout the population. Though new risks such as AIDS may arise, traditional risks will continue to be important for many years to come. Clinical judgment based on an informed assessment of individual risks will remain the primary-care physician's most important skill in the prevention and treatment of this persistent disease.

REFERENCES

1. Tuberculosis—United States, 1985—and the possible impact of human T-lymphotropic virus type III/lymphadenopathy-associated virus infection. *Morbid. Mortal. Wkly. Rep.* **35**(5):74–76, 1986.
2. Sbarbaro, J. A.: Tuberculosis: The new challenge to the practicing clinician. *Chest* **68**(suppl. 3):436–443, 1975.
3. Comstock, G. W., Livesay, V. T., and Woolpert, S. F.: The prognosis of a positive tuberculin reaction in childhood and adolescence. *Am. J. Epidemiol.* **99**:131–138, 1974.
4. Ferebee, S. H., and Mount, F. W.: Tuberculosis morbidity in a controlled trial of the prophylactic use of isoniazid among household contacts. *Am. Rev. Respir. Dis.* **85**:490–510, 1962.
5. Comstock, G. W.: Epidemiology of tuberculosis. *Am. Rev. Respir. Dis.* **125**(3, part 2):8–15, 1982.
6. Tuberculosis, in Annual Summary 1983. *Morbid. Mortal. Wkly. Rep.* **32**(54):62–65, 1984.
7. Tuberculosis—United States, 1984. *Morbid. Mortal. Wkly. Rep.* **34**:299–302, 307, 1985.
8. Chapman, J. S., and Dyerly, M. D.: Social and other factors in intrafamilial transmission of tuberculosis. *Am. Rev. Respir. Dis.* **90**:48–60, 1964.
9. Stead, W. W.: Pathogenesis of a first episode of chronic pulmonary tuberculosis in man: Recrudescence of residuals of the primary infection or exogenous reinfection? *Am. Rev. Respir. Dis.* **95**:729–745, 1967.
10. Barry, M. A., Wall, C., Shirley, L., *et al.*: Tuberculosis screening in Boston's homeless shelters. *Public Health Rep.* **101**:487–494, 1986.

11. Barrett-Connor, E.: The epidemiology of tuberculosis in physicians. *JAMA* **241:**33–38, 1979.
12. Chan, J. C., and Tabak, J. I.: Risk of tuberculous infection among house staff in an urban teaching hospital. *South. Med. J.* **78:**1061–1064, 1985.
13. Tuberculosis among Hispanics in the United States—1980. *Morbid. Mortal. Wkly. Rep.* **31:**237–239, 1982.
14. Pitchenik, A. E., Russell, B. W., Cleary, T., *et al.:* The prevalence of tuberculosis and drug-resistance among Haitians. *N. Engl. J. Med.* **307:**162–165, 1982.
15. Nolan, C. M., Aitken, M. L., Elarth, A. M., *et al.:* Active tuberculosis after isoniazid chemoprophylaxis of Southeast Asian refugees. *Am. Rev. Respir. Dis.* **133:**431–436, 1986.
16. Powell, K. E., Brown, E. D., and Farer, L. S.: Tuberculosis among Indochinese refugees in the United States. *JAMA* **249:**1455–1460, 1983.
17. Enarson, D., Ashley, M. J., and Grzybowski, S.: Tuberculosis in immigrants to Canada. *Am. Rev. Respir. Dis.* **119:**11–18, 1979.
18. Reichman, L. B., and O'Day, R.: Tuberculous infection in a large urban population. *Am. Rev. Respir. Dis.* **117:**705–712, 1978.
19. Bates, J. H.: Tuberculosis: Susceptibility and resistance. *Am. Rev. Respir. Dis.* **125**(3, part 2):20–24, 1982.
20. Stead, W. W.: The pathogenesis of pulmonary tuberculosis among older persons. *Am. Rev. Respir. Dis.* **91:**811–822, 1965.
21. Ferebee, S. H.: Controlled chemoprophylaxis trials in tuberculosis: A general review. *Adv. Tuberc. Res.* **17:**28–106, 1970.
22. Sutherland, I., Svandora, E., and Radhakrishna, S.: The development of clinical tuberculosis following infection with tubercle bacilli. *Tubercle* **63:**255–268, 1982.
23. Stead, W. W.: Does the risk of tuberculosis increase in old age? *J. Infect. Dis.* **147:**951–955, 1983.
24. Grzybowski, S., and Allen, E. A.: The challenge of tuberculosis in decline. *Am. Rev. Respir. Dis.* **90:**707–720, 1964.
25. Styblo, K.: Recent advances in epidemiological research in tuberculosis. *Adv. Tuberc. Res.* **20:**1–63, 1980.
26. Horwitz, O., Wilbek, E., and Erickson, P. A.: Epidemiological basis of tuberculosis eradication. *Bull. WHO* **41:**95–113, 1969.
27. Edwards, L. B., Acquaviva, F. A., and Livesay, V. T.: Identification of tuberculosis infected: Dual tests and density of reaction. *Am. Rev. Respir. Dis.* **108:**1334–1339, 1973.
28. Comstock, G. W., and Palmer, C. E.: Long-term results of BCG vaccination in the Southern U.S. *Am. Rev. Respir. Dis.* **93:**171–183, 1966.
29. Edwards, L. B., Livesay, V. T., Acquaviva, F. A., *et al.:* Height, weight, tuberculous infection and tuberculous disease. *Arch. Environ. Health* **22:**106–112, 1971.
30. Al-Arif, L. I., Goldstein, R. A., Affronti, L. F., *et al.:* HLA-BW15 and tuberculosis in a North American black population. *Am. Rev. Respir. Dis.* **120:**1275–1278, 1979.
31. Hwang, C. H., Khan, S., Ende, N., *et al.:* The HLA-A, -B and -DR phenotypes and tuberculosis. *Am. Rev. Respir. Dis.* **132:**382–385, 1985.
32. Bailey, W. C., Byrd, R. B., Glassroth, J. L., *et al.:* National Consensus Conference on Tuberculosis: Preventive treatment of tuberculosis. *Chest* **87**(2, suppl. 10):128S–132S, 1985.
33. Hudolin, V.: Tuberculosis and alcoholism. *Ann. NY Acad. Sci.* **252:**353–364, 1975.
34. Smith, F. E., and Palmer, D. L.: Alcoholism, infection and altered host defenses: A review of clinical and experimental observations. *J. Chronic Dis.* **29:**35–49, 1976.
35. Milne, R. C.: Alcoholism and tuberculosis in Victoria. *Med. J. Austr.* **2:**955–960, 1970.
36. Olin, J. S., and Grzybowski, J.: Tuberculosis and alcoholism. *Can. Med. Assoc. J.* **94:**999–1001, 1966.
37. Burach, W. R., and Hollister, R. M.: Tuberculous peritonitis. *Am. J. Med.* **28:**510–523, 1960.
38. Kok-Jensen, A.: Pulmonary tuberculosis in well-treated alcoholics. Long-term prognosis regarding relapses compared with non-alcoholic patients. *Scand. J. Respir. Dis.* **53:**202–206, 1972.
39. Hudson, L. D., and Sbarbaro, J. A.: Twice weekly tuberculosis chemotherapy. *JAMA* **223:**139–143, 1973.
40. Lewis, J. G., and Chamberlain, D. A.: Alcohol consumption and smoking habits in male patients with pulmonary tuberculosis. *Br. J. Prev. Soc. Med.* **17:**149–152, 1963.
41. Segarra, F., and Sherman, D. S.: Relapses in pulmonary tuberculosis. *Dis. Chest.* **51:**59–63, 1967.

42. Glassroth, J., Robins, A. G., and Snider, D. E., Jr.: Tuberculosis in the 1980's. *N. Engl. J. Med.* **302**:1441–1450, 1980.
43. Luelmo, F.: BCG vaccination. *Am. Rev. Respir. Dis.* **125**(3, part 2):70–72, 1982.
44. tenDam, H. G.: Research on BCG vaccination. *Adv. Tuberc. Res.* **21**:79–106, 1984.
45. Clemens, J. D., Chuong, J. J. H., and Feinstein, A. R.: The BCG controversy: A methodological and statistical reappraisal. *JAMA* **249**:2362–2369, 1983.
46. British Thoracic Association: Effectiveness of BCG vaccination in Great Britain in 1978. *Br. J. Dis. Chest* **74**:215–227, 1980.
47. Young, T. K.: BCG vaccination among Canadian Indians and Inuit: The epidemiological bases for policy decision. *Can. J. Public Health* **76**:124–129, 1985.
48. Lotte, A., Wasz-Hockert, O., Poisson, N., *et al.*: BCG complications. *Adv. Tuberc. Res.* **21**:107–193, 1984.
49. Adult immunization: Recommendations of the Immunization Practices Advisory Committee. *Morbid. Mortal. Wkly. Rep.* **33**(15), 1984.
50. Rust, P., and Thomas, J.: A method for estimating the prevalence of tuberculous infection. *Am. J. Epidemiol.* **101**:311–322, 1975.
51. Edwards, L. B., Acquaviva, F. A., Livesay, V. T., *et al.*: An atlas of sensitivity to tuberculin, PPD-B, and histoplasmin in the United States. *Am. Rev. Respir. Dis.* **99**(suppl.):1–132, 1969.
52. Moulding, T.: Chemoprophylaxis of tuberculosis: When is the benefit worth the risk and cost? *Ann. Intern. Med.* **74**:761–770, 1971.
53. Feingold, A. O.: Cost-effectiveness of screening for tuberculosis in a general medical clinic. *Public Health Rep.* **90**:545–547, 1975.
54. Stead, W. W.: Tuberculosis among elderly persons: An outbreak in a nursing home. *Ann. Intern. Med.* **94**:606–610, 1981.
55. Stead, W. W., Lofgren, J. P., Warren, E., *et al.*: Tuberculosis as an endemic and nosocomial infection among the elderly in nursing homes. *N. Engl. J. Med.* **312**:1483–1487, 1985.
56. Tuberculosis in a nursing care facility—Washington. *Morbid. Mortal. Wkly. Rep.* **32**:121–122, 1983.
57. Tuberculosis in a nursing home—Oklahoma. *Morbid. Mortal. Wkly. Rep.* **29**:465–467, 1980.
58. Stead, W. W.: Undetected tuberculosis in prison. *JAMA* **240**:2544–2547, 1978.
59. American Thoracic Society: The tuberculin skin test. *Am. Rev. Respir. Dis.* **124**:356–363, 1981.
60. Sokal, J. E.: Measurement of delayed skin-test responses. *N. Engl. J. Med.* **293**:501–502, 1975.
61. Snider, D. E., Jr.: The tuberculin skin test. *Am. Rev. Respir. Dis.* **125**(3, part 2):108–118, 1982.
62. Bass, J. B., Sanders, R. V., and Kirkpatrick, M. B.: Choosing an appropriate cutting point for conversion in annual tuberculin skin testing. *Am. Rev. Respir. Dis.* **132**:379–381, 1985.
63. Snider, D. E., Jr.: Bacille Calmette-Guérin vaccinations and tuberculin skin tests. *JAMA* **253**:3438–3439, 1985.
64. Comstock, G. W., Edwards, L. B., and Nabangxang, H.: Tuberculin sensitivity eight to fifteen years after BCG vaccination. *Am. Rev. Respir. Dis.* **103**:572–575, 1971.
65. Kent, D. C., and Schwartz, R.: Active pulmonary tuberculosis with negative tuberculin skin reactions. *Am. Rev. Respir. Dis.* **95**:411, 1967.
66. Holden, M., Dubin, M. R., and Diamond, P. H.: Frequency of negative intermediate-strength tuberculin sensitivity in patients with active tuberculosis. *N. Engl. J. Med.* **285**:1506–1509, 1974.
67. Rooney, J. J., Crocco, J. A., Kramer, S., *et al.*: Further observations on tuberculin reactions in active tuberculosis. *Am. J. Med.* **60**:517–522, 1976.
68. Comstock, G. W.: False tuberculin test results. *Chest* **68**(3, suppl.):465–469, 1975.
69. Chaparas, S. D., Vandiviere, H. M., Melvin, I., *et al.*: Tuberculin test: Variability with the Mantoux procedure. *Am. Rev. Respir. Dis.* **132**:175–178, 1985.
70. Thompson, N. J., Glassroth, J. L., Snider, D. E., Jr., *et al.*: The booster phenomenon in serial tuberculin testing. *Am. Rev. Respir. Dis.* **119**:587–597, 1979.
71. Ferebee, S. H., and Mount, F. W.: Evidence of booster effect in serial tuberculin testing. *Am. Rev. Respir. Dis.* **88**:118–119, 1963.
72. Lunn, J. A.: Tuberculin tine tests: Effect of variations in dried tuberculin coating. *Tubercle* **62**:241–248, 1981.
73. Osborn, T. W.: Some factors influencing the tuberculin tine test. *Tubercle* **63**:45–54, 1982.

74. Lunn, J. A., Johnson, A. J., and Fry, J. S.: Comparison of multiple puncture liquid tuberculin test with Mantoux test. *Lancet* **1**:695–698, 1981.
75. Rudd, R. M., Gellert, A. R., and Venning, M.: Comparison of Mantoux, tine and "Imotest" tuberculin tests. *Lancet* **2**:515–518, 1982.
76. Lunn, J. A., and Johnson, A. J.: Comparison of the tine and Mantoux tuberculin tests. *Br. Med. J.* **1**:451–1453, 1978.
77. Sinclair, D. J. M., and Johnston, R. N.: Assessment of tine tuberculin test. *Br. Med. J.* **1**:1325–26, 1979.
78. Donaldson, J. C., and Elliott, R. C.: A study of co-positivity of three multipuncture techniques with intradermal PPD tuberculin. *Am. Rev. Respir. Dis.* **118**:843–846, 1978.
79. British Thoracic Association—Research Committee: Reproducibility of the tine tuberculin test. *Br. J. Dis. Chest* **76**:75–78, 1982.
80. Kearns, T. J., Cole, C. H., Farer, L. S., *et al.*: National Consensus Conference on Tuberculosis. Public health issues in control of tuberculosis: Surveillance techniques and the role of health care providers. *Chest* **87**(2, suppl.):135S–138S, 1985.
81. Sbarbaro, J. A.: The FDA's final decision concerning the tuberculin multiple puncture test. *Am. Rev. Respir. Dis.* **120**:1390–1391, 1979.
82. Daniel, T. M., Debanne, S. M., van der Kuyp, F.: Enzyme-linked immunosorbent assay using *Mycobacterium tuberculosis* antigen 5 and PPD for the serodiagnosis of tuberculosis. *Chest* **88**:388–392, 1985.
83. Zeiss, C. R., Kalish, S. B., Erlich, K. S., *et al.*: IgG antibody to purified protein derivative by enzyme-linked immunosorbent assay in the diagnosis of pulmonary tuberculosis. *Am. Rev. Respir. Dis.* **130**:845–848, 1984.
84. Bass, J. B., Jr., Farer, L. S., Hopewell, P. C., *et al.*: Treatment of tuberculosis and tuberculosis infection in adults and children. *Am. Rev. Respir. Dis.* **134**:355–363, 1986.
85. Comstock, G. W., Ferebee, S. H., and Hammes, L. H.: A controlled trial of community-wide isoniazid prophylaxis in Alaska. *Am. Rev. Respir. Dis.* **95**:935–943, 1967.
86. International Union Against Tuberculosis Committee on Prophylaxis: Efficacy of various durations of isoniazid preventive therapy for tuberculosis: Five years of follow-up in the IUAT trial. *Bull. WHO* **60**:555–564, 1982.
87. Ferebee, S. H., Mount, F. W., Murray, F. J., *et al.*: A controlled trial of isoniazid prophylaxis in mental institutions. *Am. Rev. Respir. Dis.* **88**:161–175, 1963.
88. Farer, L. S.: Chemoprophylaxis. *Am. Rev. Respir. Dis.* **125**(3, part 2):102–107, 1982.
89. Comstock, G. W., Baum, C., and Snider, D. E., Jr.: Isoniazid prophylaxis among Alaska Eskimos: A final report of the Bethel isoniazid studies. *Am. Rev. Respir. Dis.* **119**:827–830, 1979.
90. Dash, L. A., Comstock, G. W., and Flynn, J. P. G.: Isoniazid preventive therapy: Retrospect and prospect. *Am. Rev. Respir. Dis.* **121**:1039–1044, 1980.
91. Kopanoff, D. E., Snider, D. E., Jr., and Caras, G. J.: Isoniazid-related hepatitis: A U.S. Public Health Service cooperative surveillance study. *Am. Rev. Respir. Dis.* **117**:991–1001, 1978.
92. Comstock, G. W., and Edwards, P. Q.: The competing risks of tuberculosis and hepatitis for adult tuberculin reactors. *Am. Rev. Respir. Dis.* **111**:573–577, 1975.
93. Taylor, W. C., Aronson, M. D., and Delbanco, T. L.: Should young adults with a positive tuberculin test take isoniazid? *Ann. Intern. Med.* **94**:808–813, 1981.
94. Rose, D. N., Schechter, C. B., and Silver, A.: The age threshold for isoniazid chemoprophylaxis: A decision analysis for low-risk tuberculin reactors. *JAMA* **256**:2709–2713, 1986.
95. Comstock, G. W.: Evaluating isoniazid preventive therapy: The need for more data. *Ann. Intern. Med.* **94**:817–819, 1981.
96. Comstock, G. W.: Prevention of tuberculosis among tuberculin reactors: Maximizing benefits, minimizing risks. *JAMA* **256**:2729–2730, 1986.
97. Byrd, R. B., Horn, B. R., Solomon, D. A., *et al.*: Toxic effects of isoniazid in tuberculosis chemoprophylaxis. *JAMA* **241**:1239–1241, 1979.
98. Falk, A., and Fuchs, G. F.: Prophylaxis with isoniazid in inactive tuberculosis. *Chest* **73**:44–48, 1978.
99. Snider, D. E., Jr., Caras, G. J., and Koplan, J. P.: Preventive therapy with isoniazid: Cost-effectiveness of different durations of therapy. *JAMA* **255**:1579–1583, 1986.
100. Sachs, J. J., Brenner, E. R., Breeden, D. C., *et al.*: Epidemiology of a tuberculosis outbreak in a South Carolina junior high school. *Am. J. Public Health* **75**:361–365, 1985.

101. Houk, V. N., Baker, J. H., Sorensen, K., *et al.*: The epidemiology of tuberculosis infection in a closed environment. *Arch. Environ. Health* **16**:26–35, 1968.
102. Stead, W. W., Kerby, G. R., Schlereter, D. P., *et al.*: The clinical spectrum of primary tuberculosis in adults. *Ann. Intern. Med.* **68**:731–745, 1968.
103. Khan, M. A., Kovnat, D. M., Bachus, B., *et al.*: Clinical and roentgenographic spectum of pulmonary tuberculosis in the adult. *Am. J. Med.* **62**:31–38, 1977.
104. Farer, L. S., Lowell, A. M., and Meador, M. P.: Extrapulmonary tuberculosis in the United States. *Am. J. Epidemiol.* **109**:205–217, 1979.
105. Alvarez, S., and McCabe, W. R.: Extrapulmonary tuberculosis revisited: A review of experience at Boston City and other hospitals. *Medicine* **63**:25–55, 1984.
106. Weir, M. R., and Thornton, G. F.: Extrapulmonary tuberculosis: Experience of a community hospital and review of the literature. *Am. J. Med.* **79**:467–478, 1985.
107. Page, M. I., and Lunn, J. S.: Experience with tuberculosis in a public teaching hospital. *Am. J. Med.* **77**:667–670, 1984.
108. Pitlik, S. D., Fainstein, V., and Bodey, G.: Tuberculosis mimicking cancer—A reminder. *Am. J. Med.* **76**:822–825, 1984.
109. MacGregor, R. R.: A year's experience with tuberculosis in a private urban teaching hospital in the post sanatorium era. *Am. J. Med.* **58**:221–228, 1975.
110. Bobrowitz, I. D.: Active tuberculosis undiagnosed until autopsy. *Am. J. Med.* **72**:650–658, 1982.
111. D'Esopo, N. D.: Clinical trials in pulmonary tuberculosis. *Am. Rev. Respir. Dis.* **125**(3, part 2):85–93, 1982.
112. Stead, W. W., and Dutt, A. K.: Chemotherapy for tuberculosis today. *Am. Rev. Respir. Dis.* **125**(3, part 2):94–101, 1982.
113. Fox, W.: The chemotherapy of pulmonary tuberculosis: A review. *Chest* **76**(suppl. 6):785–796, 1979.
114. Snider, D. E., Jr., Long, M. W., Cross, F. S., *et al.*: Six-months isoniazid–rifampin therapy for pulmonary tuberculosis. *Am. Rev. Respir. Dis.* **129**:573–579, 1984.
115. National Consensus Conference on Tuberculosis: Standard therapy for tuberculosis 1985. *Chest* **87**(suppl. 2):117S–124S, 1985.
116. Addington, W. W.: Patient compliance: The most serious remaining problem in the control of tuberculosis in the United States. *Chest* **76**:741–743, 1976.
117. Sbarbaro, J. A.: Compliance: Inducements and enforcements. *Chest* **76**:750–755, 1979.
118. National Consensus Conference on Tuberculosis: Non-drug issues related to the treatment of tuberculosis. *Chest* **87**(2, suppl.):125S–127S, 1985.
119. Grzybowski, S.: Chemoprophylaxis in inactive tuberculosis: Long-term evaluation of a Canadian trial. *Can. Med. Assoc. J.* **114**:607–611, 1976.
120. LaForce, F. M., Huher, G. L., and Fahey, J. M.: The focality of urban tuberculosis. *Am. Rev. Respir. Dis.* **108**:553–558, 1973.
121. Drug-resistant tuberculosis among the homeless—Boston. *Morbid. Mortal. Wkly. Rep.* **34**(28):429–431, 1985.
122. McAdam, J., Brickner, P. W., Glicksman, R., *et al.*: Tuberculosis in the SRO/homeless population, in Brickner, P. W., Scharer, L. K., Conanan, B., *et al.* (eds.): *Health Care of Homeless People*. Springer, New York, pp. 155–175.
123. Nardell, E., McInnis, B., Thomas, B., *et al.*: Exogenous reinfection with tuberculosis in a shelter for the homeless. *N. Engl. J. Med.* **315**:1570–1575, 1986.
124. Koplan, J. P., and Farer, L. S.: Choice of preventive treatment for isoniazid-resistant tuberculous infection. *JAMA* **244**:2736–2740, 1980.
125. Tuberculosis: Cases of specified notifiable diseases, United States, weeks ending Dec. 27, 1986 and Dec. 28, 1985. *Morbid. Mortal. Wkly. Rep.* **35**:799–801, 1987.
126. Tuberculosis and acquired immunodeficiency syndrome—Florida. *Morbid. Mortal. Wkly. Rep.* **35**(37):587–590, 1986.
127. Pitchenik, A. E., Cole, C., Russell, B. W., *et al.*: Tuberculosis, atypical mycobacteriosis, and the acquired immunodeficiency syndrome among Haitian and non-Haitian patients in South Florida. *Ann. Intern. Med.* **101**:641–645, 1984.
128. Sunderam, G., McDonald, R. J., Maniatis, T., *et al.*: Tuberculosis as a manifestation of the acquired immunodeficiency syndrome (AIDS). *JAMA* **256**:362–366, 1986.

129. Curran, J. W., Morgan, W. M., Hardy, A. M., *et al.*: The epidemiology of AIDS: Current status and future prospects. *Science* **229**:1352–1357, 1985.
130. Diagnosis and management of mycobacterial infection and disease in persons with human T-lymphotropic virus type III/lymphadenopathy-associated virus infection. *Morbid. Mortal. Wkly. Rep.* **35**(28):448–452, 1986.
131. Disseminated *Mycobacterium bovis* infection from BCG vaccination of a patient with acquired immunodeficiency syndrome. *Morbid. Mortal. Wkly. Rep.* **34**(16):227–228, 1985.

9

Sexually Transmitted Diseases

Joseph C. Chan

1. INTRODUCTION

Historically, society ignored the problems of sexually transmitted diseases (STDs) and, if forced to confront them, placed the blame on a small element of the population: prostitutes. The medical profession often contributed to this moralistic view and considered all STDs proper punishment of our sins.[1] By the turn of the century, the social hygiene movement changed some of these attitudes in this country, and physicians began to assume more responsibility for the detection and treatment of STDs. During World War I, military commanders on both sides were forced to deal with the alarming presence of STDs among their troops. In the United States, STDs constituted the most frequent cause of rejection of draftees by the Selective Service. In 1918, Congress passed the Chamberlain–Kahn Act, creating the venereal disease control division within the U.S. Public Health Service.[2] Efforts to control STDs dwindled rapidly after the war and remained in the doldrums for about 20 years. Efforts were again intensified during World War II and were again dismantled with the discovery of penicillin and an initial success in reducing gonorrhea and syphilis. At present, the United States has one of the highest rates for these two diseases in the world.

Although private physicians provide more than half the care to STD patients in this country, many of these physicians still relegate the responsibility for controlling these diseases to health departments. Such views by private physicians often resulted in replacing their much-needed, concerted efforts by apathy and neglect. This lack of interest is also paralleled in our medical education. A 1980 survey showed that only about 15% of our medical schools offer any STD clinic training to medical students. The resulting lack of clinical expertise and interest in prevention by practitioners is often cited as a major reason why STD rates are higher in this country than in the United Kingdom.[3]

2. EPIDEMIOLOGY

Reportable STDs in the United States still include only five diseases—gonorrhea, syphilis, chancroid, lymphogranuloma venereum, and granuloma inguinale. Only the

Joseph C. Chan • Department of Medicine, University of Miami School of Medicine, Miami, Florida 33101.

acquired immune deficiency syndrome (AIDS) has recently been added to the list of reportable diseases. Other new STDs, such as those caused by herpes simplex virus (HSV) and *Chlamydia trachomatis*, though easily recognizable clinically, are still excluded from the national surveillance programs. Accurate epidemiological data are lacking for the latter diseases. Complicating the picture even further are agents that can be transmitted by modes other than sexual contacts. These agents include hepatitis B virus, cytomegalovirus, group B *Streptococcus*, and many enteric pathogens. The proportion of infections transmitted sexually by these agents has no doubt increased recently; however, reliable data regarding this route of transmission of these agents are not available.

2.1. Incidence of STDs

The incidence of STDs is unevenly distributed across various demographic subgroups of the population. The important demographic determinants of STD incidence include age, gender, marital status, sexual preferences, race, and ethnic background.

The highest infection rates for most STDs are observed in the 20-to-24-year-old age group, followed by 25–29 and 15-to-19-year-old age groups.[4] However, among sexually active teenagers, incidence of STD is highest in those who are youngest. The overall morbidity rates of STDs are higher for men than for women. This difference is usually attributed to a higher level of promiscuity and the more obvious clinical manifestations in men. Single, divorced, and separated persons are known to have a higher rate than married people. Disease rates are higher among homosexual men compared to heterosexual men, and homosexual men tend to have more severe morbidity.[5]

In the United States, higher rates of sexual STDs are found among blacks compared to other ethnic groups. This observation cannot be explained simply by the difference in their socioeconomic status or sexual behavior. It may also be related to their general perception of health and illness.[6]

Most of the incidence figures are based on reported number of cases and are therefore dependent on the accuracy of reporting. It is clear that a substantial proportion of STDs are seen by private physicians, and few of these cases are reported. The composition of private cases almost certainly differs from the reported cases by age, race, sex, sexual preference and so forth. The extent of this underreporting confounds the analysis of STD incidence in relation to various demographic determinants.

The gonorrhea prevalence rate reached a peak in 1946, following World War II. After 1946, rates decreased until 1957 and increased again thereafter. Since 1975, the rate has declined each year from 473 per 100,000 in 1975 to 418 per 100,000 in 1982.[7]

The incidence of syphilis peaked in 1942 and then declined until 1977. Since then, the incidence of all forms of syphilis has risen slightly. The number of new cases rose from 21,656 in 1978 to 33,673 in 1982.[7] The distribution of syphilis cases underwent several key changes between 1967 and 1979. The most important of these included (1) a twofold increase in the male-to-female ratio; (2) an increase in cases among men reported by public clinics; and (3) an increase in the percentage of white men who reported at least one male sex partner.[8]

Since 35–40% of all nongonococcal urethritis (NGU) is caused by *C. trachomatis*, the incidence of NGU can be used to estimate the incidence of genital *C. trachomatis* infections. Such data are most reliably reported from England and Wales, and the incidence of NGU there increased steadily from 135 cases per 100,000 in 1966 to 350 cases per 100,000 in 1979. In the United States, the Centers for Disease Control (CDC) estimated that approximately 2.5 million cases of NGU occurred in 1981.[9]

Genital herpes still occurs at less than one-tenth the reported incidence of gonorrhea in England and Wales, but it is catching up rapidly. Genital herpes is the fastest increasing STD in that region of the world.

In the United States, the frequency of gonorrhea, genital herpes, and NGU seems to vary widely among patients attending different STD clinics. A study of seven public STD clinics showed that NGU is the most common STD in men. This is followed by gonorrhea, pubic lice *(Phthirus pubis),* venereal warts, and genital herpes, in that order. For women the most common STD is gonorrhea, followed by trichomoniasis, nonspecific vaginitis, venereal warts, pubic lice, and genital herpes. However, among heterosexual patients at the Seattle–King County STD clinic, NGU, genital herpes, and gonorrhea occur in roughly comparable frequencies.[10]

2.2. Factors Influencing STD Trends

Despite intensive control efforts, the transmission of gonorrhea and syphilis has not declined recently owing to a myriad of social and demographic factors. These factors include changes in the age composition and the spatial distribution of our population, changes in the institutions of marriage and family, and changes in nonmarital sexual behavior.[11]

The post-World War II "baby boom," contrary to common belief, did not peak until 1957 and extended into the early 1960s. Thus the number of young adults in the 18-to-29 age group, which experiences the highest infection rates of STDs, has just peaked.[12] This group was estimated to reach a maximum of 49.2 million in 1983 and then the number would decline slowly to a minimum of 40.5 million by 1995. This estimate indicates that the baby boom will continue to affect the STD rates well into the 1990s.

During the last two decades, the proportion of the U.S. population living in urban areas has increased. This trend exposes larger proportions of people to the higher risks of STD transmission that come with urban living.

The number of single, divorced, or separated individuals has increased at an unprecedented pace. The composition of American households has also changed drastically. Two-person households composed of unrelated adults of the opposite sex represent the fastest-expanding living arrangement. The number of households composed entirely of unrelated individuals is increasing, and a greater number of families are being maintained by persons without a spouse, especially women.[11]

In most western industrialized countries, the rate of premarital and extramarital intercourse has increased manyfold. In the United States between 1967 and 1974, the premarital intercourse rate for white women rose by about 300%. Furthermore, the median age at first coitus has decreased and the number of sex partners has increased. In 1979, half of all metropolitan-area teenage women were sexually active before marriage.[13] This change in sexual behavior in young women has a tremendous impact on the magnitude of the STD problem in this country since women and infants bear the heaviest burden of complications caused by STDs.

2.3. Magnitude of the STD Problem

Data estimated from special surveys conducted in specific health facilities and by using random surveys of health care encounters showed a cumulative annual figure of 10 million visits by persons with STD to private physicians' offices and public STD clinics. The private sector provides half the care to these persons, i.e., five million visits.

In the United States, total costs for STD exceeded the billion-dollar mark annually, and costs resulting from gonococcal infection alone totaled more than $770,000,000 in 1976. Financial costs are often misleading because they tend to underestimate human suffering caused by STDs.

The most serious complications caused by STDs are those suffered by women and children: pelvic inflammatory disease (PID), fetal wastage, and mental retardation. More than one million episodes of PID occur annually, resulting in an estimated two and a half million visits, a quarter million hospitalizations, and 150,000 surgical procedures.[14] With the increasing number of women who have had salpingitis, the number of ectopic pregnancies and the incidence of involuntary infertility also increase. The number of ectopic pregnancies increased from 13,200 in 1967 to 41,100 in 1977. Each ectopic pregnancy represents one fetal death. Excluding the costs of fetal death, the direct and indirect costs attributable to salpingitis have been estimated to be $1.25 billion for 1979.[14]

HSV infection of the newborn is associated with a case fatality rate of 60%, and at least half of the survivors have significant neurological or ocular sequelae or both.[15] The incidence of congenital syphilis correlates with the incidence of early syphilis (less than 1 year); the ratio is approximately 1.5–1.8 cases per 100 cases, respectively. Fortunately, the number of new cases of congenital syphilis has declined from 463 in 1977 to 259 in 1982.[7] Finally, the contribution of maternal STD infection to prematurity is not known. Regardless of the methods used for estimation, the magnitude of the STD problem is appalling.

3. TRANSMISSION OF STD AGENTS

The probability that an uninfected individual will become infected may be estimated by the number of infectious exposures and the risk of transmission after each exposure. The number of infectious exposures is a product of the number of sexual partners and the prevalence of infection among these partners. The risk of acquiring an infection after each exposure is determined by many factors—sex of the person and also of his or her partner, the agent involved, and the anatomical sites exposed.

The risk of acquiring urethral gonorrhea for a man following a single vaginal exposure with an infected woman is about 20%. The risk increases to about 60–80% after four exposures.[16] The risk for a woman acquiring gonorrhea from an infected man is up to 90%; however, the latter estimate did not control for number of exposures. Nevertheless, single-exposure transmission rate seems to be higher from male to female.

Transmission of syphilis by sexual contact requires exposure to infectious lesions; therefore, the individual is most infectious during the first year after infection. The rate of acquisition from an infected partner has been estimated at about 30%.[17] Women can transmit infection to their fetus shortly after onset of infection, and if untreated, they remain potentially infectious to the fetus for about 8 years.

The infection rate of male partners of women with chlamydial cervicitis was found to be about 28% after each sexual exposure, but transmission from men to women was about 45%.[18] Although gonorrhea seems to be more transmissible than *C. trachomatis*, we must take into account the difference in incubation periods and efficiency of isolation of these two agents.

The risk of development of genital herpes in a woman after exposure to an infected man has been estimated to be 80–90%.[19] Many questions regarding risk factors associated with transmission of herpes remain unanswered. Does an infected but asymptomatic sexual partner pose the same risk as one with overt disease? How long after overt lesions disappear does the risk remain high? Are there host factors associated with viral acquisition other than the sexual contact?

4. PREVENTION OF STDS

Prevention "requires anticipatory action based upon knowledge of the natural history to make the onset or further progress of disease unlikely."[20] It was in communicable-disease control that the epidemiological approach to prevention arose. There are three levels of prevention in all communicable diseases, and this divisional scheme applies very well to STDs.

Primary prevention aims at preventing infection through health promotion and specific protection. Secondary prevention has to do with early detection and prompt treatment of infections, thereby minimizing the risk of transmission and disability. Tertiary prevention is essentially rehabilitation to improve disability once occurred. Many devastating communicable diseases, such as smallpox, diphtheria, and polio myelitis, have been dealt with successfully in the past by applying these strategies of intervention. Private physicians participated and contributed significantly in every level of prevention. We should all hope that such accomplishments can be repeated with STDs.

4.1. Primary Prevention

4.1.1. Health Promotion

The principal aim of educational intervention is to encourage behavior that will ultimately reduce the impact of STDs in the community. Dissemination of information is not enough. According to a recent panel of experts of the World Health Organization, health promotion activities should include the following activities:

1. To promote discriminative sexual intercourse by avoiding multiple and/or casual sexual partners

2. To promote the use of the condom or other prophylactic methods in at-risk situations
3. To promote prompt attendance for screening examination after exposure
4. To promote early attendance for medical examination when symptomatic
5. To promote compliance with treatment and rescreening
6. To facilitate other interventions such as referral of sexual partners[21]

Individual sexual behavior is often implicated as the sole determinant of infection, and physicians often feel uncomfortable about addressing such issues with their patients. Physicians should understand that it is mainly proper health and illness behavior that they are attempting to promote and not sex education. Numerous pamphlets, booklets, and audiovisual aids are available through private foundations, professional associations, pharmaceutical companies, and governmental agencies. These materials help physicians to communicate effectively the above messages to their patient population at risk. There is no reason why pediatricians, family practitioners, and gynecologists cannot show their patients an STD educational program in addition to the other commonly shown programs dealing with hypertensions, diabetes, and natural childbirth.

In order to modify the sexual behavior of our young population who are at high risk for STDs, the most effective educational strategies seem to be those derived from the health action model (Fig. 1). This model emphasizes the importance of drives (e.g., sex drive), facilitating factors (e.g., peer pressure to perform), and inhibiting factors (e.g., fear of contracting venereal disease). These factors influence whether an intended action

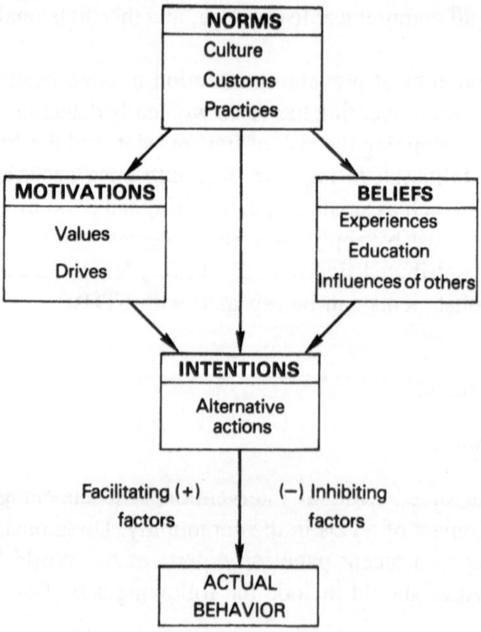

Figure 1. The heatlh action model. (Modified from Ref. 21.)

is finally translated into actual behavior.[21,22] Every level of influence should be a target of education; however, short-term gains are usually obtained through dissemination of information and emphasis on inhibiting factors. The recent decrease in gonorrhea rates in certain localities seems to be a consequence of intensive media coverage of AIDS.[23]

4.1.2. Primary Prevention—Specific Protection

Specific protection for communicable diseases can be provided through routine immunization, quarantine of infected individuals, and satisfactory vector control. Other than hepatitis B, for which an effective vaccine is available, none of these actions can be applied to other STDs. Therefore, specific protection can only be accomplished through individual prophylaxis. For practical purposes there are three methods of prophylaxis: mechanical barrier, locally acting measures, and systemic chemotherapy.

4.1.2a. Mechanical Barrier—The Condom. Condoms are effective in preventing STDs that are transmitted within the area of protection. Several studies have indicated that the condom has prophylactic value: (1) among Australian troops in Vietnam, none of the 55 consistent condom users contracted STD, compared to 35% of 191 inconsistent users or nonusers[24]; (2) among male college students, *Ureaplasma urealyticum* (a member of the Mycoplasmatales that is commonly isolated from genital tract and is transmissible through sexual activities) was detected in only 14% of condom users compared to 43% of nonusers[25]; (3) CDC reported a gonorrhea rate of 9% among women who use barrier methods for birth control, whereas 21% of all others were infected.

4.1.2b. Locally Acting Measures. These measures include such activities as washing after intercourse, urination, topically applied chemical agents, and antibiotic preparations. Studies of the clinical effectiveness of any of these methods are difficult to perform.[26] The available evidence suggests that the protective effect, if any, is minimal. Any positive effect may be biased because individuals engaging in these activities probably have a different perspective about health and illness compared to those who do not. Just as they do not use the condom, patients who are at greatest risk of infection are least likely to use any of these measures.

4.1.2c. Systemic Chemotherapy. Systemic antibiotics offer an effective protection against STDs. Oral sulfathiazole given before and after each sexual exposure reduced gonorrhea rate among troops during World War II.[27] Oral penicillin was later shown to be effective when given within a few hours after exposure. However, oral penicillin is inadequate to prevent syphilis.[28] Oral minocycline given to sailors after exposure reduced the gonorrhea rate by 58%.[29]

From the community viewpoint, such indiscriminant use of antibiotic prophylaxis should be discouraged.[30] Emergence of resistant organisms may precede any reduction in infection rate. Such an event might have taken place in other countries where penicillinase-producing *Neisseria gonorrhoeae* have been detected in high frequency. Furthermore, no single antibiotic is effective against all STDs.

4.2. Secondary Prevention

4.2.1. Disease Detection

Disease detection in STD can be accomplished at two different levels, the community and the individual. Mass screening, often performed by public health control programs, attempts to separate infected individuals from the uninfected. If mass screening is followed by prompt effective treatment, potential STD complications and potential transmitters can be eliminated from the infected pool. Unlike noncommunicable diseases, where screening inevitably reduces the prevalence of undisclosed disease, screened individuals with STDs can become reinfected and disease continues to be generated in the unscreened pool. Therefore, a decrease in prevalence does not necessarily follow mass screening and treatment in STD.[31]

In contrast, case finding by use of individual screening often takes place in a physician's office (e.g., a VDRL test for all women seeking prenatal care). Depending on the prevalence of disease in the population served by the physician, the yield of individual screening can be very low. As prevalence decreases, costs rise sharply for each case detected (cost-effectiveness). Furthermore, in low-prevalence population, the utility of a test drops significantly despite a very high specificity. For instance, the sensitivity and specificity of the VDRL test, as a premarital screening test, are reported to be 86% and 97% respectively.[32] The positive predictive value of the VDRL test in this low-prevalence situation is much smaller than those percentages (see Chapter 3, "Screening for Early Disease"). In the 44 states where premarital VDRL test is mandatory, only 453 cases of infectious syphilis were found after screening of four million individuals. The overall case-finding rate is only 0.012%.[33] Physicians should be aware of all these considerations before they begin any routine individual screening in their patients.

Physicians should recognize that the value of detecting primary syphilis in a pregnant woman is vastly different from that of detecting latent syphilis in an elderly man. From a control viewpoint, the value of locating a promiscuous, infected, asymptomatic man differs significantly from that of detecting gonorrhea in a monogamous, married woman. The most important lesson to be learned here is that the target of individual screening should be selected with considerable care. This is especially ture when effective treatment is not available, as is the case with AIDS.

4.2.2. Secondary Prevention—Prompt Treatment

Treatment regimens for patients with any confirmed STDs are widely available in many standard clinical textbooks and journals.[34,35] To facilitate successful treatment for any specific STD, the U.S. Public Health Service has published treatment guidelines periodically as a standard part of its control strategy.[36] These recommendations represent a consensus among a group of expert clinicians in STDs. Detailed discussion of these treatment guidelines is beyond the scope of this chapter. Table I provides some treatment regimens selected for some common STDs. What should be emphasized in clinical preventive medicine are contact tracing and patient counseling, as well as epidemiological treatment.

4.2.2a. Contact Tracing and Patient Counseling. A component of proper case management is prevention of reinfections. Studies have shown that the source of most of these reinfections can be traced to the person who was the source of the original infection. In a Milwaukee study, over 50% of recurrent gonorrheal infections in women were due to failure to treat their sexual partners.[37] The process of identifying and treating sexual partners is generally known as contact tracing.

Contact tracing is often viewed by private physicians as time consuming and a breach of privacy with their patients. However, neither of these assumptions is true if the referral of sexual partners is facilitated by patient counseling. Effective patient counseling also ensures compliance with both treatment and follow-up. At the time of treatment, physicians should communicate to their patients the following:

1. Results of all tests
2. The name of the patient's disease and its importance
3. The names of the medications and how they are used
4. The expected outcome of treatment
5. Potential side effects of treatment
6. The necessity for tests of cure
7. The consequences to the health of the patient and partner(s) if not treated
8. The necessity of abstaining from sex until all partners have sought appropriate care
9. The likelihood of asymptomatic infection
10. A plan of action for each sexual partner

Before discussing referral of sexual partners with their patients, physicians may select the referral method most suitable to that particular patient. There are three types of referral options:

1. Self-referral—total patient responsibility: provide appointment cards to patients for distribution to sexual partners.
2. Formal tracing—total physician responsibility: obtain names and addresses of sexual partners, locate these partners, and offer them examination and treatment.
3. Conditional self-referral—shared responsibility: obtain names and addresses of sexual partners, allow patients the option of referring partners within specified time; formal tracing will take place if the patient fails.

Conditional self-referral may provide patients the opportunity to discuss their mutual disease problem with their partners. If the patient was well prepared by the counseling effort, the success rate can be quite satisfactory. Contact tracing is clearly less productive if the sexual partners are anonymous or are too far away (e.g., in foreign countries). Physicians can also refer formal tracings to the disease intervention specialist at their local health department.

4.2.2b. Epidemiological Treatment. Epidemiological treatment refers to antibiotics administered when a diagnosis is considered likely on clinical or epidemiological grounds, but before the results of confirmatory laboratory tests are known. The CDC recommend prompt treatment of sexual partners if the patient has any of the following STDs: gonorrhea, syphilis, chancroid, lymphogranuloma venereum, NGU, PID, tri-

Table I. Treatment Guidelines for Some Common Sexually Transmitted Diseases in Adults[a]

Disease	Recommended treatment: Dosage	Route[b]	Duration (days)	Partner
Chancroid	Ceftriaxone, 250 mg	i.m.	SD[c]	Yes
Chlamydial infection[d]	Doxycycline, 100 mg twice daily	p.o.	7	Yes
Localized gonococcal infection[e]	Ceftriaxone, 250 mg	i.m.	SD	Yes
Disseminated gonococcal infection[f]	Ceftriaxone, 1 g once daily	i.v.	7	Yes
Herpes progenitalis				
First episode[g]	Acyclovir, 200 mg 5 times daily	p.o.	10	No
Recurrence[h]	Acyclovir, 200 mg 5 times daily	p.o.	5	No
Lymphogranuloma venereum	Doxycycline, 100 mg twice daily	p.o.	14	Yes
Syphilis, early	Penicillin G, 2.4×10^6 u[i]	i.m.	SD	Yes
Syphilis, late	Penicillin G, 2.4×10^6 u	i.m.	21[j]	No
Neurosyphilis	Penicillin G, 20×10^6 u[k]	i.v.	10	No
Trichomoniasis	Metronidazole, 2 g once	p.o.	SD	Yes
Vaginosis (bacterial)	Metronidazole, 500 mg once daily	p.o.	7	No

[a]Only one of the many recommended treatment regimens is presented here. These regimens were selected because of their ease of administration and their efficacy.
[b]i.m., intramuscularly; i.v., intravenously; p.o., orally.
[c]Single dose.
[d]Chlamydial urethritis, endocervicitis, and proctitis.
[e]Gonococcal urethritis, endocervicitis, proctitis, and pharyngitis.
[f]Gonococcal arthritis/dermatitis syndrome, not including endocarditis or meningitis.
[g]Treatment should be initiated within 6 days of onset; delayed treatment may not be beneficial.
[h]Within 2 days of onset.
[i]Benzathine penicillin G, 2.4 million units intramuscularly.
[j]Above regimen given once weekly for 3 consecutive weeks.
[k]Aqueous penicillin G, 12–24 million units intravenously in six divided doses.

chomoniasis, or mucopurulent cervicitis.[36] Every effort to establish the diagnosis in partners should be made; however, such treatment should be administered even before the confirmatory laboratory tests are available. Epidemiological treatment short-circuits the time required for confirmation, thereby reducing the duration of disease and the risk of further transmission. It offers health providers one of the most powerful preventive approaches at their disposal.

The academic debate over epidemiological treatment has been continuing since 1954. Clinicians often hesitate to accept this public health primacy over the concept of accurate diagnosis before treatment. In the United States, epidemiological treatment has long been accepted among STD clinics because of federal influence.

Although data supporting epidemiological treatment for other STDs are not strong, the arguments for gonorrhea are quite convincing. The culture and gram-stained smear are the principal criteria used for the diagnosis of gonorrhea. False-positive results are uncommon, but false negative results can be higher than 15%. Using decision analysis, Johnson has estimated that without epidemiological treatment, 12–30% of women and 4–13% of men seeking care as contacts would be infected and untreated.[38]

Efficacy of epidemiological treatment depends on patient compliance and the effectiveness of the chosen regimen. Compliance with single-dose therapy is usually excellent. Before choosing a particular regimen, physicians must balance the importance between the likelihood of coexisting STDs (e.g., 45% of patients with gonorrhea also have *C. trachomatis* infection) and the likelihood of patient compliance (e.g., a 7-day course of oral tetracycline). For minor STDs such as trichomoniasis and bacterial vaginosis, confirming the diagnosis in male sexual partners is not important; epidemiological treatment can be carried out using the patient as the medication courier without actually examining the sexual partners.

4.3. Tertiary Prevention—Rehabilitation

This level of prevention in STDs is the least desirable and most costly. Tertiary prevention is necessary when the control efforts have failed. Examples of rehabilitating activities for STDs are (1) *in vitro* fertilization for women with involuntary infertility due to salpingitis; and (2) special care and education for children who are mentally retarded because of congenital or neonatal STDs.

5. PREVENTION OF STDS IN NEWBORNS

STDs in newborns are often devastating diseases. Newborns can acquire their diseases from their mothers either congenitally (e.g., *Treponema pallidum* and cytomegalovirus) or neonatally (e.g., herpes simplex, *N. gonorrhoeae*, group B *Streptococcus*, and *C. trachomatis*). All measures to reduce the incidence of STDs in pregnant women will simultaneously reduce neonatal morbidity and mortality. The continuous decline in the number of cases of congenital syphilis indicates that syphilis control in pregnant women has been successful.

C. trachomatis infections in neonates can result in severe conjunctivitis and/or pneumonia. Pregnant women with genital infections due to *C. trachomatis* should be given a 7-day course of oral erythromycin.[39] Neonatal conjunctivitis due to either *C. trachomatis* or *N. gonorrhoeae* can be prevented with the application of 0.5% erythromycin ophthalmic ointment immediately postpartum.[40]

Group B *Streptococcus* is one of the most common causes of neonatal sepsis. Although this organism does not cause symptomatic genital infections in adults similar to classical STDs, it is transmitted between sex partners, and a higher genital colonization rate is found among promiscuous individuals.[41] These genital colonizations in pregnant women are quite prevalent (20–30%), and vertical transmission during parturition to mucosal membranes of neonates occurs 60–70% of the time. However, only about 1% of genital carriers deliver infants who will develop symptomatic infection. Interruption of this vertical transmission of colonization has been successful with intravenous ampicillin during labor.[42] Such intrapartum ampicillin prophylaxis has recently been shown to prevent early-onset neonatal group B streptococcal disease.[43] Such prophylactic treatment is recommended only for women with positive cultures at the time of labor, and only if they have premature labor or prolonged rupture of amniotic membranes.

Neonatal herpes simplex infection has a high case-fatality rate for the infant (see above). The number of new cases of neonatal HSV infection has been estimated to be between 1:2,500 and 1:10,000 deliveries per year. The women with a history of genital herpes or with a sexual partner who has genital lesions should be identified for serial virological and clinical evaluations. Beginning at 34 weeks of gestation, weekly cultures or Papanicolaou cytological studies (less sensitive) should be performed. Cesarean section is the procedure of choice for women with active viral shedding and intact membranes at delivery. The value of cesarean section is less clear if the membranes have been ruptured longer than 12 hr.[44] Better understanding of the epidemiology and immunology of maternal–neonatal HSV infection is necessary so that preventive methods in the future can avoid major surgery.

The incidence of *in utero* cytomegalovirus (CMV) infection ranges from 0.2 to 2.2% among all live births; however, only an estimated 10% of these infants are symptomatic at birth. Of the 90% of infants with no clinical manifestations at birth, 5–15% are at risk for some abnormalities within the first 2 years. Primary maternal CMV infection can result in infection of up to 40% of fetuses. Maternal immunity to CMV does not prevent virus reactivation, and recurrent maternal CMV infections can lead to 1.5% intrauterine infections. Although maternal immunity is not completely protective, congenital infections that result from recurrent infections are less likely to produce fetal damage than those resulting from primary infections. At present, there are no reliable, practical ways to determine intrauterine transmission and fetal disease. Virological and serological testing should not be routinely performed in pregnant women as they may cause unnecessary worry.[45]

6. PREVENTION OF STDS IN HOMOSEXUALS

During the past two decades, it has become apparent that homosexually active men are at an increased risk for a variety of STDs. Other than chlamydial urethritis, homosexuals have a higher prevalence in all other conventional STDs compared to their heterosexual counterparts. In addition, they also have a greater prevalence of other infectious conditions such as amebiasis, giardiasis, shigellosis, and hepatitis. These enteric infections were not considered to be sexually transmitted previously. Although this epidemic of STDs has been active for many years within the gay communities, it has received world attention only recently with the emergence of AIDS.

This STD epidemic is associated with a subpopulation of promiscuous urban homosexual men. Many of their worst offenders often appear to be indifferent about their health. It is the contention of most health care providers who are familiar with the homosexual population that education is the key to the control of STDs.[5] Educational effort should stress health consciousness. The language used to communicate health issues should be nonjudgmental and positive.

From the standpoint of a private practitioner, health education on STDs should be incorporated into the initial interview with the patient. Together with the usual questioning of the patient's sexual history, risk factors of acquiring STDs unique to that patient should be identified. Gathering of these risk factors can generate a risk profile that can be used by that patient to make informed decisions regarding his future sexual activities.[46]

Risk factors are often arbitrarily divided into high, medium, and low categories. Examples of some of the high-risk factors are:

1. Large number of sexual partners, such as more than 10 different monthly partners
2. Type of sexual encounter, such as anonymous contact
3. Location of sexual encounter, such as public bath houses
4. Nature of sexual activities, such as active anilingus and passive fist fornication

Homosexual patients should be taught how to examine themselves routinely. Penile, pharyngeal, and anal inspections should be done routinely before or after showers. These patients should be encouraged to seek help early with any signs or symptoms suggestive of STDs. They should also learn how to tactfully discuss the recent health of their potential partners prior to sex. Preventive measures effective for the male heterosexual population, such as those mentioned in previous sections in this chapter, are also applicable to the homosexual patient.

During the initial visit, testings for syphilis, gonorrhea, and hepatitis B should be carried out. Other diagnostic tests can be ordered according to medical indications. Subsequent testings should be carried out at intervals appropriate for the risk profile of the patient. Monthly testing is suggested for those at high risk, quarterly for those at medium risk, and annually for those at low risk. Detailed guidelines to help the clinicians are available from multiple sources; these are usually obtainable by mail.*

REFERENCES

1. Adler, M.W.: The terrible peril: A historical persepctive on the venereal diseases. *Br. Med. J.* **281**:206–211, 1980.
2. Selvin, M.: Changing medical and societal attitudes toward sexually transmitted diseases: A Historical overview, in Holmes, K. K., Mardh, P., Sparling, P. F., and Wiesner, P. J. (eds.): *Sexually Transmitted Diseases*, McGraw-Hill, New York, 1984, pp. 3–19.
3. Holmes, K. K.: Sexually transmitted diseases: An overview and perspectives on the next decade. *Sexually Transmitted Diseases, 1980 Status Report*. NIH publication No. 81-2213, Washington, DC, 1981, pp. 3–20.
4. Aral, S. O. and Holmes, K. K.: Epidemiology of sexually transmitted diseases, in Holmes, K. K., Mardh, P., Sparling, P. F., and Wiesner, P. J. (eds.): *Sexually Transmitted Diseases*. McGraw-Hill, New York, 1984, pp. 126–141.
5. Ostrow, D. G., and Altman, N. L.: Sexually transmitted diseases and homosexuality. *Sex. Trans. Dis.* **10**:(4):208–215, 1983.
6. Darrow, W. W.: Social stratification, sexual behavior and the sexually transmitted diseases. *Sex. Trans. Dis.* **6**:(3):228–230, 1979.
7. Centers for Disease Control: *Sexually Transmitted Disease Statistical Letter*, U.S. Department of Health and Human Services, Atlanta, 1982.
8. Centers for Disease Control: Syphilis—United States, 1983. *Morbid. Mortal. Wkly. Rep.* **33**(30):433, 1984.
9. Thompson, S. E., and Washington, A. E.: Epidemiology of sexually transmitted *Chlamydia trachomatis infections*. *Epidemiol. Rev.* **5**:96–123, 1983.

*Bay Area Physicians for Human Rights, BAPHR-GUIDELINES, P.O. Box 14546, San Francisco, CA 94114.

10. Wiesner, P. J.: Magnitude of the problem of sexually transmitted diseases in the United States. *Sexually Transmitted Diseases, 1980 Status Report*. NIH publication No. 81-2213, Washington, DC, 1981, pp. 21–31.
11. Aral, S. O., Johnson, R. E., Zaidi, A. A., Fichtner, R. R., and Reynolds, G. H.: Demographic effects on sexually transmitted diseases in the 1970's: The problem could be worse. *Sex. Trans. Dis.* **10**:(2):100–101, 1983.
12. Bureau of the Census: Current population reports: Population estimates and projections. *Projections of the Population of the United States: 1977–2050*. Series P25, No. 704, U.S. Department of Commerce, Washington, D.C., 1977.
13. Zelnik, M., and Kantner, J. F.: Sexual activity, contraceptive use and pregnancy among metropolitan-area teenagers: 1971–1979. *Fam. Planning Perspect.* **12**:230–237, 1980.
14. Curran, J. W.: Economic consequences of pelvic inflammatory disease in the United States. *Am. J. Obstet. Gynecol.* **138**:848–851, 1980.
15. Committee on Fetus and Newborn, Committee on Infectious Diseases: Perinatal herpes simplex virus infections. *Pediatrics* **66**(1):147–149, 1980.
16. Hooper, R. R., Reynolds, G. H., and Jones, O. G.: Cohort study of venereal disease. I. The risk of gonorrhea transmission from infected women to men. *Am. J. Epidemiol.* **108**:136–144, 1978.
17. Schroeter, A. L., Turner, R. H., and Lucas, J. B.: Therapy for incubating syphilis: Effectiveness of gonorrhea treatment. *JAMA* **218**:711–713, 1971.
18. Lycke, E., Löwhagen, G. B., and Hallhagen, G.: The risk of transmission of genital *Chlamydia trachomatis* infection is less than that of genital *Neisseria gonorrhoeae* infection. *Sex. Trans. Dis.* **7**:6–10, 1980.
19. Straus, S. E., Rooney, J. F., and Sever, J. L.: Herpes simplex virus infection: Biology, treatment and prevention. *Ann. Intern. Med.* **103**:404–418, 1985.
20. Leavell, H. A., and Clark, G. E.: *Preventive Medicine for the Doctor in His Community: An Epidemiologic Approach*. McGraw-Hill, New York, 1965.
21. *Control of Sexually Transmitted Diseases*. World Health Organization, Geneva, 1985.
22. Green, L. W.: Modifying and developing health behavior. *Annu. Rev. Public Health* **5**:215–236, 1984.
23. Judson, F. N.: Fear of AIDS and gonorrhea rates in homosexual men. *Lancet* **2**:159, 1983.
24. Hart, G.: Factors influencing venereal infections in a war environment. *Br. J. Vener. Dis.* **50**:68–72, 1974.
25. McCormack, W. M., Lee, Y., and Zinner, S. H.: Sexual experience and urethral colonization with genital mycoplasmas. *Ann. Intern. Med.* **78**:696–698, 1973.
26. Stone, K. M., Grimes, D. A., and Magder, L. S.: Primary prevention of sexually transmitted diseases. A primer for clinicians. *JAMA* **225**:1763–1766, 1986.
27. Loveless, J. A., and Denton, W.: The oral use of sulfathiazole as a prophylaxis for gonorrhea. *JAMA* **121**:827–828, 1943.
28. Eagle, H., Gude, A. V., and Beckmann, G. E.: Prevention of gonorrhea with penicillin tablets. *JAMA* **140**:940–943, 1949.
29. Harrison, W. O., Hooper, R. R., and Wiesner, P. J.: A trial of minocycline given after exposure to prevent gonorrhea. *N. Engl. J. Med.* **300**:1074–1078, 1979.
30. Sack, R. B.: Prophylactic antibiotics? The individual versus the community. *N. Engl. J. Med.* **300**:1107–1108, 1979.
31. Hart, G.: Screening to control infectious diseases: Evaluation of control programs for gonorrhea and syphilis. *Rev. Infect. Dis.* **2**:701–712, 1980.
32. Haskell, R. J.: A cost-benefit analysis of California's mandatory premarital screening program for syphilis. *West. J. Med.* **141**:538–541, 1984.
33. Felman, Y. M.: Repeal of mandatory premarital test for syphilis: A survey of state health officers. *Am. J. Public Health* **71**:155–159, 1981.
34. Holmes, K. K., Mardh, P., Sparling, P. F., and Wiesner, P. J. (eds.): *Sexually Transmitted Diseases*. McGraw-Hill, New York, 1984.
35. Washington, A. E., Mandell, G. L., and Wiesner, P. J. (eds.): Treatment of sexually transmitted diseases. *Rev. Infect. Dis.* **4**(suppl):S27-S890, 1982.
36. Centers for Disease Control: STD treatment guidelines. *Morbid. Mortal. Wkly. Rep.* **34**(4S, suppl):75S–108S, 1985.
37. Parra, W. C., Wiesner, P. J., and Drotman, D. P.: Patient counseling, in Holmes, K. K., Mardh, P.,

Sparling, P. F., and Wiesner, P. J. (eds.): *Sexually Transmitted Diseases*. McGraw-Hill, New York, 1984, p. 957.
38. Johnson, R. E.: Epidemiologic and prophylactic treatment of gonorrhea: A decision analysis review. *Sex. Trans. Dis.* **6**:159–167, 1979.
39. Schachter, J., Sweet, R. L., and Grossman, M.: Experience with the routine use of erythromycin for chlamydial infections in pregnancy. *N. Engl. J. Med.* **314**:276–279, 1986.
40. Thompson, S. E., III, and Dretler, R. H.: Epidemiology and treatment of chlamydial infections in pregnant women and infants. *Rev. Infect. Dis.* **4**(suppl):S747–S757, 1982.
41. Baker, C. J., Zabriskie, J. B., and Hill, H. R.: Group B Streptococcal Infections: Nature and extent of the problem. *Sexually Transmitted Diseases, 1980 Status Report*. NIH Publication no. 81-2213, Washington, DC, April 1981, p. 145.
42. Yow, M. D., Mason, E. O., and Leeds, L. J.: Ampicillin prevents intrapartum transmission of group B streptococcus. *JAMA* **241**:1245–1247, 1979.
43. Boyer, K. M., and Gottoff, S. P.: Prevention of early-onset neonatal group B streptococcal disease with selective intrapartum chemoprophylaxis. *N. Engl. J. Med.* **314**:1665–1669, 1986.
44. Stagno, S., and Whitley, R. J.: Herpes virus infection of pregnancy: Part II: Herpes simplex virus and varicella–zoster virus infections. *N. Engl. J. Med.* **313**:1327–1330, 1985.
45. Stagno, S., and Whitley, R. J.: Herpes virus infections of pregnancy: Part I: Cytomegalovirus and Epstein–Barr virus infections. *N. Engl. J. Med.* **313**:1270–1274, 1985.
46. Bolan, R. K.: Sexually transmitted diseases in homosexuals: Focusing the attack. *Sex. Trans. Dis.* **8**:293–297, 1981.

10

AIDS

Gordon M. Dickinson

1. INTRODUCTION

Since its recognition in 1981 the acquired immunodeficiency syndrome (AIDS) has become the most striking disease of the 20th century. It is a fatal disease that results in the death of virtually all affected patients within 3 years of diagnosis. Initially described in homosexual men and intravenous drug users,[1–3] AIDS is now recognized as a disease that also affects hemophiliacs, children born to infected mothers, and, through blood transfusions or sexual contact with infected persons, virtually anyone. The recognition of the human immunodeficiency virus (HIV)—formerly named human T-lymphotrophic virus-type III (HTLV-III), lymphadenopathy-associated virus, or AIDS-related virus—as the causative agent of AIDS was followed by the development of an antibody test and detection of asymptomatic infections that greatly outnumber cases of AIDS. The actual number of infected persons in the United States is unknown. Estimates range from 1,000,000 to 1,500,000. How many infected persons will eventually develop AIDS is also unknown. Studies of homosexual men with HTLV-III antibody have found that 7–34% developed AIDS during the 12–72 months of observation from the time HTLV-III antibody was detected.[4–7] The observation that immunological abnormalities are progressive over time in infected persons suggests that the number who eventually develop AIDS may be much higher.[8,9]

AIDS is a disease of variable clinical manifestations that appear to be largely related to secondary infections and malignancies. Some patients remain healthy for many months after their initial diagnosis, although the typical patient experiences multiple, recurrent, and persistent infections that require frequent hospitalizations. Many patients are dependent on extensive nursing care in the latter stages of the disease. The expense in dollars for medical care of a patient with AIDS is enormous—yet insignificant compared to the cost in lost productivity. The AIDS patient is often a young adult who is just beginning his or her career. Years of potential life lost (YPLL) before age 65 is one measure of premature mortality that highlights the effects of AIDS. For single men aged 25–44 years, AIDS ranked close to cancer in YPLL for the United States as a whole and surpassed YPLL due to accidents, homicides, and suicide in Manhattan and San Francisco in 1984.[10]

Gordon M. Dickinson • Department of Medicine, University of Miami School of Medicine, Miami Veterans Administration Medical Center, Miami, Florida 33101.

The use of zidovudine (azidothymidine) for treatment of persons with AIDS or symptomatic HIV infection and low T-helper cells has offered some hope to persons with HIV infection.[11,12] The drug is considered palliative rather than curative, and its long-term effects are unknown at this time. A vaccine would appear to be the most practical means to prevent the spread of HIV infection, but an effective, safe vaccine may require many years for development. It is clear that prevention of HIV infection must play a major role in controlling AIDS. A necessary step in the prevention of AIDS is the education of not only patients with HIV infection and persons at high risk for infection but also health care workers and the general public. Physicians must be familiar with all aspects of HIV infection and be able to effectively counsel patients about avoiding or transmitting this infection. This chapter reviews the epidemiology and modes of transmission of HIV virus, the means by which the diagnosis of HIV infection is established, the counseling of both patients with infection and persons with perceived or actual risk for infection, and finally, the recommended protective precautions for health care workers.

2. EPIDEMIOLOGY

2.1. Risk Characteristics

Patients with AIDS generally have exhibited certain behaviors characteristics that have been associated with acquisition of this syndrome. These risk characteristics, recognized early in the epidemic, are present in the majority of persons with AIDS (Table I). The percentages of reported cases with the different risk factors has changed very little over the past 4 years, although it is clear that increasing number of persons outside these risk groups are now being reported. The primary means of transmission of HIV is either through infusion or inoculation of infected blood or blood products or by intimate contact between an infected and a susceptible person that involves passage of body fluids and/or blood from one to the other.

2.2. Male Homosexuality

Studies of HIV infection in homosexual men have demonstrated a correlation between the number of different sexual partners and the risk for infection: the greater the number of partners, the greater has been the risk for infection. Sexual practices associated with mucosal trauma also appear to correlate with increased risk.[13–16] Men who practice

Table I. Groups at Risk for AIDS

1.	Homosexual/bisexual men
2.	Intravenous drug users
3.	Hemophiliacs
4.	Blood transfusion recipients, 1978–1985
5.	Sexual partners of one of the above
6.	Neonates born to mothers with HIV infection

primarily receptive anal intercourse tend to have a higher rate of infection than those who practice insertive anal intercourse.[14] These observations suggest not only that the quantity of exposure is important, but also that the intensity of exposure carries increased risk of transmission, particularly exposure associated with direct inoculation of infected fluids through traumatized tissue. In an area with a low incidence of HIV infection among homosexual men, sexual contact with a person from an area with a high rate of infection is a risk factor.[17]

2.3. Intravenous Drug Use

The rate of infection among intravenous drug users is extremely high in some urban areas: surveillance studies have reported seropositivity rates as high as 60% in New York City.[18] The rapid spread of HIV infection in intravenous drug addicts is related to the common practice of sharing needles and syringes. For some addicts this sharing is a matter of need, whereas for others it may be an integral factor in the culture of illicit drug use.

2.4. Heterosexual Transmission

Transmission of HIV infection occurs among heterosexual couples, and AIDS must be recognized as a sexually transmitted disease.[19] Female sexual partners of men with HIV infection are now accounting for increasing numbers of cases of AIDS in women in the United States. Anal intercourse or fellatio is not necessary for transmission. Transmission from man to woman has occurred among couples whose sexual activity includes only vaginal intercourse. The number of men in the United States who are thought to have acquired their infection from women is relatively small. However, studies of HIV infection in Haitian immigrants in the United States have found that a history of multiple sexual female partners, including prostitutes, was commonly elicited from infected men who denied homosexual activity.[20] HIV infection in Africa occurs in both men and women in approximately a 1:1 ratio. Intravenous drug use or receipt of blood products does not account for transmission in these countries. Infected men tend to be older than infected women, a pattern consistent with sexual activity, and in the absence of alternative explanations, sexual transmission is the most plausible explanation for the equal distribution of HIV infection among the sexes. Experience accumulating in the United States indicates that HIV will be readily transmissible by vaginal intercourse.[21,22] Ongoing studies will clarify this issue.

2.5. Nonsexual Contact

Transmission of HIV to close contacts of infected persons is a very rare event in the absence of sexual intercourse. Studies of families with an infected member have demonstrated transmission between sexually active spouses and between mothers and their newborn infants, but have not found secondary cases in other household members.[21–23] A mother who acquired an infection after providing intensive nursing care, including management of intravenous catheters and wound care, over many months to her infant child is an exception.[24] Because of the intensity of her exposure and her failure to take any precautions, her infection does not contradict the wider experience gained in the studies mentioned earlier.

2.6. Health Care Workers

Concerns that health care workers would be at significant risk for acquiring infection from patients have not proven justified, although several apparent instances of transmission attributed to accidental inoculation with contaminated needles and one instance of possible transmission due to a mucosal splash have occurred.[25–29] Several studies of health care workers exposed to blood or other body fluids of persons with AIDS, including a multicenter study involving more than 900 health care workers, have detected only three possible and one probable instance of transmission.[26,30–33] Of interest are two health care workers who acquired hepatitis B virus and *Cryptococcus neoformans* infection, respectively, from patients with AIDS through accidental needle punctures. These two workers failed to acquire HIV infection.[34,35] The infrequency of HIV infections in health care workers who have had documented transcutaneous and mucous membrane exposures to blood or body fluids of infected patients and the infrequency of HIV infections in workers with close contact with patient with AIDS over the past 5 years confirm that transmission to health care workers is a rare event. The infrequency of transmission via needle stick injuries is not surprising in view of the low level of infectious units in the blood of persons with AIDS.

2.7. Blood Transfusions and Blood Products

The risk for acquiring HIV infection from blood transfusions or blood products has been reduced to nearly zero since screening for all blood donations was introduced in early 1985. Factor VIII concentrate, the source of HIV infection in many hemophiliacs, is now heat-treated and no longer a threat to recipients.

2.8. Vectors and Environmental Factors

Concerns have been expressed in the lay press about the potential for transmission of HIV by other means, particularly by insect vectors and inanimate objects in the environment. Although it is true that secondary modes of transmission may exist and not be easily recognized in the early stages of epidemics, it appears highly unlikely that new modes of transmission of HIV will be identified that represent any significant risk to the general population.

3. DIAGNOSIS OF HIV INFECTION

3.1. Diagnostic Criteria and Classification

The Centers for Disease Control surveillance criteria for AIDS (Table II) continue to be used in the United States for data collection purposes with only minor modifications

Table II. Surveillance Criteria for Diagnosis of AIDS

A. Occurrence of a disease moderately predictive of a defect in cell-mediated immunity occurring in a person with no known cause for that immune deficiency.
1. Kaposi's sarcoma in patients less than 60 years of age, or
2. One of the following opportunistic infections:
   Pneumocystis carinii pneumonia
   Cryptosporidiosis > 4 weeks' duration
   Herpes simplex virus > 5 weeks mucocutaneous ulceration
   Cryptococcosis
   Toxoplasma encephalitis
   Mycobacterium avium intracellulare
   Progressive multifocal leukoencephalopathy

B. Occurrence of one of the following if the patient has a positive serological or virological test for HIV
1. Disseminated histoplasmosis
2. Isosporiasis with diarrhea > 4 weeks
3. Bronchial or pulmonary candidiasis
4. Non-Hodgkin's lymphoma of high-grade pathological type (diffuse, undifferentiated) and of B-cell or unknown immunological phenotype
5. Kaposi's sarcoma in patients who are 60 years old or older
6. Histologically confirmed diagnosis of chronic lymphoid interstitial pneumonitis in a child under 13 years of age

since first published in 1981.[36,37] Continued use of clinical criteria for the reporting of AIDS excludes some individuals who have symptoms and a disease process that is clearly AIDS in all but name, but it preserves the continuity of data collection and rarely will lead to a false diagnosis of AIDS. HIV infection, however, is often not associated with symptoms; it can be identified by culture and serological methods in the absence of other laboratory or clinical abnormalities.[33,38] The manifestations of HIV infection range from asymptomatic infection to a severe wasting syndrome associated with multiple opportunistic infections. HIV infections can be categorized in a number of ways.[39–41] One proposed classification system is shown in Table III.[41] These classification systems are helpful for research and epidemiology, but have limited use in determining prognosis for an individual patient. The laboratory is an important adjunct to the clinical evaluation, particularly for asymptomatic patients and those without a clear diagnosis.

3.2. Diagnosis: Laboratory Methods

The ultimate criterion for diagnosis of HIV infection is the isolation of HIV from blood or tissue. First achieved by researchers at the Pasteur Institute[42] and at the National Cancer Institute,[38] culture of HIV is now performed by many research laboratories. Because isolation of HIV is tedious and expensive, it is not practical for routine diagnosis. The presence of antibody against HIV correlates well with infection, and several methods for antibody detection have been described that are much simpler to perform than viral

Table III. Classification System for Human Immunodeficiency Virus Infection[a]

Group I			Acute infection
Group II			Asymptomatic infection
Group III			Persistent generalized lymphadenopathy
Group IV			Other disease
	Subgroup A		Constitutional disease
	Subgroup B		Neurological disease
	Subgroup C		Secondary infectious deseases
		Category C-1	AIDS defining infections
		Category C-2	Other infections:
			Hairy leukoplakia
			Multidermal herpes zoster
			Recurrent *Salmonella* bacteremia
			Nocardiosis
			Tuberculosis
			Oral candidiasis
	Subgroup D		Secondary cancers (Kaposi's sarcoma, non-Hodgkin's lymphoma, primary lymphoma of the brain)

[a]From Ref. 41.

culture. These include a radioimmunoprecipitation assay,[43] an immunofluorescent assay,[44] a Western blot assay,[45] and enzyme-linked immunosorbent assay (ELISA).[45] The Western blot and ELISA methods are the most widely used today.

The ELISA method is now available from a number of manufacturers in kit form and is the method used to screen donated blood and for diagnostic purposes. An enzymatic-induced color reaction of a test serum is compared to the background color of known negative sera, and a ratio or index is calculated. The interpretation of what constitutes a positive or negative test depends on the characteristics of that particular test. These tests are relatively sensitive and specific. There are occasional false positive results, and a small percentage of results fall in the borderline zone. False positive results in a technically satisfactory test are probably due to the presence of antibodies to cellular debris from the cell cultures in which the HIV used for antigen were grown. Most false positive tests are weakly positive or borderline.[46] A review of results from the initial screening of donated blood noted a positive rate of 0.89%.[47] Confirmatory tests found that only 0.25% were true positives, however. The commercially available ELISA have been refined, and the incidence of false positive is now about 0.2%.[48] A positive assay should always be confirmed by another assay, unless the diagnosis is clear on another basis.

The Western blot assay is a supplementary test that is often used to confirm a positive ELISA. It uses purified disrupted virus that is fractionated by electrophoresis and transferred to a nitrocellulose sheet. Antibodies against two or more viral proteins are indicative of a true positive serum. Because of the time and work the Western blot test entails, it is used primarily just for research or confirmation of a positive ELISA assay.

The presence of HIV antibody correlates closely with isolation of virus, although antibodies confer no apparent protection to the infected patient. They are diagnostically useful in the evaluation of persons with symptoms suggestive of HIV infection and for detection of asymptomatic infection in patients with a history of exposure. When used in conjunction with a clinical assessment, they can establish the diagnosis of HIV infection. It is well to remember, however, that in a population with a low incidence of HIV infection a positive assay will have a low predictive value for actual infection.

The presence of antibody is generally not necessary to establish a diagnosis of AIDS, except in those persons with complicating infections or tumors not definitely predictive of immunodeficiency (Table II). These tests for antibody should be used with the recognition of the potential impact a positive test carries. The social, economic, and personal implications are enormous. Loss of friends, employment, and refusal of insurance are real concerns and have occurred because of the fear of AIDS engendered by a positive test for antibody.

3.3. Clinical Evaluation

3.3.1. History

The evaluation of a patient in whom a diagnosis of HIV infection is considered should include a careful history about past activities that are associated with HIV infection. Homosexual contacts, intravenous drug use with sharing of needles, reception of blood transfusions, and sexual contact with persons in a risk group are all potential sources of infection. A man who frequently has sex with a prostitute, or a person who has a sexual partner who in turn has multiple partners is also at risk for infection. Because of the social stigma that may be associated with homosexuality, intravenous drug use, or sexual intercourse with prostitutes, questions about these activities must be asked in a nonjudgmental manner. The early symptoms of persons developing immunodeficiency are often sufficient to suggest the diagnosis, not because any one symptom is specific for the diagnosis, but because their temporal pattern, their setting (in a person at risk), and their association with other symptoms are so characteristic of evolving HIV infection. Malaise, chronic diarrhea, unexplained fevers, uninduced weight loss, enlarged lymph nodes, and fatigability are some of the symptoms that have been noted in persons developing AIDS. Patients should be questioned about these symptoms if they are not volunteered. Some patients will not admit to a life-style that places them at risk, but their past medical history may suggest it. For example, hepatitis B is common in drug users and homosexual men, and multiple or recurrent venereal diseases, rectal disease, and intestinal parasites are often a consequence of male homosexual activity.

3.3.2. Physical Examination

The physical examination should include careful attention to the patient's skin, oral cavity, eyes, lymph nodes, and rectum. Kaposi's sarcoma may first appear at any point on the body and may be unnoticed by the patient. Thus, the patient should completely disrobe for a careful viewing of his or her skin quite literally from the top of the head to the tips of the toes. The typical Kaposi's sarcoma of the skin is an oval indurated reddish-purple lesion that may be flat or raised. Some may have the appearance of a bruise. In black-skinned persons the lesions appear as hyperpigmented nodules or plaques. Many persons with evolving immunodeficiency will develop pruritic papular lesions that they scratch and excoriate. These lesions are commonly seen in the tropics and warmer climates in the United States. They resemble insect bites, but their etiology is unknown. Examination of the oral cavity may detect lesions of Kaposi's sarcoma, the white plaques of oral candidiasis, or white plaques of hairy leukoplakia on the tongue. White plaques should be scraped and examined with a microscope to confirm the presence of the hyphal elements of *Candida*. The etiology of hairy leukoplakia has been attributed to an Epstein–Barr virus infection. Ophthalmoscopic examination may detect white "cotton-wool spots" or areas of retinitis caused by opportunistic pathogens such as *Toxoplasma gondii* or cytomegalovirus even before the patient's vision has been appreciably affected. Generalized lymphadenopathy is a frequent consequence of HIV infection, and all regional nodes should be examined. Perirectal condyloma, ulcers of herpes simplex, fissures, mucosal induration, and lax sphincter muscles suggest the practice of receptive anal intercourse.

3.3.3. Laboratory

The laboratory evaluation should begin with basic studies: a complete blood count may show the characteristic lymphopenia, and a battery of skin tests (mumps, *Candida,* tetanus, *Trichophyton,* for example) may detect defects in cellular immunity. Serum proteins are frequently elevated because of a polyclonal increase in the immunoglobulins, and the serum albumin may be decreased because of malnutrition. Antibody against HIV is the best marker for infection and is a key factor in the evaluation of possible HIV infection. A positive ELISA for HIV in a person with symptoms and/or laboratory studies suggestive of immunodeficiency does not require confirmation with a Western blot test. On the other hand, a person with antibody detected by ELISA in the absence of other evidence of infection should not be considered antibody positive until a confirmatory test is performed.

3.3.4. Evaluation of Patients according to Clinical States

Further evaluation of the patient with HIV infection will depend on the status of the patient's health. The patient who is asymptomatic and is normal on physical examination requires no further study but should be counseled (see Section 4) and advised to have periodic checkups and an evaluation if symptoms develop.

The patient with HIV infection and lymphadenopathy should be evaluated for other potential causes of the lymphadenopathy. Syphilis is always a consideration in sexually active adults. In some populations, disseminated tuberculosis involving lymph nodes may develop in advance of other infectious complications. These patients are typically febrile and complain of night sweats, fatigue, and malaise. Other infectious causes are encountered less frequently, but may be suggested by a history of travel, specific exposure to a known agent, or the past medical history. Lymphomas and Kaposi's sarcoma may initially present as lymphadenopathy, and striking adenopathy in one group of nodes is an indication for biopsy. The patient with generalized lymphadenopathy in the absence of other symptoms may be followed periodically without biopsy once the initial evaluation has been completed.

Some patients with HIV infection present with a number of symptoms and abnor-

Table IV. Symptoms of AIDS-Related Complex (Prodromal Symptoms)

1.	Generalized lymphadenopathy
2.	Uninduced weight loss
3.	Chronic diarrhea not attributed to a specific pathogen
4.	Oral candidiasis
5.	Chronic fever
6.	Night sweats
7.	Chronic fatigue

malities indicative of marked immunodeficiency with potential for complications but do not satisfy the criteria for a diagnosis of AIDS. The term AIDS-related complex (ARC) has been used to describe the abnormalities shown in Table IV. The patient who has symptoms and signs consistent with a diagnosis of ARC may be quite ill and in imminent risk of developing a severe opportunistic infection. Because ARC is a poorly defined diagnosis, it includes persons who are relatively healthy, as well as persons with multiple problems and an immunodeficiency as pronounced as if AIDS were present. These patients need a thorough evaluation and investigation of any complaints or abnormalities suggestive of an evolving infection. Fever, chronic cough, and diarrhea with progressive weight loss are complaints that particularly warrant an investigation to determine their etiology since these are frequently caused by specific infectious agents. In the absence of specific infections these patients should be followed closely and advised to report any new symptoms promptly. Most opportunistic infections are more easily controlled if treatment is instituted early than if begun after the infection is severe or the patient is in poor condition.

4. COUNSELING PATIENTS

Counseling patients with HIV infection is an integral part of their management. It should encompass two subjects: precautions for the prevention of transmission of HIV to others and the implications of the diagnosis for the patient's life.

4.1. Prognosis

The prognostic implications of HIV infection will depend on the stage of the patient's infection. A diagnosis of AIDS carries a grave prognosis, and at the time of this writing it must be considered a fatal disease that will run its course within 2–3 years in all but an occasional patient. If the diagnosis is based on Kaposi's sarcoma alone, the prognosis is better than if it is based on an opportunistic infection. The drug zidovudine clearly improves survival of persons with AIDS and ARC over 6 months[11] to 1 year, and it is possible that it may prolong survival indefinitely. Until the long-term effects of zidovudine are known, however, its potential benefits must be described cautiously.

Counseling a patient about his or her prognosis should be individualized, but it must provide the facts necessary for the patient to cope intelligently with the infection. The majority of patients will be aware of the fatal nature of AIDS, and many will be fearful, anxious to the point of panic, and depressed. Some may be unable to function because of anxiety and depression, and formal psychiatric consultation may be needed. The diagnosis and prognosis must be discussed with great care to assure the patient is fully informed yet not left without hope. Persons with asymptomatic HIV infection or lymphadenopathy alone are not necessarily going to develop AIDS. Persons with AIDS may enjoy many months of good health. However, patients with AIDS and also those with ARC should be alerted to the importance of symptoms that may be early indications of new infections. Fever, respiratory tract complaints, headaches, diarrhea, and other new symptoms should be mentioned to their physician. Practically speaking, timely recognition of a new infection is frequently difficult. The onset is often insidious, and the presence of chronic, preexistent symptoms may obscure those caused by a new infection. Both the patient and the physician should realize this and be alert for subtle changes.

Patients with AIDS should be told that because of the unpredictable nature of their disease, they should put their personal affairs in order at the earliest convenient time. This might include writing a will, completing unfinished business matters, making arrangements for stopping work, clarifying insurance benefits, and informing family and close friends of their disease. A diagnosis of AIDS qualifies an eligible person for social security benefits. Because of inescapable delays that attend the start of social security benefits, application should be made as soon as a diagnosis is established. Other benefits may be available. If local support groups have been formed, the patient should be referred to them. These groups may be very helpful to a newly diagnosed patient. Many persons with AIDS are in relatively good condition and physically able to continue to work. They should be encouraged to do so since continued activity is often psychologically and physically beneficial. The prognosis for persons with asymptomatic HIV infection and those with chornic lymphadenopathy is not clear at the present time. The incubation period, defined as the time from infection to the onset of AIDS, is greater than 5 years for some. An analysis of data accumulated from studies of transfusion-related infections estimates that the mean time to onset of AIDS is 1.97 years for children less than 5 years of age, 7.97 years for persons 5 to 59 years of age, and 5.5 years for persons 60 years or older.[49] It is clear that more experience will be needed before the natural history of HIV infection is fully defined. It is likely that a larger proportion will develop AIDS over a longer period.

4.2. Precautions

All infected patients must be informed that their infection is probably lifelong and that they are potentially infectious for other persons. The potential routes of transmission should be discussed and appropriate precautions advised. Obviously, they should refrain from donating blood, plasma, sperm, or other body tissues or fluids. If the person uses intravenous drugs, he or she should not share needles or syringes with other drug users.

Sexual intercourse must be identified as a major mode of transmission. Total abstinence is the only absolutely safe method to avoid acquiring sexually transmitted diseases, including HIV. If abstinence is not possible, so called "safe sex" practices should be adopted. Safe sex is defined as sexual contact without transfer of body fluids. Safe sex may be a misnomer, however, and patients must realize that elimination of all risk cannot be assured. Barrier contraceptives (condoms) may offer some protection, but foam, spermicidal jellies, and diaphragms are unlikely to reliably diminish risk of infection. Condoms have been widely recommended. Experimentally they have been shown to be impervious to other viruses,[50,51] but condoms may tear, slip, or leak, and patients should know that they do not provide absolute protection. The threat attendant upon kissing appears to be insignificant, but passage of saliva should be prevented. Implements that could be contaminated with blood, e. g., toothbrushes and razors, should not be shared. Surfaces or objects contaminated with blood or other body fluids should be carefully cleaned. Household bleach freshly diluted with 10 parts water to one part bleach is highly active against HIV, inexpensive, and readily available. Implements that have punctured skin should be sterilized before reuse or safely discarded in a manner that will avoid injury to those disposing of waste. Patients who seek medical or dental attention should notify the professional of their infection before care is given. Finally, they should notify those persons with whom they have had sexual contact in the recent past of their infection.

Contact that does not involve transfer of body secretions or blood (casual contact) is not associated with transmission of infection but is often of great concern to friends and family as well as patients. It is appropriate to assure them that daily casual contact with a person with HIV infection does not represent a threat to the noninfected. It is prudent for infected persons to avoid kissing if saliva may be transferred, and they should not share food or dining utensils that have been contaminated with saliva. On the other hand, a separate set of dishes for the infected person is not necessary, provided dishes are thoroughly washed in hot soapy water after use, nor is it necessary to launder the patient's clothing separately. Good hygienic practices based on common sense and recognition of the known routes of HIV transmission will avoid virtually all potential threats of infection.

If the patient and his or her family are carefully advised, unnecessary isolation of the patient can be avoided without compromising safety. Many irrational fears and concerns can be dispelled by counseling. Because AIDS is a difficult disease in all aspects, unnecessary precautions waste valuable resources and should be avoided whenever possible.

4.3. Measures to Maintain Health

Patients often want to know what they can do to maintain their health and avoid infections. There are many hypotheses about the value of high-dose vitamin intake, selected diets, and a variety of folk remedies. These are to be expected with any disease that is incurable. Unfortunately, there are few data to support most of the dietary and vitamin theories, and the patients need to know that virtually all of them are unproven therapies. Some may be harmful, and most entail expense or discomfort.

The patients can be told that good nutrition is important, and that they should make a special effort to eat a balanced diet. A one-a-day multivitamin is reasonable, though of unproven value. Because alcohol and some recreational drugs are known to depress cellular immunity, their use should be avoided. On the other hand, it is unlikely that an occasional alcoholic beverage has any significant effect.

Patients not infrequently express concern about exposure to infections they may incur by visiting friends, walking in crowds, dining in public restaurants, or attending movies. They should be assured that it is unlikely that appearing in public represents any risk to their health since most agents that cause disease in patients with AIDS are ubiquitous and cannot be specifically avoided. In fact, most disease probably represents activation of latent infection. On the other hand, some activity probably should be avoided. For example, travel to an underdeveloped area where sanitation is poor and the risk of acquiring an infection high would not be appropriate. Exploring caves in which *Histoplasma capsulatum* might be encountered would be unwise. Eating uncooked meat probably carries some risk and should be avoided.

Patients often raise questions about the potential risk animals represent as a source of opportunistic pathogens. Although certain pathogens may be acquired from animals—*T. gondii* from cats, *Salmonella* species from turtles, and *Cryptosporidia* from farm livestock, for example—there are no data to suggest that domestic pets, particularly if they have been with the patient prior to the diagnosis of HIV infection, represent a significant risk. Intense exposure to large numbers of cats, birds, swine, or cattle, as occurs with the activities of a veterinarian, abattoir worker, or farmer, theoretically represents some risk, and the patients should be so advised.

Physical activity to maintain good conditioning is appropriate if the patient is able to perform it. The psychological benefits probably equal the physical benefit of exercise.

Zidovudine is now the only drug with proven benefit in the treatment of AIDS and ARC. Although this drug is toxic,[12] does not fully or permanently reverse the immunologic abnormalities or erradicate the virus, and does not prevent the onset of opportunistic infections, it does prolong survival and improve the well-being of most patients.[11] It should be offered to patients who have symptoms suggestive of ARC and less than 200 T helper cells (the currently approved indications for the drug).

Patients should be warned about attempting to treat themselves with unproven drugs. These are typically expensive, potentially harmful, and, at best, of doubtful value. However, since some patients will pursue these self-treatments regardless of medical advice, they should be gently admonished and encouraged to fully divulge which medication they administer so appropriate care can be provided.

5. COUNSELING PERSONS AT RISK FOR HIV INFECTION

It now appears that all sexually active persons who have intercourse with multiple partners (or a single partner who has other sexual contacts), regardless of their sexual preference, are at some risk for acquiring HIV infection. The risk is undoubtedly small for most heterosexual persons, but real. HIV infection is a sexually transmitted disease that can be acquired, just as syphilis, herpes, or gonorrhea is acquired. Before becoming sexually involved with a new acquaintance, persons should inquire about the acquaintance's background and past sexual activity. Although the safety provided by use of condoms should not be considered to be absolute, their use should be the rule.

Homosexual men and sexual partners of persons in a high-risk group are at great risk for infection. Simply limiting sexual contact to a few men is not adequate at a time when HIV infection may be present in the majority of homosexual men. Homosexual men need to be informed of their risk and given the advice about sexual activity noted earlier.

Patients often ask about being tested for the presence of antibody. The implications of a positive test are great, and an asymptomatic person should be tested only if he or she fully understands these implications. For instance, he or she may be refused employment or insurance on the basis of a positive test. Absolute confidentiality is difficult to achieve, and the results may become known to family or aquaintances the patient would not want to inform. Alternative test sites are available in many large metropolitan areas that provide antibody testing at a reasonable charge with confidentiality guaranteed by use of identifier codes only. The patient obtains the results only when he or she gives the site the identifer code. Names are never revealed. If the test is requested only out of curiosity, it should not be ordered. On the other hand, if the patient is going to make decisions and changes based on whether or not he or she has HIV antibody, it is appropriate to perform it. The physician who orders the test must be prepared to discuss the results in detail. The physician should also be prepared to deal with an emotionally overwrought patient if the result is positive.

6. PRECAUTIONS FOR HEALTH CARE WORKERS

As noted earlier, the risk that HIV infection poses to health care workers is negligible. Extensive guidelines for protective precautions have been periodically published by the public health service,[52–58] and adherence to these guidelines should eliminate any risk. The basic precautions are those used for the management of patients with hepatitis B. Fortunately, the risk of transmission of HIV is much less than for hepatitis B. The guidelines appropriate to a doctor's office are shown in Table V. The only significant danger to a health care worker would be an accident in which a patient's blood or infected body fluid is introduced into an open wound or actually inoculated. Thus, of equal importance to the precautions is the need for good technique whenever an invasive procedure is performed on the patient or infected material is handled. For example, it is inappropriate to allow an inexperienced phlebotomist to draw blood from infected patients until the phlebotomist has demonstrated proficiency in his or her work.

Table V. Precautions to Prevent Acquisition of HIV Infection by Staff in a Doctor's Office

1. Handle all sharp items (needles, scalpel blades) as potentially infective.
2. Disposable sharp items should be placed into puncture-resistant containers at the work site immediately after use.
3. Do not recap contaminated needles before disposal.
4. If the possibility of exposure to blood or other body fluids exists, appropriate precautions should be employed:
   Gloves alone for handling contaminated specimens or equipment
   Gowns, masks, and eye coverings if splatter or aerosolization may occur
5. Have available ventilation devices for use in place of emergency mouth-to-mouth resuscitation.
6. Educate staff at regular intervals about protective precautions.
7. Dispose of contaminated waste in accordance with local regulations.

A health care worker who is infected but otherwise healthy should be able to safely work with patients,[58] unless the worker has open cuts or dermatitis that might lead to the patient coming into contact with the worker's blood or serum. An infected health care worker probably should not be involved in the performance of invasive procedures in which minor trauma to the worker might readily lead to a significant exposure for the patient.

REFERENCES

1. Gottlieb, M. S., Schroff, R., Schauker, H. M., *et al.*: *Pneumocystis carinii* pneumonia and mucosal candidiasis in previously healthy homosexual men: Evidence of a new acquired cellular immunodeficiency. *N. Engl. J. Med* **305:**1425–1431, 1981.
2. Masur, H., Michelis, M. A., Greene, J. B., *et al.*: An outbreak of community-acquired *Pneumocystis carinii* pneumonia: Initial manifestations of cellular immune dysfunction. *N. Engl. J. Med.* **305:**1431–1438, 1981.
3. Siegal, F. P., Lopez, C., Hammer, G. S., *et al:* Severe acquired immunodeficiency in male homosexuals, manifested by chronic peri and ulcerative herpes simplex lesions. *N. Engl. J. Med.* **305:**1439–1444, 1981.
4. Curran, J. W.: The epidemiology and prevention of the acquired immunodeficiency syndrome. *Ann. Intern. Med.* **103:**657–662, 1985.
5. Feorino, R. M., Jaffe, H.W., Palmer, E., *et al.*: Transfusion-associated acquired immunodeficiency syndrome: Evidence for persistent infection in blood donors. *N. Engl. J. Med.* **312:**1293–1296, 1985.
6. Jaffe, H. W., Darrow, W. W., Echenberg, D. F., *et al.*: The acquired immunodeficiency syndrome in a cohort of homosexual men: A 6-year follow-up study. *Ann. Intern. Med.* **103:**210–214, 1985.
7. Goldert, J. J., Biggar, R. J., Weiss, S. H., *et al.*: Three year incidence of AIDS in five cohorts of HTLV-III infected risk group members. *Science* **231:**992–995, 1986.
8. Eyster, M. E., Gordert, J. J., Sarngadharan, M. G., *et al.*: Development and early natural history of HTLV-III antibodies in persons with hemophilia. *JAMA* **253:**2219–2223, 1985.
9. Melbye, M., Biggar, R. J., Ebbesen, P., *et al.*: Long-term seropositivity for human T-lymphotrophic virus type III in homosexual men without the acquired immunodeficiency syndrome's development of immunologic and clinical abnormalities. *Ann. Intern. Med.* **104:**496–500, 1986.
10. Curran, J. W., Morgan, W. M., Hardy, A. M., *et al.*: The epidemiology of AIDS: Current status and future prospects. *Science* **229:**1351–1357, 1985.
11. Fischl, M. A., Richman, D. D., Grieco, M. H., *et al.*: The efficacy of azidothymidine (AZT) in the treatment of patients with AIDS and AIDS related complex. A double-blind, placebo controlled trial. *N. Engl. J. Med* **317:**(4):185–191, 1987.
12. Richman, D. D., Fischl, M. A., Grieco, M. H., *et al.*: The toxicity of azidothymidine (AZT) in the treatment of patients with AIDS and AIDS related complex. *N. Engl. J. Med.* **317:**(4):192–197, 1982.
13. Jaffe, H. W., Choi, K., Thomas, F. A., *et al.*: National case control study of Kaposi's sarcoma and *Pneumocystis carinii* pneumonia in homosexual men: Part 1, Epidemiologic results. *Ann. Intern. Med.* **99:**145–151, 1983.
14. Goldert, J. J., Sarngadharan, M. G., Biggar, R. J., *et al.*: Determinants of retrovirus (HTLV-III) antibody and immunodeficiency conditions in homosexual men. *Lancet* **2:**711–716, 1984.
15. Marmor, M., Friedman-kein, A. E., Zolla-Pazner, S., *et al.*: Kaposi's sarcoma in homosexual men: A seroepidemic case control study. *Ann. Intern. Med.* **100:**809–815, 1984.
16. Groopman, J. E., Mayer, K. H., Sarngadharan, M. G., *et al.*: Seroepidemiology of human T-lymphotrophic virus type III among homosexual men with the acquired immunodeficiency syndrome or generalized lymphadenopathy and among asymptomatic controls in Boston. *Ann. Intern. Med.* **102:**334–337, 1985.
17. Melbye, M., Biggar, R. J., Ebbesen, R., *et al.*: Seroepidemiology of HTLV-III antibody in Danish homosexual men: Prevalence, transmission, and disease outcome. *Br. Med. J. (Clin. Res.)* **289:**573–575, 1984.
18. Melbye, M.: The natural history of human T lymphotrophic virus infection: The cause of AIDS. *Br. Med. J.* **292:**5–12, 1986.
19. Clameck, N., Sonnet, J., Taelman, H., *et al.*: Acquired immunodeficiency syndrome in African patients. *N. Engl. J. Med.* **310:**492–497, 1984.

20. Collaborative Study Group of AIDS in Haitian Americans: Risk factors for the acquired immunodeficiency syndrome (AIDS) among Haitians residing in the United States: Evidence of heterosexual transmission. *JAMA* **257**:635–639, 1986.
21. Fischl, M., Dickinson, G. M., Scott, G., *et al.*: Heterosexual and household transmission of the human T-lymphotrophic virus type III. International Conference on AIDS (Communication 175:S22C). Paris, France. June 23–25, 1986.
22. Redfield, R. R., Markham, P. D., Salahuddin, S. Z., *et al.*: Frequent transmission of HTLV-III among spouses of patients with AIDS-related complex and AIDS. *JAMA* **253**:1571–1573, 1985.
23. Friedland, G. H., Saltzman, B. R., Rogers, M. F., *et al.*: Lack of transmission of HTLV-III/LAV infection to household contacts of patients with AIDS or AIDS-related complex with oral candidiasis. *N. Engl. J. Med.* **314**:344–349, 1986.
24. Centers for Disease Control: Apparent transmission of human T-lymphotrophic virus type III/lymphadenopathy-associated virus from a child to a mother providing health care. *Morbid. Mortal. Wkly. Rep.* **35**:76–79, 1986.
25. Anonymous: Needlestick transmission of HTLV-III from a patient in Africa. *Lancet* **2**:1376–1377, 1984.
26. McCray, E.: The cooperative needlestick surveillance group. Occupational risk of the acquired immunodeficiency syndrome among health care workers. *N. Engl. J. Med.* **314**:1127–1132, 1986.
27. Stricof, R. L., and Morse, D. L.: HTLV-III/LAV seroconversion following a deep intramuscular needlestick injury. *N. Engl. J. Med.* **314**:1115, 1986.
28. Oksenhendler, E., Harzic, M., Le Roux, J. M., *et al.*: HIV infection with seroconversion after a superficial needlestick injury to the finger. *N. Engl. J. Med.* **315**:582, 1986.
29. Centers for Disease Control: Update: Human immunodeficiency virus infections in health-care workers exposed to blood of infected patients. *Morbid. Mortal. Wkly. Rep.* **36**:285–289, 1987.
30. Hirsch, M. S., Wormser, G. P., Schooley, R. T., *et al.*: Risk of nosocomial infection with human T-cell lymphotrophic virus III (HTLV-III). *N. Engl. J. Med.* **312**:1–4, 1985.
31. Update: Evaluation of human T-lymphotrophic virus type III/lymphadenopathy-associated virus infection in health care personnel—United States. *Morbid. Mortal. Wkly. Rep.* **34**:575–578, 1985.
32. Weiss, S. H., Saxinger, W. C., Rechtman, D., *et al.*: HTLV-III infection among health care workers: Association with needlestick injuries. *JAMA* **254**:2089–2093, 1983.
33. Schupbach, J., Popovic, M., Gildan, R. V., *et al.*: Serological analysis of a subgroup of human T-lymphotrophic retroviruses (HTLV-III) associated with AIDS. *Science* **224**(4648):503–505, 1984.
34. Gerberding, J. L., Hopewell, P. C., Kaminsky, L. S., and Sande, M. A.: Transmission of hepatitus B without transmission of AIDS by accidental needlestick. *N. Engl. J. Med.* **312**:56, 1985.
35. Glaser, J. B., Garden, A.: Inoculation of cryptococcosis without transmission of the acquired immunodeficiency syndrome. *N. Engl. J. Med.* **313**:266, 1985.
36. Centers for Disease Control: Update on acquired immune deficiency syndrome (AIDS)—United States. *Morbid. Mortal. Wkly. Rep.* **31**:507–514, 1982.
37. Centers for Disease Control: Revision of the case definition of acquired immunodeficiency syndrome for national reporting—United States. *Morbid. Mortal. Wkly. Rep.* **34**:373–375, 1985.
38. Gallo, R. C., Salahudden, S. Z., Popovic, M., *et al.*: Frequent detection and isolation of cytopathic retroviruses (HTLV-III) from patients with AIDS and at risk for AIDS. *Science* **224**:500–503, 1984.
39. Haverkos, H. W., Gottlieb, M. S., Killen, J. Y., and Edelman, R.: Classification of HTLV-III/LAV-related diseases (Letter). *J. Infect. Dis.* **152**:1095, 1985.
40. Redfield, R. R., Wright, D. C., and Tramont, E. C.: The Walter Reed staging classification for HTLV-III/LAV infection. *N. Engl. J. Med.* **314**:131–132, 1986.
41. Centers for Disease Control: Classification system for human T-lymphotrophic virus type III/Lymphadenopathy-associated virus infections. *Ann. Intern. Med.* **105**:234–237, 1986.
42. Barre-Sinoussi, F., Chermann, J. C., Rey, F., *et al.*: Isolation of a T-lymphotrophic retrovirus from a patient at risk for acquired immune deficiency syndrome (AIDS). *Science* **220**:868–871, 1983.
43. Barin, F., McLane, M. F., Allan, J. S., *et al.*: Virus envelope protein of HTLV-III represents major target antigen for antibodies in AIDS patients. *Science* **228**:1094–1096, 1985.
44. Levy, J. A., Hoffman, A. D., Kramer, S. M., *et al.*: Isolation of lymphocytopathic retrovirus from San Francisco patients with AIDS. *Science* **225**:840–842, 1984.
45. Sarngadharan, M. G., Popovic, M., Bruch, L., *et al.*: Antibodies reactive with human T-lymphotrophic retrovirus (HTLV-III) in the serum of patients with AIDS. *Science* **224**:506–508, 1984.

46. Weiss, S. H., Goedert, J. J., Sarngadharan, M. G., *et al.* Screening test for HTLV-III (AIDS agent) antibodies. *JAMA* **253**:221–225, 1985.
47. Centers for Disease Control: Results of human T-lymphotrophic virus type III test kits reported from blood collection centers—United States, April 22–May 19, 1985. *Morbid. Mortal. Wkly. Rep.* **34**:375–376, 1985.
48. Ward, J. W., Grindon, A. J., Feorino, P. M., *et al.*: Laboratory and epidemiologic evaluation of an enzyme immunoassay for antibodies to HTLV-III. *JAMA* **256**:357–361, 1986.
49. Medley, G. F., Anderson, R. M., Cox, D. R., and Billard, L.: Incubation period of AIDS in patients infected via blood transfusion. *Nature* **328**:719–721, 1987.
50. Conant, M. A., Spicer, D. W., and Smith, C. D.: Herpes simplex virus transmission: Condom studies. *Sexually Transmitted Diseases* **11**(2):94–95, 1984.
51. Katznelson, S., Drew, W. L., and Mintz, L.: Efficacy of the condom as a barrier to the transmission of cytomegalovirus. *J. Infect. Dis.* **150**:155–157, 1984.
52. Centers for Disease Control: Acquired immune deficiency syndrome (AIDS): Precautions for clinical and laboratory staffs. *Morbid. Mortal. Wkly. Rep.* **31**:577–580, 1982.
53. Centers for Disease Control: Acquired immunodeficiency syndrome (AIDS): Precautions for health care workers and allied professionals. *Morbid. Mortal. Wkly. Rep.* **32**:450–452, 1983.
54. Centers for Disease Control: Recommendations for preventing possible transmission of human T-lymphotropic virus type III/Lymphadenopathy-associated virus from tears. *Morbid. Mortal. Wkly. Rep.* **34**:533–534, 1985.
55. Centers for Disease Control: Recommendations for preventing transmission of infection with human T-lymphotropic virus III/Lymphadenopathy-associated virus in the workplace. *Morbid. Mortal. Wkly. Rep.* **34**:681–686, 691–696, 1985.
56. Centers for Disease Control: Recommendations for preventing transmission of infection with human T-lymphotropic virus type III/Lymphadenopathy-associated virus during invasive procedures. *Morbid. Mortal. Wkly. Rep.* **35**:221–223, 1986.
57. Centers for Disease Control: Recommended infection-control practices for dentistry. *Morbid. Mortal. Wkly. Rep.* **35**:237–242, 1986.
58. Centers for Disease Control: Recommendation for prevention of HIV transmission in health-care settings. *Morbid. Mortal. Wkly. Rep.* **36**:(25):35–185, 1987.

11

Coronary Artery Disease

Arthur M. Fournier

1. INTRODUCTION

Although there has been a steady decline in the incidence of coronary artery disease over the past two decades, it is still the most common cause of death in this country. Almost one million deaths occurred in 1980 due to heart and blood vessel disease. Of these, 350,000 were sudden deaths. One million patients had a myocardial infarction and 3.4 million suffer from chronic atherosclerotic heart disease. The estimated cost of caring for this disease is 57 billion dollars.

The decline in coronary artery disease recently is striking. The age-adjusted cardiovascular death rate fell by 31% in the decade that ended in 1980 and appears to be continuing to fall. The rate of decline in cardiovascular death rates is twice that of all other causes. This decline in coronary artery disease mortality has been attributed to the following reasons:

1. Reductions in populations levels of hypertension and cigarette smoking and dietary intake of cholesterol.[1]
2. Improved medical care after the onset of clinical atherosclerotic disease.

Evidence points to the first reason as being the one responsible for the greater reduction in cardiovascular mortality rates. Death rates from sudden death have fallen to a much greater degree than those for acute myocardial infarction.[2] This implies that primary as opposed to secondary intervention has had the greatest impact. Most of the efforts in primary prevention have occurred at the level of public health policy and strategies and not in physicians' offices.[3] The initial lead in public policy came at the initiative of cardiologists and cardiovascular researchers with the publication of *Statement on Arteriosclerosis, the Main Cause of Heart Attacks and Strokes,* which was published as a brochure in 1959. This brochure was distributed widely and called attention to hypertension, hypercholesterolemia, cigarette smoking, obesity, and a positive family history as contributing factors to atherosclerotic disease. In 1960 the American Heart Association issued its first statement on cigarette smoking and cardiovascular disease. A year later the

Arthur M. Fournier • Department of Medicine, University of Miami School of Medicine, Miami, Florida 33101.

same organization implicated dietary intake of cholesterol and saturated fat in the pathogenesis of atherosclerotic heart disease. In 1964 the famous *Report of the Advisory Committee to the Surgeon General on Smoking and Health*[4] marked the first involvement of the federal government in an effort to prevent coronary heart disease. More and more reduction of cardiovascular mortality has become federal policy. In 1973 the Secretary of Health, Education, and Welfare launched a major effort directed at hypertension. These changes in public policy seem to a certain extent to have captured the popular imagination and lead to a positive change in lifestyles, at least with regard to cigarette smoking, dietary intake of cholesterol, blood pressure identification and treatment, and abandonment of a sedentary lifestyle.[5]

The kind of primary prevention that occurs in physicians' offices is known as case identification and risk factor modification. This sort of primary preventive approach has been underdeveloped compared to the public health policy approach just outlined. As a generalization, physicians have tended to emphasize secondary prevention or acute medical management. What timely primary prevention has been advocated has centered mainly on medication treatment for lipid disorders and hypertension. This pattern of behavior is reinforced by reimbursement patterns that compensate for acute care, but not for preventive health measures.

A much better job of primary prevention in physicians' offices could be achieved if the epidemiological principle of "risk factors" were modified and used in a preventive health philosophy applied to the individual patient.[5]

The remainder of this chapter outlines the "risk factor" concept and details the preventive strategies that may be applied to the physician's practices.

2. *RISK FACTORS FOR CORONARY ARTERY DISEASE*

The "cause" of atherosclerosis is still unknown. In 1961 the Framingham Study introduced the concept of risk factors for the development of coronary artery disease.[6] This concept was based on the observation that no one factor could be identified as the cause of atherosclerotic heart disease but that a statistical correlation with cardiovascular risk existed for several clinical and laboratory features. Risk factors currently mean different things to different people. A risk factor may represent only a statistical correlation, such as finding that ear-lobe creases correlate with coronary artery disease,[7] or it may reflect a predisposition to the disease or, occasionally, a causal relationship. A risk factor is a characteristic of a person (demographic, psychological, anatomical, or physiological) that increases the likelihood of that person developing coronary artery disease. Criteria for risk factors include the following:

1. The association must be consistent.
2. The association must be strong.
3. There must be biological plausibility.
4. A temporal relationship between the risk factor and the disease must be present.
5. There may be a dose–response gradient.[8]

Ideally, a risk factor should imply the potential for intervention. Thus, although advancing age, male sex, and a positive family history have been shown to have a statistical correlation with coronary artery disease, we shall spend little time discussing them, since they are not modifiable. Modifiable risk factors include:

1. Cigarette smoking
2. Hypertension
3. Diabetes
4. Serum lipids
5. Obesity

For the most part these risk factors can be quantitated by epidemiological studies[9] and a relative risk determined (see Table I for an example of how this can be done). In the following sections we shall discuss each potentially modifiable risk factor in more detail. These classical risk factors have been recognized since the Framingham study. It is important to remember, however, that the Framingham study could explain only one-half of cardiovascular risk by the risk factors they identified. New risk factors may yet be identified, and important mechanisms in the pathogenesis of atherosclerosis still need to be elucidated.

2.1. Cigarette Smoking

The risk for coronary artery disease associated with cigarette smoking is more closely related to the number of cigarettes smoked per day than the duration of the habit. The effect is probably reversible, since individuals who quit smoking have only half the risk for myocardial infarction of those who continue to smoke. Several mechanisms by which cigarette smoking can accelerate atherogenesis and provoke myocardial infarction have been proposed. Two major noxious agents are nicotine and carbon monoxide. Nicotine stimulates catecholamine release, increases myocardial irritability and heart rate, and causes vascular constriction. It also increases platelet aggregability. Concomitantly, carbon monoxide buildup reduces the oxygen available to the myocardium.[10]

One can conceptualize cigarette smoking as a risk factor that will operate most forcibly in persons with an already compromised circulation, favoring sudden thrombosis, coronary spasm, or occlusion of the circulation to the heart and promoting potentially lethal arrhythmias. At any given level of coronary artery atherosclerosis cigarette smoking promotes more myocardial infarctions and more sudden deaths. The risk of cigarette smoking is most independent of the levels of other cardiovascular risk factors. Conversely, in populations with a low incidence of coronary heart disease there is little relationship between cigarette smoking and coronary heart disease mortality.

Cigarette smoking is therefore a major reversible contributor to cardiovascular morbidity and mortality. Statistically, the risk of cigarette smoking on cardiovascular mortality is less strong than its association with lung cancer and chronic pulmonary disease. Coronary artery disease is so much more prevalent an illness, however, that elimination of smoking would save more lives from coronary heart disease than it would from lung cancer.

Table I. Relative Risk of Developing Coronary Artery Disease in 4 Years according to Quantifiable Risk Factors (Women Aged 50–70 Years)[a]

	Systolic blood pressure 120 mm Hg							Systolic blood pressure 135 mm Hg						
LDL-C	100	120	140	160	180	200	220	100	120	140	160	180	200	220
HDL-C														
25	1.6	1.8	2.1	2.5	2.8	3.2	3.7	1.9	2.2	2.5	2.9	3.3	3.8	4.3
35	1.1	1.2	1.4	1.6	1.9	2.2	2.5	1.3	1.5	1.7	1.9	2.2	2.6	2.9
45	0.7	0.8	0.9	1.1	1.2	1.4	1.6	0.8	0.9	1.1	1.3	1.5	1.7	1.9
55	0.4	0.5	0.6	0.7	0.8	0.9	1.1	0.5	0.6	0.7	0.8	0.9	1.1	1.3
65	0.3	0.3	0.4	0.4	0.5	0.6	0.7	0.3	0.4	0.5	0.5	0.6	0.7	0.8
75	0.2	0.2	0.3	0.3	0.3	0.4	0.5	0.2	0.3	0.3	0.3	0.4	0.5	0.5
85	0.1	0.1	0.2	0.2	0.2	0.3	0.3	0.1	0.2	0.2	0.2	0.3	0.3	0.4

	Systolic blood pressure 150 mm Hg							Systolic blood pressure 165 mm Hg						
LDL-C	100	120	140	160	180	200	220	100	120	140	160	180	200	220
HDL-C														
25	2.3	2.6	3.0	3.4	3.9	4.5	5.1	2.7	3.1	3.6	4.1	4.6	5.2	5.9
35	1.5	1.7	2.0	2.3	2.6	3.1	3.5	1.8	2.1	2.4	2.7	3.1	3.6	4.1
45	1.0	1.1	1.3	1.5	1.8	2.0	2.3	1.2	1.4	1.6	1.8	2.1	2.4	2.8
55	0.6	0.7	0.8	1.0	1.2	1.3	1.5	0.8	0.9	1.0	1.2	1.4	1.6	1.8
65	0.4	0.5	0.6	0.6	0.7	0.9	1.0	0.5	0.6	0.7	0.8	0.9	1.1	1.2
75	0.3	0.3	0.4	0.4	0.5	0.6	0.6	0.3	0.4	0.4	0.5	0.6	0.7	0.8
85	0.2	0.2	0.2	0.3	0.3	0.4	0.4	0.2	0.2	0.3	0.3	0.4	0.4	0.5

	Systolic blood pressure 180 mm Hg							Systolic blood pressure 195 mm Hg						
LDL-C	100	120	140	160	180	200	220	100	120	140	160	180	200	220
HDL-C														
25	3.2	3.7	4.2	4.7	5.4	6.1	6.8	3.8	4.3	4.9	5.5	6.2	7.0	7.8
35	2.2	2.5	2.8	3.3	3.7	4.2	4.8	2.6	2.9	3.4	3.8	4.4	4.9	5.6
45	1.4	1.6	1.9	2.2	2.5	2.9	3.3	1.7	1.9	2.3	2.6	2.9	3.4	3.9
55	0.9	1.1	1.2	1.4	1.6	1.9	2.2	1.1	1.3	1.5	1.7	2.0	2.3	2.6
65	0.6	0.7	0.8	0.9	1.1	1.3	1.4	0.7	0.8	1.0	1.1	1.3	1.5	1.7
75	0.4	0.4	0.5	0.6	0.7	0.8	0.9	0.5	0.5	0.6	0.7	0.8	1.0	1.1
85	0.3	0.3	0.3	0.4	0.5	0.5	0.6	0.3	0.4	0.4	0.5	0.5	0.6	0.7

[a]LDL-C, low-density cholesterol; HDL-C, high-density cholesterol.

2.2. Hypertension

At any age and in both sexes the risk of heart attack and stroke is proportional to both systolic and diastolic blood pressure. The risk associated with hypertension varies widely depending on whether there is evidence for hypertensive heart disease at the time hypertension is discovered and according to the number of associated other risk factors.[11] As detailed in the following sections, the association between hypertension, diabetes, abnormal serium lipids, and obesity may be more than just statistical. Women are no less immune to the effects of hypertension than men are. The steady increase in the incidence of hypertension that is usually seen with age in both sexes in Western countries does not seem to be inevitable, since in some study populations rise in blood pressure with age is not seen at all. The impact of hypertension on cardiovascular risk does not decrease with advancing age. Cardiovascular mortality is three times greater in the hypertensive elderly compared to normotensive individuals of the same age. The elderly are particularly prone to systolic hypertension. The mechanisms for this variety of hypertension may be different from those of diastolic hypertension and our ability to treat it with currently available medication is limited. This does not negate the fact, however, that isolated systolic hypertension has clearly been shown to be associated with an increased risk for coronary heart disease.

Because of the high prevalence of systolic hypertension with advancing age it is not logical to accept the usual level of blood pressure in the elderly as "normal." In the case of both systolic and diastolic hypertension the ability to modify these risk factors is still somewhat controversial and will be dealth with in the appropriate section.[12,13]

2.3. Diabetes

Diabetes is a curious risk factor for coronary artery disease. It is not quantifiable in terms of either degree of hyperglycemia or duration of diabetes. Its presence implies a greater risk for women than men, and the risk appears to antedate the clinical onset of diabetes.[14] Diabetes is also highly correlated with the risk factors of abnormal lipids, hypertension, and obesity. However, multivariate analyses that take these other risk factors into account reveal that diabetes is itself an independent risk factor. The issue has been raised whether diabetes is causally related to atherogenesis or merely a statistical association. One group of authors has suggested that the gene for type II diabetes and the gene for accelerated atherogenesis may be closely linked on the same chromosome but not related causally.[15] An alternative hypothesis is that hyperinsulinemia and not hyperglycemia *per se* is the causally related risk factor. Patients with clinical diabetes would represent only the tip of the iceberg with a larger population at risk. This theory is attractive since there is also evidence relating hyperinsulinemia in the absence of hyperglycemia (a phenomenom known as "relative insulin resistance") to hypertension and lipid abnormalities. Thus, hyperinsulinemia may link diabetes mechanistically with hypertension, lipid disorders, and obesity.[16]

There is currently no evidence to indicate that treatment of diabetes when it is clinically apparent modifies cardiovascular risk. Although a multifactorial risk factor intervention program appears to be the most attractive alternative dealing with diabetes as a risk factor, there may be practical problems with this approach. Many of the drugs used in the treatment of hypertension and hyperlipidemia have untoward effects on diabetic patients. Therefore, in our section on preventive strategies we shall emphasize factors that will prevent or forestall clinical diabetes and perhaps hyperinsulinemia, rather than treatment of diabetes *per se*.

2.4. Lipid Abnormalities

As association between cholesterol and coronary artery disease was well established by the Framingham study and has been confirmed by clinical and interpopulation studies.

Recently the concept of lipid abnormalities as a risk for atherogenesis has been refined. Whereas previous theories focused on dietary intake of cholesterol and saturated fats, the current theory regards atherogenesis as an imbalance between intake and excretion of dietary cholesterol. Accordingly, low-density-lipoprotein (LDL) cholesterol represents the dietary intake of cholesterol packaged for transport in the blood, whereas high-density-lipoprotein (HDL) cholesterol, which is a much more hydrophilic and therefore soluble lipoprotein, is the body's way of packaging cholesterol for the excretion through the biliary system. Thus, the ratio of HDL to LDL cholesterol has shown to have an even greater predictive value of cardiovascular risk than simple cholesterol determinations.[17] Further refinements of lipid abnormalities involving HDL subfractions and apoprotein concentrations are currently being elucidated (i.e., HDL_2, HDL_3, and apoprotein subfactions), but these are of more value to the investigator trying to sort through the details of cholesterol metabolism than they are of practical value to the clinician caring for patients. As a general rule, the majority of HDL is in the form of HDL_2 and factors that increase HDL such as dietary modification and exercise increase the HDL_2 subfraction. The exception to this generality is alcohol, which increases total HDL but predominantly as the HDL_3 subfraction. Figures 1 and 2 show the magnitude of the effect of lipid abnormalities on cardiovascular risk. As mentioned earlier, lipid abnormalities are frequently seen in conjunction with diabetes, obesity, and hypertension.

2.5. Obesity

There is little argument that obesity promotes insulin resistance, increased insulin production, glucose intolerance, hypertension, and reduced HDL cholesterol. Until recently, there was debate as to whether obesity could qualify as an independent contributor to cardiovascular risk if all other established risk factors were taken into consideration.[18,19] These arguments become specious if obesity leads to insulin resistance and hyperinsulinemia, which in turn affects blood pressure and lipid concentrations, as mentioned earlier.

Although it is true that moderate obesity unaccompanied by any of the other risk factors carries little cardiovascular risk, few people gain weight without a worsening of associated atherogenic traits. This observation was made originally during the Fra-

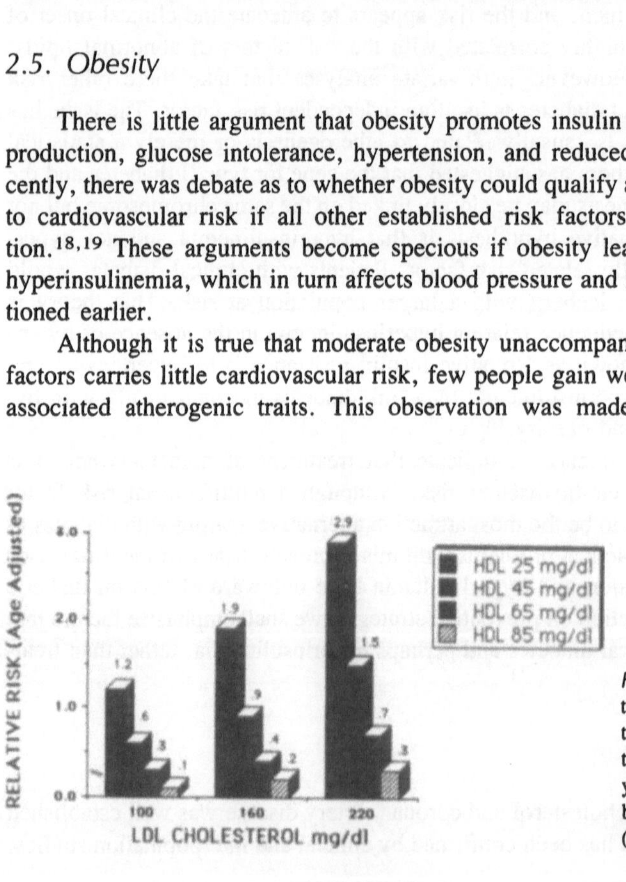

Figure 1. The interrelationship between LDL and HDL cholesterol in terms of relative risk for coronary artery disease in men aged 50–70 years—Framingham study systolic blood pressure of 135 mm Hg. (Source: Ref. 30.)

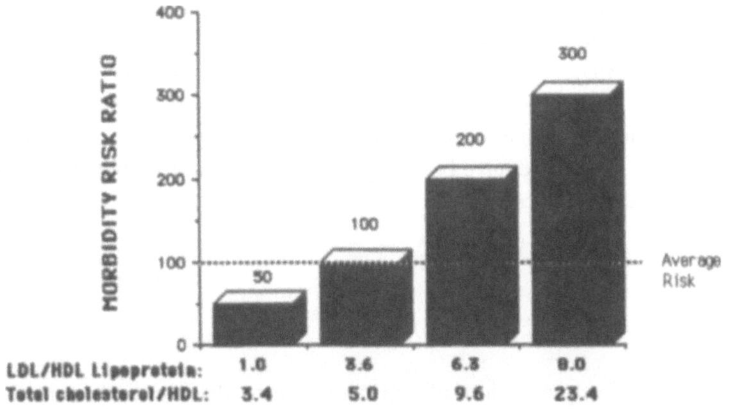

Figure 2. The impact of LDL/HDL or total cholesterol/HDL ratios on the 4-year relative risk for coronary heart disease in men aged 50–79 years. (Source: Adapted from the Framingham study.)

mingham study. Weight gain reduced the HDL-to-LDL ratio and tended to lead to hypertension and more diabetes. Conversely, weight loss is accompanied by a corresponding reduction in the levels of associated risk factors.

2.6. Other Potentially Modifiable Risk Factors

Several other risk factors for coronary artery disease have been proposed, but they are either difficult to modify or the association is not the same order of magnitude as the major risk factors we have already mentioned. These risk factors include personality type, sedentary lifestyle, and platelet abnormalities.

"Type A" personality is characterized by the following characteristics:

1. Striving for achievement
2. Easily provoked impatience
3. Time urgency
4. Abrupt gestures and speech
5. Excess drive and hostility

This coronary-prone personality ("striving without joy") has recently been challenged as a risk factor. It certainly seems a paradox that coronary artery disease is as frequent in occurrence in the lower and upper classes as it is in the middle class, whereas type A personality is predominantly a middle-class trait. In spite of recent criticism of the type A personality as a risk factor for coronary artery disease, there does seem to be evidence linking life satisfaction and stress to an increased risk for coronary artery disease.[20]

Evidence linking sedentary occupations and lifestyles to coronary risks is indirect. Controlled studies on the effect of exercise on lipids and other risk factors are lacking. It seems that the lack of daily exercise is an independent risk factor but of a lower order of magnitude than the other risk factors mentioned. If exercise is to be used as an intervention, it must be habitual, vigorous, and continuous. A controlled prospective trial of graded exercise as an intervention is clearly needed.[21]

Several of the major risk factors adversely influence platelet function. Platelet-induced thrombosis may well be the final event leading to sudden death or a myocardial infarction in a patient who has been undergoing degenerative atherogenic changes for years. However, to date there have been no studies demonstrating platelet abnormalities as a primary risk factor for coronary artery disease.[10]

3. RATIONALE FOR PREVENTION

The rationale for prevention of coronary artery disease is based on the epidemiological evidence mentioned earlier. Preventive strategies can be divided into two groups. Primary prevention is aimed at preventing or delaying the development of disease. Secondary prevention is aimed at limiting the morbidity and mortality of disease once it has become clinically apparent. As a generalization, the greatest benefit is gained by primary preventive strategies since they can be directed at large populations for relatively little cost. Public health policy is directed more toward primary prevention, whereas most clinicians deal to a large extent with secondary prevention. This is not meant to imply that primary prevention cannot be carried out in a physician's office. Much can be done on an individual basis for primary prevention, as discussed in the following section. One further paradox: although primary preventive strategies are simple and less costly, secondary preventive strategies are more easily reimbursed by insurance companies. It is impossible to avoid the conclusion that the yield in terms of decreased morbidity and mortality is much less utilizing secondary preventive strategies than if the equivalent amount of time and money were spent on primary prevention. Specifically with regard to coronary artery disease, the primary preventive measures are simple and not terribly expensive. Screening tests include blood pressure, blood sugar, HDL and LDL cholesterol determinations, and sequential weights. These tests should be included as a package in any general medical examination.

It should be clear from the discussion concerning risk factors that it would be foolish to focus on a single risk factor, but that rather all potentially modifiable risk factors should be addressed. In addition, individual physicians should go beyond "case finding" and support more general educational and public health programs. The most treatable risk factors are cigarette smoking, hypertension, and lipid abnormalities. More difficult to manage, but still potentially treatable risk factors include obesity and physical inactivity. Currently available strategies for modifying personality, ameliorating the risk associated with diabetes, or identifying and treating platelet or clotting abnormalities are in their infancy. Because so many risk factors are interrelated, however, treatment of one frequently has a beneficial effect on others. This positive feedback effect is helpful in encouraging patients to maintain the prescribed treatment regimen. The details of these treatment regimens are outlined in the next section.

Once coronary artery disease has become clinically apparent, the impact of addressing primary risk factors is markedly diminished.[3] The exception to this statement is stopping cigarette smoking, which has clear and immediate benefits even after patients have suffered myocardial infarction. For the most part, however, our discussion of strategies for secondary prevention will focus on the efficacy of noninvasive screening with specific regard to its ability to identify patients with high risk for reinfarction and sudden death and the use of medication to prevent recurrent infarction or death.

4. OFFICE STRATEGIES

4.1. Primary Prevention

The foundation of primary office prevention is patient education. The first way to teach patients about prevention is to set a good example. Physicians who continue to smoke, stay overweight, and lead sedentary lifestyles have a difficult time convincing their patients to do otherwise.

A risk factor analysis should be undertaken for each patient, followed in a continuity of care practice, and updated periodically. Risk factors should be divided into those that have been proven to be modifiable, those that are potentially modifiable, and those which, although they carry a risk, cannot be changed. Potentially modifiable risk factors include hypertension, cigarette smoking, and lipid abnormalities. Less modifiable risk factors are obesity, diabetes, and sedentary lifestyle. Age, sex, and family history are nonmodifiable. Major effort should be spent in correcting the risk factors that are most easily modifiable. However, nonmodifiable factors also need to be identified in order to accurately assess risk. A method for calculation of relative cardiovascular risk has been well publicized.[9] This method can easily be adapted to individual patients and followed from visit to visit by applying microcomputer technology. Programs are now being evolved that can be easily coupled with patinet self-assessment questionnaires to provide individualized quantification of risk and patient education.

Strategies for dealing with individual risk factors will be dealt with in more detail in Chapters 13, 22, and 23. However, our current understanding of the pathophysiologyof coronary artery disease (see Section 2) suggests that the greatest benefit could be achieved with two simple modifications:

1. Assisting patients who smoke cigarettes to quit.
2. Dietary modification that leads to a decrease in weight, a decrease in total cholesterol, and an increase in HDL-to-LDL cholesterol ratio. This dietary modification is particularly important given the links that have been established between obesity, lipid abnormalities, diabetes, and hypertension.[22]

The only pharmacological agent that has been shown to be efficacious for primary prevention in a large, randomized double-blind study is cholestyramine. This drug binds cholesterol in the gastrointestinal tract and hastens its excretion, thereby lowering total and LDL cholesterol. The population studied was a large cohort of middle-aged men with hypercholesterolemia and a type II hyperlipoprotein lipid profile. Expense, poor taste, and frequent dose requirements limit the applicability of this treatment modality.[23]

4.2. Secondary Prevention

Coronary artery disease can present clinically as either angina pectoris, myocardial infarction, or sudden death. With regard to coronary artery disease, anatomy is destiny. That is, mortality depends more on the coronary artery or arteries involved than the clinical presentation. Left main coronary artery disease has a much higher mortality for each clinical presentation than the other types of coronary artery disease. Moreover, the mortality of patients with left main disease who present as angina pectoris (commonly thought of as a more benigh disease than myocardial infarction) is greater than the mortality of patients presenting with myocardial infarction with less strategic vessels involved. Therefore, secondary prevention is aimed at decreasing overall morbidity and mortality and also identifying patients with left main disease.[24] Achievement of these goals requires a combination of diagnostic tests and appropriate medical and occasionally surgical therapy.

There is a great need for noninvasive tests with high sensitivity and specificity for presence of both coronary artery disease and, in particular, disease of the left main coronary artery. Even this theoretically "ideal" test would have little predictive value unless clinical judgment is exercised with regard to who is tested and who is not (see Chapter 3). Conventional exercise testing lacks the predictive value necessary to be applied as a broad screening test prior to cardiac catheterization.[22] Two diagnostic modalities are currently being evaluated to fill this need. The first is thallium imaging and the second 24-hr ambulatory monitoring, not for arrhythmias, but for ST-segment and T-wave abnormalities. The latter technology is still in the developmental stages. Enough experience has been derived from thallium stress testing so that patients who undergo this procedure and show a defect in the anterior distribution should be treated much more aggressively with regard to catheterization and possible surgery than patients in whom the defect is shown in the inferior or posterior views. Although thallium imaging coupled with stress testing seems to be an advance over conventional exercise testing, it still cannot be applied as a mass screening test in asymptomatic populations because of its expense and because of the fact that even relatively specific tests lack predictive value when applied to populations in which the pretest incidence of disease is relatively low.

The predictive value of "ministress" testing after myocardial infarction with regard to predicting recurrent infarction or sudden death is currently being evaluated. The statistical associations derived from these evaluations are frequently difficult to apply to individuals. At this point there is no clear consensus among cardiologists as to how to use this test as a practical guide to secondary prevention. Its greatest usefulness may be as a guide to post-myocardial infarction rehabilitation.

A variety of therapeutic interventions have been evaluated as secondary prevention for coronary artery disease.[23] These include risk factor reduction, exercise, and a variety of pharmacological agents, including antiarrhythmics, anticoagulants, antiplatelet drugs, beta blockers, calcium antagonists, inotropic agents, and antihypertensive medications. To date, no controlled studies have been able to evaluate the effects of calcium antagonists, inotrophic agents, or antihypertensive medicines. Fairly strong evidence shows positive benefits to exist for the use of beta blockers, physical exercise, and perhaps antiplatelet therapy (aspirin). No benefit has been shown for classical antiarrhythmics such as quinidine or procainamide or for anticoagulation therapy.

It is not clear whether the benefit of beta-blocking agents is related to their intrinsic antiarrhythmic properties or their positive effects on the ratio of myocardial oxygen supply versus demand. The beneficial effects seem to be present for beta-blocking agents as a class and not for individual agents.[25] They should be prophylactically started on all patients who survive myocardial infarction without evidence of congestive heart failure prior to discharge. For reasons that are not clear, the benefit of beta blockade does not seem to be present if they are started more than 6 weeks after infarction. When beta blockers are started in hospital, it is estimated that mortality can be reduced by approximately 20–25% in post-myocardial infarction patients.[27] Patients evaluated for the effects of physical exercise are relatively selected. Allowing for this referral bias, however, positive benefits of physical training seem to reduce risk for further myocardial infarction on the order of magnitude of 25%. The numbers involved in these studies, however, are relatively small, and the traditional end point of mortality was not used. The duration of the study was also relatively short-lived, and therefore the long-term benefits of a daily exercise program and secondary prevention are difficult to assess.[22]

The results of several studies evaluating aspirin therapy in patients who have suffered myocardial infarction are conflicting.[28,29] If the data from several studies are pooled, it seems that some benefit from aspirin therapy can be expected. However, this reduction in risk is at best 10%, and this modality of therapy has to be considered of secondary importance at this time. If aspirin therapy is chosen, the current theory favors low-dose (1 baby aspirin per day) over high-dose aspirin therapy because of the differential effect of aspirin in low doses on thromboxane synthetase compared to cycloperoxidase activity. A recent study, however, showed a significant reduction in mortality of patients with unstable angina using 1200 mg aspirin per day in divided doses.[26]

Lowering lipid levels by using pharmacological agents has not been shown to have obvious benefit with regard to secondary prevention.

To summarize, at the time of clinical onset of coronary artery disease patients should be carefully evaluated for the presence of left main coronary disease. This may be suspected on the basis of clinical criteria, such as areas involved with electrocardiographic changes on routine cardiogram or with chest pain. The younger the patient, the greater the functional impairment, and the greater the suspicion of left main disease, the more aggressively the primary-care physician should pursue cardiac catheterization with a thought to the possibility of bypass surgery. Patients who are found not to have left main disease should initially be treated medically. Primary risk factor reduction can be applied. The benefits are small, but so are the risks. In the absence of congestive heart failure, patients should be started on beta-blocking agents regardless of the clinical presentation of coronary artery disease, since these agents have been shown to reduce both sudden death and recurrence of infarction. Patients should be advised to stop smoking and should be started on a gradually increasing exercise program. This exercise program is probably improved when guided by exercise testing. Benefits of antiplatelet therapy may be small, but again carry very little risk.

REFERENCES

1. Stern, M. P.: The recent decline in ischemic heart disease mortality. *Ann. Intern. Med.* **91**:630–640, 1979.
2. Gillum, R. F., Folsom, A. R., and Blackburn, H.: Decline in coronary heart disease mortality. *Am. J. Med.* **76**:1055–1065, 1984.

3. Borhani, N.O.: Primary prevention of coronary heart disease: A critique. *Am. J. Cardiol.* **40**:251–259, 1977.
4. Report of the Advisory Committee to the Surgeon General on Smoking and Health. U.S. Gov't Press, 1964.
5. Stamler, J.: Primary prevention of coronary heart disease: The last 20 years. *Am. J. Cardiol.* **47**:722–735, 1981.
6. Kannel, W. B., Dawber, T. R., Kagan, A., *et al.*: Factors of risk in the development of coronary heart disease—six year follow-up experience: The Framingham study. *Ann. Intern. Med.* **55**:33–50, 1961.
7. Elliott, W. J.: Ear lobe crease and coronary artery disease. *Am. J. Med.* **75**:1024–1032, 1983.
8. Kannel, W. B., and Schatzkin, A.: Risk factor analysis. *Prog. Cardiovasc. Dis.* **4**:309–332, 1983.
9. Gordon, T., and Kannel, W. B.: Multiple risk functions for predicting coronary heart disease: The concept, accuracy, and application. *Am. Heart J.* **103**:1031–1069, 1982.
10. Mehta, J., and Mehta, P.: Role of blood platelets and prostaglandins in coronary artery disease. *Am. J. Cardiol.* **48**:366–373, 1981.
11. Goldman, G. J., and Pichard, A. D.: The natural history of coronary artery disease: Does medical therapy improve the prognosis? *Prog. Cardiovasc. Dis.* **25**(6):513–545, 1983.
12. Hypertension Detection and Follow-up Program Cooperative Group: Five year findings of the hypertension detection and follow-up program: I. Reduction of mortality of persons with high blood pressure including mild hypertension. *JAMA* **242**:2572, 1979.
13. Hypertension Detection and Follow-up Program Cooperative Group: Five year findings of the hypertension detection and follow-up program: II. Mortality by race, sex and age. *JAMA* **242**:2572, 1979.
14. Garcia, M. J., McNamara, R. M., Gordon, T., and Kannell, W. B.: Morbidity and mortality in diabetics in Framingham population. *Diabetes* **3**:105–111, 1974.
15. Jarrett, R. J.: Type 2 (non-insulin-dependent) diabetes mellitus and coronary heart disease—Chicken, egg or neither? *Diabetologia* **26**:99–102, 1984.
16. Modan, M., Halkin, H., Shiomo, A., Lusky, A., Eshkol, A., Shefi, M., Shitrita, A., and Fuchs, Z.: Hyperinsulinemia—A link between hypertension, obesity and glucose tolerance. *J. Clin. Invest.* **75**:809–817, 1985.
17. Gordon, T., Castelli, W., Hiortland, M., Kannell, W., and Dawbert, T.: High density lipoprotein as a protective factors against coronary heart disease. *Am. J. Med.* **62**:707–714, 1977.
18. Garrison, R. J., Wilson, P. W., Castelli. W. P., *et al.*: Obesity and lipoprotein cholesterol in the Framingham offspring study. *Metabolism* **29**:1053–1060, 1980.
19. Barrett-Conner, E. L.: Obesity, atherosclerosis and coronary artery disease. *Ann. Intern. Med.* **103**:1010–1019, 1985.
20. Siltanen, P.: Psychosomatic factors in coronary heart disease. *Ann. Clin. Res.* **16**:142–155, 1984.
21. Oberman, A.: Exercise and the primary prevention of cardiovascular disease. *Am. J. Cardiol.* **55**:10D–20D, 1985.
22. Lewis, B.: Dietary prevention of ischaemic heart disease—A policy for the 80's. *Br. Med. J.* **281**:177–180, 1980.
23. The Lipid Research Clinics Coronary Primary Prevention Trial results. *JAMA* **251**(3):351–363, 1984.
24. Kornitzer, M.: Primary coronary risk and secondary prevention of coronary heart disease. *Adv. Cardiol.* **31**:162–167, 1982.
25. Harris, P. J., Harrell, T. E., Jr., Lee, K. L., *et al.*: Survival in medically treated coronary artery disease. *Circulation* **60**:1259, 1979.
26. Morris, S. N., and McHenry, P. L.: Role of exercise stress testing in healthy subjects and patients with coronary heart disease. *Am. J. Cardiol.* **42**:659–666, 1978.
27. Singh, B. N., and Venkatesh, N.: Prevention of myocardial reinfarction of sudden death in survivors of acute myocardial infarction: Role of prophylactic B-adrenoceptor blockade. *Am. Heart J.* **107**:189–200, 1984.
28. May, G. S., Eberlein, K. A., Furberg, C. D., Passamani, E. R., and DeMets, D. L.: Secondary prevention after myocardial infarction: A review of long-term trials. *Prog. Cardiovasc. Dis.* **4**:331–352, 1982.
29. Cairns, J. A., Gent, M., Singer, J., *et al.*: Aspirin, sulfinpyrazone, or both in unstable angina. Results of a Canadian mutlicenter trial. *N. Engl. J. Med.* **313**(22):1369–1374, 1985.
30. Coronary Risk Handbook. American Heart Association, Dallas, 1973.

12

Diabetes

Jay M. Sosenko

1. INTRODUCTION

Diabetes is a major source of morbidity and mortality. It can lead to a number of complications including retinopathy, kidney failure, and neuropathy. Diabetic patients have a propensity for the development of atherosclerosis and they are at high risk for myocardial infarction. In addition to these chronic complications, acute complications such as ketoacidosis, nonketotic hyperosmolar coma, and hypoglycemia can present major problems.

There are approximately 5.8 million people with diabetes in the United States. Diabetes is one of the 10 most common underlying causes of death in the United States and is frequently reported as a contributing cause of death. Diabetic patients are more frequently work-disabled in comparison with the general population. For example, in 1978 diabetic individuals were 3.8 times more likely to be severely work-disabled (33.7%) than the general population for individuals 20–64 years of age.[1] Thus, diabetes has major health and economic impact.

Diabetes is generally subdivided into type 1 (insulin-dependent) and type 2 (non–insulin-dependent). Patients who have type 1 diabetes are ketosis-prone without the administration of insulin. Formerly called juvenile-onset diabetes, type 1 diabetes usually occurs before age 20. Patients with type 2 diabetes are not ketosis-prone, and their hyperglycemia can often be controlled with diet or oral medication. A significant proportion still require insulin to adequately control glucose levels. This form of diabetes was previously called maturity-onset diabetes and occurs mostly in adults; however, occasionally it occurs in adolescents and even in young children. Obese individuals are at especially high risk for type 2 diabetes.

The importance of prevention in the care of the diabetic patient has become increasingly apparent in recent years. New information suggests that the complications of diabetes are not inevitable and that measures can be undertaken to prevent or significantly delay them. The practitioner should thus be aware of current knowledge concerning prevention in diabetes.

Jay M. Sosenko • Department of Medicine, University of Miami School of Medicine, Miami, Florida 33101

2. CONCEPTS CONCERNING DIABETES PREVENTION

It is now evident that genetic factors are involved in the etiology of type 1 diabetes. Several markers on the sixth chromosome have been identified that are associated with an increased risk for the development of type 1 diabetes. The DR 3 and DR 4 alleles are especially associated with excess risk for type 1 diabetes,[2] and it is theorized that these markers are proximal to another locus that is a determinant of an immunological susceptibility to diabetes.

There are also data to suggest that environmental factors are critical for the expression of type 1 diabetes. In one case report a virus was isolated from the pancreas of a child with new-onset diabetes.[3] The onset of diabetes has a seasonal variation, with the highest occurrence rates in the winter months.[2] In addition, an appreciable percentage of patients have a history of infection just prior to onset.[2]

A report from Canada suggested that a prolonged remission could be obtained with the administration of cyclosporine A to newly diagnosed type 1 patients.[4] The data from that study are consistent with evidence that immunological factors are critical to the pathogenesis of type 1 diabetes. Controlled clinical trials are currently being conducted to determine whether cyclosporine A and other interventions are in fact beneficial in newly diagnosed type 1 patients.

Type 2 diabetes is often familial; however, genetic markers have not been clearly established. This disorder is strongly associated with obesity, which leads to insulin resistance and ultimately to hyperglycemia. Weight loss tends to be associated with improvement in glucose tolerance.[5,6] Thus, obesity is a potentially modifiable risk factor for type 2 diabetes.

3. PREVENTION OF ACUTE COMPLICATIONS

3.1. Diabetic Ketoacidosis

This condition appears most commonly in children and adolescents. Mortality estimates vary, but most series indicate a rate of 5–10%. Death can occur from cerebral edema, although the mechanism for this is not fully understood.

Ketoacidosis tends to occur in certain clinical settings. It is often present at the onset of type 1 diabetes. Patient with type 1 diabetes who develop infections have increased insulin requirements and they are also at high risk for ketoacidosis. A number of patients with ketoacidosis are noncompliant and omit insulin injections. These patients may be difficult to differentiate from those who are brittle and particularly prone to the development of ketoacidosis.

The prevention of ketoacidosis at the onset of diabetes is dependent on the knowledge of both the child's primary physician and the child's family. Children often present with polyuria and polydipsia. If these indicators are missed, severe ketoacidosis can develop. Thus, it is important for both physicians and parents to be aware of the warning signals of diabetes.

In patients with known diabetes, education is also critical in the prevention of ketoacidosis. Both families and physicians should be aware that infections often lead to a need for increased insulin and hydration. Regular urine testing for ketonuria can alert the patient to impending ketoacidosis. Urine testing should especially be performed in individuals with infections or other stresses. Testing should be performed frequently in patients who have recurrent ketoacidosis.

3.2. Hyperosmolar Hyperglycemic Nonketotic Diabetic Coma

Diabetic patients may develop severe hyperglycemia and ensuing hyperosmolar coma. It tends to occur in elderly diabetic patients and can even occur in some patients who have no prior history of diabetes. The mortality rate has been reported to vary from 40 to 70%. Patients with hyperosmolar coma often have precipitating factors, including infections, chronic renal failure, gastrointestinal bleeding, acute pancreatitis, and parenteral hyperalimentation. Certain drugs (e.g., glucocorticoids) also can contribute to hyperosmolar coma. Evidence of polyuria, polydipsia, and dehydration in the setting of the above conditions should lead to the suspicion of impending hyperosmolar coma. Early therapeutic interventions based on these indicators should lower the mortality rate.

3.3. Hypoglycemia

Hypoglycemia is not a function of the diabetic state itself, but is the result of the therapies for diabetes. It is the most common acute complication and is especially common in those on insulin therapy. Although hypoglycemia may occur somewhat less frequently in patients on oral agents, it can be more severe and enduring in these patients. Hypoglycemic reactions may lead to seizures, permanent neurological damage, and even death; however, fortunately these consequences are unusual.

There are several settings in which hypoglycemic reactions tend to occur. New-onset type 1 patients who are entering their remission (honeymoon) phase may be prone to hypoglycemia. Increments in the dosage of medication, exercise, and dieting can all provoke hypoglycemia. Elderly patients who have an inadequate diet may also be susceptible to hypoglycemia. If they are on long-acting oral agents, the hypoglycemia can be prolonged. It is important to recognize that there is a fine line between being in good metabolic control and being at high risk for severe reactions.

The vast majority of reactions are mild and only a nuisance to patients. Usually there are symptoms that indicate a mild degree of hypoglycemia. These include headache, tremor, sweating, and hunger, and the ingestion of carbohydrate quickly resolves the hypoglycemia. However, if these warning signals are ignored, more marked hypoglycemia can develop, with potentially severe consequences. Patients with autonomic neuropathy and those taking beta blockers may lack the normal physiological responses to hypoglycemia. Thus, they may not recognize mild hypoglycemia and severe reactions can develop.

In general, frequent small meals and snacks are helpful in preventing reactions. High-risk patients (see above) must be carefully monitored. Patients with frequent hypoglycemia may require a change in therapy. Laboratory evidence of hypoglycemia, even in the absence of clinical symptoms, may also necessitate a modification of therapy.

Significant hypoglycemia is preventable in most cases. New-onset diabetic patients should be taught the early warning symptoms of hypoglycemic reactions and measures to take when they occur. They should be instructed to carry sucrose (sugar or candy) which can be quickly ingested. Patients should have adequate carbohydrate ingestion prior to engaging in vigorous physical activity. Since patients with severe reactions may be unable to eat, family members and close acquaintances should have glucagon available and be instructed in its use.

4. PREVENTION OF CHRONIC COMPLICATIONS

4.1. Introduction

The major complications of diabetes include retinopathy, nephropathy, neuropathy, and atherosclerotic disorders. It is still unclear as to the extent to which the pathogenesis of these complications overlap, and because of this, there is confusion with regard to classification. Traditionally, complications have been grouped into those which are either microvascular or macrovascular. Retinopathy and nephropathy have been included among the microvascular complications, since these disorders are associated with pathology of small vessels. Although there is some evidence for vascular disease in diabetic neuropathy, its pathogenesis is thought to be distinct from that of other complications. The term macrovascular generally refers to disorders associated with atherosclerosis.

There has been a great deal of controversy concerning the etiology of diabetic complications.[7,8] It has been argued that the complications of diabetes are not necessarily the result of metabolic aberration, but they are perhaps constitutionally or genetically associated with the occurrence of diabetes itself. However, there is now substantial evidence to indicate that retinopathy, nephropathy, and neuropathy are at least in part the result of the metabolic abnormalities of diabetes.[9] It is still possible, however, that genetic and constitutional factors are important in influencing complications. We have reported evidence indicating that height may be a risk factor for diabetic peripheral neuropathy.[10]

Recent developments have made the prevention of diabetic complications more feasible. There has been substantial improvement in the treatment of metabolic abnormalities. Also, potentially modifiable risk factors for the occurrence and progression of complications are being identified. The preventive measures are summarized in Table I.

4.2. Retinopathy

4.2.1. Overview

Diabetic retinopathy is the leading cause of new-onset legal blindness in adults between the ages of 20 and 74 years. Of all new cases of legal blindness in the United States, at least 10% are the result of diabetic retinopathy.[11]

Diabetic retinopathy is generally classified into two categories: background retinopathy and proliferative retinopathy. Background retinopathy is the less severe form and is commonly manifested by the presence of microaneurysms, hemorrhages, and exudates. Patients with proliferative retinopathy have an abnormal growth of retinal vessels. These

Table I. Suggested Measures for the Prevention of Chronic Diabetic Complications

Retinopathy	Foot ulceration
Glucose control	Detection of neuropathy
Blood pressure control	Appropriate footwear
Regular eye examinations	Regular inspection of feet
Nephropathy	Avoidance of trauma
Glucose control	Avoidance of high-pressure loads
Blood pressure control	Atherosclerosis
Hyperglycemia during pregnancy	Glucose control
Adequate screening	Blood pressure control
Glucose control	Optimization of serum lipid levels
Frequent eye examinations	Avoidance of smoking
Peripheral neuropathy	Weight control
Glucose control	Exercise
Avoidance of ethanol consumption (?)	

are fragile and can lead to vitreous hemorrhage with eventual retinal detachment and severe visual loss.

4.2.2. Risk Factors

Numerous studies have been performed to examine the association between retinopathy and glycemia; however, it has been difficult to definitively show this association. Until recently investigators had been unable to adequately assess glucose levels over time. However, the advent of both the glycosylated hemoglobin measurement and home blood glucose monitoring has resulted in the improved assessment of glycemia. Most studies show an association between retinopathy and glycemia[9]; however, a precise risk function has not been defined.

Diabetes duration has also been shown to be a major risk factor for retinopathy. The estimation of the association varies from study to study, which is at least in part related to differences in diagnostic techniques for retinopathy. It does appear, however, that the cumulative incidence of any form of retinopathy is at least 10% after 10 years of diabetes.[12] In one study the prevalence of proliferative retinopathy was observed to be greater than 20% in females and greater than 40% in males after 20 years' duration.[13] There is some evidence that blood pressure is also a risk factor for the occurrence of retinopathy.[14,15] Otherwise, no other risk factors for diabetic retinopathy have been clearly established. It should be noted, however, that few studies have specifically examined nonmetabolic risk factors. With a broader view toward the etiology and pathogenesis of diabetic retinopathy, it is possible that more risk factors will be identified.

4.2.3. Prevention

Most diabetologists concur that normalization of the metabolic state would prevent diabetic retinopathy. Attempts should be made to optimize glycemic control, and new therapeutic modalities make this more feasible. Home blood glucose monitoring provides a great deal of information for both the physician and the patient in regulating blood glucose levels. New oral agents have been introduced that at the least provide a greater variety of treatment possibilities for hyperglycemia. External insulin infusion pumps have been developed which can lead to a marked improvement in blood glucose levels. However, insulin pumps have limited current usage. A number of patients find them inconvenient. Also, a high frequency of equipment malfunctions leading to an interruption of insulin flow has been reported. This may contribute to the occurrence of ketoacidosis, which has been observed in some of the pump-treated patients.[16] Ultimately, these problems should be circumvented by improved technology.

Blood pressure control may be an important means for the prevention of diabetic retinopathy. Although it is difficult to define an exact goal, it should not necessarily be assumed that blood pressure has the same risk function for retinopathy as it does for cardiovascular disorders.

The ophthalmologist plays a critical role in the prevention of the progression of retinopathy and the maintenance of visual function. There have been major advances in the therapy of diabetic retinopathy which can prevent loss of vision; these are discussed elsewhere.

4.3. Nephropathy

4.3.1. Overview

One-fourth of the cases of end-stage renal disease in the United States can be attributed to diabetes.[17] Renal dysfunction is often progressive, and renal failure usually develops within 10 years following its onset. The loss of function is often preceded by mild proteinuria. Proteinuria can become substantial, and the nephrotic syndrome is associated with diabetic nephropathy.

4.3.2. Risk Factors

As is the case with retinopathy, there appears to be an association between nephropathy risk and glycemia. In Pirart's extensive prospective study,[18] patients in poorest glycemic control were at the highest risk for nephropathy. Also, there was a clear association between diabetic nephropathy and duration in that study, with a prevalence of approximately 10% after 10 years of diabetes. Other risk factors have been less well defined; however, blood pressure appears to influence the progression of diabetic nephropathy.[19]

Recently new methodologies have been developed that can sensitively measure small amounts of albuminuria.[20,21] Since microalbuminuria appears to be an early indicator for the occurrence of nephropathy, it may be useful in the assessment of risk factors for diabetic nephropathy. Thus, new risk factors may be identified in the near future.

4.3.3. Prevention

The same measures undertaken to prevent retinopathy should be utilized for the prevention of nephropathy. These especially include the optimization of blood glucose and blood pressure control. The latter may be especially important in delaying the progression of renal impairment.

4.4. Neuropathy

4.4.1. Overview

A number of neuropathic disorders are associated with diabetes. These include autonomic neuropathy, mononeuropathies, mononeuropathy multiplex, diabetic amyotrophy, the carpal tunnel syndrome, and peripheral neuropathy. The latter is the most common form of neuropathy, and most of the following discussion deals with aspects of this particular disorder.

Peripheral neuropathy has several manifestations. Patients can have severe and even intolerable pain. Motor dysfunction can be equally troublesome. Although patients may complain less about lack of sensation, hypesthesia can lead to major consequences such as foot ulceration, burns, and trauma.

Most of the evidence for the etiology of diabetic neuropathy points toward metabolic factors. Sorbitol deposition in the nerve is thought by some to be an important contributor to neuropathy by causing osmotic damage.[22] Decreased myoinosotol in the nerve has also been implicated as contributing to diabetic neuropathy.[23] Protein glycosylation in the nerve is another potentially pathogenetic metabolic factor.[24] Although there is some evidence that vascular factors contribute to the pathogenesis of diabetic neuropathy,[25] most attention has been focused on metabolic causes.

4.4.2. Risk Factors

Few epidemiological studies have been undertaken to investigate risk factors for diabetic neuropathy. In the study of Pirart,[18] there was an association between the occurrence of neuropathy and the level of glycemia. In that study diabetes duration was also found to be an important risk factor. Several clinical studies also indicate the importance of glycemia as a risk factor. An association between the peroneal motor nerve conduction velocity and glycosylated hemoglobin has been observed in newly diagnosed patients.[26] Also, there was evidence of improvement in velocity with improved blood glucose control following treatment.[27]

Other factors may also be important. We observed a strong association between abnormal vibratory perception and body stature.[10] For patients in the lower, middle, and upper thirds of the height distribution, the prevalance of absent vibratory perception in at least one of the great toes was 0.05, 0.08, and 0.40, respectively.

There are few data concerning ethanol use as a risk factor for neuropathy. However, in our study we found that diabetic patients with past and/or present ethanol use had a much higher prevalence of sensory impairment. It is of interest that there was no association between neurological impairment and ethanol intake in a group of nondiabetic control subjects. These are preliminary data, however, and further studies must be performed before firm conclusions can be drawn concerning ethanol consumption.

4.4.3. Prevention

Since there is substantial evidence for an association between peripheral neuropathy and glycemia, blood glucose control is an important preventive measure. It may also be important in preventing the progression of neuropathy and perhaps even in its reversal.[28] Since ethanol is a potential neurotoxin, it should probably be avoided.

Over the past decade aldose reductase inhibitors have been developed. These are thought to prevent the accumulation of sorbitol in the nerve, and they may have therapeutic efficacy in the treatment of neuropathy.[29] Although most studies have examined their effect in patients with severe neuropathy, it is possible that this class of agents may also be useful in the prevention of the occurrence of neuropathy or the progression of mild neuropathy.

4.5. Foot Ulceration

4.5.1. Overview

Diabetic foot ulceration is usually not though of as a major complication of diabetes; however, it can be extremely troublesome for patients. Foot ulcers are often slow in healing and they are the most common cause of gangrene and amputation in diabetic patients. It has been estimated that 20% of hospital admissions for diabetic patients are caused by foot ulcers.[30]

4.5.2. Risk Factors

Foot ulceration in diabetic patients has been attributed to both neuropathy and vascular disease. We performed a case-control study to assess the relative importance of these factors.[31] Diabetic patients with foot ulcers were compared to diabetic patients who had no history of foot ulcers. The study results revealed a strong association between foot ulceration and diminished vibratory perception. With increasing severity of vibratory perception abnormality (quantitated with the Bio-Thesiometer), there was a greater risk for foot ulceration (Table II). However, there was little association between foot ulceration and vascular insufficiency (as measured by the Doppler stethoscope). Although vascular factors may still be important for the development of diabetic foot ulceration, it is clear that hypesthesia is extremely important. Data indicate that diabetic patients with hypesthesia tend to put large pressure loads on their feet, which can then lead to the development of foot ulcers.

Table II. Odds Ratio Estimates according to Severity of Vibratory Perception Abnormality[a]

Vibratory perception threshold	Foot ulcer: Present (n = 86)	Foot ulcer: Absent (n = 49)	Odds ratio
<25.0 (reference category)	11	30	—
25.0–32.9	9	7	3.51
33.0–41.9	16	6	7.27
>42.0	50	6	22.73

[a]Chi-square test for trend p value <0.001.

4.5.3. Prevention

Patients with hypesthesia may not be fully aware of it. Thus, it is important to examine patients for neuropathy. All diabetic patients should be informed and educated with regard to the prevention of foot ulcers. Measures include avoidance of tight shoes, avoidance of "thongs" and other potentially irritating footwear, not walking on bare feet, and frequent foot inspection. Patients with hypesthesia should also be informed about ways of avoiding burns from such common sources as scalding water and radiators. Since the quantitative assessment of vibratory perception is simple and inexpensive, it is not unreasonable to perform this measurement on a yearly basis.

4.6. Macrovascular Disease

4.6.1. Overview

Atherosclerotic involvement of the large vessels is common in diabetic patients. It has been clearly shown in several epidemiological studies that diabetes is a major risk factor for coronary heart disease,[32,33] and among diabetic individuals, coronary heart disease is the leading cuase of death. The basis for accelerated atherosclerosis has not been clearly determined, however.

4.6.2. Risk Factors

Numerous studies have examined lipid levels in diabetic patients with conflicting results, which may result from differences in the populations under study. The abnormality in glucose metabolism of type 1 patients differs markedly from that of type 2 patients. Even among type 2 patients, the pathogenesis of hyperglycemia can vary greatly. Differences in the level of insulin and the degree of insulin resistance in type 2 patients could lead to differences in lipid levels.

Most studies indicate that low-density-lipoprotein cholesterol (LDL-C) tends to be elevated in diabetic patients.[34,35] This could be related to overall blood glucose control, since a correlation between LDL-C and glycosylated hemoglobin has been observed.[34] Studies of high-density-lipoprotein cholesterol (HDL-C) have been conflicting. However, HDL-C has been shown in various studies to be normal in young, type 1 patients,[34] normal or increased in adult, insulin-treated patients,[36] and normal or decreased in type 2 patients.[37] In general, studies have shown little association between HDL-C and glycemia among diabetic subjects.[34,36]

Epidemiological evidence suggests that there is a higher prevalence of hypertension in diabetic patients.[38] The mechanism for this elevation is not clear; however, recent studies have shown an association between blood pressure and insulin levels in nondiabetic individuals.[39,40] Also, insulin appears to influence the reabsorption of sodium in the proximal tubules of the kidney in dogs.[41] Thus, it is possible that insulin is involved in the pathogenesis of hypertension in type 2 diabetic patients, who frequently have elevated insulin levels.

Epidemiological studies generally show that the relative risk for coronary disease in diabetic women is greater than that for diabetic men.[42] The more marked effect of diabetes in women may be related to the apparently greater impact of diabetes on lipid levels in women[43]; however, other risk factors may also be critical.

Investigators from the Framingham study assessed whether the greater risk of coronary disease in diabetic patients could be explained by abnormalities of known risk factors.[38] In the multivariate analyses, these risk factors could not account for all of the excess risk in diabetic patients. Thus, other unknown risk factors could be extremely important for the causation of coronary disease. For example, there is evidence that insulin itself[44] could contribute to the occurrence of coronary disease.

4.6.3. *Prevention*

In general, diabetic patients should follow the same measures as the general population for the prevention of coronary disease. These include attention to diet, exercise, weight control, control of blood pressure, control of lipids, and the avoidance of smoking. As it is possible that abnormal glucose metabolism may influence the occurrence of coronary disease, every attempt should be made to maintain as normal a metabolic state as possible. Diabetic patients are especially prone to having asymptomatic coronary disease. Thus, there should be close surveillance of diabetic patients, which entails obtaining periodic electrocardiographic tracings and careful attention to any symptomatology that may develop.

5. DIABETES AND PREGNANCY

Overt diabetes has been estimated to be present in 0.3% of pregnant women in the United States. The offspring of pregnant women with established diabetes are at greater risk for prematurity, macrosomia, hypoglycemia, congenital malformations, the respiratory distress syndrome, and hyperbilirubinemia.[45] Pregnant women with type 1 diabetes are at higher risk for ketoacidosis, and those with either type of diabetes may have an accelerated progression of chronic complications. In addition, toxemia appears to be associated with diabetic pregnancies.[46] Gestational diabetes develops in about 2–3% of pregnancies in the United States.[47] It usually occurs during the second or third trimester and may go undetected in a sizable number of women. This condition also jeopardizes fetal outcome in that macrosomia, hypoglycemia, hypocalcemia, and hyperbilirubinemia can occur as a result.[48]

Data suggest that the outcome of the diabetic pregnancy is at least partly determined by the level of metabolic control. Hypoglycemia and macrosomia appear to be related to hyperinsulinemia in the fetus which is the result of maternal hyperglycemia.[49,50] Also, there is evidence that congenital malformations are associated with glycosylated hemoglobin values in early pregnancy.[51] It is thus clear that the control of hyperglycemia is an important goal in the care of diabetic pregnant women. Home blood glucose monitoring and the self-adjustment of insulin are perhaps most successful during the diabetic pregnancy. Pregnant diabetic women are highly motivated and they often achieve excellent blood glucose control. Pregnant women should be carefully observed for chronic complications, especially the acceleration of diabetic retinopathy.

Unless there is careful screening, the diagnosis of gestational diabetes may be missed. Several risk factors have been identified that may aid in detection. These are age greater than 25, a history of an infant weighing more than 9 lb, a previous stillbirth or congenital malformation, and a family history of diabetes.[52] Some advocate that all pregnant women should be screened for gestational diabetes. This may not be feasible in certain settings and the above risk factors may be useful in these circumstances.

It is recommended that a glucose challenge be administered between the 24th and 28th weeks of gestation, and specific diagnostic criteria have been proposed.[52] In women who are at a particularly high risk for gestational diabetes, it is recommended that screening be performed when pregnancy is diagnosed, and if negative, at 24 weeks' gestation.

6. CONCLUSION

Knowledge concerning risk factors is increasing. For example, individuals with high ratios of waist to hip circumferences appear to be at greater risk for type 2 diabetes.[53] Thus, adipose distribution may be an important factor in the causation of type 2 diabetes. In addition, new data suggest that a predisposition for essential hypertension may be a risk factor for diabetic nephropathy.[54] Although these findings do not lead directly to prevention strategies, they may ultimately improve diabetes prevention.

The major current problems in diabetes prevention are the still limited therapies and, perhaps more important, the lack of patient compliance. The latter can only be achieved through proper patient awareness of the risks for complications. Thus, the practitioner should not take the patient's knowledge concerning diabetes for granted. The education of the diabetic patient should be viewed as an ongoing process and not simply as a "crash course" at the time of diagnosis.

Diabetes care is tied to prevention as much as in any other major illness. In fact, prevention of acute and chronic complications is the main rationale for vigilance over glycemia levels. Advances in the basic sciences, therapeutics, epidemiology, and clinical medicine should markedly accelerate our ability to improve prevention in diabetes.

REFERENCES

1. Drury, T. F.: Disability among adult diabetics, in *Diabetes in America.* NIH Publication no. 85-1468, XXVII-7, Washington, DC, 1985.
2. Tajima, N., LaPorte, R. E., Hibi, I., Kitagawa, T., Fujito, H., and Drash, A.: A comparison of the epidemiology of youth-onset insulin-dependent diabetes mellitus between Japan and the United States (Allegheny County, Pennsylvania). *Diabetes Care* **8**(suppl 1):17–23, 1985.
3. Yoon, J., Austin, M., Onodera, T., and Notkins, A. L.: Virus-induced diabetes mellitus: Isolation of a virus from a child with diabetic ketoacidosis. *New Engl. J. Med.* **300:**1173–1179, 1979.
4. Stiller, C. R., Dupre, J., Gent, M., *et al.:* Effects of cylcosporine immunosuppresion in insulin-dependent diabetes mellitus of recent onset. *Science* **223:**1362–1367, 1984.
5. Newburgh, L. H.: Control of hyperglycemia of obese "diabetics" by weight reduction. *Ann. Intern. Med.* **17:**935–942, 1942.
6. Osserman, K. E., and Dolger, H.: Obesity in diabetes: A study of therapy with anorexigenic drugs. *Ann. Intern. Med.* **34:**72–79, 1951.
7. Cahill, G. F., Etzwiler, D. D., and Freinkel, N.: "Control" and diabetes. *N. Engl. J. Med.* **294:**1004–1005, 1976.

8. Siperstein, M. D., Foster, D. W., Knowles, H. C., Jr., Levine, R., Madison, L. L., and Roth, J.: Control of blood glucose and diabetic vascular disease. *N. Engl. J. Med.* **296**:1060–1063, 1977.
9. Skyler, J. S.: Complications of diabetes mellitus: Relationship to metabolic dysfunction. *Diabetes Care* **2**:499–509, 1979.
10. Sosenko, J. M., Gadia, M. T., Fournier, A. M., O'Connell, M. T., Aguiar, M. D., and Skyler, J. S.: Body stature as a risk factor for diabetic sensory neuropathy. *Am. J. Med.* **80**:1031–1034, 1986.
11. Herman, W., Halpern, M., Pack, B. E., Beasley, J., and Callaghan, C.: Improving eye care for persons with diabetes mellitus—Michigan. *Morbid. Mortal. Wkly. Rep.* **34**:697–699, 1985.
12. Dwyer, M. S., Melton, J., Ballard, D. J., Palumbo, P. J., Trautmann, J. C., and Chu-Pin, C.: Incidence of diabetic retinopathy and blindness: A population-based study in Rochester Minnesota. *Diabetes Care* **8**:316–322, 1985.
13. Klein, R., Klein, B. E. K., and Moss, S. E.: A population-based study of diabetic retinopathy in insulin using patients diagnosed before 30 years of age. *Diabetes Care* **8**(suppl 1):71–76, 1985.
14. Knowler, W. C., Bennett, P. H., and Ballintine, E. J,: Increased incidence of retinopathy in diabetics with elevated blood pressure. *N. Engl. J. Med.* **302**:645–650, 1980.
15. West, K. M., Erdreich, L. J., and Stober, J. A.: A detailed study of risk factors for retinopathy and nephropathy in diabetes. *Diabetes* **29**:501–508, 1980.
16. Mecklenberg, R. S., Guinn, T. S., Sannar, C. A., and Blumenstein, B. A.: Malfunction of continuous subcutaneous insulin infusion systems: A one-year prospective study of 127 patients. *Diabetes Care* **9**:351–355, 1986.
17. Herman, W. H., and Teutsch, S. M.: Kidney disease associated with diabetes, in *Diabetes in America*. NIH Publication no. 85-1468, XIV-1, Washington, DC, 1985.
18. Pirart, J.: Diabetes mellitus and its degenerative complications: A prospective study of 4,400 patients observed between 1947 and 1973. *Diabetes Care* **1**:168–188, 1978.
19. Mogensen, C. E.: Long-term antihypertensive treatment inhibiting progression to diabetic nephropathy. *Br. Med. J.* **285**:685–688, 1982.
20. Mogensen, C. E.: Microalbuminuria predicts clinical proteinuria and early mortality in maturity-onset diabetes. *N. Engl. J. Med.* **310**:356–360, 1984.
21. Viberti, G., and Keen, H.: The patterns of proteinuria in diabetes mellitus. Relevance to pathogenesis and prevention of diabetic nephropathy. *Diabetes* **33**:686–692, 1984.
22. Gabbay, K. H.: The sorbitol pathway and the complications of diabetes. *N. Engl. J. Med.* **288**:831–836, 1973.
23. Greene, D. A., DeJesus, P. V., and Winegrad, A. I.: Effects of insulin and dietary myoinositol on impaired peripheral motor nerve conduction velocity in acute streptozotocin diabetes. *J. Clin. Invest.* **55**:1326–1336, 1975.
24. Vlassava, H., Brownlee, M., and Cerami, A.: Nonenzymatic glycosylation of peripheral nerve protein in diabetes mellitus. *Proc. Natl. Acad. Sci. USA* **78**:5190–5192, 1981.
25. Sugimura, K., and Dyck, P. J.: Multifocal fiber loss in proximal sciatic nerve in symmetrical distal diabetic neuropathy. *J. Neurol. Sci.* **53**:501–509, 1982.
26. Graf, R. J., Halter, J. B., Pfeiffer, M. A., *et al.*: Nerve conduction abnormalities in untreated maturity onset diabetes: Relation to fasting plasma glucose and glycosylated hemoglobin. *Ann. Intern. Med.* **90**:298–303, 1979.
27. Graf, R. J., Halter, J. B., Pfeiffer, M. A., *et al.*: Glycemia control and nerve conduction abnormalities in non-insulin-dependent diabetic subjects. *Ann. Intern. Med.* **94**:307–311, 1981.
28. Boulton, A. J. M., Drury, J., Clarke, B., and Ward, J. D.: Continuous subcutaneous insulin infusion in the management of painful diabetic neuropathy. *Diabetes Care* **5**:386–390, 1982.
29. Judzewitsch, R. G., Jaspan, J. B., Polonsky, K. S., *et al.*: Aldose reductase inhibition improves nerve condition velocity in diabetic patients. *N. Engl. J. Med.* **308**:119–125, 1983.
30. Levin, M. E.: Diabetic peripheral vascular disease, in Rifkin, H., and Raskin, P. (eds.): *Diabetes Mellitus*, Vol. V. Robert J. Brady, Bowie, MD, 1982, pp. 281–290.
31. Boulton, A. J. M., Kubrusly, D. B., Bowker, J. H., *et al.*: Impaired vibratory sensation and diabetic foot ulceration. *Diabetic Med.* **3**:335–337, 1986.
32. Ostrander, L. D., Jr., Frances, T., Jr., Hayner, N. S., Kjelsberg, M. O., and Epstein, F. H.: Relationship of cardiovascular disease to hyperglycemia. *Ann. Intern. Med.* **62**:1188–1198, 1965.

33. Kannel, W. B., and McGee, D. L.: Diabetes and glucose tolerance as risk factors for cardiovascular disease: The Framingham study. *Diabetes Care* **2:**120–126, 1979.
34. Sosenko, J. M., Breslow, J. L., Miettinen, O. S., and Gabbay, K. H.: Hyperglycemia and plasma lipid levels. A prospective study of young insulin-dependent diabetic patients. *N. Engl. J. Med.* **302:**650–654, 1980.
35. Schonfeld, G., Birge, C., Miller, J. P. Kessler, G., and Santiago, J.: Apolipoprotein B levels and altered lipoprotein composition in diabetes. *Diabetes* **23:**827–834, 1974.
36. Nikkila, E. A., and Hormila, P.: Serum lipids and lipoproteins in insulin treated diabetes: demonstration of increased high density lipoprotein concentrations. *Diabetes* **27:**1078–1086, 1978.
37. Howard, B. V., Savage, P. J., Bennion, L. J., and Bennett, P. H.: Lipoprotein composition in diabetes mellitus. *Atherosclerosis* **30:**153–162, 1978.
38. Garcia, M. J., McNamara, P. M., Gordon, T., and Kannel, W. B.: Morbidity and mortality in diabetics in the Framingham population. *Diabetes* **23:**105–111, 1974.
39. Modan, M., Halkin, H., Shiomo, A., *et al.:* Hyperinsulinemia—A link between hypertension, obesity and glucose intolerance. *J. Clin. Invest.* **75:**809–817, 1985.
40. Fournier, A. M., Gadia, M. T., Kubrusly, D. B., Skyler, J. S., and Sosenko, J. M.: Blood pressure, insulin, and glycemia in nondiabetic subjects. *Am. J. Med.* **80:**861–864, 1986.
41. DeFronzo, R. A.: The effect of insulin on renal sodium metabolism. *Diabetologia* **21:**165–171, 1981.
42. Barrett-Connor, E., and Wingard, D. L.: Sex differential in ischemic heart disease mortality in diabetics: A prospective population-based study. *Am. J. Epidemiol.* **118:**489–496, 1983.
43. Walden, C. E., Knopp, R. H., Wahl, P. W., Beach, K. W., and Strandness, E., Jr.: Sex differences in the effect of diabetes mellitus on lipoprotein triglyceride and cholesterol concentrations. *N. Engl. J. Med.* **311:**953–959, 1984.
44. Pyorala, K.: Relationship of glucose tolerance and plasma insulin in the incidence of coronary heart disease: Results from two population studies in Finland. *Diabetes Care* **2:**131–141, 1979.
45. Freinkel, J., Metzger, B. E., and Potter, J. M.: Pregnancy in diabetes, in Ellenberg, M., and Rifkin, H. (eds.): *Diabetes Mellitus: Theory and Practice.* Medical Examination Publishing Co., New York, 1983, pp. 689–714.
46. Freinkel, N., Dooley, S. L., and Metzger, B. E.: Current concepts: Care of the pregnant woman with insulin-dependent diabetes mellitus. *N. Engl. J. Med.* **313:**96–101, 1985.
47. Sepe, S. J., Connell, F. A., Geiss, L. S., and Teutsch, S. M.: Gestational diabetes: Incidence, maternal characteristics, and perinatal outcome. *Diabetes* **34** (suppl 2):13–16, 1985.
48. Landon, M. B., and Gabbe, S. G.: Antepartum fetal surveillance in gestational diabetes mellitus. *Diabetes* **34** (suppl 2):50–54, 1985.
49. Sosenko, I. R., Kitzmiller, J. L., Loo, S. W. H., Blix, P., Rubenstein, A. H., and Gabbay, K. H.: The infant of the diabetic mother: Correlation of increased cord C-peptide levels with macrosomia and hypoglycemia. *N. Engl. J. Med.* **301:**859–862, 1979.
50. Sosenko, J. M., Kitzmiller, J. L., Fluckinger, R., Loo, S. W. H., Younger, D. M., and Gabbay, K. H.: Umbilical cord glycosylated hemoglobin in infants of diabetic mothers: Relationships to neonatal hypoglycemia, macrosomia, and cord serum C-peptide. *Diabetes Care* **5:**566–570, 1982.
51. Miller, E., Hare, J. W., Cloherty, J. P., *et al.:* Elevated maternal hemoglobin A_{1C} in early pregnancy and major congenital anomalies in infants of diabetic mothers. *N. Engl. J. Med.* **304:**1331–1334, 1981.
52. Summary and Recommendations of the Second International Workshop-Conference on Gestational Diabetes Mellitus. *Diabetes* **34** (suppl 2):123–126, 1985.
53. Larson B., Svardsudd K., Welin L., *et al.*: Abdominal adipose tissue distribution, obesity and risk of cardiovascular disease and death: 13 year follow-up of participants in the study of men born in 1913. *Br. Med. J.* **288:**1401–1404, 1984.
54. Krolewski A. S., Canessa M., Warram J. H., *et al.*: Predisposition to hypertension and susceptibility to renal disease in insulin-dependent diabetes mellitus. *N. Engl. J. Med.* **318:**140–145, 1988.

13

Hypertension

Mark T. O'Connell

1. INTRODUCTION

Because of the large number of affected individuals and the well-established cardiovascular risks, high blood pressure is quantitatively the largest single risk for premature death and disability in the Western world. Although the working definition of hypertension varies from source to source, most surveys reveal that between 15 and 25% of adult, western populations have significantly elevated systemic arterial blood pressures.[1] Effective treatment of hypertension has had a significant impact on its associated morbidity and mortality. In the 1960s less than one-half of individuals found to have high blood pressure had been previously diagnosed, and less than one-sixth were adequately treated. This situation improved significantly during the 1970s. Thanks to both government and private efforts to increase the public's awareness, by the late 1970s approximately two-thirds of hypertensive patients had been diagnosed and nearly one-half were being adequately treated.

These efforts at improved control of high blood pressure have had impressive results. Since 1968 there has been a steady decrease in cardiovascular mortality, greater in proportion than the decline seen in noncardiovascular death rates (Fig. 1). Incidence and mortality rates of strokes and coronary events have both declined, and these declines are in large part responsible for the 3-year increase in life expectancy for U.S. adults that has been realized since 1970.

Although the pathophysiological mechanisms responsible for essential hypertension are not well characterized, many modifiable risk factors associated with increased blood pressure have been identified. Sodium intake, obesity, alcohol use, sedentary life-style, and stress have all been associated with chronically increased blood pressure. Modification of these factors could be expected to have a significant effect on an individual's, as well as a population's, risk of cardiovascular morbidity and mortality, in large part through a decrease in blood pressure. It has been estimated that moderation of sodium intake in our country, causing a 2–3 mm Hg lowering of the U.S. population's distribution of blood pressure, would reduce the overall risks of hypertension as effectively as would the active treatment of all persons with diastolic blood pressure greater than 104

Mark T. O'Connell • Department of Medicine, University of Miami School of Medicine, Miami, Florida 33101.

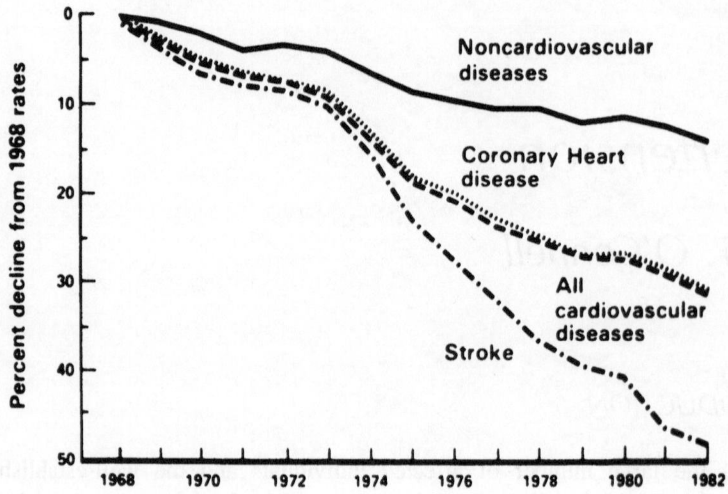

Figure 1. Percent decline in age-adjusted mortality rates for noncardiovascular and cardiovascular diseases in the United States. (Source: Feinleib.[99])

mm Hg.[2] Obviously, efforts to modify some of these risk factors are potentially worthwhile and easily justifiable. Primary-care providers should be aware of these associations and should attempt to implement preventive as well as therapeutic treatment whenever possible. More will be said later regarding this approach to the management of hypertension.

In the following sections this chapter will discuss measurement and definitions of hypertension, the epidemiology of hypertension, the attendant cardiovascular risks of elevated blood pressure, the evidence that lowering blood pressure improves cardiovascular morbidity and mortality, the controversy surrounding the appropriate treatment of mild hypertension, the usefulness of nonpharmacological methods to lower blood pressure, and a rational approach to the workup and treatment of the individual patient with essential hypertension.

2. MEASUREMENT OF BLOOD PRESSURE

Indirect measurement of systemic arterial blood pressure is a routine and frequently performed task. Rarely is any other physical examination data of such importance in identifying or predicting systemic disease. An awareness of the proper methodology and the sources of potential error in blood pressure measurement is important if accurate and timely decisions in patient care are to be provided. The proper equipment and techniques and the sources of variation in recording blood pressure are well described in the American Heart Association's excellent monograph.[3]

An adequate sphygmomanometer and stethoscope are required. Significant research has been done on the proper cuff and bladder size, and recommendations are now fairly standardized. The width of the bladder must be appropriate for the size of the patient's arm. If the bladder is too narrow, the blood pressure reading will be erroneously high; if the bladder is too wide, the reading may be erroneously low. Recommended bladder size is related to patient arm size: "the width of the bladder should be 40% of the circumference of the midpoint of the limb (or 20% wider than the diameter) on which it is to be used."[3] The length of the bladder also has an influence on the accuracy of blood pressure measurements. The current recommendation is that the bladder's length should be twice its width (80% of the arm circumference). Several investigators have shown that longer bladders (35–40 cm for average adult size) provide a closer approximation of intraarterial diastolic blood pressure and a reduction in random error.[4–6] These data have not been substantially corraborated, and their improved accuracy has not been shown to be clinically valuable.

In the absence of arterial disease, blood pressure can be accurately measured in the thigh, lower leg, or forearm. With the use of an appropriate-sized cuff, pressures in the lower extremities are only several mm Hg higher than those in the arm.

Arterial blood pressure is a dynamic entity with a great deal of variability within any individual. Studies have shown that in the same individual, blood pressure measured on separate occasions differs by an average of 9.1 mm Hg for systolic and 7.2 mm Hg for diastolic pressure. For multiple readings on the same occasion the standard deviation of the differences was 7.1 and 5.9 mm Hg for the systolic and diastolic pressures, respectively.[7]

In spite of this lability, single, "casual" blood pressure readings have been shown to correlate with predicted cardiovascular mortality and morbidity in many epidemiological studies. Yet, it is still important that health care providers be cognizant of this variability, especially when contemplating therapeutic or diagnostic interventions.

This variation can be of two overall sources: biological variation due to factors within the patient or measurement variation due to problems with the observer.[8] Twenty-four-hour intraarterial blood pressure measurements reveal a great deal of natural variation. Some of the factors accounting for this biological variability include diurnal variation, especially related to sleep cycles; recent physical activity; emotional and physical stress; recent tobacco use; recent feeding; ambiant temperature; and even the season and altitude. Many of these sources of variation are not controllable but must still be acknowledged. Measurement variation is more easily controlled. Examples of these types of observation errors include faulty equipment, improper arm position, inappropriate cuff size or placement, inattention to the auscultatory gap, too rapid deflation of the cuff bladder, too much pressure over the stethoscope bell, the presence of arrythmia or clinical shock, and rounding off of numbers or "digit preference."

3. DEFINITIONS OF HYPERTENSION

Systemic arterial blood pressure is a numerical quantity with a continuous distribution within a population. As Sir George Pickering stated, "There is no dividing line [between normal and high blood pressure]. The relationship between arterial pressure and mortality is quantitative; the higher the pressure, the worse the prognosis. Arterial pressure is a quantity and the consequences numerically related to the size of that quantity."[9]

It is artificial to create a cutoff that attempts to distinguish ''normal'' from ''elevated'' blood pressure. Cardiovascular risk can be shown to increase steadily with diastolic blood pressure greater than 76 mm Hg. For all ages and both sexes life expectancy can be shown to decrease when the diastolic blood pressure is higher than 90 mm Hg. An operational definition of hypertension is that level of blood pressure at which the benefits of action exceed those of inaction. Large clinical studies have documented the efficacy of treatment when the diastolic blood pressure is greater than 104 mm Hg. The utility of treating diastolic blood pressure in the 90–104 mm Hg range is less clear. Treatment of diastolic blood pressure in the 90–104 mm Hg range is currently a topic of intense debate. Data regarding the results of treatment of this population of patients will be reviewed later.

Although it is artificial to set limits on normal and elevated blood pressure, health care providers need specific criteria on which to base the diagnosis and recommended treatment of increased arterial pressure. The various guidelines set forth by the World Health Organization and the Joint Committee on Detection, Evaluation and Treatment of High Blood Pressure of the National Heart, Lung and Blood Institute (JNC) provide a practical framework for diagnosis and treatment.

The World Health Organization criteria are widely accepted and often used as the ''official'' definition of hypertension (Table I). The use of a ''borderline'' classification has been criticized, as this level of blood pressure has a definite associated increased cardiovascular morbidity and mortality. In addition, there is no consideration of the age and sex of the individual patient in this definition.

The JNC modified their consensus stand on the definition and management of hypertension in 1984 (JNC-III).[10] They have recommended the used of five categories of hypertension pertaining to the diastolic blood pressure (normal, high–normal, mild, moderate, and severe) and three categories of hypertension pertaining to the systolic blood pressure (normal, borderline, and isolated systolic) (Table II).

Recommendations for follow-up (Table III) as well as diagnostic and therapeutic guidelines are also contained in this report, and all health care providers who treat hypertension are encouraged to read this document. The JNC-III definition of hypertension is a reasonable standard to accept. As stated earlier, the increased risk of cardiovascular events due to blood pressure is a continuum, identifiable at levels of diastolic blood pressure > 76 mm Hg. Active treatment of the milder elevations of blood pressure in the ''high–normal'' and ''mild'' groups is a separate and controversial issue which will be addressed later in this chapter.

Table I. World Health Organization Criteria for Classifying Hypertension[a]

Normotension	SBP < 140 mm Hg and DBP < 90 mm Hg
Borderline	SBP 140–160 mm Hg and DBP 90–95 mm Hg
Hypertension	SBP > 160 mm Hg and/or DBP > 95 mm Hg

[a]SBP = systolic blood pressure; DBP = diastolic blood pressure.

Table II. Blood Pressure Classification[a,b]

Diastolic blood pressure	Systolic blood pressure		
	Less than 140	140–159	160 or greater
Less than 85	Normal	Borderline systolic hypertension	Systolic hypertension
85–89	High–normal	Same as above	Same as above
90–104	Mild hypertension	Mild hypertension	Mild hypertension
105–114	Moderate hypertension	Moderate hypertension	Moderate hypertension
115 or greater	Severe hypertension	Severe hypertension	Severe hypertension

[a]Individuals 18 years or older, average of two or more measurements, pressure in mm Hg.
[b]Source: The 1984 Report of the Joint National Committee on Detection, Evaluation, and Treatment of High Blood Pressure.[10]

4. EPIDEMIOLOGY AND RISK

As stated earlier, hypertension is the greatest risk factor for premature death and disability in Western society. Depending on the definition of hypertension, in the United States alone approximately 15–20% of individuals, or nearly 50,000,000 people, suffer from this disorder. Other epidemiological factors associated with hypertension and its cardiovascular risks are discussed in Section 6 (Table IV).

Many cross-sectional studies of large populations reveal a continuous increase in the blood pressure as age increases. Several longitudinal studies reveal the same direct relationship. Nearly one-third of persons older than 65 years have isolated systolic hypertension. Controlling for all other risk factors, a certain level of blood pressure carries similar risks for young and old alike. A younger person has a longer time to suffer any conse-

Table III. Follow-up Criteria for Blood Pressure Measurements[a,b]

Diastolic blood pressure	Systolic blood pressure		
	Less than 140	140 to 199	200 or greater
Less than 85	Recheck in 1–2 years	Confirm within 2 months, then evaluate and treat	Evaluate and treat
85–89	Recheck in 1 year	Criteria same as above	Criteria same as above
90–104	Confirm within 2 months, then evaluate and treat	Confirm within 2 months, then evaluate and treat	Confirm within 2 months, then evaluate and treat
105–114	Evaluate and treat	Evaluate and treat	Evaluate and treat
115 or greater	Immediately evaluate and treat	Immediately evaluate and treat	Immediately evaluate and treat

[a]Individuals 18 years or older, average of two or more measurements, pressure in mm Hg.
[b]Source: The 1984 Report of the Joint National Committee on Detection, Evaluation, and Treatment of High Blood Pressure.[10]

Table IV. Factors Associated with Hypertension

	Epidemiological	
Age	Ethnicity	Caffeine
Sex	Family history	Nicotine
Race	Body-weight index	Alcohol
	Diseases and other factors	
Diabetes	Menopause	Osteoarthritis
Hyperuricemia	Uterine fibroids	Blood type A1
Polycythemia vera	Increased intraocular pressure	Pseudoxanthoma elasticum

quences of elevated blood pressure and a longer time for the blood pressure to increase even further, while older persons suffer a higher incidence of cardiovascular sequelae.

As a population, women have lower blood pressure than men. They also tolerate their blood pressure better with less mortality for a given pressure[11] (Fig. 2). After menopause, women seem to develop more hypertension than similarly aged men. Blacks

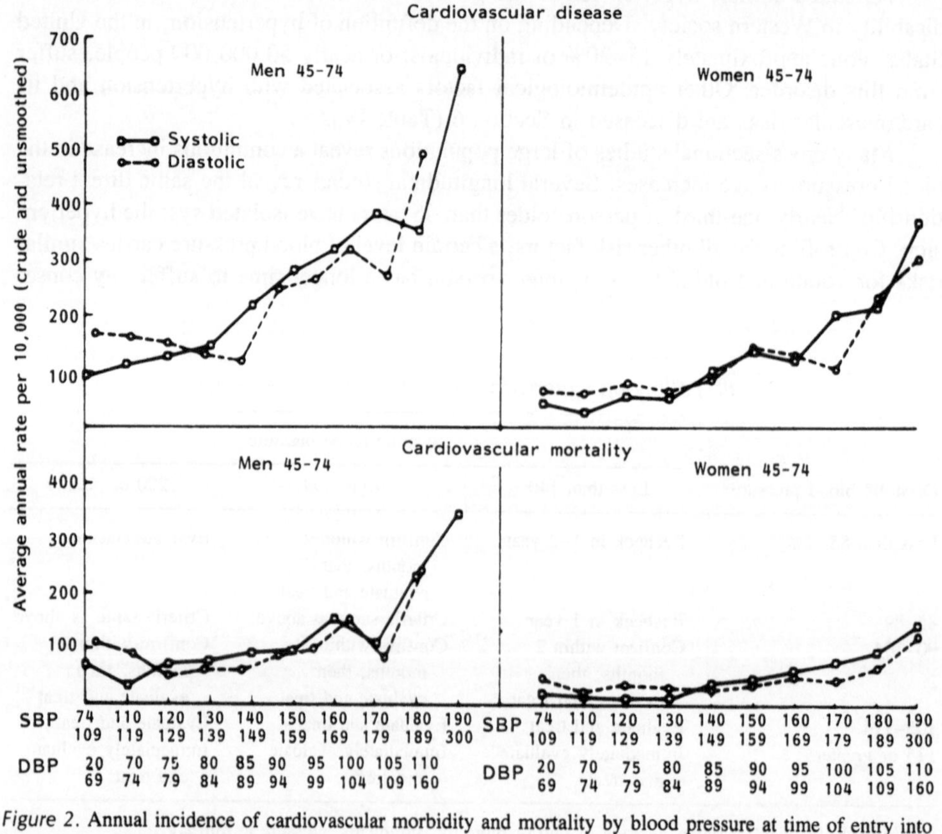

Figure 2. Annual incidence of cardiovascular morbidity and mortality by blood pressure at time of entry into Framingham Study. (Source: Ref. 47.)

have higher blood pressure than whites and suffer more morbidity and mortality, especially that related to strokes, renal damage, and congestive heart failure.[12] Mortality from hypertensive disease is 6–10 times higher in young blacks (35–54 years old) compared to whites. This is not due solely to poorer access to the health care system or to socioeconomic differences. Hispanics probably have a lower prevalence of hypertension compared to Anglos.[13] American Indians, compared to Anglos, have a similar prevalence of hypertension.[14] Many hypotheses exist to explain this difference, with a genetic difference in physiological responses to dietary sodium ingestion receiving most favor. Familial as well as racial patterns of hypertension exist. Hypertension is found twice as frequently in individuals with a hypertensive parent compared to those with normotensive parents.[15]

Body size and the body-weight index are directly correlated with blood pressure. In a population and in an individual, weight gain is associated with an increase in blood pressure.[16–18] Physical and emotional stress, in populations as well as individuals, directly correlates with increased blood pressure. Animal experiments, as well as epidemiological surveys in humans, support this association.[19–22] An often-quoted example is the 5.6 times higher annual incidence of hypertension in air traffic controllers, as compared to well-matched nonprofessional pilots. Stress is felt to increase the sympathetic nervous system's activity, leading to a higher cardiac output and vascular resistance.

Many minerals are related to hypertension. Most notably, sodium intake is directly correlated with the prevalence of hypertension in populations and the level of blood pressure in individuals.[23–25] Much weaker associations have been described between other minerals and blood pressure: decreased calcium intake, decreased serum potassium, decreased serum magnesium, increased serum lead, and increased red cell zinc are all associated with an increased prevalence of hypertension and increased blood pressure levels.

The acute effects of caffeine and nicotine use cause an elevation of blood pressure. However, chronic caffeine users have blood pressures similar to those of nonusers.[26] Habituated smokers have no increase in the prevalence of hypertension although their overall cardiovascular risk is greatly increased, and the mortality ascribed to hypertension is significantly greater.[27] Alcohol use, in mild amounts (less than three or four drinks per day), is actually associated with decreased blood pressure. Heavier use of alcohol, or complete abstinence, is associated with an increased prevalence of hypertension.[28]

Quantitative analysis of the cardiovascular risks of hypertension comes from several types of studies: large-scale observational databases such as insurance industry-generated actuarial data; the Framingham Study[29]; The Pooling Project[30]; and also the control groups from several large interventional studies such as the VA Co-operative Study (VA Co-op),[31,32] the U.S. Public Health Service Hospital Study (USPHS), the Hypertension Detection and Follow-Up Project (HDFP),[34] the Oslo Trial,[35] the Australian Therapeutic Trial (ATT),[36] and the Multiple Risk Factor Intervention Trial (MRFIT).[37] Although methodologies differ among these studies, making direct comparisons inappropriate, valid generalizations regarding the cardiovascular risk of hypertension can be drawn. Essential hypertension usually has its onset between the ages of 20 years and 50 years, with the mean age of onset in the mid-30s. The incidence of all forms of cardiovascular disease increases with each increment of either the systolic or diastolic blood pressure. This increased morbidity can be detected at diastolic blood pressure greater than 80 mm Hg and rises progressively faster as the blood pressure increases further (Fig. 2). Overall, 20-year mortality rates double when the diastolic blood pressure is greater than 100 mm Hg. This increased cardiovascular morbidity and mortality is greater for men than women. As the level of blood pressure increases, stroke becomes relatively more common. The specific rates of cardiovascular events are dependent on many factors all of which can be used to calculate an individual's total cardiovascular risk profile, discussed below.

Clearly, the risk of a cardiovascular morbid event or death increases exponentially with increasing blood pressure in the individual patient. The higher the blood pressure, the higher the frequency of stroke, myocardial infarction, congestive heart failure, renal failure, and aortic aneurysm. But for the total population, this direct relationship between blood pressure and cardiovascular risk is less meaningful. As the HDFP study revealed, the majority of cardiovascular morbidity and mortality in our population occurs in those with mild elevations of blood pressure. Even though the risk of death is much lower in an individual with mild hypertension, so many more persons are exposed to this risk that the absolute number of deaths is greater than in persons with severe hypertension. As Fig. 3 shows, nearly 60% of the excess deaths attributable to hypertension in the United States occur in persons with diastolic blood pressure between 90 and 104 mm Hg. However, pharmacological treatment of this group of patients has not been shown to be definitely efficacious, and treating this group of hypertensives is currently the topic of much debate among experts in the field.

5. EFFICACY OF TREATMENT

Prior to the 1950s there was little effective treatment for hypertension, but since that time many effective and safe compounds have been developed. Today's practitioner has

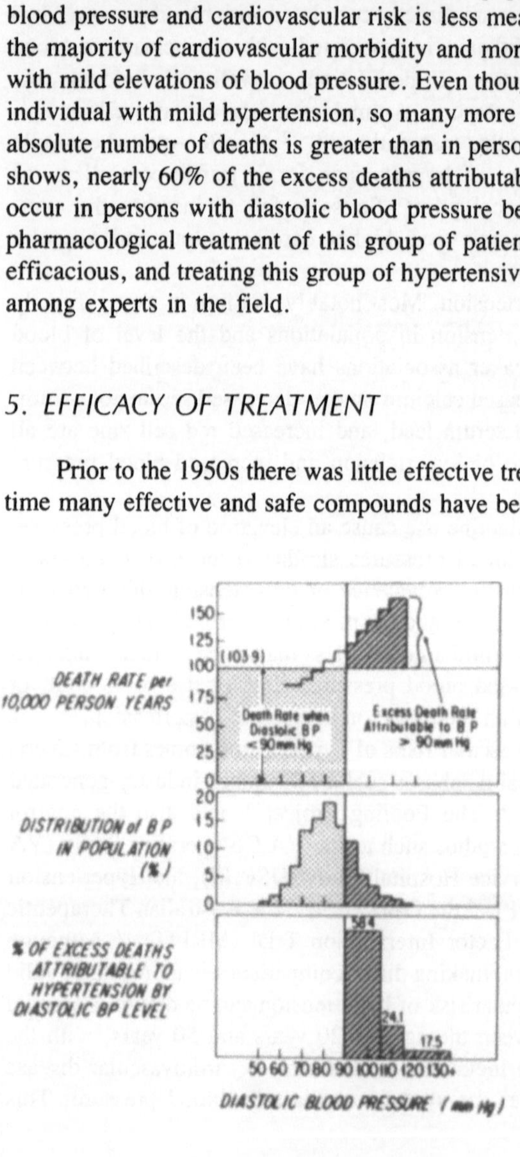

Figure 3. Excess deaths attributable to diastolic pressure above 90 mm Hg. (Source: Hypertension Detection and Follow-up Program.[48])

over 30 different medications available and approved for the treatment of hypertension. The relationship of increased blood pressure and cardiovascular disease has been known since the early 20th century. It was only after the availability of effective treatments that the efficacy of lowering the blood pressure could be proven.

The evidence is convincing that blood pressure can be lowered with pharmacological and nonpharmacological interventions. This evidence will be addressed separately for severe (diastolic blood pressure ≥ 115 mm Hg), moderate (diastolic blood pressure 105–114 mm Hg), and mild (diastolic blood pressure 90–104 mm Hg) ranges of hypertension.

The first evidence that lowering blood pressure affected survival appeared in the late 1950s and addressed malignant hypertension. Prior to effective drug treatments, malignant hypertension carried an 80% 1-year mortality rate and a 97% 5-year mortality. The first 5-year treatment studies appeared in 1958 showing a 34% 1-year and 67% 5-year mortality. Obviously a significant improvement! The VA Co-op,[31] begun in 1963 and published in 1967, offered the first definite and dramatic proof that blood pressure-lowering treatments were effective. A total of 143 hospitalized men with severe, nonmalignant hypertension (diastolic blood pressure 115–129 mm Hg) were studied. It took only one and one-half years until a significant difference in morbidity and mortality between the 70 control patients and 73 treated (hydrochlorothiazide, reserpine, and hydralazine) patients was observed. Mortality and morbidity rates were 5.7% and 32.9%, respectively, in the placebo group versus 0.0% and 2.7%, respectively, in the treated group (Table V).

This same study also enrolled 380 men with diastolic blood pressure between 90 and 114 mm Hg.[32] After an average follow-up of 3.3 years there was a significant difference in mortality and morbidity between the placebo and treated groups (Table VI). This difference was highly significant for the 210 patients with moderate hypertension (diastolic blood pressure 105–114 mm Hg) but only suggestive for the 170 patients with mild elevation of the diastolic blood pressure (90–104 mm Hg) (Table VII).

The results of the VA Co-op are conclusive and well accepted with respect to the utility of the treatment of moderate and severe hypertension (diastolic blood pressure > 104 mm Hg). The results of this same study, in patients with mild hypertension, are not nearly as definitive. Indeed, there have been several large, expensive multicenter studies addressing the question of the efficacy of treatment of mild hypertension (diastolic blood

Table V. VA Co-operative Study: Diastolic Blood Pressure 115–129 mm Hg[a]

	Treatment	Placebo
Total patients	70	73
Deaths	0	4
Accelerated hypertension	2	23
Stroke	1	4
Coronary disease	0	2
Congestive heart failure	0	2
Renal damage	0	2

[a]Source: VA Co-operative Study.[31]

Table VI. VA Co-operative Study: Diastolic Blood Pressure 90–114 mm Hg[a]

	Treatment	Placebo
Total patients	186	194
Stroke	5 (1 fatal)	20 (7 fatal)
Coronary disease	11 (6 fatal)	13 (11 fatal)
Congestive heart failure	0	11
Accelerated hypertension	0	4
Renal damage	0	3
Ruptured aortic aneurysm	1 (1 fatal)	2 (1 fatal)

[a]Source: VA Co-operative Study.[32]

pressure 90–104 mm Hg). The results of these studies are variable and their conclusions sometimes contradictory, especially for the group of patients with diastolic blood pressure between 90 and 100 mm Hg. The key elements of these studies are shown in Table VIII. These studies are impossible to compare directly with each other. They all have unique study designs and patient populations. Nevertheless, there are useful positive and negative findings in each. The VA Co-op showed significant protection with treatment, but only in men over 50 years old or those who had preexisting cardiovascular disease. The USPHS[33] trial showed no significant reduction in the atherosclerotic complications of hypertension [e.g., myocardial infarction (MI), sudden death]. The HDFP[34] showed a 20% reduction in cardiovascular mortality in patients with diastolic blood pressure between 90 and 104 mm Hg, but its design compared special comprehensive care to usual community care. It did not directly address the usefulness of treatment *per se*. Other findings of note from the HDFP study include the following: women and patients under 50 years of age showed no beneficial effect of treatment; there was a 13% decrease in noncardiovascular mortality as well, suggesting that some factor other than treatment of hypertension was at work; many of the patients in this mild hypertension group were already on drug treatment and actually had more severe hypertension. The ATT[36] did compare the drug treatment with placebo treatment of mild hypertension in patients with no evidence of end-organ disease. After 3 years a 30% reduction in cardiovascular disease endpoints was shown for the treated group. But closer analysis of the data revealed that placebo-treated patients with diastolic blood pressure less than 100 mm Hg had less morbidity than the actively treated patients. The Oslo Trial[35] showed results similar to the ATT, i.e., protection from cardiovascular

Table VII. VA Co-operative Study: Morbidity and Level of Diastolic Blood Pressure

	Treatment group			Control group		
	At risk	No.	%	At risk	No.	%
DBP 90–104 mm Hg	86	14	16.3	84	21	25.0
DBP 105–114 mm Hg	100	8	8.0	110	35	31.8

Table VIII. Key Clinical Studies of Mild Hypertension

Trial name	Number pts	Entry DBP (mm Hg)	Study design	Follow-up (mean years)
VA (1972)	170	90–104	Placebo vs step-care	3
USPHS (1977)	389	90–104	Placebo vs step-care	7
HDFP (1979)	7825	90–104	Referred care vs step-care	5
Australian (1980)	3427	95–109	Placebo vs step-care	4
Oslo (1980)	785	95–109	No Rx vs step-care	6
MRFIT (1982)	8012	90–114	Usual care vs special care	7
MRC (1985)	17,354	95–109	Placebo vs diuretic or beta blocker	5.5

disease by treatment of diastolic blood pressure > 100 mm Hg but no advantage to treating diastolic blood pressure less than 100.

The MRFIT trial[37] yielded some of the most alarming and controversial findings. Males with diastolic blood pressure of 90–94 mm Hg, treated aggressively with drugs, had higher coronary rates and total mortality than those treated less intensively. There was no difference in patients with diastolic blood pressure 95–99, while those with diastolic blood pressure > 100 mm Hg fared better with aggressive treatment. Of special note is the higher coronary death rate seen in patients treated aggressively who had abnormal baseline electrocardiograms (EKG) (2.92 versus 17.7 deaths per 1000 in the usual care and special intervention groups, respectively). The British Medical Research Council Trial (MRC)[38] showed a decrease in stroke and total cardiovascular events but no difference in coronary events or total mortality with the active treatment of mild hypertension.

In summary, there is strong, well-accepted evidence that drug treatment of moderate and severe hypertension (diastolic blood pressure > 105 mm Hg) improves survival and decreases the incidence of cardiovascular events. There is reasonable evidence that similar advantages are derived from the treatment of diastolic blood pressure > 100 mm Hg. Although this is less conclusive, it is still the accepted standard of practice in the United States today. Major controversy still exists regarding the proper management of the patient with diastolic blood pressure between 90 and 100 mm Hg. Yet, as was demonstrated earlier, it is this level of blood pressure that is responsible for nearly 60% of the excessive mortality associated with hypertension. Thus the question is important, both to the management of the individual patient, to our population's health as a whole, and to our health care system's resources.

There is no well-accepted explanation for this relative failure of drug treatment of mild hypertension, especially when the diastolic blood pressure is below 100 mm Hg. Although unlikely, it may be an inaccurate observation due to the lack of control of unidentified confounding variables or other methodological flaws. But even the earliest studies, done on more severe hypertension, have either shown a mild effect or no effect of treatment on the atherosclerotic complications of high blood pressure, especially ischemic coronary heart disease (i.e., MI, angina, sudden death). When the MRFIT data revealed a significantly worse outcome for mild hypertensives treated aggressively with drugs, it forced a critical evaluation of the question. The increased mortality in the aggressively treated patients in the MRFIT study was most significant in those who had an abnormal baseline EKG. The major proportion of this increased death rate was due to coronary heart disease. Immediately, attention turned to the electrolyte abnormalities associated with diuretic therapy, the form of antihypertensive treatment most often used in the United States today. Hypokalemia is well known to predispose to ventricular arrythmias, especially in an ischemic setting. Studies have documented an inverse relationship not only between potassium levels and ventricular fibrillation but also between potassium levels and survival in cardiac care unit patients.[39,40] These associations are strongest for serum K^+ levels less than 2.5 meq/liter but also hold true for levels in the "normal" range. Diuretic-induced magnesium depletion has also been implicated in this explanation. On a less acute basis, drug-induced changes in lipid profiles, glucose tolerance, and uric acid levels have also been examined. Glucose intolerance and hyperlipidemia can be precipitated by diuretics. Diuretics and many beta blockers increase total cholesterol and decrease high-density lipoprotein cholesterol. Although not responsible for decreased survival due to acute ischemic events, these changes in cholesterol have significant implications for an individual's as well as a population's overall cardiovascular risk. It has been shown that a diuretic will, on the average, lower diastolic blood pressure 10–15 mm Hg and raise the total cholesterol 20 mg%. In a young, mildly hypertensive individual without other risk factors these changes can actually increase the overall total cardiovascular risk.

It is no longer appropriate to approach all patients with hypertension in a cookbook fashion. Stepped care is being replaced with an individualized approach, often stressing the use of a single drug, or monotherapy, and addressing the patient's total cardiovascular risk profile, not just the level of blood pressure.

6. NONPHARMACOLOGICAL TREATMENT

This chapter does not deal with the multitude of drugs currently available for the treatment of hypertension. Excellent reviews of these compounds and their proper use exist and the reader is referred to them for this information. Here we review the usefulness of nonpharmacological therapy and a rational approach to the patient with mild hypertension.

There are many reasons for the recent renewed interest in the nonpharmacological treatment of hypertension. As has been discussed, there is growing concern over the evidence that patients with mild hypertension do not universally benefit from drug-induced lowering of the blood pressure. It has long been observed that the morbidity and mortality due to coronary heart disease is not improved to the same degree by treatment as other hypertensive disease endpoints such as cerebrovascular accidents, congestive heart failure, and renal failure. Several studies have even suggested an alarming increase in coronary heart disease mortality and morbidity in mildly hypertensive patients treated aggressively with drug therapy (e.g., MRFIT). Experts have implicated the changes in electrolytes and lipid profiles induced by antihypertensive drugs as possible explanations of these findings. In addition, many patients with mild hypertension will have a spontaneous decrease in blood pressure over 3–6 months' time. For these reasons the nonpharmacological strategies listed in Table IX are receiving renewed popularity in research efforts as well as clinical practice. A brief overview of these modalities is presented next.

6.1.1. Sodium Restriction

The average American diet contains 10–20 g of salt per day (170–350 mg Na^+). On the average, one-third of this amount is added from a salt shaker during cooking or at the table. This amount is far in excess of any physiological need for sodium. Many experts feel this high sodium intake, in the presence of an inherited inability to efficiently excrete this sodium load via the kidneys, is integral to the development of essential hypertension. Epidemiological studies have demonstrated a direct association between a culture's sodium intake and the prevalence of hypertension.[41–46] Members of a low-sodium culture who increase the salt content of their diet sustain an increase in the prevalence of hypertension.[43,45,49]

It has been known since the 1940s that dietary sodium restriction can lower the blood pressure in most subjects.[50] More recent reports have demonstrated the efficacy of moderate sodium restriction hypertension.[51–55] In general, a diet containing approximately 5 g of sodium can be expected to decrease the blood pressure by 10/5 mm Hg in the majority of patients with mild hypertension. This level of sodium intake can usually be obtained with the following guidelines: (1) No added salt to cooking or at table, (2) avoid milk and milk products, (3) avoid processed and fast foods as much as possible, (4) avoid obviously salty foods, and (5) read packaging labels of all foods for sodium content.

6.1.2. Weight Reduction

Obesity is not an independent predictor of cardiovascular disease. However, it is strongly associated with the presence or development of hypertension. Although there is a great deal of suggestive data, a direct cause-and-effect association between obesity and

Table IX. Nondrug Interventions for Hypertension[a]

1.	Dietary sodium restriction	Effective
2.	Weight reduction in the obese	Effective
3.	Regular exercise	Effective
4.	Relaxation techniques	Effective
5.	Stopping cigarettes	Possibly effective
6.	Potassium supplementation	Possibly effective
7.	Increased polyunsaturated fat in diet	Possibly effective
8.	Calcium supplementation	Possibly effective
9.	Limited (<60 oz/month) ethanol	Possibly effective

[a]Source: Kaplan.[95]

hypertension is not universally accepted. Actuarial and epidemiological data show not only that obese individuals have a higher prevalence of hypertension but also that further weight gain is associated with up to 8 times the incidence of hypertension compared to that of nonobese persons.[18] The Framingham study showed that men who lost 15% of their body weight dropped their systolic blood pressure by 10% and those who gained 15% of their weight raised their systolic blood pressure by 18%.[56]

More recently controlled trials of weight loss in hypertension patients have shown that weight loss lowers the blood pressure significantly in mildly, moderately, or severely obese hypertensive patients.[57–60] This observation holds true for the majority of hypertensive patients, regardless of the degree of hypertension or the use of concomitant antihypertensive drugs. In general, for each kilogram of weight loss, the blood pressure falls by 2.5/1.5 mm Hg.[61] This effect is independent and synergistic with simultaneous sodium restriction.

6.1.3. Exercise

There is controversial evidence that regular, aerobic exercise decreases cardiovascular mortality and coronary artery disease morbidity. It has been suggested that, in part, this effect may be mediated by a chronic decrease in blood pressure. In normotensives, isotonic, aerobic exercise causes an acute decrease in diastolic blood pressure while in hypertensive subjects the diastolic blood pressure increases acutely. Nevertheless, many investigators have attempted to show that regular exercise can cause a sustained decrease in blood pressure. Both vigorous[62,63] and milder exercise regimens[64–67] have shown significant decreases in resting blood pressure. Regimens of mild walk–jog or calisthenics (70–80% maximum predicted heart rate) 3 times a week have shown decreases in blood pressure of up to 20/15 mm Hg after 3 months. This antihypertensive effect disappears after cessation of the exercise program. Many of these studies are critized because they do not adequately control for changes in weight or sodium ingestion. But those that do control for these confounding variables have still shown a beneficial effect of exercise alone. It is not contested that the combination of sodium restriction, weight loss, and regular mild aerobic exercise is useful in most patients and can lower the blood pressure by up to 20/10 mm Hg. Sustained compliance with these life-style changes is the limiting factor.

6.1.4. Relaxation Therapy

Physical and emotional stress has been associated with sustained hypertension in both experimental animal models and human epidemiological studies. Skeletal muscle relaxation has been known to lower blood pressure since the 1940s.[68] Since then, hundreds of reports have investigated the usefulness of relaxation techniques (transcendental meditation, yoga, psychotherapy) and biofeedback for lowering blood pressure. Most investigators have shown a significant decrease in blood pressure (5–10/5–10 mm Hg) in subjects adequately motivated in these techniques. Reviewers of these many reports have reached varying conclusions.[69,70] In general, the techniques of relaxation and biofeedback can be of utility in some subjects and are worth trying in these individuals. The potential for gain is real and the costs and risks are minimal.

6.1.5. Dietary Lipids

Epidemiological data have shown an association between vegetarian diets and lower blood pressure.[71] Specifically, diets with a high polyunsaturated-to-saturated fats ratio have been shown to lower the blood pressure of both normotensive and hypertensive subjects. These interventions have used the substitution of foodstuffs (margarine, skim milk, lean meats, low-fat cheese, vegetable oils) as well as pills containing polyunsaturated fats or placebo.[72–75]

Studies have shown a decrease in blood pressure of up to 12/11 mm Hg with these interventions over 4–6 weeks. They have attempted to control for total caloric intake, weight, and sodium intake. Hypothetically, these polyunsaturated fats are the metabolic precursors of vasodilatory and saluretic prostaglandins and may increase the production of these compounds. Large-scale and long-term controlled studies are needed to further address this point. In the interim, it is easily justifiable to recommend these sorts of dietary changes because of their additional advantageous effect on other cardiovascular risk factors such as lipid profiles and weight.

6.1.6. Potassium Intake

Since the early 1930s potassium has been known to have an effect on the regulation of blood pressure.[76] The success of the Kempner rice diet has been partially ascribed to its high potassium as well as its low sodium content. Epidemiological studies have documented a significant association between high potassium intake and lower blood pressure, which is independent of sodium's effect.[77–80] Both serum potassium and total body potassium has been found to be lower in hypertensives compared to normotensives.[81] Interventional studies have been less conclusive but highly suggestive of potassium's usefulness in helping lower blood pressure in mildly hypertensive patients.[82–87] Theoretically, potassium may improve blood pressure through several mechanisms: (1) potassium has a direct saluretic effect on the kidney, (2) potassium increases baroreceptor sensitivity, and (3) potassium prevents the increase in catechols seen with sodium restriction.[88]

Prospective, controlled studies are required to further define the role of potassium supplementation in hypertensives, including those on diuretic therapy. Meanwhile, the use of potassium-containing salt substitutes to improve compliance with dietary sodium restriction should probably be encouraged, but only in patients without evidence of renal insufficiency or potassium-sparing diuretic use.

6.1.7. Calcium Intake

Calcium is also involved in the regulation of arterial pressure. Its relation to blood pressure is not well understood. Hypercalcemia is well known to cause hypertension, and hypertensives have a higher incidence of primary hyperparathyroidism. But increased dietary calcium is also epidemiologically associated with lower blood pressure and a lower prevalence of cardiovascular disease. This relationship has been identified through studies looking at the hardness of water (increased calcium),[89] urinary calcium levels, and dietary recall.[90] Increased ionized calcium levels and decreased parathyroid hormone levels have also been found in some surveys of hypertensive individuals.[91]

Interventional studies controlling calcium intake have not been impressive in changing the blood pressure.[92,93] The small decrements in blood pressure reported (1–5 mm Hg) are not highly significant for an individual but if achieved in a large population would have major effects on overall cardiovascular risk. At this time one cannot strongly recommend calcium supplementation to hypertensive patients. But the common recommendation to decrease dairy products as part of sodium restriction may have a slightly detrimental effect since nearly two-thirds of our dietary calcium comes from this source.

7. EVALUATION OF HYPERTENSION

Initial evaluation of the hypertensive patient is directed toward three main objectives: (1) to rule out the presence of secondary, curable hypertension, (2) to assess the presence and degree of target organ damage caused by hypertension, and (3) to fully evaluate the overall risk of significant cardiovascular disease. These three objectives can be met without extensive cost in nearly all cases.

Curable, secondary hypertension is much rarer in the general population than the literature from 15–20 years ago initially indicated. This is probably due to the tertiary, referral center nature of the institutions reporting these data. Of 5485 patients in the HDFP stepped-care group evaluated for secondary hypertension with history, physical, routine laboratory work, and, where indicated, more extensive tests, approximately 1% were found to have possibly curable secondary hypertension.[94] In fact, only nine patients were cured of their hypertension, six by stopping oral estrogen use and three by surgical repair of renovascular lesions.

With this low prevalence of specifically curable causes of secondary hypertension, the routine use of sophisticated and relatively expensive screening tests in all patients with high blood pressure becomes especially hazardous. The ability of a test to accurately establish the presence or absence of a disease, i.e., its predictive value, is directly related to its specificity and sensitivity and the prevalence of the disease in the tested population. The routine use of the rapid-sequence intravenous pyelogram (IVP) in evaluating all hypertensives for the presence of renovascular hypertension has been essentially abandoned because of its limited predictive value. For example, if the IVP has an 85% sensitivity and specificity in diagnosing renovascular hypertension, and if the prevalence of this cause of hypertension were 2%, a patient with a positive IVP would still have only a 10% chance of truly having renovascular hypertension. Even with a 10% prevalence of renovascular hypertension, a positive IVP is indicative of only a 39% chance of a true renovascular etiology.

This concept has major socioeconomic implications in developing recommendations for screening hypertensive patients for the relatively rare causes of secondary hypertension. In fact, the history and physical examination will be able to exclude most causes of secondary hypertension.[95] With the addition of a simple and inexpensive laboratory database, nearly all cases of secondary hypertension can be detected. These tests include a complete blood count, serum electrolytes, a blood urea nitrogen and creatinine, a complete urinalysis, and an EKG. Additional studies should be reserved for those who demonstrate features of unusual hypertension, such as young or old age of onset (less than

20 years or more than 50 years), severe or resistant hypertension, significant end-organ damage [left ventricular hypertrophy (LVH), renal insufficiency, grade III or IV retinopathy], hypokalemia, diastolic abdominal bruit, or highly variable pressure and symptoms of tachycardia, diaphoresis, and headaches. These further tests are outlined briefly in Table X.

End-organ damage can be assessed with minimal extra cost or discomfort to the patient or physician. This evaluation yields information that is integral to the physician's ability to determine the severity of the patient's hypertensive disorder, the need for therapy, and the prognosis. The organ systems evaluated are those most susceptible to the effects of hypertension: the eyes, brain, heart, arterial system, and kidneys.

Funduscopic examination reveals the presence and extent of hypertensive damage to the microvasculature. The milder changes (KW grade I and II) can be directly related to risk for coronary artery disease and stroke[96] and most likely represent generalized atherosclerosis. More severe funduscopic changes reflect direct effects of the elevated blood pressure.

Cardiac damage usually results in ischemic events or sudden death and less frequently in congestive failure. Changes are often evident long before the occurrence of these events. The physical examination, chest x-ray (CXR), and EKG are useful in detecting changes in cardiac size but are insensitive. Although echocardiography is much more sensitive than these modalities, its role in the routine evaluation of left ventricular size and function in hypertension is not well established. Because of the strong association between LVH and premature death, especially sudden death,[97] and the increasing evidence that certain drug treatments are more effective than others in reversing LVH, the echocardiogram may some day become an important resource in the workup of hypertension.

There is presently no effective means of evaluating the early effects of hypertension on the cerebral vasculature. Magnetic resonance imaging and positron emission tomography may someday play a role here. Renal involvement is usually quantitated through the use of a urinalysis and serum and urine measurements of renal function.

Determination of the overall cardiovascular risk of a patient with high blood pressure is crucial to the effective management of hypertension and to the preventive health care

Table X. Diagnostic Tests for Secondary Hypertension[a]

Disease	Tests
Chronic renal failure	Urinalysis, BUN, creatinine, sonography; consider renin assay, renal biopsy, IVP
Renovascular disease	Plasma renin, renal vein renin
Coarctation of the aorta	Blood pressure in legs, aortogram
Primary aldosteronism	Plasma potassium; consider plasma renin and/or aldosterone, urinary potassium
Cushing's syndrome	Dexamethasone suppression testing
Pheochromyoctoma	Spot urine metanephrine; consider urinary catechols and vanillylmandelic acid, plasma catechols

[a]Source: Kaplan.[95]

mission of the primary-care provider. The overall risk is derived from epidemiological data, especially the Framingham Study. The factors usually considered are age, sex, systolic or diastolic blood pressure, lipoprotein levels, the presence of diabetes, LVH by EKG, and a history of cigarette smoking. Booklets[98] and hand-held calculators are available to determine the risk.

This exercise of risk specification has several benefits. Although the blood pressure is usually the easiest risk factor to control, any other significant causes of increased risk and their contributions to the overall risk ratio can also be identified. This sort of analysis can greatly influence the level of aggressiveness and areas of emphasis in a physician's management of his patient. In a young, mildly hypertensive patient with no other risk factors, observation and nondrug therapy can be attempted without undo concern, since the 8-year risk of a cardiovascular event is less than 5%. In an older individual with multiple risk factors in addition to mild hypertension, other recommendations would be made and the blood pressure lowered aggressively since this person's 8-year risk can be as high as 70%.

Hypertension is a common problem for the primary-care physician and is often approached in a glib manner. The era of "cookbook" stepped-care management is over. The modern physician must have an understanding and appreciation of this disorder and the repurcussions its management can have on the individual patient as well as on the population as a whole. In the young mildly hypertensive patient, nonpharmacological therapy can be effective not only in lowering the blood pressure but also in improving other factors related to the increased risks of cardiovascular and cerebrovascular disease.

REFERENCES

1. National Center for Health Statistics: *Monthly Vital Statistics Rep.* **29:**1–9, 1981.
2. Rose, G.: Strategy of prevention: Lessons from cardiovascular disease. *Br. Med. J.* **282:**1847–1850, 1981.
3. Kirkendall, W. M., Feinleib, M., Freis, E. D., *et al.: Recommendations for Human Blood Pressure Determination by Sphygmomanometers.* American Heart Association, New York, 1980.
4. Simpson, J. A., Jamieson, G., Dickhaus, D. W., *et al.:* Effect of size of cuff bladder on accuracy of measurement of indirect blood pressure. *Am. Heart J.* **70:**208–211, 1965.
5. Karvonen, M. J., Telivuo, L. J., and Jarnieven, E. J. K.: Sphygmomanometer cuff size and the accuracy of indirect measurement of blood pressure. *Am. J. Cardiol.* **13:**688–691, 1964.
6. King, G. E.: Taking the blood pressure. *JAMA* **209:**1902, 1969.
7. Armitage, P., Fox, W., and Rose, G.: The variability of measurements of casual blood pressure. *Clin. Sci.* **30:**337–340, 1966.
8. Marshall, A. J., and Barrit, D. W. (eds.): *The Hypertensive Patient.* Pitman Medical Press, Kent, 1980.
9. Pickering, G.: Hypertension. Definitions, natural histories and consequences. *Am. J. Med.* **52:**570–577, 1972.
10. The 1984 Report of the Joint National Committee on Detection, Evaluation, and Treatment of High Blood Pressure. *Arch. Intern. Med.* **144:**1045–1057, 1984.
11. Lerner, D. J., and Kannel, W. B.: Patterns of coronary heart disease morbidity and mortality in sexes: A 26-year follow-up of the Framingham population. *Am. Heart J.* **111:**383–387, 1986.
12. Neaton, J. D., Kuller, L. H., Wentwork, D., *et al.:* Total and cardiovascular mortality in relation to cigarette smoking, serum cholesterol concentration, and diastolic blood pressure among black and white males followed up for five years. *Am. Heart J.* **108:**759–766, 1984.
13. Franco, L. J., Stern, M. P., Rosenthal, M., *et al.:* Coffee consumption, diet, and lipids. *Am. J. Epidemiol.* **121:**684–687, 1985.

14. DeStefano, F., Coulehan, J. L., and Wlant, M. K.: Prevalence, detection, and control of hypertension in a biethnic community. *Am. J. Epidemiol.* **109**:335–340, 1979.
15. Stamler, R., Stamler, J., Reidlinger, W. F., *et al.*: Family (parental) history and prevalence of hypertension. *JAMA* **241**:43–48, 1979.
16. Dustan, H. P.: in Lauer, R. M., and Shehelle, R. B. (eds.): *Childhood Prevention of Atherosclerosis and Hypertension.* Raven Press, New York, 1980.
17. Havlik, R. J., Hubert, H. B., Fabsitz, R. R., *et al.*: Weight and hypertension. *Ann. Intern. Med.* **98**:855–859, 1983.
18. Paul, O. (ed.): *Epidemiology and Control of Hypertension.* Stratton Intercontinental, New York, 1975.
19. Cobb, S., and Rose, R. M.: Hypertension, peptic ulcer, and diabetes in air traffic controllers. *JAMA* **224**:489–493, 1973.
20. Sever, P. S., Gordon, D., Peart, W. S., *et al.*: Blood pressure and its correlates in urban and tribal Africa. *Lancet* **2**:60–61, 1980.
21. Monk, M.: Psychologic status and hypertension. *Am. J. Epidemiol.* **112**:200–203, 1980.
22. Dworkin, B. R., Filearich, R. J., Miller, N. E., *et al.*: Baroreceptor activation reduces reactivity to noxious stimulation: Implications for hypertension. *Science* **205**:1299–1300, 1979.
23. Freis, E. D.: Salt, volume and the prevention of hypertension. *Circulation* **53**:589–593, 1976.
24. Garcia-Palmieri, M. R., Costas, R., Cruz-Vidal, M., *et al.*: Milk consumption, calcium intake, and decreased hypertension. *Hypertension* **6**:322–326, 1984.
25. Tobain, L.: The relationship of salt to hypertension. *Am. J. Clin. Nutr.* **32**:2739–2741, 1979.
26. Robertson, E., Wade, D., Workman, R., *et al.*: Tolerance to the humoral and hemodynamic effects of caffeine in man. *J. Clin. Invest.* **67**:1111–1113, 1981.
27. Doll, R., and Peto, R.: Mortality in relation to smoking: 20 years observations on male British doctors. *Br. Med. J.* **2**:1525–1528, 1976.
28. Harburg, E., Ozgoren, F., Hawthorne, V. W., *et al.*: Community norms of alcohol usage and blood pressure: Tecumseh, Michigan. *Am. J. Public Health* **70**:813–816, 1980.
29. Castelli, W. P.: Epidemiology of coronary heart disease: The Framingham Study. *Am. J. Med.* **76**(2A):4–8, 1984.
30. The Pooling Project Research Group: Final report of the Pooling Project. *J. Chronic Dis.* **31**(4):201–206, 1978.
31. VA Co-op: Effects of treatment on morbidity in hypertension. Results in patients diastolic blood pressures averaging 115 through 129 mm Hg. *JAMA* **202**:1028–1031, 1967.
32. VA Co-op: Effects of treatment on morbidity in hypertension. Results in patients diastolic blood pressure averaging 90 through 11 mm Hg. *JAMA* **213**:1143–1146, 1970.
33. Smith, W. M.: Treatment of mild hypertension: Results of a ten-year intervention trial. *Circ. Res.* **40** (suppl 1):98–101, 1977.
34. Hypertension Detection and Follow-up Program Cooperative Group: Five year findings of hypertension detection and follow-up program. II. Reduction in stroke incidence among persons with high blood pressure. *JAMA* **247**:633–635, 1982.
35. Helgeland, A.: Treatment of mild hypertension: A five year controlled drug trial. *Am. J. Med.* **69**:725–727, 1980.
36. Management Committee: The Australian therapeutic trial in mild hypertension. *Lancet* **1**:1261–1263, 1980.
37. Multiple Risk Factor Intervention Trial Research Group: Risk factor changes and mortality results. *JAMA* **248**:1465–1472, 1982.
38. Medical Research Council Working Party: MRC trial of treatment of mild hypertension: Principal results. *Br. Med. J.* **291**:97–99, 1985.
39. Nordrehaug, J. E., Johannesseen, K. A., and von-der-Lippe, G.: Serum potassium concentration as a risk factor of ventricular arrhythmias early in acute myocardial infarction. *Circulation* **71**:645–648, 1985.
40. Dyckner, T., Helmers, C., and Webster, P. O.: Cardiac dysrhythmias in patients with acute myocardial infarction. Relation to serum potassium level and prior diuretic therapy. *Acta Med. Scand.* **216**:127–142, 1984.
41. Oliver, W. J., Cohen, E. L., Neel, J. V., *et al.*: Blood pressure sodium intake and sodium related hormones in the Yanomamo Indians, a "no salt" culture. *Circulation* **52**:146–151, 1975.
42. Lowenstein, F. W.: Blood pressure in relation to age and sex in the tropics and subtropic. A review of the literature and an investigation in two tribes of Brazil Indians. *Lancet* **1**:389–390, 1961.

43. Prior, A. M., Evans, J. G., Harvey, H. P. B., *et al.*: Sodium intake and blood pressure in two Polynesian populations. *N. Engl. J. Med.* **279**:515–518, 1968.
44. Sinnet, P. F., and Whyte, H. M.: Epidemiologic studies in the total highland population, Tukisenta, New Guinea. *J. Chronic Dis.* **26**:265–269, 1973.
45. Maddocks, I.: Blood pressure in Melanesians. *Med. J. Aust.* **1**:1123–1124, 1967.
46. Dahl, L. K.: Salt and hypertension. *Am. J. Clin. Nutr.* **25**:231–238, 1972.
47. Genest, J., Koiw, E., and Kuchel, O. (eds.): *Hypertension: Physiopathology and Treatment.* McGraw-Hill, New York, 1977.
48. Hypertension Detection and Follow-up Program. *Circ. Res.* **40**(suppl):106, 1977.
49. Sever, P. S., Gordon, D., Peart, W. S., *et al.*: Blood pressure and its correlates in urban and tribal Africa. *Lancet* **2**:60–62, 1980.
50. Kempner, W.: *Am. J. Med.* **4**:545–548, 1948.
51. Parijs, J., Joossens, J. V., Van der Linden, L., *et al.*: Moderate sodium restriction and diuretics in the treatment of hypertension. *Am. Heart J.* **85**:22–34, 1973.
52. Morgan, T., Gillies, A., Morgan, G., *et al.*: Hypertension treated by salt restriction. *Lancet* **1**:227–230, 1978.
53. MacGregor, G. A., Markandu, N. D., Best, F. E., *et al.*: Double-blind randomized crossover tiral of moderate sodium restriction in essential hypertension. *Lancet* **1**:235–351, 1982.
54. Watt, G. C. M., Edwards, C., Hart, J., *et al.*: Dietary restriction for mild hypertensives in general practice. *Br. Med. J.* **286**:432–436, 1983.
55. Morgan, T. O., and Myers, J. B., Hypertension treated by sodium restriction. *Med. J. Aust.* **2**:396–397, 1981.
56. Kannel, W. B., Brund, N., Skinner, J. J., *et al.*: The relation of adiposity to blood pressure and development of hypertension. *Ann. Intern. Med.* **67**:48–52, 1967.
57. Reisen, E., Abel, R., *et al.*: Effect of weight loss without salt restriction on the reduction of blood pressure in overweight hypertensive patients. *N. Engl. J. Med.* **298**:1–6, 1978.
58. Tuck, M. L., Sowers, J., Modan, M., *et al.*: The effect of weight reduction on blood pressure plasma renin activity, and plasma aldosterone levels in obese patients. *N. Engl. J. Med.* **304**:930–933, 1981.
59. Reisen, E., Frohlich, E. D., Dornfeld, L., *et al.*: Cardiovascular changes after weight reduction in obesity hypertension. *Ann. Intern. Med.* **98**:315–319, 1983.
60. Maxwell, M. H., Kushiro, T., Dornfeld, L. P., Messerli, F. H., *et al.*: Blood pressure changes in obese hypertensive subjects during rapid weight loss. Comparison on restricted vs unchanged salt intake. *Arch. Intern. Med.* **144**:1581–1584, 1984.
61. McMahon, F. G.: *Management of Essential Hypertension; the New Low Dose Era.* Futura, New York, 1984, p. 46.
62. Choquette, G., and Ferguson, R. J.: Blood pressure reduction in "borderline" hypertensives following physical training. *Can. Med. Assoc. J.* **108**:699–702, 1973.
63. Cade, R., Mars, D., Wagemaker, H., *et al.*: Effect of aerobic exercise training on patients with systemic arterial hypertension. *Am. J. Med.* **77**:785–789, 1984.
64. Boyer, J. L., and Kasch, F. W.: Exercise therapy in hypertensive men. *JAMA* **211**:1668–1671, 1970.
65. Bonanno, J. A., and Lies, J. E.: Effects of physical training on coronary risk factors. *Am. J. Cardiol.* **33**:760–764, 1974.
66. Roman, O., Camuzzi, A., Villalon, E., *et al.*: Physical training program in arterial hypertension: A long-term prospective follow-up. *Cardiology* **67**:230–243, 1981.
67. Krotkiewski, M., Mandroukas, K., Sjostrom, L., *et al.*: Effects of long-term physical training on body fat, metabolism, and blood pressure in obesity. *Metabolism* **28**:650–658, 1979.
68. Jacobson, E.: Variation of blood pressure with skeletal muscle tension and relaxation. *Ann. Intern. Med.* **12**:1194–1212, 1939.
69. Black, H. R.: Nonpharmacologic therapy for hypertension. *Am. J. Med.* **66**:837–842, 1979.
70. Agras, W. S.: Behavioral approaches to the treatment of essential hypertension. *Int. J. Obesity* **5**:100–106, 1981.
71. Ophir, O., Peer, G., Gilad, J., *et al.*: Low blood pressure in vegetarians: The possible role of potassium. *Am. J. Clin. Nutr.* **37**:755–759, 1983.
72. Puska, P., Iacono, J. M., *et al.*: Controlled, randomized trial of the effect of dietary fat on blood pressure. *Lancet* **1**:1–5, 1983.

73. Rouse, I. L., Beilin, L. J., Armstrong, B. K., *et al.:* Blood pressure-lowering effect of a vegetarian diet: Controlled trial in normotensive subjects. *Lancet* **1**:5–10, 1983.
74. Iacono, J. M., and Marshall, M. W.: Reduction in blood pressure associated with high polyunsaturated fat diets that reduce blood cholesterol in man. *Prev. Med.* **4**:426–443, 1975.
75. Rao, R. H., Rao, U. B., and Srikantia, S. G.: Effect of polyunsaturated-rich vegetable oils on blood pressure in essential hypertension. *Clin. Exp. Hypertension* **3**(1):27–38, 1981.
76. Addison, W. T. L.: The use of sodium chloride, potassium chloride, sodium bromide, and potassium bromide in cases of arterial hypertension. *Can. Med. Assoc. J.* **18**:281–288, 1928.
77. Reed, D., McGee, Yano, K., *et al.:* Diet, blood pressure, and multicollinearity. *Hypertension* **7**:405, 1985.
78. Staessen, J., Bulpitt, C., Fagard, R., *et al.:* Four urinary cations and blood pressure-a population study of two Belgian towns. International Symposium on Potassium, Blood Pressure and Cardiovascular Disease. Excerpta Medica, Amsterdam, 1983.
79. Khaw, K. T., and Rose, G.: Population study of blood pressure and associated factors in St. Lucia, West Indies. *Int. J. Epidemiol.* **11**:372–377, 1982.
80. Walker, W. C., Whelton, P. K., Saito, H., *et al.:* Relation between blood pressure and renin, renin substrate, angiotension II, aldosterone, and urinary sodium and potassium in 574 ambulatory subjects. *Hypertension* **1**(3):287–291, 1979.
81. Ericsson, F., Clarkmark, B., Elliasson, K., *et al.:* potassium in whole body and skeletal muscle in untreated primary hypertension. International Symposium on Potassium, Blood Pressure and Cardiovascular disease. Excerpta Medica, Amsterdam, 1983.
82. Parfrey, P. S., Vandenburg, M. J., Wright, P., *et al.:* Blood pressure and hormonal changes following alteration in dietary sodium and potassium in mild essential hypertension. *Lancet* **1**:59–63, 1981.
83. MacGregor, G. A., Smith, S. J., Markandu, N. D., *et al.:* Moderate potassium supplementation in essential hypertension. *Lancet* **2**:567–570, 1982.
84. Khaw, K. T., and Thorn, S.: Randomized double-blind crossover trial of potassium on blood pressure in normal subjects. *Lancet* **2**:1127–1129, 1982.
85. Iimura, O., Kyima, T., Kikuchi, K., *et al.:* Studies on the hypotensive effect of high potassium intake in patients with essential hypertension. *Clin. Sci.* **61**:77–90, 1981.
86. Mazzola, C., and Guffanti, E.: Cardiovascular modifications after K^+ supplementation in hypertensive patients. International Symposium on Potassium, Blood Pressure, and Cardiovascular Disease. Excerpta Medica, Amsterdam, 1983.
87. Kaplan, N. M., Carnegie, A., Raskin, P., *et al.:* Potassium supplementation in hypertensive patients with diuretic-induced hypokalemia. *N. Engl. J. Med.* **312**:746–749, 1985.
88. Skrabal, F., Auboch, J., and Hortnagl, H.: Low sodium/high potassium diet for prevention of hypertension: Probable mechanisms of action. *Lancet* **2**:895–900, 1981.
89. Shaper, A. G.: Soft water, heart attacks, and stroke. *JAMA* **230**:130–134, 1974.
90. McCarron, D. A., Morris, C. D., and Cole, C.: Dietary calcium in human hypertension. *Science* **217**:267–269, 1982.
91. McCarron, D. A.: Low serum concentrations of ionized calcium in patients with hypertension. *N. Engl. J. Med.* **307**:226–228, 1982.
92. Belzian, J. M., Villar, J., Pineda, O., *et al.:* Reduction of blood pressure with calcium supplementation in young adults. *JAMA* **249**:1161–1165, 1983.
93. McCarron, D. A., and Morris, C. D.: Blood pressure response to oral calcium in persons with mild to moderate hypertension. A randomized, double-blind, placebo-controlled, crossover trial. *Ann. Intern. Med.* **103**:825–829, 1985.
94. Lewin, A., Blaufox, D., Castle, H., *et al.:* Apparent prevalence of curable hypertension in the Hypertension Detection and Follow-up Program. *Arch. Intern. Med.* **145**:424–429, 1985.
95. Kaplan, N. M. (ed.): *Clinical Hypertension,* 4th ed. Williams & Wilkins, Baltimore, 1986.
96. Svardsudd, K., Wedel, H., Aurell, E., *et al.:* Hypertensive eye ground changes. Prevalence, relation to blood pressure and prognostic importance. The study of men born in 1913. *Acta Med. Scand.* **204**:159–163, 1978.
97. Schatzkin, A., Cupples, L. A., Heeren, T., *et al.:* The epidemiology of sudden unexpected death: Risk factors for men and women in the Framingham Heart Study. *Am. Heart J.* **107**:1300–1308, 1984.
98. *Coronary Risk Handbook.* American Heart Association, New York, 1973.

99. Feinleib. M.: The magnitude and the nature of the decrease in coronary heart disease mortality rate. *Am. J. Cardiol.* **54** (suppl): 2c–10c, 1984.

14

Thromboembolism

Daniel M. Becker

There are numerous approaches to the prevention of primary and recurrent thromboembolism. Before outlining specific preventive treatments, the need for prevention will be clarified by describing who is at risk, the frequency of the problem, diagnostic approaches, and the consequences of thromboembolism.

1. EPIDEMIOLOGY

1.1. Frequency

Accurate estimates of the incidence and prevalence of thromboembolic disease are not available. The clinical spectrum of disease is variable, ranging from asymptomatic events to sudden death. Accurate diagnosis is difficult. Clinical, laboratory, and radiological evaluation may be nonspecfic, and invasive testing is often necessary. Not infrequently pulmonary embolism is a postmortem diagnosis. Less than 10% of autopsy-proven pulmonary emboli are diagnosed before death.[1] To estimate the overall frequency of thromboembolic disease, it has been necessary to extrapolate from various types of data: clinical and pathological, prospective and retrospective. Despite the difficulty of these estimates, various investigators have arrived at remarkably similar figures.

Estimates of the incidence of pulmonary embolism rest largely on autopsy information.[2] Rates of pulmonary embolism found at autopsy vary from 6% to 64%, depending on the population studied and the effort of the pathologist. Meticulous dissection led to evidence of pulmonary embolism in 64% of 61 consecutive autopsies at a general hospital.[3] The presence of pulmonary embolism at postmortem does not necessarily mean that the embolic event was clinically significant. Based on pathological judgments that the embolism was the sole or major contributing cause of death, several studies suggest that 15% of deaths in acute general hospitals result from this problem.[4,5]

From such data, crude as they are, it is possible to estimate the number of deaths resulting from pulmonary embolism.[2,6,7] Such calculations assume that more than 15% of nursing-home or chronic hospital deaths are from pulmonary embolism, and that much

---

Daniel M. Becker • Department of Internal Medicine, University of Virginia School of Medicine, Charlottesville, Virginia 22908.

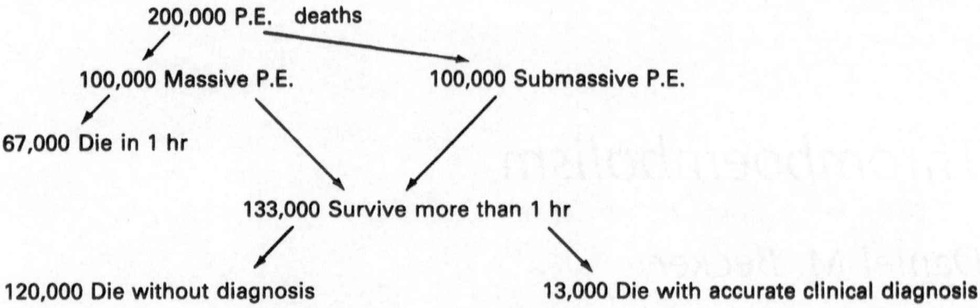

Assume: 50% of overall deaths from massive P.E.
Majority (67%) of massive P.E. survive less than 1 hr
Accurate premortem diagnosis in 10%
30% mortality for undiagnosed patients[8]
120,000 undiagnosed P.E. deaths represent 400,000 P.E.
8% mortality for diagnosed patients[9]
13,000 diagnosed P.E. deaths represent 163,000 P.E.

Total P.E. = Undiagnosed PE (400,000) + diagnosed P.E. (163,000) + sudden death (67,000) = 630,00

Figure 1. Pulmonary embolism: incidence and mortality. P.E., pulmonary embolism. (Source: adapted from Dalen and Alpert.[2])

less than 15% of sudden deaths outside hospitals are due to pulmonary embolism. This type of arithmetic leads to an estimate of 200,000 deaths annually attributable to pulmonary embolism. Similar calculations can be extended to reach an estimate of the overall incidence (fatal and nonfatal events) of pulmonary embolism (Fig. 1). By these estimates, 630,000 episodes of pulmonary embolism account for 67,000 immediate deaths and 133,000 delayed deaths per year in the United States.

Prospective data are available to estimate the incidence and prevelance of venous thrombosis in the United States.[7] These data are from a longitudinal study of health and disease in Tecumseh, Michigan. In this study the diagnosis of venous thrombophlebitis was based only on historical information or physical examination. The community data were extrapolated to 1970 U.S. census figures. The national estimates include 24 million people with varicose veins; 6–7 million people with venous stasis changes; 400,000–500,000 people with a stasis ulcer or a history of a stasis ulcer; an annual incidence of deep venous thrombosis of 250,000; and an annual incidence of superficial phlebitis of 128,000.

1.2. *Morbidity*

Accepting the limitations of these estimates of disease frequency and mortality, it is clear that thromboembolism is a common disease with a significant mortality. In addition, among the survivors there can be long-term morbidity. Although only rare patients develop pulmonary hypertension and cor pulmonale as a complication of recurrent pulmonary embolism, it is not unusual to demonstrate persistent changes in the pulmonary circulation after a single epidode of pulmonary embolism.[10] The clinical consequences of decreased pulmonary capillary blood volume or decreased pulmonary diffusion capacity are not known. The morbidity of deep-vein thrombosis is easier to demonstrate. Patients with thrombotic obstruction of the deep veins of the lower extremity can develop chronic venous insufficiency. The majority of such patients, treated with heparin, have chronic venographic abnormalities. Such patients followed prespectively are at high risk for developing chronic dependent edema and venous ulceration.[11] The economic and personal costs of this complication are high.[12]

1.3. Risk Factors

Virchow's triad of venous stasis, hypercoagulability, and altered venous endothelium, described in 1856, still best explains the development of venous thrombosis. For most high-risk situations, venous stasis is the obvious pathophysiological change. Hypercoagulability can be inferred but is rarely proven. Assessment of coagulation activity is imprecise, difficult, expensive, and generally not available. Although the endothelial surface contributes to platelet and plasminogen activation, its clinical importance in thrombus genesis is usually uncertain.

With the development of sensitive and specific tests for the early diagnosis of venous thrombosis, selective patient groups could be prospectively evaluated. In large part these studies confirmed clinical and pathological observations. Before reviewing the risks for specific clinical settings, some general factors should be stressed.[13,14] For medical as for surgical patients, risk increases with age. Some studies suggest that thrombosis occurs more commonly in women. For any patient, immobility increases the chance of thrombosis formation. Bed rest and inactivity promote venous stasis and dilatation, thereby allowing clot development. Obesity may increase the risk of thromboembolism. Obese patients are generally less mobile. In addition, they may have impaired fibrinolysis.[15]

1.3.1. Surgical Patients

The thromboembolic complications of patients undergoing surgery have been carefully studied. Leg scanning using [^{125}I]fibrinogen has been used to estimate specific surgical risks as well as to clarify the natural history of postoperative venous thrombosis. Previous history of thrombosis, varicose veins, obesity, malignancy, and old age are associated with thromboembolic surgical complications.[16] Other studies have examined type of operation and length of surgery. Major procedures have increased risk, and general anesthesia seems to carry a greater risk than regional anesthesia. Total hip and knee replacement, repair of hip fracture, open prostatectomy, and hysterectomy for gynecological malignancy have the highest incidence of thrombosis.[13,14] Table I summarizes these data.

The incidence of thromboembolism following trauma has been more difficult to study. The risk is particularly high following lower-extremity fracture or amputation. Femur fracture, tibial fracture, and leg amputation carry risks of thromboembolism comparable to that for hip fracture.[13] The diagnosis of thromboembolism is more difficult in patients with multiple organ and limb damage, and thus prospective data are not readily available. Autopsy studies suggest that such patients are at increased risk. Acute spinal

Table I. Incidence of Postoperative Deep-Venous Thrombosis[a]

General surgery[b]	30%
Urology	
Transurethral prostatectomy	10%
Transvesical prostatectomy	40%
Gynecology	
Simple hysterectomy	10%
Major cancer surgery	35%
Orthopedic surgery	
Fractured hip	50%
Hip, knee arthroplasty	60%
Neurosurgery	30%

[a]Diagnosis by [^{125}I] fibrinogen leg scan.[13,14]
[b]Major abdominal surgery.

cord injury with paralysis creates one of the highest risk settings. Prospective data in these patients consistently show an incidence greater than 50%.[17] Patients with severe burns are prone to thromboembolism.[18,19]

Venous thrombosis can remain asymptomatic or lead to pulmonary embolism and death. In a classic study, Kakkar *et al.* followed the natural history of postoperative venous thrombosis using fibrinogen scanning and venography.[20] Among 40 patients with postoperative positive leg scans, the clot persisted for more than 72 hr in 26. Only 7 of the 26 persistent clots later showed radiographic evidence of proximal propagation. Of those with proximal thrombosis, four patients (approximately 50%) then developed pulmonary embolism by clinical criteria. Thus, the initial thrombus usually begins in the calf, advances into the thigh less than 20% of the time, and once above the knee is likely to embolize. In patients with hip trauma, the femoral vein can be involved initially.

In addition to leg scans, pulmonary perfusion scans have been used to screen surgical populations. The incidence rate of pulmonary embolism in mixed surgical populations by this technique is 10–20%.[14] Despite abnormal lung scan results, most of these patients remain asymptomatic. The false positive rate of perfusion lung scan screening is likely to be high. In one study pulmonary angiography was used extensively to diagnose pulmonary embolism following leg amputation, and results were positive in 10 of 70 patients.[21]

Based on autopsy data from multiple studies, the incidence of fatal postoperative pulmonary embolism is 0.2–1.2%.[14] However, rates as high as 10% have been shown following hip fracture or hip surgery.[13] Fatal postoperative pulmonary embolism can occur after a significant delay. The overall period of risk is not known, but fatal pulmonary embolism has occurred up to 2 months following the injury.[22]

1.3.2. Medical Patients

The incidence of deep-vein thrombosis has been carefully studied in patients with acute myocardial infarction.[23,24] Various studies using leg-scanning techniques have shown that approximately one-third of acute myocardial infarction patients develop a venous thrombosis. This high rate may explain why the routine use of anticoagulant drugs in cardiac-care-unit patients has saved lives in some studies.[25] Patients with heart failure are also at increased risk for thromboembolism. In patients with myocardial infarction complicated by congestive heart failure, the frequency of leg vein thrombosis is increased two or three times relative to uncomplicated myocardial infarction patients.[13]

Patients with hemiplegia, quadriplegia, or paraplegia are at increased risk for thromboembolism.[17,26] In these patients immobility and loss of muscular tone reduce venous flow. The overall incidence of thrombosis in this population is approximately 50%. The frequency of pulmonary embolism following an acute stroke is approximately 10%, and there is evidence of pulmonary emboli in 50% of stroke patients who undergo postmortem examination.[27] The incidence of venous thrombosis in paraplegic or quadriplegic patients is higher than 50%. In a postmortem study 29% of paraplegic or quadriplegic patients had evidence of pulmonary emboli.[18] The risk of fatal pulmonary embolism within 2–3 months of spinal cord injury is 2–16%.[17] As expected, a high rate of thromboembolism occurs in patients with other forms of paralysis such as Guillain-Barré syndrome.[28]

Cardiac and neurological disease predispose to thromboembolism mainly because of associated venous stasis. Abnormal coagulation can lead to thromboembolism in a large and heterogeneous group of patients (Table II).[29] It is not always possible to distinguish abnormal vessels from abnormal coagulation; hence diseases such as vasculitis and homocystinuria are included in Table II. Many of these diseases are rare, and quantitative estimates of risk are not available. For patients with recurrent thromboembolism and without clear predisposing factors, it may be worthwhile to look for laboratory evidence of hypercoagulation.

Some of the secondary hypercoagulable disorders are common. Trousseau in 1865 described the association between malignancy and thrombosis. Malignancies of the pancreas, stomach, lung, colon, ovaries, and gallbladder have the highest rates.[30] The incidence of thrombosis in pancreatic carcinoma approaches 50%.[31] Factors contributing to the association of thrombosis and malignancy include laboratory evidence of clotting activation, surgery, venous stasis due to immobility or tumor compression, and tumor-produced or associated procoagulant substances.

Thromboembolism has been associated with pregnancy and, in particular, the puerperium.[32] The risk for thromboembolism is highest in women following cesarean section or confined to bed with preeclampsia or eclampsia. The overall risk of thromboembolism after delivery is increased approximately 49 times relative to nonpregnant women.[33] The

Table II. Hypercoagulable States

Antithrombin III deficiency	Pregnancy
Protein C deficiency	Estrogens
Protein S deficiency	Nephrotic syndrome
Plasminogen deficiency	Myeloproliferative disorders
Abnormal plasminogen	Paroxysmal nocturnal hemoglobinuria
Plasminogen activator deficiency	Vasculitis
Factor XII deficiency	Homocystinuria
Lupus anticoagulant	Hyperviscosity states
Malignancy	Thrombotic thrombocytopenic purpura

increased rate of thromboembolism is explained by increased plasma viscosity, reduced venous flow due to mechanical factors, increased fibrin production with decreased removal, increased clotting factors (VII, VIII, IX, X, XII) and gradually decreasing antithrombin III during pregnancy.

Thromboembolic and cardiovascular complications of oral contraceptives have been extensively documented.[33] Estrogens used for other clinical purposes have similar risks. The coagulant effect of estrogens in pharmacological doses is similar to that of the latter stages of pregnancy. The thrombotic effect of estrogens is dose related. Thus lower-estrogen contraceptives seem to be safer.

2. TESTS FOR THROMBOEMBOLISM

Much of what is known about the epidemiology and natural history of thromboembolism has been learned as sensitive and specific diagnostic techniques have developed. A variety of tests are now available to assist the clinician in confirming or excluding thromboembolism. Because of the increased mortality of untreated disease and the problems associated with anticoagulation, both an early and specific diagnosis is important. However, the clinical diagnosis is difficult. In prospective studies on high-risk patients using leg scans, the presence of thrombosis by scan was suspected clinically only 50% of the time.[16] The signs and symptoms of pulmonary embolism are also nonspecific. It occurs commonly in patients with preexisting cardiac and pulmonary disease. The added effect of pulmonary embolism on such patients is difficult to decipher.

2.1. Venous Thrombosis

There are radiological and nonradiological methods for diagnosing venous thrombosis.[34,35] Fibrinogen leg scanning has already been mentioned. Following the intravenous injection of [^{125}I]fibrinogen, radioactivity at various points along the leg is measured daily. As a clot develops, the labeled fibrinogen is incorporated and radioactivity at that site increases. This technique is sensitive and specific for venous thrombosis in the calf, but it is nonspecific for proximal thrombi. False positives occur over hematomas, wounds, or areas of inflammation. The technique is most useful for prospective testing of high-risk patients. It may also be useful in patients with chronic venous insufficiency to distinguish new thrombosis amid a background of chronic symptoms.

Impedance plethysmography (IPG) and Doppler ultrasound are noninvasive tests that are useful in diagnosis of proximal-vein thrombosis. They are both relatively insensitive to calf thrombi. Compared to the Doppler method, IPG is easier to learn and to use reliably. IPG works by relating changes in venous outflow via the deep-venous system to changes in electrical resistance across the calf. The Doppler technique is based on changes in frequency between incident and reflected ultrasound beams according to velocity of blood flow.

If IPG and Doppler studies are normal, proximal-vein (but not calf vein) thrombosis is effectively excluded. False positives occur in low-venous-flow states, such as congestive heart failure, constrictive pericarditis, severe arterial peripheral vascular disease, hypotension, and external (e.g., tumor) venous compression. Doppler ultrasound is more specific than IPG for these low-flow states. It can also be used for patients who have their legs in traction or casts.

Although ascending contrast venography is the most occurate test for venous thrombosis, it should not be used for screening purposes. Its drawbacks include cost, risks associated with contrast pain at the ejection site, extravasation of dye resulting in skin damage, and venogram-induced phlebitis. This last problem is estimated to occur less than 10% of the time if dilute contrast medium is used.[36]

For some patients contrast studies are excessively dangerous. For these situations it is possible to substitute IPG and fibrinogen scanning for venography. It has been shown that therapeutic decisions based on this noninvasive approach are safe and accurate.[37] Table III summarizes the sensitivity and specificity of various diagnostic strategies.

2.2. Pulmonary Embolism

Most patients with clinically suspected pulmonary embolism require radiological confirmation. Perfusion lung scanning is widely used. A normal perfusion study effectively excludes pulmonary embolism. Abnormal perfusion studies can be interpreted more precisely if they are matched with ventilation studies.[38] Large perfusion defects that ventilate normally are considered high probability for pulmonary embolism and have a positive predictive value of more than 90%. Therapeutic decisions based on normal or high-probability scans can be made. Between these extremes a range of abnormal but nonspecific results can occur. Large perfusion defects with matched ventilatory defects can represent embolism, as can small unmatched defects.[39]

Because ventiliation–perfusion lung scans often give imprecise results, more invasive testing using pulmonary angiography or contrast venography is frequently necessary. In experienced hands pulmonary angiography is a safe procedure. Major risks include acute exacerbation of pulmonary hypertension, contrast complications, and arrythmias. Morbidity is less than 1% and mortality less than 0.5%.[40] Selective injection into pulmonary artery branches reduces the overall risk. Considering the hazards of missing the diagnosis or overtreating with anticoagulants, the use of pulmonary angiography for diagnostic specificity seems justified.[41]

In patients with suspected pulmonary embolism but nondiagnostic lung scans, it may be useful to use venography or impedance plethysmography before angiography. Finding

Table III. Tests for Venous Thrombosis

Test	Thrombus location	Sensitivity	Specificity
[^{125}I] fibrinogen scan	Calf	94%	93%
IPG[a]	Thigh	90%	90%
Doppler	Thigh	90%	93%
Fibrinogen and IPG	Calf and thigh	94%	91%
Venography	Calf and thigh	>95%	>95%

[a]IPG = impedance plethysmography.

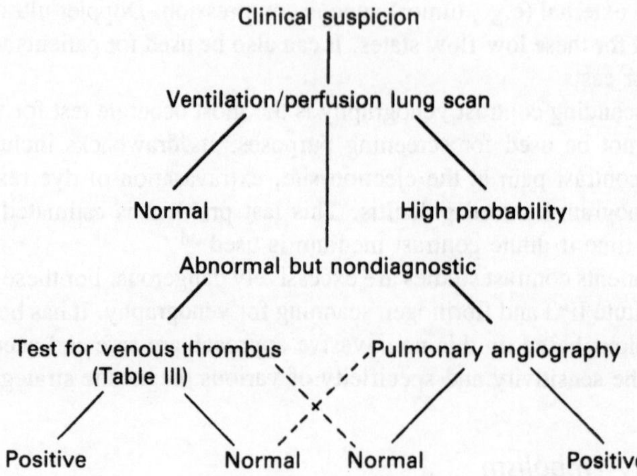

Figure 2. Diagnostic strategy for pulmonary embolism.

thrombosis in the extremity allows treatment to proceed. However, negative studies do not rule out pulmonary embolism and angiography may still be necessary. Similarly, a suspicious but equivocal angiogram may necessitate tests for venous thrombosis.[39] Figure 2 outlines the decision-making process in diagnosing pulmonary embolism.

3. PREVENTION

Methods for preventing thromboembolism vary from simple maneuvers for increasing venous flow to complicated pharmacological and surgical treatments.

3.1. Mechanical Methods

Mechanical methods for preventing deep venous thrombosis include leg elevation, active ankle flexion, electrical calf muscle stimulation, compression stockings, motorized foot mover, intermittent external calf compression, and rotating treatment tables (in lieu of hospital bed). These techniques attempt to increase venous flow. Their prophylactic effects, determined by prospective controlled studies, are variable.[42]

The effect of leg elevation is uncertain.[43] In a nonrandomized study of hip surgery patients, leg evaluation was shown to be beneficial, but the rate of thrombosis in the treated group was high (20%).[44] Active physical therapy does not appear helpful. Compression stockings are probably useful. In an early controlled but nonrandomized study of hospitalized medical and surgical patients, there were 50% fewer deaths due to pulmonary embolism in the treated group.[45] Stockings with graded compression decreasing proximally seem to be more effective.[46] Patients at particular risk, such as those with malignant disease or after hip surgery, are less likely to benefit. A motorized device that maintains continuous foot movement during surgery has been shown to be effective in one study.[47] Combining simple mechanical interventions may yield additive benefits. In a randomized trial, a combined preventive treatment (elastic stockings, leg elevation, passive and active dorsal and plantar flexion of the feet, and early ambulation) was effective.[48]

Electrical stimulation of the calf muscles has been tried with variable results. In addition to stimulating venous flow, it may activate the fibrinolytic system. This method is limited because it is painful. It may have a role in the immediate postoperative period while the patient is still anesthetized.

Intermittent calf external muscle compression is probably the most promising of the mechanical methods of prophylaxis. Several varieties of pumps are available, differing in compression pattern and sequence of compression. Efficacy in general surgery patients without malignancy has been demonstrated. Benefits have been shown following orthopedic surgery[49] and surgery for gynecological malignancy.[50] Among various studies the preventive effect is remarkably consistent despite variation in flow increasing effect. External calf compression may work by activating fibrinolysis or by emptying valve pockets of incipient thrombi. Complications of external compression are minimal. Mild discomfort and rarely skin blistering have been reported. Unfortunately, intermittent compression cannot be used after hip surgery. Following neurosurgery, when even minimal bleeding would be hazardous, this method has distinct advantages.

Rotating treatment tables, used in some centers for neurosurgery patients, may prevent thromboembolism. These tables are used in lieu of conventional hospital beds when immobilization is important for maintaining neurological integrity. These beds rotate along their axis in a 70° arc, thereby allowing even distribution of ventilation, preventing pressure sores, and facilitating general nursing care.[51] In a small clinical trial they have also been shown to reduce venous thrombosis in acute spinal cord injury patients,[52] perhaps by reducing venous stasis in the paralyzed extremities.

3.2. Pharmacological Methods

Various medications are useful in preventing venous thrombosis. The available agents have been used in different dosages and combinations to increase preventive effects while reducing risks. Commonly used medications include vitamin K antagonists, heparin, antiplatelet drugs, and dextran. Several fibrinolytic agents have been studied as well. Ancrod, a thrombinlike substance derived from Malayan pit viper venom, has undergone clinical trials. Anabolic steroids activate fibrinolysis and may have preventive value. Further experience and research are necessary before these fibrinoloytic methods can be recommended. It is possible to improve venous flow pharmacologically as well as retard hemostasis. An ergot derivative, dihydroergotamine, has been shown to be clinically valuable for this purpose.

3.2.1. Vitamin K Antagonists

Vitamin K antagonists or oral anticoagulants are commonly used to prevent thromboembolic disease either in the immediate postoperative setting or for patients at risk for recurrent disease. In fact, the first modern study of thromboembolism prophylaxis (1959) showed that oral anticoagulants reduced the incidence of fatal pulmonary embolism following surgery for hip fracture.[53] There are two classes of drugs in this category: the coumarins and the indonediones. Warfarin, a coumarin derivative, is the most commonly used oral anticoagulant. These agents interfere with vitamin K–dependent gamma carboxylation of clotting factors II, VII, IX, and X, thus inhibiting calcium and phospholipid binding during the clotting process.

The preventive value of oral anticoagulants has been studied in a variety of surgical patients. Hip surgery patients seem to benefit, particularly if the anticoagulant is given early. For elective hip surgery, two-step warfarin therapy has been used.[54] Low doses are given prior to surgery, and the dose is increased postoperatively. Bleeding can be minimized by this approach. In addition to hip surgery, an oral anticoagulant effect has been shown for general surgery patients, chest surgery patients, and gynecology patients. In high-risk settings, the incidence of thrombosis while on vitamin K antagonists remains approximately 20%.

Oral anticoagulants are the treatment of choice for preventing recurrent thromboembolism following the acute episode. Their efficacy has been shown in retrospective and prospective studies.[55–57] In two studies by Hull *et al.* comparing warfarin to varying doses of heparin,[56,57] the recurrence rate of thrombosis for the warfarin-treated patients was very low (0%, 2%, respectively). Oral anticoagulant therapy is guided by monitoring the extrinsic clotting pathway using the prothrombin time. Therapeutic doses of oral anticoagulants prolong the prothrombin time from 1½ to 2 times the normal value.

It is not clear how long secondary prevention with anticoagulants should be continued. The probability of recurrence is highest soon after the initial event.[58] Patients with multiple previous recurrences or chronic medical risk factors (congestive heart failure, malignancy, neurological disorders) may require prolonged treatment. Other risk factors, such as pregnancy, orthopedic injury, and acute myocardial infarction, are temporary. Prophylaxis for thromboembolism in these settings can be achieved with 3 months of anticoagulation. In the clinical trials mentioned, Hull and others continued to follow their patients following the 3-month treatment period. After treatment for calf vein thrombosis, there were no recurrences. After treatment of proximal vein thrombosis, recurrence was rare (less than 5%) and usually associated with either a chronic risk factor (paralysis, cancer) or shortened compliance with the early treatment.

Hemorrhage limits the prophylactic value of oral anticoagulants. Bleeding into a surgical wound can be hemodynamically trivial but nonetheless significant. Following total hip or knee replacement, a wound hematoma can easily lead to infection. A spontaneous central nervous system, joint, bowel wall, or retroperitoneal bleed can be clinically dramatic without a major change in hemoglobin or hematocrit. In perioperative settings, bleeding is worse if the oral anticoagulant was started before surgery. The reported incidence of bleeding complications for surgical patients varies considerably. In one series of 63 elderly patients with hip fractures treated with anticoagulants, there were two fatal hemorrhages and three serious hemorrhages.[59] Anticoagulants in this study were started before surgery, and a relatively intense regimen was prescribed. Other studies suggest that oral anticoagulants are less dangerous. Coon and Willis retrospectively reviewed their experience with a large series of medical and surgical patients.[60] Bleeding occurred in 6.8% of treatment courses. For surgical prophylaxis, the bleeding rate was 7.3%. This was comparable to the rate for patients with congestive heart failure (5.2%) and acute stroke (6.9%). Bleeding rates during prolonged anticoagulation at different therapeutic ranges (15 sec versus 20 sec for prothrombin time using rabbit brain thromboplastin) have been studied prospectively. The less intense regimen has less bleeding (4% versus 22%) while effectively preventing recurrent venous thrombosis.[61]

Aside from hemorrhage, complications of oral anticoagulants are rare and include various dermatological conditions, allergy, and fetal effects. The most distinctive and serious skin reaction is a necrotizing process with small vessel thrombosis occurring early in treatment involving skin with abundant subcutaneous fat. Women are usually affected.

Oral anticoagulants can cross the placenta, where they can lead to fetal bleeding or malformation. They are contraindicated in pregnancy, but breast feeding by mothers on oral anticoagulants is possible. Although the anticoagulant is secreted in the maternal milk, coagulation in the infant is usually not affected.

3.2.2. Heparin

Heparin is widely used for treating thromboembolism. It is useful for initial therapy and for both primary and secondary prevention. Its pharmacological effects are due to its interaction with antithrombin III (AT III or heparin cofactor). When heparin binds to AT III, it induces a conformational change that markedly accelerates the inhibitory affects of AT III on those activated clotting factors which are serine proteases (XII, XI, IX, X). Activated factor X is particularly sensitive to heparin-induced inhibition. Because heparin is selective for this intermediate point in the clotting cascade, low doses can inhibit thrombin formation with a multipled effect. Clot formation can thus be slowed while a safe range of hemostatis is preserved. Heparin effects are measured by the activated partial thromboplastin time (APTT), which reflects activity in the intrinsic clotting pathway. Large doses of heparin can markedly prolong the APTT and thus protect patients with acute pulmonary embolism or deep-venous thrombosis from further clot formation. At less than full dosage, careful clinical trials have shown heparin to be useful in a variety of preventive situations.

Low-dose heparin, given as 5000 international or U.S.P. units subcutaneously every 12 hr, is effective prophylaxis for most surgical patients.[62] For patients undergoing general abdominal, thoracic, and urological operations, the incidence of venous thrombosis by leg scan is about 7% in heparin-treated patients compared to 25% for controls. In addition, fatal pulmonary embolism is significantly reduced in the heparin group. However, low-dose heparin is less effective for patients undergoing hip surgery, knee surgery, and pelvic cancer surgery.

Modifications of the low-dose regimen have been made in order to increase its efficacy for higher-risk surgical patients. The APTT can be slightly prolonged by small adjustments (+500/unit) of the standard low dose. Following total hip replacement, patients treated with an adjusted low dose of heparin (partial thromboplastin time 31.5–36 sec) had a 13% rate of thrombosis compared to a rate of 39% for patients on fixed low-dose heparin.[63] This result is promising, but laboratory monitoring before dosage decisions seems cumbersome. Further research and clinical experience are needed before this approach can be promoted.

Low-dose heparin can be used for prolonged prophylaxis in pregnant patients or patients with severe coumarin reactions. As discussed, Hull and others compared both fixed and adjusted low-dose heparin to warfarin in 3-month clinical trials following proximal vein deep-venous thrombosis.[56,57] The adjusted regimen was as effective as warfarin for preventing recurrence.

Low-dose heparin is also useful for preventing thromboembolism in patients with medical illnesses. This has been shown in prospective randomized trials of patients with specific clinical problems (acute myocardial infarction, acute stroke, suspected myocardial infarction) and patients admitted to a general medical service.[64–67] The latter study used death as an endpoint and showed that heparin improved surival.

Even at low dosages heparin has some significant side effects. Bleeding can occur. For secondary prevention in the Hull study, patients receiving adjusted heparin had significantly less bleeding than the warfarin group (2% versus 17%). Major hemorrhage, from previously unknown sites of pathology, occurs rarely. In multicenter trials transfusion requirements were not increased in heparin-treated patients.[62] However, wound hematomas were more common. Heparin at any dose can lead to thrombocytopenia by inducing platelet aggregation or through a more troublesome immunological mechanism. Paradoxically, patients with severe heparin-induced thrombocytopenia can develop new arterial and venous thrombi as aggregated platelets settle in small vessels. Long-term use of heparin, such as in pregnancy, can cause osteoporosis. Since heparin is acidic, bone mass is reduced as bone-buffering capacity is tapped.

3.2.3. Antiplatelet Agents

Antiplatelet agents offer the simplest means of preventing thromboembolism. Dosing is easy, therapeutic monitoring is not necessary, and safety can generally be assumed. Four types of platelet-active agents have been studied: aspirin, dipyridimole, sulfinpyrazone, and hydroxychloroquine. The results are generally disappointing. Dipyridimole and sulfinpyrazone are not effective when used alone. The combination of dipyridimole and aspirin has been used effectively to prevent thrombosis in general-surgery patients but not in higher-risk groups.[68] There is limited evidence that this combination may be useful for patients with recurrent venous thrombosis who have failed to improve on standard oral anticoagulant therapy.[69] Hydroxychloroquine has antiplatelet properties in addition to its antimalarial and antiinflammatory effects. It can reduce postoperative thrombosis in general surgery patients[70] but not following hip surgery.[71] Aspirin has been extensively studied. In general it has not been effective. In one study of patients following total hip arthroplasty, men but not women were protected by aspirin.[72] On the arterial side of the circulation, antiplatelet agents have been more consistently beneficial for cerebrovascular disease and peripheral vascular disease. This therapeutic difference underscores the different pathophysiology of venous and arterial thrombosis.

3.2.4. Dextran

Dextran has been used successfully to prevent thromboembolism.[73] It is a polysaccharide with variable molecular weight. Because dextran is relatively inert and exerts high oncotic pressure, it is useful as a plasma substitute. It actually has multiple physiological effects. Low-molecular-weight dextran reduces red blood cells and thereby reduces blood viscosity. Flow is improved due to hemodilution, capillary dilation from oncotic changes, and effects on red-cell aggregation. Dextran can coat both vessel endothelium and red cells. Red-cell electronegativity is increased, perhaps from the coating affect, and thus red-cell aggregation is diminished. Platelet adhesion and aggregation are reduced. There are inconsistent effects on fibrin formation and the thrombolytic system. Factor XIII antigenicity decreases, and as a consequence, in experimental models, thrombi are easier to lyse. It should be clear that these myriad changes might be clinically useful in preventing thrombus formation.

The benefits are clearest in patients with hip fracture, where dextran seems to be as effective as warfarin. In a multicenter study of mixed surgical patients with fatal pulmonary embolism as an endpoint, low-dose heparin and dextran had similar preventive efficacy. Within 30 days of surgery there was a 1.9% incidence of fatal pulmonary embolism for each group.[74]

Dextran use is limited by the accompanying volume expansion and risk of congestive heart failure. Bleeding complications are possible but are clinically unimportant. The low-molecular-weight dextran (dextran 40) has been reported to cause acute renal failure, particularly in volume-depleted or hypotensive patients. Rarely (0.3% of patients treated), dextran can provoke an anaphylactic reaction.

Dextran is available for clinical use in several sizes and concentrations: dextran 70 (molecular weight 70,000) as a 6% or 10% solution; dextran 40 in a 10% solution. Generally 500–1000 ml is given during surgery with repeated infusions every other postoperative day until the patient is fully ambulatory. No specific laboratory monitoring is necessary. Careful attention to volume status, urine output, and bleeding is mandatory.

3.3. Combination Treatment

Various combinations of preventive measures have been tested. One of the more promising combines low-dose heparin with dihydroergotamine (DHE). DHE reduces venous stasis in the lower extremity by causing venoconstriction of the capacitance vessels. Large clinical trials in Europe and the United States have demonstrated the efficacy of this combination.[75,76] In these studies bleeding was not a serious problem. Compared to low-dose heparin alone, the combination was significantly better. For high-risk patients there are limited data. The incidence of thrombosis following elective hip arthoplasty in heparin–DHE-treated patients is approximately 25%.[75,77] This is considerably less than no preventive treatment, and further studies are warranted. Careful patient selection is necessary to prevent DHE-induced vascular complications. One death in the U.S. study was due to bowel infarction in a DHE patient.[76]

Another encouraging method uses external pneumatic compression and dextran. This was studied following total hip replacement and compared to aspirin at two dosages.[78] The combination of external pneumatic compression and dextran reduced the incidence of postoperative thrombosis to 20%, compared to 60% for both low- and high-dose aspirin.

4. COSTS, RISKS, BENEFITS

Because of the significant morbidity and mortality of thromboembolism, the case for prevention is strong. However, there are many choices facing the clinician, and the decision is not necessarily clear cut. Table IV presents clinical situations and the choices for effective prophylaxis. Risks related to the setting, available resources, and the individual patient must be factored into the decision. Bleeding must be considered whenever

Table IV. Recommended Prophylaxis

Setting	Method
Medical	Low-dose heparin[a]
General surgery	Low-dose heparin
Thoracic surgery	Low-dose heparin
Pelvic surgery (routine GU, GYN)	Low-dose heparin
Major cancer surgery	Heparin–dihydroergotamine[b]
	External pneumatic compression
Noncancer surgery (with risk factors)	Heparin–dihydroergotamine
Neurosurgery/spinal cord injury	External pneumatic compression
	Rotating treatment table
Hip arthroplasty/hip fracture	Adjusted low-dose heparin[c]
	Two-step warfarin[d]
	Dextran/external compression[e]
	Heparin–dihydroergotamine

[a]5000 units s.c. every 8–12 hr; first dose 2 hr before surgery.
[b]5000 units of heparin plus 0.5 mg DHE s.c. every 12 hr; first dose 2 hr before surgery.
[c]Beginning with heparin, 3500 units every 8 hr; dose adjusted by ±500 units to keep activated partial thromboplastin time at 31–36 sec.
[d]Preoperative prothrombin time 1.5–3.0 sec prolonged; postoperative prothrombin time approximately 5.0 sec prolonged (1.5 times control).
[e]10 ml/kg of dextran 40 given during surgery and 7.5 ml/kg for 2 days thereafter; external pneumatic compression 10–14 days postoperatively.

anticoagulants are used. Fortunately, there are effective mechanical methods for patients who cannot tolerate any hemorrhage (ophthalmological, neurosurgical). Underlying vascular disease might prohibit use of heparin–DHE even in a patient at high risk for thromboembolism. Even though the proper prophylaxis may not be obvious, the concerned well-informed physician is able to reduce the risk of thromboembolic complications in almost any clinical setting.

Questions regarding the efficacy of thromboembolism prevention involve overall costs as well as the clinical balance of risks and benefits. Decision theory has been applied to the preventive treatment of deep-vein thrombosis in the coronary care unit.[79] After weighing of various risks (fatal pulmonary embolism, fatal hemorrhage from heparin, deep-vein thrombosis with or without pulmonary embolism), treatment allocation rules were developed. Preventive treatment using low-dose heparin for patients older than 70 years reduces overall mortality in this analysis. Bentley and Kakkar suggest that low-dose heparin postoperative prophylaxis reduces fatal pulmonary embolism by 88% while increasing wound hematomas by 2.1%.[80] Finally, Salzman and Davies compared the cost of various preventive strategies.[81] For general-surgical patients, low-dose heparin and external pneumatic compression are similar in terms of cost and potential lives saved. Careful surveillance of all patients at risk is slightly more effective in terms of mortality, but is more than five times as expensive as preventive treatment.

Analyzing the cost and benefits of various preventive methods is interesting, but the results are limited when the supporting data are so variable. Regardless of what clinical trials or formal decision analyses suggest, practitioners rely on their own experience and local opinion in deciding to use preventive treatment. In 1974, a survey of practicing orthopedists showed that the overall use of prophylaxis was low and at variance with recommendations from the published literature.[82] This reluctance says something about the perceived value of the methods available for prophylaxis at the time of the survey. Fortunately, the last decade has brought significant advances in the preventive management of thromboembolism. Epidemiological research has clarified the natural history of untreated disease, and clinical trials have evaluated the many available therapies. Presently, for the individual patient, the risk for thromboembolism can be accurately assessed, and the decision about prevention can then be tailored to the particular setting.

REFERENCES

1. Coon, W. W.: Epidemiology of venous thromboembolism. *Ann. Surg.* **186:**149–164, 1977.
2. Dalen, J. E., and Alpert, J. S.: Natural history of pulmonary embolism. *Prog. Cardiovasc. Dis.* **17:**259–270, 1975.
3. Freiman, D. G., Suyemoto, J., and Wessler, S.: Frequency of pulmonary thromboembolism in man. *N. Engl. J. Med.* **272:**1278–1280, 1965.
4. Morrell, M. T., and Dunnill, M. S.: The post-mortem incidence of pulmonary embolism in a hospital population. *Br. J. Surg.* **55:**347–352, 1968.
5. Uhland, H., and Goldberg, L. M.: Pulmonary embolism: A commonly missed clinical entity. *Dis. Chest* **45:**533–536, 1964.
6. Hume, M., Sevitt, S., and Thomas, D. P.: *Venous Thrombosis and Pulmonary Embolism.* Commonwealth Fund/Harvard University Press, Cambridge, MA, 1970, p. 4.
7. Coon, W. W., Willis, P. W., III, and Keller, J. B.: Venous thromboembolism and other venous disease in the Tecumseh community health study. *Circulation* **48:**839–846, 1973.
8. Barritt, D., and Jordan, S.: Anticoagulant drugs in treatment of pulmonary embolism: A controlled trial. *Lancet* **1:**1309–1312, 1960.
9. The urokinase pulmonary embolism trial. *Circulation* **47**(suppl II)**:**1–108, 1973.
10. Sharma, G., Burleson, V., and Sasahara, A.: Effect of thrombolytic therapy on pulmonary capillary volume in patients with pulmonary embolism. *N. Engl. J. Med.* **303:**842–845, 1980.
11. Arneson, H., Hoiseth, A., and Ly, B.: Streptokinase or heparin in the treatment of deep venous thrombosis. *Acta Med. Scand.* **211:**65–68, 1982.
12. O'Donnell, T. F., Browse, N. L., Burnand, K. G., and Thomas, M. L.: The socioeconomic effects of an iliofemoral venous thrombosis. *J. Surg. Res.* **22:**483–488, 1977.
13. Hirsh, J., Genton, E., and Hull, R.: *Venous Thromboembolism.* Grune & Stratton, New York, 1981, pp. 19–41.
14. Bergqvist, D.: *Postoperative Thromboembolism: Frequency, Etiology, Prophylaxis.* Springer-Verlag, Berlin, 1983, pp. 6–32.
15. Almer, L., and Janzon, L.: Low vascular fibrinolytic activity in obesity. *Thromb. Res.* **6:**171–175, 1975.
16. Kakkar, V., Howe, C., Nicolaides, A., *et al.:* Deep vein thrombosis of the leg: Is there a high risk group? *Am. J. Surg.* **20:**527–530, 1970.
17. Todd, J. W., Frisbie, J. M., Rossier, A. B., *et al.:* Deep venous thrombosis in acute spinal cord injury: A comparison of 125I-fibrinogen leg scanning, impedance plethysmography, and venography. *Paraplegia* **14:**50–57, 1976.
18. Coon, W. W.: Risk factors in pulmonary embolism. *Surg. Gynecol. Obstet.* **143:**385–390, 1976.
19. Sevitt, S., and Gallagher, N.: Venous thrombosis and pulmonary embolism: A clinico-pathological study in injured and burned patients. *Br. J. Surg.* **48:**475–489, 1960.
20. Kakkar, V., Howe, C., Flanc, C., *et al.:* Natural history of postoperative deep-vein thrombosis. *Lancet* **1:**230–233, 1972.
21. Williams, J. W., Britt, L. G., Eades, T., *et al.:* Pulmonary embolism after amputation of the lower extremity. *Surg. Gynecol. Obstet.* **140:**246–248, 1975.

22. Sevitt, S.: Venous thrombosis and pulmonary embolism: Their prevention by oral anticoagulants. *Am. J. Med.* **33**:703–716, 1962.
23. Murray, T., Lorimer, A., Cox, F., *et al.*: Leg-vein thrombosis following myocardial infarction. *Lancet* **2**:792–793, 1970.
24. Miller, R., Lies, J., Carretta, R., *et al.*: Prevention of lower extremity venous thrombosis by early ambulation. *Ann. Intern. Med.* **84**:700–703, 1976.
25. Goldman, L., and Feinstein, A.: Anticoagulants and myocardial infarction: The problems of pooling, drowning, and floating. *Ann. Intern. Med.* **90**:92–94, 1979.
26. Warlow, C., Oston, D., and Douglas, A. S.: Deep venous thrombosis after strokes: Incidence and predisposing factors. *Br. Med. J.* **1**:1178–1182, 1976.
27. Warlow, C., Oston, D., and Douglas, A. S.: Deep venous thrombosis after strokes: Natural history. *Br. Med. J.* **1**:1181–1183, 1976.
28. Raman, K., Blake, J. A., and Harris, T. M.: Pulmonary embolism in Landry-Guillian-Barré-Strohl syndrome. *Chest* **60**:555–557, 1971.
29. Schafer, A. I.: The hypercoagulable states. *Ann. Intern. Med.* **105**:814–828, 1985.
30. Rickels, F. R., and Edwards, R. L.: Activation of blood coagulation in cancer: Trousseau's syndrome revisited. *Blood* **62**:14–31, 1983.
31. Bick, R. L.: Alterations of hemostasis associated with malignancy. *Semin. Thromb. Hemost.* **5**:1–26, 1978.
32. Treffers, P. E., Heidekoper, B. L., Weenink, G. M., *et al.*: Epidemiological observations of thromboembolic disease during pregnancy and in the puerperium in 56,022 women. *Int. J. Gynecol. Obstet.* **21**:327–331, 1983.
33. Siegel, D. G.: Pregnancy, the puerperium, and the steroid contraceptive. *Milbank Mem Fund A* **50**(suppl 2):15–23, 1972.
34. Hirsh, J., and Hull, R.: Comparative value of tests for the diagnosis of venous thrombosis. *World J. Surg.* **2**:27–38, 1978.
35. Hirsh, J., and Gallus, A. S.: Diagnosis of venous thromboembolism: Limitations and applications, in Madden, J. L., and Hume, M. (eds.): *Venous Thromboembolism: Prevention and Treatment.* Appleton-Century-Crofts, New York, 1976, pp. 183–213.
36. Bettman, M. A., and Paulin, S.: Leg phlebography: The incidence, nature, and modification of undesirable side effects. *Radiology* **122**:101–104, 1977.
37. Hull, R., Hirsh, J., Sackett, D., *et al.*: Replacement of venography in suspected venous thrombosis by impedance plethysmography and I-125 fibrinogen leg scanning. *Ann. Intern. Med.* **94**:12–15, 1981.
38. McNeil, B. J.: A diagnostic strategy using ventiliation–perfusion studies in patients suspect for pulmonary embolism. *J. Nucl. Med.* **17**:613–616, 1976.
39. Hull, R. B., Hirsh, J., Carter, C. J., *et al.*: Pulmonary angiography, ventilation lung scanning, and venography for clinically suspected pulmonary embolism with abnormal perfusion lung scan. *Ann. Intern. Med.* **98**:891–899, 1983.
40. Bell, W. R., and Simon, T. L.: A comparative analysis of pulmonary perfusion scans with pulmonary angiograms. *Am. Heart J.* **92**:700–706, 1976.
41. Robin, E. D.: Overdiagnosis and overtreatment of pulmonary embolism: The emperor may have no clothes. *Ann. Intern. Med.* **87**:775–781, 1977.
42. Bergqvist, D.: *Postoperative Thromboembolism: Frequency, Etiology, Prophylaxis.* Springer-Verlag, Berlin, 1983, pp. 65–161.
43. Browse, N. L., Jackson, B. T., Mayo, M. E., *et al.*: The value of mechanical methods of preventing postoperative calf vein thrombosis. *Br. J. Surg.* **61**:219–223, 1974.
44. Hartman, J. T., Altner, P. C., and Freeark, R. J.: The effect of limb elevation in preventing venous thrombosis: A venographic study. *J. Bone Joint Surg.* **52A**:1618–1622, 1970.
45. Wilkins, R. W., and Stanton, J. R.: Elastic stockings in the prevention of pulmonary embolism. *N. Engl. J. Med.* **248**:1087–1090, 1953.
46. Turner, G. M., Cole, S. E., and Brocks, J. H.: The efficacy of graduated compression stockings in the prevention of deep vein thrombosis after major gynecological surgery. *Br. J. Obstet. Gynecol.* **91**:588–591, 1984.
47. Scurr, J. H., Robbe, I. J., Ellis, H., and Goldsmith, H. S.: Simple mechanical method for decreasing the incidence of thromboembolism. *Am. J. Surg.* **141**:582–585, 1981.

48. Tsapogas, M. J., Goussous, H., Peabody, R. A., *et al.:* Post operative venous thrombosis and the effectiveness of prophylactic measures. *Arch. Surg.* **103:**561–567, 1971.
49. Hull, R., Delmore, T. J., Hirsh, J., *et al.:* Effectiveness of intermittent pulsatile elastic stockings for the prevention of calf and thigh vein thrombosis in patients undergoing elective knee surgery. *Thromb. Res.* **16:**37–45, 1979.
50. Clarke-Pearson, D. L., Synan, I. S., and Hinshaw, W. M.: Prevention of postoperative venous thromboembolism by external pneumatic compression in patients with gynecologic malignancy. *Obstet. Gynecol.* **63:**92–97, 1984.
51. Keane, F. X.: New appliance: Ruto-rest. *Br. Med. J.* **3:**731–733, 1967.
52. Becker, D. M., Gonzalez, M., Gentili, A., *et al.*: Prevention of deep venous thrombosis in patients with acute spinal cord injuries: Use of rotary treatment tables. *Neurosurg.* **20:**675–677, 1987.
53. Sevitt, S., and Gallagher, N. G.: Prevention of venous thrombosis and pulmonary embolism in injured patients. *Lancet* **2:**982–989, 1959.
54. Francis, C. W., Marder, V. J., Evarts, M., *et al.:* Two step warfarin therapy: Prevention of postoperative venous thrombosis without excessive bleeding. *JAMA* **249:**374–378, 1983.
55. Coon, W. W., Willis, P. W., III, and Symons, M. J.: Assessment of anticoagulant treatment of venous thromboembolism. *Ann. Surg.* **170:**559–567, 1969.
56. Hull, R., Delmore, T., Genton, E., *et al.:* Warfarin sodium versus low dose heparin in the long term treatment of venous thrombosis. *N. Engl. J. Med.* **301:**855–858, 1979.
57. Hull, R., Delmore, T., Carter, C., *et al.:* Adjusted subcutaneous heparin versus warfarin sodium in the long term treatment of venous thrombosis. *N. Engl. J. Med.* **306:**189–194, 1982.
58. Coon, W. W., and Willis, P. W., III: Recurrence of venous thromboembolism. *Surgery* **73:**823–827, 1973.
59. Bergqvist, E., Bergqvist, D., Bronge, A., *et al.:* An evaluation of early thrombosis prophylaxis following fracture of the femoral neck. *Acta Chir. Scand.* **138:**689–693, 1972.
60. Coon, W. W., and Willis, P. W., III: Hemorrhagic complications of anticoagulant therapy. *Arch. Intern. Med.* **133:**386–392, 1974.
61. Hull, R., Hirsch, J., Jay, R., *et al.:* Different intensities of oral anticoagulant therapy in the treatment of proximal-vein thrombosis. *N. Engl. J. Med.* **307:**1676–1681, 1982.
62. Kakkar, V. V.: The current status of low dose heparin in the prophylaxis of thrombophlebitis and pulmonary embolism. *World J. Surg.* **2:**3–18, 1978.
63. Leyvraz, P. F., Richard, J., Bachman, F., *et al.:* Adjusted versus fixed dose subcutaneous heparin in the prevention of deep vein thrombosis after total hip replacement. *N. Engl. J. Med.* **309:**954–958, 1983.
64. Warlow, C., Terry, G., Kenmore, A. C., *et al.:* A double blind trial of low doses of subcutaneous heparin in the prevention of deep vein thrombosis after myocardial infarction. *Lancet* **2:**934–936, 1973.
65. McCarthy, S. T., Turner, J. J., Robertson, D., *et al.:* Low dose heparin as a prophylaxis against deep vein thrombosis after acute stroke. *Lancet* **2:**800–801, 1977.
66. Gallus, A. S., Hirsh, J., Tuttle, R. J., *et al.:* Small subcutaneous doses of heparin in prevention of venous thrombosis. *N. Engl. J. Med.* **288:**545–551, 1973.
67. Halkin, M., Goldberg, J., Modan, M., *et al.:* Reduction of mortality in general medical inpatients by low dose heparin prophylaxis. *Ann. Intern. Med* **96:**561–565, 1982.
68. Renney, J. T., O'Sullivan, E. F., and Burke, P. F.: Prevention of post operative deep vein thrombosis with dipyridamole and aspirin. *Br. Med. J.* **1:**992–994, 1976.
69. Steele, P.: Trial of dipyridamole-aspirin in recurring venous thrombosis. *Lancet* **2:**1328–1329, 1980.
70. Wu, T. K., Tsapogas, M. J., and Jordan, F. R.: Prophylaxis of deep vein thrombosis by hydroxychloroquine sulfate and heparin. *Surg. Gynecol. Obstet.* **145:**714–718, 1977.
71. Cook, E. D., Dawson, M. H., and Ibbotson, R. M.: Failure of orally administered hydroxychloroquine sulphate to prevent venous thromboembolism following elective hip operations. *J. Bone Joint Surg.* **59A:**496–499, 1977.
72. Harris, W. H., Salzman, E. W., Athanasoulis, C. A., *et al.:* Aspirin prophylaxis of venous thromboembolism after total hip replacement. *N. Engl. J. Med.* **297:**1246–1249, 1977.
73. Bergqvist, D.: Dextran, in *Postoperative Thromboembolism: Frequency, Etiology, Prophylaxis.* Springer-Verlag, Berlin, 1983, pp. 129–145.
74. Gruber, F., Saldeen, T., Brokop, T., *et al.:* Incidences of fatal postoperative pulmonary embolism after

prophylaxis with dextran 70 and low-dose heparin: An international multicentre study. *Br. Med. J.* **280**:69–72, 1980.
75. Kakkar, V. V., Stamatakis, J. D., and Bentley, P. G.: Prophylaxis for postoperative deep vein thrombosis: Synergistic effect of heparin and dihydroergotamine. *JAMA* **241**:39–42, 1979.
76. Multicenter Trial Committee: Dihydroergotamine–heparin prophylaxis of postoperative deep vein thrombosis. *JAMA* **251**:2960–2966, 1984.
77. Kakkar, V. V., Fok, P. J., Murray, W. J., *et al.*: Heparin and dihydroergotamine prophylaxis against thromboembolism after hip arthroplasty. *J. Bone Joint Surg.* **67A**:538–542, 1985.
78. Harris, W. H., Athanasoulis, C. A., Waltman, A. C., *et al.*: Prophylaxis of deep-vein thrombosis after total hip replacement: Dextran and external pneumatic compression compared with 1.2 or 3.0 grams of aspirin daily. *J. Bone Joint Surg.* **67A**:57–62, 1985.
79. Teather, D., Emerson, P. A., and Handley, A. J.: Decision theory applied to the treatment of deep vein thrombosis. *Meth. Inform. Med.* **13**:92–97, 1974.
80. Bentley, P. G., and Kakkar, V. V.: Advances in the prevention of venous thromboembolic disease. *Adv. Exp. Med. Biol.* **164**:81–83, 1984.
81. Salzman, E. W., and Davies, G. C.: Prophylaxis of venous thromboembolism: Analysis of cost effectiveness. *Ann. Surg.* **191**:207–215, 1980.
82. Simon, T. L., and Stengle, J. M.: Antithrombotic practice in orthopedic surgery. *Clin. Orthop.* **102**:181–187, 1974.

15

Nephrolithiasis

Laurence B. Gardner

1. INTRODUCTION

Nephrolithiasis is a common, painful, and costly condition which afflicts approximately 2–3% of the total population of the United States and western Europe.[1] The risk of recurrence in an individual who has had a single episode of nephrolithiasis has been estimated to be 20–50%.[1,2] Thus, except in the rare instances of familial types of nephrolithiasis, the physician must wait for the first episode and then practice secondary prevention (that is, prevention of recurrent stone disease).

The rationale for prevention of recurrent nephrolithiasis lies in the reduction of morbidity (pain and infection) and mortality (the progression to chronic renal failure). In addition, frequent hospitalizations or visits to the emergency room result in loss of work and significant costs to the patient. If risk reduction can be adequately achieved, these economic losses can be minimized. Even with the introduction of ultrasonic lithotripsy,[3,4] a technique that, when applicable, avoids the morbidity of surgery, all would agree that prevention is far preferable to treatment in nephrolithiasis.

1.1. Diagnosis

Screening for persons at risk for nephrolithiasis is usually not practical except when a strong history of a known familial cause of kidney stones is present. On occasion asymptomatic hypercalcemia or hyperuricemia, discovered on routine chemical profile evaluations, may indicate that the patient is at increased risk for stone formation.

In general, the following diagnostic approach is applicable for all types of renal stones. First, the physician must delineate the stone composition, and this is best done by analysis of a passed stone. This is an inexpensive, accurate, and extremely cost-effective measure. Patients should be strongly urged to strain their urine through cheesecloth or some other suitable filter during a suspected episode of nephrolithiasis. If direct stone analysis is impractical because the stone was not retrieved or retained, then a metabolic evaluation to identify the most likely cause of nephrolithiasis is mandatory. (See Table I.)

If a known etiology for nephrolithiasis is identified, then specific treatment in most

Laurence B. Gardner • Department of Medicine, University of Miami School of Medicine, Miami, Florida 33101.

instances is available. These treatments are discussed in detail in the following sections of this chapter. On the other hand, if no cause is clearly identified, then the decision as to whether or not to treat a patient with "idiopathic stone formation" is a difficult one. Many of the drugs employed carry with them a significant risk of idiosyncratic or dose-related reactions, and these risks must be balanced against the risk of recurrent stone formation.

1.2. Metabolic Evaluation of the Patient with Nephrolithiasis

If direct analysis of the stone is not possible or if there is some reason to doubt the accuracy of such an analysis, detailed analysis of blood and urine samples in patients with stone disease is virtually mandatory in planning a program of prophylaxis. The following outline of evaluative steps represents the consensus of several prominent investigators in this field regarding an adequate evaluation.[2,5]

2. PREDISPOSING FACTORS

2.1. Oxalate Stones

Calcium oxalate stones are by far the most common and constitute approximately 65% of all renal stones. Predisposing metabolic factors for these types of stones include

Table I. Metabolic Evaluation for Stone Disease[a]

Laboratory test	Stone composition	No. of daily studies
Serum Ca	Ca oxalate; Ca phos	4
Serum phosphate	Ca oxalate; Ca phos	1
24-hr urine Ca	Ca oxalate; Ca phos	2[b]
Serum electrolytes	Ca phosphate	1[c]
Cystine screening	Cystine	1[d]
Serum uric acid	Uric acid; Ca oxalate	4
24-hr urine urate	Uric acid; Ca oxalate	2
Serum creatinine	All	4
24-hr urine creatinine	All	2[e]
Urinalysis	All	1
Urine culture	All	1

[a]Adapted from Maffly[2] with permission and Coe and Favus[1] with permission.
[b]If hypercalciuria is present, a calcium tolerance test should be performed.[6]
[c]A picture of hyperchloremic acidosis will require evaluation for renal tubular acidosis, including several urine pH determinations and an acid-loading test if appropriate.[7]
[d]Only if hexagonal crystals, staghorn calculi, a family history, or other index of suspicion is present.
[e]Used to assess adequacy of collection as well as renal function.

Table II. Pathogenetic Mechanisms in Calcium Stone Formation[a,b]

Primary hyperparathyroidism	5.2%
Idiopathic hypercalciuria	32%
A. Absorptive	
B. Renal leak	
C. Normocalcemic hyperparathyroidism	
Hyperuricosuria	26%
Renal tubular acidosis	3.7%
Hyperoxaluria	4.6%
Idiopathic[c]	28.5%

[a]Adapted from Coe[16] with permission.
[b]Based on studies of 460 patients.
[c]May contain a significant number of patients with idiopathic hypocitraturia.[15]

hypercalciuria, hypercalcemia with hypercalciuria, hyperoxaluria, and hypocitraturia (see Table II).

Hypercalciuria (>4 mg/kg body weight per day with a normal serum calcium concentration) is the most common predisposing metabolic factor and is found in approximately one-third of patients with calcium oxalate stones. It is now generally agreed that there are three basic types of hypercalciuria. The first, absorptive hypercalciuria, is markedly dependent on oral calcium intake and is seen in idiopathic and secondary forms. Sarcoidosis and hypervitaminosis D are two common examples of acquired hypercalciuria of the absorptive type. A second variety of hypercalciuria, called "renal leak" hypercalciuria, apparently represents a tubular defect in the nephron, the consequences of which are the failure to adequately and completely reabsorb calcium.[8–10] Finally, and perhaps most rare, is a type of hypercalciuria that has been attributed to "normocalcemic hyperparathyroidism."[8] In the latter entity, the parathyroid hormone excess is not sufficient to raise the serum calcium to distinctly abnormal levels but is sufficient to increase the filtered load of calcium and result in hypercalciuria.

Hypercalcemic hypercalciuria occurs more commonly in hyperparathyrodism than normocalcemic hypercalciuria and accounts for approximately 5–7% of all calcium oxalate stones. Thus, careful evaluation of the serum calcium (see above) is indicated in patients who pass calcium oxalate or radiopaque stones.

Hyperoxaluria is seen in two forms and is responsible for a small fraction of calcium oxalate stones: a very rare primary hyperoxaluria that is inherited by an autosomal recessive mechanism[11,12] and the much more common, secondary enteric forms of hyperoxaluria.[13,14] The latter variety is seen in diseases involving the small bowel and associated with steatorrhea. Current thinking suggests that the excess fat in the stool in these patients complexes with the calcium component of calcium oxalate, allowing the free oxalate salt to be absorbed into the bloodstream along with a sodium cation. In the particular instance of enteric secondary hyperoxaluria, restriction of dietary calcium may lead to enhanced intestinal oxalate absorption and increased stone formation.

Recent studies by Pak and Fuller[15] have identified a subgroup of calcium oxalate stone formers without hyperoxaluria or hypercalciuria who demonstrate a deficiency of urinary citrate. These patients respond dramatically to citrate supplementation (see Section 3.2.2).

Another important segment of the calcium oxalate stone-forming population exhibits hyperuricosuria not necessarily associated with hypercalciuria. The exact mechanisms whereby hyperuricosuria causes calcium oxalate stone formation are not clear, but absorption of inhibitors of calcium oxalate crystal growth has been proposed as a possible mechanism.[1]

Finally, and perhaps most frustrating for the physician and patient, is the fact that approximately 20% of calcium oxalate stones occurs for reasons that are not yet understood. These patients are referred to as "idiopathic stone formers." By definition, these patients excrete normal quantities of calcium and have no other identifiable metabolic abnormalities. Empirical therapy (see Section 3.3) has been somewhat successful in treating this group of patients.

2.2. *Magnesium Ammonium Phosphate (Struvite) and Calcium Phosphate (Apatite)—"Triple-Phosphate Stones"*

These stones are extremely common and account for approximately 20% of all renal stones. They are frequently large, not uncommonly bilateral, and may present as staghorn calculi. Triple-phosphate stones form in the presence of a persistently alkaline urine, a consequence of chronic urinary infection with urea-splitting organisms (*Proteus, Klebsiella, Pseudomonas*, etc.). These stones are frequently discovered as part of a routine evaluation for chronic or recurrent urinary tract infections and represent one of the most serious complications of such infections.

2.3. *Calcium Phosphate Stones*

Stones consisting predominantly of calcium phosphate account for approximately 7.5% of all episodes of nephrolithiasis. As in the case of other phosphate stones, a persistently alkaline urine is felt to play an important part in the pathogenesis of calcium phosphate stone formation.[2] Patients suffering from renal tubular acidosis (of the distal or classic variety),[7,17] those treated with certain oral antacids, and those receiving chronic carbonic anhydrase inhibitory therapy are all at increased risk for calcium phosphate nephrolithiasis.[2]

In addition, primary hyperparathyroidism may be associated with calcium phosphate stone formation as well as calcium oxalate stone formation.

2.4. *Uric Acid Nephrolithiasis*

Uric acid stones account for approximately 5% of all renal stones. Hyperuricosuria due to overproduction of uric acid or, more commonly, to a high purine intake is an easily identified and treated (see Section 3.6) precipitating factor for uric acid nephrolithiasis. Unfortunately, excess excretion of uric acid is present in the minority of patients who form uric acid stones (approximately 26% in one study[18]) and of these considerably less than half were hyperuricemic.[18] The majority of patients have normal uric acid excretion but a persistently acid urine, which is thought to result at least in part from a deficiency of ammonia buffer, a substance ordinarily required for complete and efficient acid elimination.[19] Other authors have yet additional explanations for uric acid lithiasis in patients with normal serum uric acid concentrations and normal uric acid excretion. Suffice it to say that this area is still undergoing active study.

2.5. Cystine Stones

Cystine stones are quite rare and result from the inherited metabolic defect known as cystinuria (not to be confused with cystinosis). This represents an extremely unusual cause of stone formation and accounts for no more than 1–2% of all episodes of nephrolithiasis. Cystine stones tend to be bilateral and staghorn in nature. They are the only non-calcium-containing stones that are radiopaque on plain films of the abdomen and kidneys. The radiopacity is somewhat less than that seen with calcium-containing stones and can be attributed to the high concentration of sulfur atoms within cystine.

2.6. Summary

Thus, calcium oxalate, triple-phosphate, calcium phosphate, uric acid, and cystine stones make up the spectrum of human nephrolithiasis. Application of general preventive measures or specific prophylaxis demands that the stone type and underlying disorder, if identifiable, be known. (See Table III.)

3. PREVENTION: GENERAL PRINCIPLES AND SPECIFIC THERAPIES

3.1. General Principles

As has been emphasized thus far in this chapter, identification of the specific stone type and etiological factor, if any, makes it easier for physicians and patients to prevent recurrence. The two general therapeutic principles applied to all stone formation are: (1) decrease the concentration of the agent or agents most subject to crystallization and (2)

Table III. Frequency and Characteristics of Renal Stones[a]

Stone composition	Frequency	X-ray appearance
Ca oxalate	65%	Opaque
"Triple phosphate"	20%	Opaque
Ca phosphate	7.5%	Opaque
Uric acid	5%	Lucent
Cystine	1–2%	Opaque

[a]Adapted from Maffly,[2] with permission.

simultaneously (if possible) change the solubility of those substances in the patient's urine.

The most efficacious means of decreasing the concentration of the various substances is to *increase urine volume*. This single nontoxic, noncostly prophylatic step is commonly neglected by physician and patient alike. Urine volume should be raised to a point at which the urinary concentrations of the various lithogenic salts are below saturated levels.[20] For practical purposes, one would like to see the urine volume in any given patient with nephrolithiasis in excess of 3 liters daily. This is most easily accomplished by reminding the patient to drink water whenever practical—on the job, at school, or while traveling. A patient with nephrolithiasis should be instructed never to pass a water cooler without taking a drink. In addition, the ingestion of two 12-oz glasses of water at bedtime will ensure a nocturnal awakening for urination and the opportunity for further ingestion of 24 oz of fluid at that time. Urine specific gravity can be measured at home by the patient by a variety of inexpensive techniques. This value should be kept below 1.005.[20,21]

Measures to change solubility usually relate to measures to change urinary pH. This may be important for certain types of stones and will be discussed later.

Dietary restriction is usually not effective and can occasionally prove harmful (e.g., secondary enteric hyperoxaluria).

3.2. Calcium Oxalate Nephrolithiasis

When hypercalcemia is present, the specific cause should be identified and treatment instituted. In most settings of mild hypercalcemia, nephrolithiasis does not occur. Among patients with cancer and hypercalcemia who have not responded to surgery or chemotherapy, nephrolithiasis is rarely a problem.[8]

The hypercalcemia and hypercalciuria of sarcoidosis and vitamin D intoxication (resulting from excessive absorption of calcium from the gastrointestinal tract) do lead to stone formation. These conditions may be treated by either calcium restriction (avoidance of dairy products is usually sufficient) or the administration of glucocorticoids. The latter are rather specific for these types of absorptive hypercalcemia and hypercalciuria, which result from excessive sensitivity to and increased concentrations of 1,25-dihydroxycholecalciferol.[22–24]

Primary absorptive hypercalciuria associated with nephrolithiasis should be initially treated with dietary calcium restriction. If this is unsuccessful, then two alternative approaches are available to the physician. The administration of cellulose phosphate has been shown by Pak *et al.*[24,25] to be effective in decreasing urinary calcium excretion but has been associated with a marked increase in urinary oxalate.[26–28] Treatment with thiazide and sodium restriction as outlined below is thought to be both more efficacious and safe.[24,29,30]

When absorptive hypercalciuria is associated with hypophosphatemia (presumably secondary to a renal leak of phosphate), orthophosphate (a combination of monobasic and dibasic sodium and potassium phosphates) in doses of 1.5 g/day has proven effective.[24]

Hypercalciuria due to "a renal leak" or normocalcemic hyperparathyroidism requires more specific and at times invasive therapy. Patients with these two types of hypercalciuria should be placed on hydrochlorothiazide, 50 mg daily, and modest sodium restriction.[1,24] In patients with the renal leak variety, the urinary calcium excretion can be expected to fall and the serum parathyroid hormone measured by radioimmunoassay can be expected to fall as well. In this case the elevated parathyroid hormone levels were secondary to the loss of calcium in the urine and respond to cessation of calcium loss by returning to normal.

In patients with normocalcemic hyperparathyroidism, the urinary calcium can be expected to fall in response to hydrochlorothiazide therapy coupled with modest sodium restriction, but the parathyroid hormone levels may remain unchanged and the serum calcium may begin to rise. In effect, this therapy may convert normocalcemic hyperparathyroidism into hypercalcemic hyperpathyroidism by decreasing the renal loss of calcium and exposing the excessive bone resorption resulting from parathyroid hormone excess. In these patients, careful medical follow-up and consideration for surgery are necessary. Parathyroidectomy is the treatment of choice for nephrolithiasis associated with hyperparathyroidism.[8]

The mechanism whereby mild diuretic therapy coupled with sodium restriction corrects hypercalciuria is only partially understood.[30,32] The induction of a state of modest volume depletion enhances proximal tubular calcium reabsorption and permits less calcium to escape to the distal nephron and the ascending limb of the loop of Henle where the primary leak is thought to be located.[31]

3.2.1. Hyperoxaluria

Patients with primary (genetic) hyperoxaluria require severe dietary restriction of foods high in oxalate (rhubarb, spinach, chocolate, nuts, and tea).[33] In addition, administration of pyridoxine in doses of 150–400 mg/day reduces oxalate excretion in these disorders.[2]

Patients with secondary or enteric hyperoxaluria will also respond in part to the restriction of dietary oxalate and dietary fat. They may also require the use of calcium supplementation (see Section 2.1). Finally, cholestyramine, which binds oxalate directly, has also been proven to be useful in patients with enteric hyperoxaluria. As in all types of stone formation, high fluid intake is especially important in these conditions.

There is considerable evidence to suggest that in some patients with idiopathic calcium oxalate nephrolithiasis, the coexistence of uric acid crystals may absorb inhibitors of calcium oxalate cystallization.[34] These data have derived in large part from stone analysis and from clinical studies by Coe and others.[35–37] These investigators, among others, suggest that in patients with calcium oxalate nephrolithiasis in whom hyperuricosuria coexists or in whom a defined mechanism has not been identified, treatment with allopurinol to decrease uric acid excretion may be efficacious. Natural history studies, especially those by Coe,[5,16] confirm these suggestions. Allopurinol should be employed in the patient with coexistant hyperuricosuria and calcium oxalate nephrolithiasis and may prove useful in refractory idiopathic stone formation (see Section 3.3.).

3.2.2. Hypocitraturia

Recent convincing clinical studies by Pak and Fuller[15] have suggested that in patients with calcium oxalate nephrolithiasis and hypocitraturia, chronic administration of potassium citrate in amounts of 30–80 mg/day in four divided doses will markedly decrease recurrent stone formation from 2.11 ± 5.68 to 0.28 ± 1.30 stones/patient-year with minimal or no side effects.[38]

This observation, if supported by further clinical observations, may be extremely important in the patient with seeming "idiopathic" stone formation because it defines yet another subset of calcium oxalate stone formers who are no longer in the "idiopathic" category and for whom a specific and benign form of effective therapy exists.

3.3. Prevention of Idiopathic Calcium Stones

As mentioned earlier, approximately 20% of patients with calcium oxalate nephrolithiasis have no identifiable metabolic cause for stone formation. Considerable controversy exists as to how this difficult group of patients should be treated. Naturally, high fluid intake should be prescribed for all patients with idiopathic calcium oxalate stone formation.

Orthophosphate in doses of 2 g of inorganic phosphate daily has been shown to be useful in the normocalciuric stone former.[2] Although the mechanism of action is not entirely clear, this agent is thought to act by decreasing urinary calcium excretion and by increasing urinary excretion of inorganic pyrophosphate and is much more effective than acid phosphate. This agent is not always well tolerated and may produce persistent diarrhea. Secondary hyperparathyroidism resulting from a rise in serum phosphate and a secondary fall in serum calcium, although not yet observed with this therapy, is also a theoretical concern.

The use of hydrochlorothiazide and sodium restriction with or without the addition of allopurinol represents an effective alternative if orthophosphate is not well tolerated and if stone formation continues.[1,16,30]

In summary, the patient with idiopathic stone formation should be treated with a graduated approach, depending on the severity and morbidity of the recurrent nephrolithiasis. If stone recurrence is rare, a high fluid intake and perhaps modest calcium restriction should suffice. Multiple episodes probably justify treatment with one of the two more aggressive regimens referred to earlier.

3.4. Prevention of Triple-Phosphate Stones

As mentioned in Section 2.2, triple-phosphate stones are encountered in the setting of chronic urinary tract infection. They are frequently bilateral and may result in partial or complete urinary tract obstruction. For this reason, surgical evaluation and nephrolithotomy should be considered early during the evaluation and treatment of a patient with triple-phosphate stone formation.[39]

In addition to this approach, aggressive treatment of the chronic urinary tract infection is indicated. In some instances, removal of the stones may be required before sterilization of the urinary tract can be accomplished. A new experimental urease inhibitor, acetohydroxamic acid, has been used to decrease or prevent triple-phosphate stone formation in the setting of chronic "untreatable" urinary tract infection.[40,41] This agent has been rarely associated with headache and hemolytic anemia, but preliminary clinical data are encouraging.[42]

3.5. Prevention of Calcium Phosphate Stones

These stones are among the easiest to treat in that they are most frequently associated with an identified secondary cause. For example, patients with chronic renal tubular acidosis and calcium phosphate stones are effectively treated by replacement of alkali and correction of the metabolic acidosis and resultant acidemia.

If this therapy is started early enough, stone formation can be virtually abolished. Interestingly enough, many patients with distal renal tubular acidosis have associated hypocitraturia and respond to therapy with Shohl's solution (a mixture of sodium and potassium citrate), which increases urinary citrate excretion while simultaneously correcting systemic metabolic acidosis and acidemia.

Absorbable oral antacids (e.g., calcium carbonate) may play a role in calcium phosphate nephrolithiasis. Patients with calcium phosphate stones should use nonabsorbable antacids. Dietary restriction of calcium may also be effective in this stone-forming state, and the increase in urinary oxalate excretion will not increase the risk of calcium phosphate stone formation.

3.6. Prevention of Uric Acid Nephrolithiasis

High fluid intake plays a critical role in the treatment of renal stones composed or uric acid. Modest alkalinization of the urine (to a pH greater than 6.0) has been shown to have a significant beneficial effect in this condition[2] and may be achieved through a combination of oral alkali and acetazolamide, 250 mg at bedtime. In this instance, the acetazolamide alkalinizes the urine, and the alkali prevents the resultant metabolic acidosis and acidemia.

Allopurinol should be reserved for patients with refractory stone formation, documented hyperuricosuria (greater than 1000 mg/day), or, as noted earlier, with idiopathic calcium oxalate stone formation in whom a uric acid nidus is suspected to be the root cause of the stone formation.

3.7. Prevention of Cystine Stones

High urine volume and maximum alkalinization of the urine are the mainstays of the preventive therapy of cystinuria. Acetazolamide may be used in doses up to 250 mg three times daily as long as sufficient potassium and alkali are administered to prevent hypokalemia and acidemia. A cystine concentration in the urine of less than 250 mg/liter, coupled with a urinary pH of 6.0 or greater, is usually sufficient to prevent recurrent cystine nephrolithiasis.

If these therapies are not successful, *d*-penicillamine is an effective, though potentially toxic second choice. Penicillamine in this instance combines with cystine to form a penicillamine–cysteine complex. This complex is 50 times more soluable than cystine alone. Penicillamine therapy should be a treatment of last resort and reserved for patients excreting greater than 1000 mg of cystine per day. The complications of *d*-penicillamine therapy are many and include proteinuria, skin rash, and bone marrow depression. A new agent, mercaptopropionylglycine, may act similarly and be associated with fewer side effects.[43]

3.8. Summary

Nephrolithiasis is a painful, morbid, and expensive condition that affects a large number of patients in the United States and western Europe. Identification of the specific underlying disease entity or predisposing factor is usually helpful in the prevention of recurrent stone formation.

Even in the absence of the specific diagnosis, logical general therapies and careful medical follow-up may prevent or minimize recurrent nephrolithiasis and the associated morbidity and mortality.

REFERENCES

1. Coe, F. L., and Favus, M. J.: Disorders of stone formation, in Brenner, B. M., and Rector, F. C. (eds.): *The Kidney,* 3rd ed. Saunders, Philadelphia, 1986, pp. 1403–1442.
2. Maffly, R. H.: Nephrolithiasis, in Rubenstein, E., and Federman, D. D. (eds.): *Scientific American Medicine*. Scientific American, New York, 1985.
3. Finlayson, B., and Thomas, W. C., Jr.: Extracorporeal shock-wave lithotripsy (editorial). *Ann. Intern. Med.* **101**:387, 1984.
4. Chaussy, C., Brendel, W., and Schmiedt, E.: Extracorporeally induced destruction of kidney stones by shock waves. *Lancet* **2**:1265, 1980.
5. Coe, F. L.: Prevention of kidney stones. *Am. J. Med.* **71**:514, 1981.
6. Broadus, A. E., and Thier, S. O.: Metabolic basis of renal-stone disease. *N. Engl. J. Med.* **300**:839, 1979.
7. Coe, F. L., and Parks, J. H.: Stone disease in hereditary distal renal tubular acidosis. *Ann. Intern. Med.* **93**:60, 1980.
8. Breslau, N. A., and Pak, C. Y. C.: Endocrine aspects of nephrolithiasis. *Special Topics Endocrinol. Metab* **3**:57–86, 1982.
9. Coe, F. L., Canterbury, J. M., Firpo, J. J., and Reiss, E.: Evidence for secondary hyperparathyroidism in idiopathic hypercalciuria. *J. Clin. Invest.* **52**:134–142, 1973.
10. Pak, C. Y. C., Kaplan, R. A., Bone, H., Townsend, J., and Waters, O.: A simple test for the diagnosis of absorptive, resorptive and renal hypercalciurias. *N. Engl. J. Med.* **292**:497–500, 1975.
11. Willaims, H. E., and Smith, L. H.: Primary hyperoxaluria, in Stanbury, J. P., Wyngaaden, J. B., and Fredrickson, D. S. (eds.): *The Metabolic Basis of Inherited Disease*. McGraw-Hill, New York, p. 196, 1972.
12. Hockaday, T. D. R., Fredric, E. W., Clayton, J. E., and Smith, L. H.: Studies on primary hyperoxaluria. II. Urinary oxalate, glycolate and glyoxylate measurement by isotope dilution. *J. Lab. Clin. Med.* **65**:677, 1965.
13. Chadwick, V. S., Modha, K., and Dowling, R. H.: Mechanism for hyperoxaluria in patients with ileal dysfunction. *N. Engl. J. Med.* **289**:172, 1973.
14. Smith, L. H.: Enteric hyperoxaluria and other hyperoxaluric states, in Coe, F. L., Brenner, B. M., and Stein, J. H. (eds.): *Contemporary Issues in Nephrology,* Vol VI: *Nephrolithiasis*. Churchill Livingstone, New York, p. 136, 1980.
15. Pak, C. Y. C., and Fuller, C.: Idiopathic hypocitraturic calcium–oxalate nephrolithiasis successfully treated with potassium citrate. *Ann. Intern. Med.* **104**:33–37, 1986.
16. Coe, F. L.: Treated and untreated recurrent calcium nephrolithiasis in patients with idiopathic hypercalciuria, hyperuricosuria, or no metabolic disorder. *Ann. Intern. Med.* **87**:404, 1977.
17. Brenner, R. J., Spring, D. B., Sebastian, A., *et al.*: Incidence of radiographically evident bone disease, nephrocalcinosis, and nephrolithiasis in various types of renal tubular acidosis. *N. Engl. J. Med.* **307**:217, 1982.
18. Coe, F. L.: Treated and untreated recurrent calcium nephrolithiasis in patients with idiopathic hypercalciuria, hyperuricosuria or no metabolic disorder. *Ann. Intern. Med.* **87**:404, 1977.
19. Gutman, A. B., and Uy, T. F.: Urinary ammonium excretion in primary gout. *J. Clin. Invest.* **44**:1474–1481, 1965.

20. Pak, C. Y. C., Sakhaee, K., Crowther, C., *et al.*: Evidence justifying a high fluid intake in treatment of nephrolithiasis. *Ann. Intern. Med.* **93**:36, 1980.
21. Daniel, H. W.: Urinometers as a guide to hydration (letter). *N. Engl. J. Med.* **298**:1089, 1978.
22. Frame, B., and Parfitt, A. M.: Corticosteroid-responsive hypercalcemia with elevated serum 1-alpha, 25-dihydroxyvitamin D. *Ann. Intern. Med.* **93**:449–451, 1980.
23. Zerwekh, J. E., Pak, C. Y. C., Kaplan, R. A., McGuire, J. L., Upchurch, K., Breslau, N., and Johnson, R., Jr.: Pathogenetic role of 1a,25-dihydroxyvitamin D in sarcoidosis and absorptive hypercalciuria: Different response to prednisolone therapy. *J. Clin. Endocrinol. Metab.* **51**:381–386, 1980.
24. Pak, C. Y. C., Peters, P., and Hurt, G.: Is selective therapy of recurrent nephrolithiasis possible? *Am. J. Med.* **71**:615, 1981.
25. Pak, C. Y. C., Delea, C. S., and Bartter, F. C.: Successful treatment of recurrent nephrolithiasis (calcium stones) with cellulose phospate. *N. Engl. J. Med.* **190**:175, 1974.
26. Hayasaki, Y., Kaplan, R. A., and Pak, C. Y. C.: Effect of sodium cellulose phosphate therapy on crystallization of calcium oxalate in urine. *Metabolism* **24**:1273, 1975.
27. Hautmann, R., Hering, F. J., and Lutzeyer, W.: Calcium oxalate stone disease effects and side effects of cellulose phosphate and succinate in long-term treatment of absorptive hypercalciuria or hyperoxaluria. *J. Urol.* **120**:712, 1978.
28. Backman, U., Danielson, B. G., Johansson, G., Ljunghall, S., and Widstrom, B.: Treatment of recurrent calcium stone formation with cellulose phosphate. *J. Urol.* **123**:9, 1980.
29. Coe, F. L.: Treated and untreated recurrent calcium nephrolithiasis in patients with idiopathic hypercalciuria, hyperuricosuria or no metabolic disorder. *Ann. Intern. Med.* **87**:404, 1977.
30. Yendt, E. R.: Renal calculi. *Can. Med. Assoc. J.* **102**:479, 1970.
31. Agus, Z. A., Gardner, L. B., Beck, L. H., and Goldberg, M.: Effect of parathyroid hormone on renal tubular reabsorption of calcium, sodium and phosphate. *Am. J. Physiol.* **224**:1143–1148, 1973.
32. Yendt, E. R., and Cohanim, M.: Prevention of calcium stones with thiazides. *Kidney Int.* **13**:397, 1978.
33. Pak, C. Y. C., Smith, L. H., Resnick, M. I., *et al.*: Dietary management of idiopathic calcium urolithiasis. *J. Urol.* **131**:850, 1984.
34. Pak, C. Y. C., Holt, K., and Zerwekh, J. E.: Attentuation by monosodium urate of the inhibitory effect of glycosaminoglycans on calcium oxalate nucleation. *Invest. Urol.* **17**:138–140, 1979.
35. Smith, M. J. V., Hunt, L. D., King, J. S., Jr., *et al.*: Uricemia and urolithiasis. *J. Urol.* **101**:637–642, 1969.
36. Coe, F. L., and Kavalach, A. G.: Hypercalciuria and hyperuricosuria in patients with calcium nephrolithiasis. *N. Engl. J. Med.* **291**:1344–1350, 1974.
37. Coe, F. L.: Hyperuricosuric calcium oxalate nephrolithiasis. *Kidney Int.* **13**:418, 1978.
38. Pak, C. Y. C., Sakhaee, K., and Fuller, C. J.: Physiological and physicochemical correction and prevention of calcium stone formation by potassium citrate therapy. *Trans. Assoc. Am. Physicians* **96**:294, 1983.
39. Silverman, D. E., and Stamey, T. A.: Management of infection stones: The Stanford experience. *Medicine* **62**:44, 1983.
40. Griffith, D. P.: Infection-induced renal calculi. *Kidney Int.* **21**:422, 1982.
41. Oral acetohydroxamic acid (lithostat) for staghorn calculi. *Med. Lett. Drugs Ther.* **25**:110, 1983.
42. Williams, J. J., Rodman, J. S., and Peterson, C. M.: A randomized double-blind study of acetohydroxamic acid in struvite nephrolithiasis. *N. Engl. J. Med.* **311**:760, 1984.
43. Hautmann, R., Terhorst, B., Stuhlsatz, H. W., and Lutzeyer, W.: Mercaptopropionylglycine: Progress in cystine stone therapy. *J. Urol.* **117**:628, 1977.

16

Cancer

David V. Schapira and J. Donald Temple

1. INTRODUCTION

In 1975 the likelihood that an American would develop cancer in his/her lifetime was 30%. By 1985 this had risen to 35% and by the year 2000 the risk will be 40%. During the period 1968–1978 the age-adjusted death rate due to cancer rose by 5%.[1] The rates of the other most common causes of death all fell—coronary artery disease by 22%, cerebral vascular disease by 36%, and accidents by 22%. Despite this rather alarming rise in cancer incidence, the National Cancer Institute has set a goal to reduce the mortality from cancer by 50% by the year 2000. This goal, though, is not unreasonable. It relies on the implementation of strategies for preventing cancer. Primary-care physicians will play a vital role in this effort by educating their patients and the general public.

Although impressive gains have been made in the treatment of certain tumors such as leukemias, lymphomas, testicular cancer and bone tumors, the extension of survival among patients with the more common cancers has been far shorter. Fortunately, though, the potential exists for preventing the development of a large percentage of these cancers. This can be realized by modifying those lifestyle factors among the population that are implicated in causing cancer.

The answer to reducing the number of premature deaths due to cancer lies in interrupting what appears to be an avoidable event—the conversion of a normal cell to a cancer cell. Certain substances in our diet have been shown to aid the carcinogenic process and others appear to be protective. Even knowledge of the existence of these substances in our present diet is probably still not enough to change the lifestyle of a population. Habits ingrained over the years require appreciable motivation and behavior modification if they are to be altered. It is the role of the physician to educate *all* patients, particularly patients identified as being at increased risk of developing certain cancers, as to how to decrease their own risk of developing cancer. In addition, the physicians should follow the guidelines themselves. A physician who does not himself practice a health-enhancing lifestyle is unlikely to try enthusiastically to motivate his patients.

Unfortunately, it is extremely difficult to identify individuals who are at a high risk of developing cancer. A family history of cancer is found in only 5% of women who

David V. Schapira • H. Lee Moffitt Cancer Center, University of South Florida College of Medicine, Tampa, Florida 33612. *J. Donald Temple* • Department of Medicine, University of Miami School of Medicine, Miami, Florida 33101.

develop breast cancer and 2% of all individuals who develop cancer.[2] Therefore, interventional and educational programs should be directed at the entire population. This proposition is not as unrealistic as it may appear. The general public is quite receptive to ideas about how to improve their health. If physicians can convince the public that the control of their future health lies in their own hands and then give information regarding appropriate lifestyle changes, a decrease in mortality from cancer may ensue.

There are two reasons why a successful program of public education could lead to a marked decrease in cancer mortality:

1. There is evidence that 75% of all cancers and 90% of the six most common cancers are potentially preventable.[2]
2. The public has changed its eating and exercise habits in the past in response to recommendations by the American Heart Association.

2. CARCINOGENESIS

Before addressing why most cancers are preventable, it is important to understand how a normal cell is converted to a cancer cell. There are two stages to the carcinogenic process: initiation and promotion.[3] Initiation is a one-time, irreversible event. When a normal cell is initiated, it is primed to become a cancer cell, but will not complete the conversion unless it is exposed to a promoter. Promotion is the second essential step in carcinogenesis. The process of promotion takes several years to be completed and it is somewhat reversible.

To convert a normal cell to a cancer cell may require two specific errors in cellular DNA. Let us say they need to occur at base pair 27 and 53. Initiation will produce the first error at base pair 27. If this error is not corrected by the time the cell divides, then the mistake will be carried by all daughter cells. If only a few cells had the one mistake, then the chances of a second mistake occurring at exactly the correct point in the DNA would be extremely small.

Initiated cells appear normal but, they are different from normal cells in one important respect—they can divide more quickly than normal cells if they are exposed to a promoter. This is because the gaps in the cell membrane, which are present in normal cells, are closed off after they become initiated. These gaps allow the passage of growth-controlling substances from one cell to another. When the gaps are closed off, the growth of a cell is no longer controlled by neighboring cells. It can thus divide more rapidly than normal if exposed to the appropriate stimulus. This stimulus is a promoter.

By stimulating initiated cells to divide more rapidly than normal, a promoter will produce millions more copies of the initiated cell with the one DNA error. This greatly increases the chances of a second error occuring at exactly the right location in the DNA. The lower the concentration of promoter the initiated cell is exposed to and the briefer the time of exposure, the less proliferation of initiated cells there will be and therefore the less chance there will be for a cancer cell to develop.

It is intervening in the process of promotion that holds the promise for preventing or delaying the occurrence of cancer. An excellent example of this principle is cigarette smoking. The main carcinogens in cigarette smoke are both initiators and promoters. If a person stops smoking, initiated cells in the pulmonary epithelia are no longer exposed to the promotional effects of cigarette smoke. The risk of lung cancer in ex-smokers starts falling after the first year and after 7–8 years of cessation is almost the same as in someone who has never smoked a cigarette.

3. FACTORS ASSOCIATED WITH THE DEVELOPMENT OF CANCER

The factors that have been associated with the development of cancer were investigated by Doll and Peto in a comprehensive review of existing epidemiological data.[2] The more common factors associated with the causation of cancer are listed in Table I. Many cancers are associated with multiple factors. Therefore, the values presented in Table I do not total 100%.

Although the population is most agitated over such issues as pollution, background radiation, and family history as sources of cancer, these factors actually play a minor role.

Dietary factors are associated with between 35 and 45% of all cancers. Excessive intake of dietary fat and/or total calories has been associated with the incidence of five of the six most common cancers—colorectal, breast, prostate, pancreas, and uterus.

4. EVIDENCE FOR CANCER PREVENTION

The evidence that suggests that 75% of all cancers are preventable is culled from three areas of research.

4.1. International Differences in Cancer Incidence

There are large differences in cancer incidence around the world.[4] Some striking examples are listed in Table II. If the rates of all cancers in the United States are compared to those of other countries with a lower incidence of those cancers, it is possible to estimate the percentage of cancers that are potentially preventable. Table III estimates the

Table I. Factors Associated with Development of Cancer[a]

Diet	35%
Smoking	30%
Infection	10%
Sunlight	8%
Alcohol	5%
Occupation	4%
Family history	2%
Pollution	2%
Food additives	1%
Industrial products	1%

[a]Adapted from Doll and Peto.[2]

Table II. International Differences in Cancer Incidence

Cancer site	High rate	Low rate	Ratio high:low
Lip	Canada Newfoundland	Osaka, Japan	228:1
Prostate	Alameda, U.S. (blacks)	Shanghai	125:1
Nasopharynx	Hong Kong	Niyagi, Japan	110:1
Melanoma	New South Wales, Australia	Osaka, Japan	96:1
Uterus	Alameda, U.S. (whites)	Fukouka, Japan	39:1
Cervix	Cali, Colombia	Israel	25:1

percentage of preventable cancer cases among the six most common cancers in the United States.

4.2. Migration Studies

One might argue that the international differences in cancer rates listed in Table II are due to hereditary differences between races and ethnic groups. These differences, however, appear to be due to environmental factors. When individuals migrate from their own country to another, they develop cancer at the rate that is currently prevailing in their new country.[5,6] Indeed, the rate of certain cancers may be lower than in the country from which they have just migrated (see Tables IV and V).

It can be noted from these findings that the rates of certain cancers rose dramatically in the migrants or their children. This rise in cancer rates in the migrants points to an environmental cause. The fall in stomach cancer in the Japanese may be due to their decreased intake of salted food when they adopted western eating habits. Sodium enhances the reaction between nitrites and amines to produce carcinogenic nitrosamines.

Table III. Estimated Preventability of the Six most Common Cancers in the United States

Cancer	Expected number of cancers in U.S., 1985	Country with low incidence	Ratio of incidence lower than U.S.	Number of potentially preventable cancers	Percent of potentially preventable cancers
Lung	144,000	Nigeria	35X	140,000	97
Colon/rectum	138,000	Nigeria	10X	124,000	90
Breast	119,000	Japan	5X	95,000	80
Prostate	86,000	Japan	40X	84,000	98
Uterus	52,000	Japan	30X	50,000	96
Pancreas	25,000	India	8X	22,000	88
Totals	564,000			515,000	92%

Table IV. Cancer in Japanese Migrants to the United States[a]

Site	Japan	U.S. Japanese	U.S. whites
Stomach	133	39	21
Colon	8	37	37
Prostate	1	15	34
Breast	33	122	187

[a]Values are per 100,000.

Vitamin C inhibits this reaction. The dramatic rise in colon, prostate, and breast cancer may well be due to increased dietary fat intake by the migrants as they acculturated.

4.3. Laboratory Research

An increase in total caloric intake has been shown to increase the incidence of spontaneous and carcinogen-induced cancers.[7] Increasing the percentage of fat in their diet increases the number of rodents that develop breast cancer and preneoplastic pancreatic lesions. These breast cancers develop earlier, tend to behave more aggressively, and are more resistant to hormonal manipulation when compared to the cancers developing in rats on a low-fat diet. If the percentage of fat is decreased prior to the clinical appearance of tumors, then the number of resultant cancers is decreased.

Strategies aimed at preventing cancer involve decreasing or eradicating exposure to carcinogens and increasing exposure to substances that seem to be protective.

5. ADVERSE FACTORS IN CANCER CAUSATION

5.1. Smoking

Cigarette smoking has been identified as a major cause of cancers of the lung, head and neck, and esophagus and a contributory factor in cancers of the bladder, kidney,

Table V. Cancer in Black Migrants to the United States[a]

Site	Nigerian blacks	U.S. blacks	U.S. whites
Colon	3	35	30
Liver	27	7	4
Lung	3	154	98
Breast	34	126	182

[a]Values are per 100,000.

pancreas, stomach, and uterine cervix. Unfortunately, the survival of patients developing most of these cancers is poor. The 5-year survival rates for cancers of the lung, esophagus, and pancras are 12%, 4%, and 3%, respectively, and these have barely changed in the last 30 years.

The data linking cigarette smoking with lung cancer have come from both retrospective and prospective studies. The relative risk of smoking is proportional to the number of cigarettes smoked per day and the number of years the person smoked. For a smoker of more than a pack of cigarettes per day the relative risk is increased approximately 15- to 20-fold. The risk falls after 1 year of cessation and falls to the lowest possible risk at 15 years. The increase over the past 30 years in the number of women who smoke cigarettes has led to a dramatic increase in lung cancer. In 1985, lung cancer overtook breast cancer as the most common cancer in women. Between 1950 and 1977 age-adjusted lung cancer mortality increased almost 200% in men but more than 250% in women.

Other carcinogens have been shown to have a synergistic effect with the carcinogens from cigarette smoke. Exposure to asbestos increases the incidence of lung cancer and mesothelioma fivefold among nonsmokers and 50-fold among smokers.[8] The incidence of lung cancer in uranium miners who smoke is four times higher than in smokers not exposed to uranium.

Apart from the direct action of cigarette smoke on the lung, the effect of aromatic amines absorbed has probably accounted for about 40% of bladder cancers. Studies have been done on the likelihood of nonsmokers developing cancer by being exposed passively to smoke. Studies from Japan and Greece demonstrated significant increases in lung cancer risk in the nonsmoking wives of smoking husbands, but this issue is still open to question.

5.2. Dietary Fat

An increased intake of dietary fat has been implicated in the causation of breast, colon, pancreatic, and prostate cancer. The incidence of breast cancer in a country is proportional to the gross national consumption of fat in the diet and to a certain extent to high socioeconomic status. The incidence of breast cancer is five to six times greater in the United States compared to Japan. The difference in incidence between the two populations is about threefold for premenopausal women and eightfold for postmenopausal women.

Americans consume 1000 more calories a day than the Japanese.[9] This increased intake is in the form of a threefold increased fat intake. Westernization of the Japanese diet in the last 20 years has been associated with an increased incidence of breast cancer.[10] Hormonal changes have taken place in Japanese women in conjunction with this change. Adolescent Japanese girls now start menstruating 3 years earlier than in 1950 and their height and weight are now very close to the median of their U.S. counterparts. Early menarche and increased weight have been implicated in producing breast cancer.[11] The increased consumption of dietary fat, particularly by the urban-dwelling Japanese, probably accounts for the increase in breast cancer in Japan in the past 25 years.

Using the DMBA rat model, a high-fat diet exerts its primary effect on the promotion phase of mammary carcinogenesis. Diets rich in polyunsaturated fats tend to be more effective tumor promoters than diets rich in saturated fats.[12,13] High-fat diets increase the serum prolactin in the preestrous and estrous stages of the menstrual cycle.[14,15] Prolactin produces proliferation of the cells lining the breast duct and may be important to the promotional phase of breast cancer.

6. PROTECTIVE FACTORS

Certain substances appear to exert a protective effect against the development of cancer in the animal model.

6.1. Vitamin A

Vitamin A (retinoids) appears to be essential for the normal growth of squamous epithelium (lung, bladder, cervix, skin).[16,17] If animals are fed a diet reduced in vitamin A content, they develop squamous metaplasia initially and subsequently squamous cell carcinoma. The squamous cell metaplasia can be reversed by administering vitamin A. Studies among smokers have shown that despite smoking the same number of cigarettes, the rates of small cell and squamous cell cancer of the lung and cancer of the bladder were significantly decreased for people who had a high intake of vitamin A through dietary sources, compared to those with a low intake.

Vitamin A analogs are powerful antioxidants. During normal metabolism, free radicals are generated. Free radicals are unstable substances that have an extra unpaired election. They can combine with the cell membrane causing lipid peroxidation of the membrane resulting in cell death, or they can combine with DNA and cause initiation. Antioxidants, such as vitamins A, C, E, zinc, and selenium, combine with free radicals and render them harmless.

Another interesting property of vitamin A is that it reopens the gaps in the cell membrane that have been closed off following initiation of the cell. The reopening of these gaps reinstitutes control of the cell's growth by the passage of growth-controlling substances from surrounding cells into the affected cell. Finally, vitamin A has been shown to be effective in suppressing the activity of certain oncogenes—the myc and ras oncogenes. This is an intriguing property as the activation of oncogenes is an early step in carcinogenesis.

6.2. Fiber

When a diet containing fat is eaten and bile acids are secreted, they are broken down in the colon. Two secondary bile acids—lithocolic acid and deoxycholic acid—are carcinogenic. These bile acids are thought to be promoters of colonic epithelium, and they are present in much greater amounts in the feces of Americans compared to Japanese, Chinese, or American Seventh-Day Adventists. The latter three populations eat a diet low in fat. The Hindu population eats a diet rich in cellulose, fiber, and roughage. There is virtually no colon cancer in this sect; however, the Parsi Indian community in Bombay, which eats a more westernized diet, has rates of colon and breast cancer almost equal to those of western countries.

The conversion from bile acids to secondary bile acids is enhanced by *Bacteroides* in the colon. The growth of these anaerobic bacteria is inhibited by the oxygen produced by increasing the numbers of aerobic bacteria in the colon. The fermentation process that is part of the breakdown of fiber in the colon leads to increased numbers of aerobic bacteria. In addition, the increased acidity produced by fermentation decreases the conversion of primary to secondary bile acids. It has been noted that people from countries with high rates of colon cancer (United States and Great Britain) have seven times the amount of bile acids in their feces as people from low-risk countries. There is also a 30% higher number of *Bacteroides* in the feces of individuals from countries with high rates of colon cancer, compared to individuals from countries with low rates. The fermentation of fiber produces butyrate, which has been shown to be essential for the normal differentiation of colonic epithelia and *in vitro* has been shown to slow the growth of colonic neoplasia.

Fiber also adds bulk to the stool, thus decreasing the concentration of bile acids in the stool. It also decreases the transit time of digested material from the 36–60 hr of the average person in the Western hemisphere to the 12 hr seen in Africans on high-fiber diets. If the protective effect from fiber does exist, it is not known whether this effect is due to total fiber intake or from specific constituents such as fruits, vegetables, or cereals.

6.3. Other Protective Factors

Other protective factors include the phenols, flavones, indoles, and aromatic isothiocyanates. Phenols have been shown to inhibit mutagenesis and the promotional phase of carcinogenesis. They also raise the level of the enzyme glutathione-*S*-transferase, an important enzyme that detoxifies carcinogens. The most widely known phenols are the food additives butylated hydroxyanisole and butylated hydroxytoluene.

Flavones, found in fruit and vegetables, increase the activity of aryl hydrocarbon hydroxylase. This enzyme inhibits the formation of pulmonary neoplasia. The indoles, found in the cruciferous vegetables—brussels sprouts, cabbage, broccoli, and cauliflower—increase microsomal monoxygenase oxidase activity. They can inhibit the development of pulmonary and breast neoplasia.

7. STRATEGIES FOR CANCER PREVENTION

Strategies that should reduce the incidence of cancer are outlined in the following sections.

7.1. Smoking Cessation

Smoking has been associated with cancers of the lung, head and neck area, esophagus, bladder, kidney, and pancreas. Cigarette smoking is the single major cause of cancer mortality in the United States. It is imperative that physicians explain to patients not only the fact that smoking is hazardous but also that the effects are to a large degree reversible on cessation. This effect applies to lung cancer risk and the risk of myocardial infarction. It has been shown that even a brief period of time spent by the physician is effective in influencing patients to stop smoking.

In a study in the United Kingdom, 28 physicians reported a 5.1% 1-year abstinence rate among 2138 smoking patients who were given advice, an antismoking leaflet, and a warning concerning follow-up.[18] The cessation rate was 0.3% in the nonintervention control group, 1.6% in a questionnaire-only group, and 3.3% in an advice-only group. The advice was given by the physician in his own style, in 1–2 min. It was estimated that general practitioners would see at least 18 million of the 20 million smokers at least once every 5 years, and most more often. It was estimated that this brief intervention would convert ½ million smokers each year to nonsmokers. The 5-year survival for lung cancer was 7% in 1930 and 12% in 1980. One can see that this brief intervention would be far more effective in preventing premature morbidity and mortality than lung cancer detection and treatment programs.

Unfortunately, snuff dipping (smokeless tobacco) has become very popular among young people. The risk of cancer of the cheek and gum has been shown to be 50 times greater in long-term users of snuff.

The strategy with regard to younger people who chew tobacco should be directed toward the social unacceptability of the habit, as well as the health hazard.

7.2. Dietary Changes

7.2.1. Decreasing Fat Consumption

Currently, the average American consumes 42% of calories as fat each day. To complicate matters, the daily caloric requirement figures for females and males used currently is incorrect. They are based on an estimate of calories burned with each activity multiplied by the number of hours engaged in that activity. A more direct way of measuring daily caloric expenditure has been perfected and demonstrates that the daily caloric expenditure for women (2150 cal currently) is in fact, when measured accurately, 1700 cal. This implies that the currently recommended calculated caloric and fat intake is being overcalculated by 27%.

The current recommendation from the National Cancer Institute, American Cancer Society, and National Academy of Sciences is that dietary fat should be decreased to 30% of total calories. This fat intake should consist of 10% saturated fat, 10% polyunsaturated fat, and 10% monounsaturated fat. In addition, one should eat plenty of vitamin A-containing vegetables and increase fiber to 25–30 g/day.

It will be a particularly difficult task to try to decrease the intake of fat consumed by the U.S. population for the following reasons:

1. There does not appear to be a consensus among the scientific community as to the benefits of reducing fat intake. This mixed message is hardly likely to convince the public that giving up foods they have grown to love and that are part of the American culture is worthwhile.
2. A goal of not developing cancer is not tangible enough to induce people to modify radically their behavior over the long term. This imperceptible and negative goal

does not supply enough motivation over the years. After all, the success rate of all weight loss programs at 1 year is 5%, and weight loss is a perceptible reward.

3. Instructing the public to "try and cut down" or "eat less of" or "eat more" is unlikely to be successful. Such nonspecific directions do not readily translate into everyday eating habits.
4. If someone set out to eat a diet that was less than 30% fat and comprised a ratio of 1:1:1 saturated-to-monounsaturated-to-polyunsaturated fat, that would leave very little time during the day for other activities. The recommendation is of course completely impractical. People eat food, not nutrients.
5. People tend to attribute illness to uncontrollable factors in order to protect their self-esteem. In the case of cancer causation, most of the public and indeed the medical profession attribute cancer causation to uncontrollable factors such as family history, pollution, and background radiation. At the same time they minimize the importance of controllable factors such as diet. This was illustrated in a recent survey[19] that I made of 217 physicians, nurses, and medical students assessing their knowledge of cancer prevention and nutrition. Table VI demonstrates the percentage of respondents who were aware that diet was more important than family history, pollution, radiation, and sunlight. Referring back to Table I, diet was associated with causing 35% of all cancers, sunlight 8%, pollution 2%, and family history 2%.

The percentages of respondents aware of the recommendation that 30% of calories should be derived from fat were nurses 15.2, private physicians 38.5, internal medicine house staff 51.2, family practice house staff 11.1, freshman medical students 23.8, and sophomore medical students exposed to material 2 months prior to test 53.3.

Recommendations. An increased intake of saturated fats and cholesterol has been associated with the development of atherosclerosis, which in turn has been associated with an increased mortality from coronary artery disease and strokes. Increased dietary intake of fat, probably polyunsaturated fat, has been linked with the causation of five of the six most common cancers—breast, colorectal, pancreatic, prostatic, and uterine. It seems more than reasonable for the scientific community to embark on widespread public and professional education programs that combine the recommendations of the cardiovascular

Table VI. Respondents (%) Aware that Diet Is a More Important Factor in Cancer Causation[a]

	N	PP	IM	FP	MSI	MSII
Diet versus pollution	15.2	3.8	7.0	11.1	14.3	6.7
Diet versus family history	18.2	7.7	7.0	16.7	19.0	66.7
Diet versus radiation	13.6	5.8	4.7	0.0	9.5	6.7
Diet versus sunlight	15.2	5.8	7.0	11.1	33.3	40.0

[a]N, nurses; PP, private physicians; IM, internal medicine house staff; FP, family practice house staff; MSI, freshman medical students; MSII, sophomore medical students exposed to material 2 months prior to test.

and cancer disciplines. This should result in a recommendation that will reduce total fat intake in a practical and realistic manner.

It is vital that the public understands that each individual's lifestyle will be the most important factor in his future health. One must not rely on medical technology or ineffective and expensive screening procedures such as the annual physical examination.

It is important that the public understands that interventions can drastically reduce the risk of cancer. Smoking cessation is a persuasive example. Irrespective of the length of time or number of cigarettes a person has smoked, his risk of lung cancer becomes almost the same as that of someone who never smoked, 7–8 years after stopping.

Techniques that increase a person's feeling of mastery over his health should be used. Participation in exercise programs seems to increase a sense of mastery, and the production of endorphins during exercise enhances the experience and feeling of well-being afterward.

It is unlikely that the majority of the American population will reduce their fat intake to less than 30% of total calories. However, it may be possible to reduce their intake of fat in increments as healthier foods are introduced. Public pressure and interaction between the scientific community and the food industry can result in manufacture of such foods.

Simple guidelines are required to direct the public toward healthier foods. In addition, education of the public regarding foods that are extremely high in fat is necessary. An example is the consumption of nuts, which are widely regarded as a healthy food. A handful of peanuts contains 560 cal and the nuts are 75% fat. Three handfuls of peanuts represents the total daily requirement of calories for most women, and they would have consumed 2½ times the recommended daily intake of fat.

Broad guidelines for decreasing fat intake and increasing the dietary intake of vitamin A and fiber are described in the next sections.

7.2.2. Decreasing Fat Intake

1. Eat red meat once or twice weekly at the most. Cut visible fat off red meat and drain fat off when cooking.
2. Eat more white meat such as chicken or turkey. A chicken cooked with its skin intact provides 2000 cal. If the skin is removed prior to cooking, the chicken provides 600 cal; if the skin is removed after cooking, the chicken provides 1300 cal. The 1400 cal derived from the skin are mostly fat.
3. Eat fish at least twice weekly. It is low in fat and high in the fish oils eicosapantaenoic acid and menhaden oil. The former may decrease myocardial infarctions; the latter, breast and pancreatic cancer in the animal model.
4. Drink skim or 1% milk and eat low-fat cheeses. Most cheeses are 70–80% fat and, if eaten, should be in small amounts.
5. Avoid deep frying—a baked potato is 130 cal and if converted to French fries a potato is 450 cal. The additional calories are derived from fat.
6. Avoid eating large amounts of regular potato chips, cookies, doughnuts, or chocolate as they are all high in fat. Pretzels contain no fat and one can obtain low-fat potato chips.
7. Put low-fat salad dressing on salad. Although a salad contains no fat and only a

small number of calories, a tablespoonful of salad dressing is 400 cal and extremely high in fat. Use oil-and-vinegar dressings.

7.2.3. Increasing Intake of Vitamin A

Dark-green and yellow vegetables are rich in vitamin A. The richest sources are carrots, tomatoes, and cantaloupe. Other valuable sources are broccoli, spinach, cabbage, and Brussels sprouts.

In addition to being a useful source of vitamin A, these vegetables are valuable sources of fiber.

7.2.4. Increasing Intake of Fiber

Fiber should be derived from cereals and vegetables. Approximately 25–30 g should be eaten each day. Bran cereals offer the greatest amount of fiber. A serving of Raisin Bran cereal with added fiber provides 12 g of fiber. Most of the other cereals provide only 4 g of fiber. Other sources of fiber are whole-grain breads, pancakes, and pastas. Vegetables and fruit, as well as being a valuable source of vitamins A and C, are an important source of fiber. Examples are oranges, grapefruit, apricots, cantaloupe, apples, and pears. In addition, fiber derived from fruit has cholesterol-lowering properties.

Smoking cessation and dietary change offer such enormous benefits in the reduction of cancer and cardiovascular mortality rates that the impact could be the most spectacular medical advance since the development of antibiotics. The medical profession must reevaluate its priorities and become more aware of the potential of preventive medicine. The extent to which primary-care physicians become involved in educating the public about the value of lifestyle changes will to a great extent determine what the mortality rates from cancer and cardiovascular disease will be 20 years from now.

8. EARLY DETECTION OF CANCER

Cancer will affect one of four of today's Americans. For most cancers, early detection and surgical resection offer the best hope for cure because chemotherapy and radiation therapy are ineffective at eradicating advanced or metastatic disease. The most common malignancies in this country are cancers of the lung (149,000 new cases/year), breast (124,000 cases/year), and large bowel (140,000 cases/year).[20] The cost, measured both in dollars and in human suffering, is staggering.

Most physicians are trained in the art of diagnosis and management of disease. This implies that a patient comes to the physician with a complaint referable to the underlying disease. In most cases of cancer, by the time symptoms develop the malignancy is advanced and is not likely to be "cured" with presently available therapy. Thus, in order to decrease mortality from cancer, the tumor should be detected before any symptoms develop. This is the rationale behind efforts at screening populations at risk for various malignancies.

The success or failure of an early detection program in altering mortality depends on many factors, the most important of which is the biology of the specific target malignancy. If the disease progresses in a slow, orderly, predictable fashion and remains "curable" by available means, then attempts at early detection may affect survival. A good example of this is carcinoma of the uterine cervix. If, on the other hand, the disease advances and spreads early and rapidly, such as small cell carcinoma of the lung, then attempts at early detection are unlikely to have any impact on survival.

The value of a screening test depends on its ability to separate those who have disease from those who do not (see Chapter 3). A successful screening test must not miss disease when present (i.e., it must have sensitivity). On the other hand, the test must not falsely indicate the presence of disease (it must have specificity). The most useful parameter of test utility is the *predictive value*. This is determined by the association between test specificity and the prevalence of the target disease in the population being tested.

Limiting the screening to high-risk groups will significantly improve the predictive value of any test. Unfortunately, if only high-risk groups are tested, most cancers will be missed because even when all known risk factors are considered, it is impossible to predict those who will and those who will not develop cancer. Most malignancies occur in individuals with no known risk factors. On the other hand, *knowledge* of risk factors is important to allow exceptions to the boundaries defining the target population. A good example is the need for frequent colonic examination to look for early colon cancer in young adults with ulcerative colitis.

The availability of an accurate screening test is essential to the success of an early detection program. Less obvious but equally important is the acceptability of the procedure or test to the patient. A simple and accurate serum assay would be ideal, but most available tests involve some degree of discomfort, inconvenience, risk, or expense. Each of these considerations results in an obstacle to patient compliance and compromises the success of the program, especially considering the fact that the patient is asymptomatic. In addition, the inherent lack of specificity of most available tests results in many patients being subjected to the risks and discomfort of further testing as well as the emotional trauma of a workup for cancer, only to be told that they are free of disease. Although relieved, they are unlikely to enthusiastically embrace further efforts at cancer screening.

Given the complexity of the problem, it is easy to understand the current confusion regarding recommendations for cancer screening.

8.1. Cancer of the Uterine Cervix

Cervical cancer is, in many respects, the perfect candidate for effective early detection and intervention. The anatomy of a woman's lower genital tract allows direct access to the uterine cervix via speculum examination, tissue is readily sampled through a noninvasive technique with virtually no morbidity, and the natural history of squamous cell carcinoma of the cervix is well understood and predictable.

Analysis of cervical cytology using the method of Papanicolaou (Pap smear) began in 1928. Large-scale screening programs began approximately 20 years later and continue today. Although no prospective studies have been performed, most physicians believe that the Pap smear has contributed to the decrease in cervical cancer-related mortality observed since 1950. In addition, cervical cancer has not declined in any country in which screening has not been widely used.[21]

Epidemiological studies indicate that cervical cancer is a venereally transmitted disease. It is not seen in virgins, and the incidence is affected by the number of sexual partners and the age at onset of sexual activity. Many physicians divide women into three groups. The *low-risk* group includes women who have never had sexual intercourse or who have had a hysterectomy. Sexually active women who began sexual activity after the age of 20 but have had no more than two sexual partners are considered *medium risk*. The *high-risk* group includes women who began sexual activity before the age of 20 or who have had three or more partners.

Squamous cell carcinoma of the cervix begins as a unifocal lesion at the squamocolumnar junction of the transformation zone. The term *dysplasia* has been used to describe this well-differentiated lesion. With time, the lesion grows and becomes less well differentiated. The final stage of intraepithelial involvement has been termed carcinoma *in situ* or *cervical intraepithelial neoplasia*. Prospective studies have conclusively demonstrated that virtually all patients with carcinoma *in situ* will ultimately develop invasive carcinoma unless therapy is undertaken.[22]

The rate of progression from dysplasia to carcinoma *in situ* to invasive carcinoma is slow and relatively predictable. Studies have indicated that the mean transit time of mild dysplasia to carcinoma *in situ* is 5.8 years, of moderate dysplasia 3.1 years, and of severe dysplasia 1 year. The estimated transit time from the onset of carcinoma *in situ* to invasive carcinoma is approximately 10 years. Less than 5% of patients with carcinoma *in situ* will convert to invasive carcinoma in less than 3 years.[23]

The ease of obtaining cytology, the slow progression of disease, and the effectiveness of early therapy suggest that it should be possible to predict and prevent the development of invasive carcinoma in all women regularly tested. However, in routine medical practice the false negative rate is approximately 30% (sensitivity 70%). That is, one-third of all women tested who have cervical neoplasia will test negative on a single Pap smear. The results can be improved if the cytology is obtained by highly skilled personnel, especially if a sample is obtained from the os by aspiration or cotton-tipped applicator as well as the usual cervical scraping. Most physicians, however, use the cervical scraping technique alone.

There is currently no argument regarding the effectiveness of screening for cervical cancer. There is, however, controversy concerning the appropriate screening interval. The American College of Obstetricians and Gynecologists recommends an annual Pap smear for all sexually active women. The American Cancer Society recommends screening sexually active women at least every 3 years following two negative Pap smears performed 1 year apart.[24] They also recommend that women in the previously defined high-risk group should be screened more often, but they do not specify the optimum interval. Although promiscuity certainly increases the risk of developing cancer of the cervix, it does not alter the rate of progression from dysplasia to invasive carcinoma. A 3-year interval between Pap smears offers almost the same protection against the undetected development of invasive carcinoma as a yearly interval, but the recommendation for frequent screening attempts to compensate for test insensitivity as well as patient non-compliance regarding office visits.

8.2. Breast Cancer

Breast cancer will strike 1 of 11 women in the United States.[25] Early detection is critical because surgical excision of small cancers will afford cure in a significant proportion of patients. Once metastasis has occurred, there is no available curative therapy, although hormonal manipulations, chemotherapy, and radiotherapy may allow control of the disease for a period of time.

One of the most important risk factors for breast cancer is age.[26] The incidence increases dramatically from 0.3 cases per 100,000 at age 30 to 200 cases per 100,000 at age 50. Above age 50 the incidence continues to rise but at a slower rate.

Women who have a mother or sister with breast cancer have a two- to threefold increased risk of developing the disease. Age at first pregnancy also affects risks. There is a protective effect for women whose first birth occurs below the age of 20, while there is increased risk if the first pregnancy is delayed until after age 35. Increased dietary fat content also increases risk.[27]

Unfortunately, these factors affect relative risk so little that they do not allow us to accurately predict which women will or will not develop breast cancer. Therefore, an effective program for early detection of this common disease is important so that tumors may be identified early while they are amenable to curative therapy.

Three basic forms of breast-cancer detection are readily available and extensively evaluated: breast self-examination, physical examination by the physician, and mammography.

Self-examination has been advocated by the American Cancer Society for many years. Several studies have indicated that cancers found by self-examination are usually detected at an earlier stage compared to tumors found accidentally or on routine physical examination performed by the physician.[28–33] Sixty-five percent of women with breast cancer who never practiced self-examination or other screening procedures had advanced disease at the time of diagnosis. In contrast, women whose cancer was detected by self-examination had early-stage disease (stage 1 or 2) in 82% of cases. Those discovered by the physician on routine physical examination were stage 1 or 2 in 73% of cases, while mammography detected early-stage disease in 93%. Another study clearly demonstrated that self-examination leads to earlier detection. In over 300 cases of breast cancer, the average size of the tumor in women who practiced self-examination at monthly intervals was 2 cm. For those performing self-examination at less than monthly intervals the average tumor size was 2.5 cm, and for those never performing self-examination the average size was 3.6 cm. There was a corresponding difference in nodal status and stage in each group. It has been estimated that breast cancer mortality could be reduced by 20% by monthly self-examinations.

The effectiveness of mammography as a screening tool was first demonstrated in 1963 by the Health Insurance Plan of Greater New York.[21,31] This study involved 31,000 women who were annually examined by mammography and physical examination for 4 consecutive years. They were compared with a similar group of women who did not undergo screening. At the end of 14 years of observation, there was a 23% reduction in deaths due to breast cancer in the screened population. The decrease in mortality was most marked in women over the age of 50, while no significant benefit was seen in the 40- to 49-year age group.

As in any screening program, the benefits must be weighed against any potential morbidity as well as financial costs. Neither physical examination nor mammography is 100% specific, and many women will be subjected to biopsy for benign lesions. In addition, there is concern among some patients and physicians that radiation exposure during mammography will actually increase the risk of breast cancer. There is no question that significant radiation exposure has the potential for increasing the incidence. However, this effect is seen only when exposure occurs prior to age 40, and the risk is further minimized by newer equipment that requires less than 1 rad of exposure to the breast for each two-view mammogram.[34]

Current recommendations made by the American Cancer Society call for a baseline mammogram to be performed between ages 35 and 40, followed at 1- to 2-year intervals between ages 40 and 49, and yearly thereafter.

It must be kept in mind that mammography is an important addition to physical examination, but neither modality must be relied on without the other. In the previously mentioned Health Insurance Plan study, one-third of tumors were found by mammography but were not detected by physical examination while 40% were found by physical examination but were not detected by mammography.

The role of xerography and thermography remains unclear. Neither seems to offer significant benefits over conventional mammography. Xerography is a reasonable alternative to conventional mammography and is preferred by some radiologists. The efficacy of thermography is unclear and cannot be recommended as a routine screening procedure at this time.

8.3. Lung Cancer

The effectiveness of screening for lung cancer remains controversial. Two diagnostic tests have been used: periodic chest x-rays and sputum cytology.

The New York Lung Cancer Detection Program began screening high-risk men in 1974 by evaluating the ability of annual chest x-rays to detect lung cancer at an early stage (stage I), thus allowing curative resection.[35] From 1974 through 1978, 10,040 men over the age of 45 who smoked more than one package of cigarettes daily were entered into the study. In addition to annual chest x-rays, approximately half of the men were screened with sputum cytology at 4-month intervals. A total of 114 cases were diagnosed after the initial evaluation, and approximately 40% of these were stage I and underwent resection, with almost 90% of this group remaining alive at the time of publication of study results. Only 14% of stage II or III patients remained alive during the same interval.

In 1970, the Thoracic Division of the Mayo Clinic began a study to determine whether mortality from lung cancer in high-risk patients could be reduced by screening with even more frequent examinations.[36] The patients in the Mayo Lung Project (MLP) were men over 45 years of age who smoked more than one package of cigarettes per day. They were randomized into two groups. One was followed with chest x-rays and sputum cytology examinations at yearly intervals. The other group was examined every 4 months. The MLP demonstrated that more early-stage (stage I) squamous cell carcinomas were detected in the group studied every 4 months (48%) compared to the group studied yearly (21%). There was no significant differences in the clinical stage of small cell carcinoma between the two groups. (This reflects the tendency of small cell carcinoma to metastasize at a very early stage and, thus, to be detected at an advanced stage regardless of the screening interval.) The data were inconclusive regarding large cell carcinoma or adenocarcinoma. The most important statistic of all, overall mortality, was the same in the two groups, thus demonstrating no true benefit from screening at frequent (4-month) intervals. Sputum cytology examination did not prove to be as sensitive as x-ray examination for the detection of early-stage cancer. Approximately five stage I carcinomas were detected by chest x-ray for every one diagnosed by sputum cytology. When diagnosis by cytology was made, the tumor was invariably a squamous cell carcinoma involving a major bronchus.

Neither of these studies incorporated a control population to compare survival of unscreened individuals. Clinical observations indicate that most lung cancers that are diagnosed "accidentally" or after symptoms begin are advanced and long-term survival is poor. These studies suggest, but do not prove, that early-stage tumors may be detected as a result of periodic screening in a high-risk population. However, the apparent improvement in median survival as opposed to overall mortality may be deceptive because of "lead-time bias." Any study that allows earlier diagnosis in an asymptomatic phase will increase the time measured from diagnosis to death even though there may be no true change in the progression of disease and no true prolongation of life. If screening increases the percentage of genuine cures, then the study conclusions will be valid. However, this will not be known until many years have passed. At present there is no evidence that lung cancer screening prevents lung cancer deaths, and routine screening for lung cancer is therefore not recommended.

8.4. Colorectal Cancer

Recent statistics indicate that 1 of 20 Americans will ultimately develop carcinoma of the colon or rectum. The cases are equally divided between men and women, and the 5-year survival is only 40% owing to late diagnosis in most cases. Approximately 60% of the patients have metastases by the time they become symptomatic, and the magnitude of this problem begs for accurate and effective early-detection procedures. Fecal occult blood testing and proctosigmoidoscopy can aid in the detection of asymptomatic cancers prior to the development of metastases.

The use of guaiac-impregnated cards is a simple and aesthetically acceptable method of testing for occult blood in the stool. This test, however, suffers from a lack of sensitivity and specificity. Currently available cards require approximately 20 ml of blood loss per day to register positive, and this method of testing is positive in only 50–60% of patients with proven malignancy.[37] In addition, only approximately 45% of positive tests are associated with malignancy in asymptomatic persons above the age of 50. The predictive value will be further compromised if strict guidelines regarding pretest diet, medications, and so forth are not followed. Nevertheless, studies indicate that this screening method offers high patient compliance and can result in the detection of early-stage cancer, thus allowing surgical intervention and improving the opportunity for cure.[43]

Yearly examination of the stool from three consecutive bowel movements is recommended for persons over the age of 50. An abnormal test for stool occult blood should then be evaluated by colonoscopy. This is an expensive and sometimes unpleasant procedure which is not suitable for screening the general population but offers advantages over barium enema, such as removal of polyps, which, left in place, might result in cancerous lesions.[38]

Most colorectal cancers arise from preexisting polyps. Studies indicate that removal of all benign polyps and adenomatous lesions by proctosigmoidoscopy significantly reduces the incidence of cancer.[39] Early detection of cancer by periodic proctosigmoidoscopy, a procedure that may be performed by most primary-care physicians, improves the 5-year survival rate to almost 90%.[40,41] Flexible sigmoidoscopy offers the additional advantage of extending to 40–50 cm from the anal verge, resulting in even higher yields and better results.

The optimum frequency of proctosigmoidoscopy examination and the age at the time of first examination are controversial. Current recommendations from the American Cancer Society call for proctosigmoidoscopy to be performed at age 50 and repeated 1 year later to detect missed or interval lesions. Further examinations should be performed at approximately 3-year intervals, taking into account the slow growth of most polyps.

Carcinoembryonic antigen is elevated in many cases of colorectal carcinoma. However, this test is not useful for screening purposes because of expense and low sensitivity and specificity. It is generally used to follow the clinical course or response to therapy of established cases of unresectable or metastatic disease.[42]

8.5. Prostatic Cancer

Clinically detectable cancer of the prostate accounts for 16% of all known malignancies in men in the United States, being exceeded in frequency only by lung cancer.[34] It results in 10% of all male cancer-related deaths, making it the third leading cause of cancer-related death in this patient population. The incidence increases with advancing age, and the actual incidence is not known because an estimated 90% remain asymptomatic and are detected only at portmortem examination.

Prostatic carcinoma is certainly a significant health problem in this country, and early detection might spare some of the 21,000 men who die each year from this disease. Unfortunately, the only available method of early detection remains the digital rectal examination performed by a diligent and experienced examiner. Any area of abnormal induration or the presence of a firm nodule requires further evaluation by biopsy. Of course, the success of early detection by digital examination is dependent on the skill of the examiner.

Serum acid phosphatase is elevated in many cases of prostatic carcinoma. However, it is most commonly a sign of metastatic disease and has not proven useful in the early detection of localized tumors.

The lack of sensitive, specific, and readily reproducible screening tests and the extreme variability of growth characteristics of the disease make it impossible to recommend specific screening programs other than a yearly rectal examination for men over the age of 50.

8.6. Malignant Melanoma

Only 1 in 150 persons in the United States will develop a malignant melanoma during their lifetime. This is expected to increase to 1 in 100 by the year 2000. The prognosis for cure by surgical removal of early-stage disease is excellent, yet therapy of metastatic disease is dismal. The importance of early diagnosis in this disease cannot be overemphasized because of the marked disparity in prognosis between localized and disseminated disease.

Early detection requires the physician to have a thorough knowledge of the clinical characteristics of early malignant melanoma. In addition, the physician must know the features of skin lesions that may be confused with melanoma and the characteristics of precursor lesions such as dysplastic nevi. Excellent reviews of these clinical features, including color photographs, have recently appeared in the medical literature and are helpful in distinguishing malignant from nonmalignant skin lesions.[44–48]

No specific recommendations for the screening of the population at large are currently accepted. However, any patient who is at high risk, such as those with the dysplastic nevus syndrome or with a history of chronic and excessive sun exposure, should be examined carefully at yearly intervals and should be taught to do frequent self-examinations. Periodic photographs of the skin, especially in areas of numerous nevi, allow detection of a slowly, but progressively enlarging lesion which may otherwise be overlooked.

8.7. Endometrial Cancer

The incidence of endometrial cancer in the United States is rising and accounts for 40,000 new cases and over 3000 deaths per year. Risk factors include high socioeconomic status, low parity, early menarche, late menopause, obesity, and estrogen use. Since it is a significant health problem and most cases occur in patients older than 40, it seems appropriate to screen patients at that age and at periodic intervals thereafter.

Several methods of detection have been proposed, including endometrial aspiration, endometrial lavage, suction biopsy, and others.[49] Each of these methods has been shown to accurately diagnose endometrial cancer in 75–95% of cases in *symptomatic* women as measured against the standard of accuracy attained under anesthesia by dilatation and curettage. The sensitivity and specificity have not been determined in asymptomatic women, who, of course, would represent the population to be screened. Conventional Pap smears yield a positive diagnosis in less than 50% of known cases.

The most accurate methods of diagnosis yield histological rather than cytological specimens. They are, therefore, unpleasant, expensive, and involve some risk, which makes them unsuitable for screening the general population. The American Cancer Society currently recommends examination of endometrial tissue at menopause, but there are no current recommendations regarding resampling at periodic intervals.

9. EXCEPTIONS

The preceding discussion applies, for the most part, to the population at large. Special circumstances arise, however, when the patient has a recognized condition that predisposes him to the development of cancer to such a degree that malignancy is likely. Periodic testing is required and is more properly considered surveillance rather than screening. Examples include the development of colon carcinoma associated with ulcerative colitis, malignant melanoma in patients with the dysplastic nevus syndrome, and endometrial cancer in women exposed to diethylstilbestrol *in utero*. Such situations require that testing begin at an earlier age and be repeated at more frequent intervals compared to the general population.

10. ECONOMICS

The ability of a screening test to affect morbidity or mortality in a given population is a complex issue but can be measured objectively through epidemiological studies and carefully planned clinical trials. However, the financial impact on the individual or society is more difficult to determine. Nevertheless, it is becoming an increasingly important factor in determining the feasibility of cancer screening programs.

If a screening program has been found to be effective at detecting cancer early enough so that medical intervention can affect survival, then the most cost-efficient means of delivering the program must be determined while not allowing too many cases of cancer to be missed. Four major points must be considered: the optimal frequency of testing; screening selected groups only; controlling the cost of delivering screening tests; and the proper workup of patients with a positive test.[50] In addition, it must be determined whether the dollars would be more effectively spent on prevention rather than early detection.

At first glance it seems that economic considerations coldly sacrifice lives for the saving of a few dollars. However, it must be remembered that all physicians make these decisions every day, albeit usually on an intuitive rather than a scientific basis. For example, there is no dispute that one should not recommend yearly sigmoidoscopic examinations of apparently healthy 25-year-old men to screen for colon cancer. Certainly, colon cancer is known to occur in this population, but the incidence is so low and the cost and discomfort from sigmoidoscopy are significant enough that this recommendation is clearly not justified. It is not a new activity for physicians to consider various health programs to select those that deliver the greatest net benefit. Every physician does this to some extent every day.

The actual cost of testing is not as obvious as it seems. Most patients are more aware of this than physicians. For example, the charge for an annual Pap smear may be only a few dollars, but the patient is well aware of the additional expense of transportation to the physician's office, parking, the charge for the office visit, and, in many cases, lost earnings from a missed day of work. It has been estimated that the actual cost to the patient of a Pap smear averages $100. This expense will, in many cases, affect patient compliance with physician recommendations.

The problem of cost is compounded when the testing procedure has low specificity. In the case of stool guaiac testing, most positive results are not due to malignancy, yet the finding of a positive result will launch a workup costing hundreds or even thousands of dollars.

If we are to get the most ''mileage'' out of every dollar spent on screening, thus allowing the greatest good for the greatest number, then continued efforts must be made to define whether or not a test is effective at improving the ''cure'' rate of cancer and, if so, what the most cost-effective screening interval is for a given population. In virtually every case, the latter consideration remains controversial.

REFERENCES

1. Ries, L. G., Pollock, E. S., Young, J. L., Jr.: Cancer patient survival: Surveillance, Epidemiology and End Results: Incidence and Mortality Data, 1973–1977. *JNCI* **70**:693–707, 1983.

2. Doll, R., and Peto, R.: The causes of cancer. *J. Natl. Cancer Inst.* **66:**1197–1312, 1981.
3. Boutwell, R. K.: Biochemical mechanism of tumor promotion. *Carcinogenesis* **2:**49–59, 1978.
4. Dull, R. (ed.): *Cancer Incidence in Five Continents.* Vol. IV. Springer-Verlag, 1982.
5. Buell, P.: Changing incidence in breast cancer in Japanese–American women. *J. Natl. Cancer Inst.* **51:**1473–1479, 1973.
6. Haenszel, W., and Kurihara, M.: Studies of Japanese migrants: Mortality from cancer and other diseases among Japanese in the United States. *J. Natl. Cancer Inst.* **40:**43–68, 1968.
7. Carroll, K. K., and Khor, H. T.: Dietary fat in relation to tumorigenesis. *Prog. Biochem. Pharmacol.* **10:**308–353, 1975.
8. Nicholson, W. J.: Cancer following occupational exposure to asbestos and vinyl chloride. *Cancer* **39:**1792, 1977.
9. Brewster, L., and Jacobson, M. F.: *The Changing American Diet.* Center for Science in the Public Interest, Washington, DC, 1978.
10. Hirayama, T.: Epidemiology of breast cancer with special reference to the role of diet. *Prev. Med.* **7:**178–195, 1978.
11. De Waard, E.: Breast cancer incidence and nutritional status with particular reference to body weight and height. *Cancer Res.* **35:**3351–3356, 1975.
12. Carroll, K. K., and Khor, H. T.: Effects of level and type of dietary fat on incidence of mammarv tumors induced in female Sprague–Dawley rats by 7,12 dimethyl-benz (a) anthracence. *Lipids* **6:**415–420, 1971.
13. Carroll, K. K., and Hopkins, G. J.: Dietary polyunsaturated fat versus saturated fat in relation to mammary carcinogenesis. *Lipids* **14:**155–158, 1978.
14. Shin, R. P. C., Lima, G., and Iwasiow, B.: Prolactin inducible proteins in human breast cancer cells. 7th Int. Cong. of Endocrine, 1984, p. 983.
15. Hill, P., and Wynder, E. L.: Diet and prolactin release. *Lancet* **2:**806–807, 1976.
16. Hill, D. L., and Grubbs, C. J.: Retinoids as chemopreventive and anticancer agents in intact animals. *Anticancer Res.* **2:**111–124, 1982.
17. Sporn, M. B., and Newton, D. L.: Chemoprevention of cancer with retinoids. *Fed. Proc. Fed. Am. Soc. Exp. Bio.* **38:**2528–2534, 1979.
18. Russell, M. A. H., Wilson, C., and Taylor, C., *et al.:* Effect of general practitioners' advice against smoking. *Br. Med. J.* **2:**231–235, 1979.
19. Schapira, D. V., and Pozo, C.: Physicians, nurses, and medical students knowledge of cancer prevention and nutrition. *Journal of Cancer Education* **1:**201, 1986.
20. Cancer statistics, 1985. *Ca* **36:**16–24, 1986.
21. Richart, R. M., and Barron, B. A.: Screening strategies for cervical cancer and cervical intraepithelial neoplasia. *Cancer* **47:**1176–1181, 1981.
22. Stern, E., and Neely, P. M.: Dysplasia of the uterine cervix: Incidence of regression, recurrence and cancer. *Cancer* **17:**508, 1964.
23. Barron, B. A., and Richart, R. M.: Statistical model of the natural history of cervical carcinoma. *J. Natl. Cancer Inst.* **45:**1025–1030, 1979.
24. American Cancer Society recommendations for the early detection of cancer in asymptomatic people. *Ca* **35:**199, 1985.
25. Carlile, T.: Breast cancer detection. *Cancer* **47:**1164–1169, 1981.
26. Nasca, P. C., Baptiste, M. S., and Greenwald, P.: *Issues in Cancer Screening. Cancer Prevention in Clinical Medicine.* Raven Press, New York, 1983.
27. Miller, A. B.: Breast cancer. *Cancer* **47:**1109–1113, 1981.
28. Foster, R. S., and Costanza, M. C.: Breast self-examination practices and breast cancer survival. *Cancer* **53:**999–1005, 1984.
29. Greenwald, P., Lawrence, C., Horton, J., *et al.:* Effect of breast self examination and routine physical examinations on breast cancer mortality. *N. Engl. J. Med.* **199:**271–273, 1978.
30. Feldman, J., Carter, A., Nicastri, A., *et al.:* Breast self examination: Relationship to stage of breast cancer at diagnosis. *Cancer* **47:**2740–2745, 1981.
31. Shapiro, S., Strax, P., and Venet, L.: Periodic breast cancer screening, the first two years of screening. *Arch. Environ. Health* **15:**547–553, 1967.
32. Shapiro, S.: Evidence on screening for breast cancer from a randomized trial. *Cancer* **39:**2772–2782, 1977.
33. Wertheimer, M. D., Costanza, M. E., Dodson, T. F., *et al.:* Increasing the effort toward breast cancer detection. *JAMA* **255:**1311–1315, 1986.

34. DeVita, V. T., Hellman, S., and Rosenberg, S. A. (eds.): *Cancer—Principles and Practice of Oncology*. Lippincott, Philadelphia, 1985, pp. 1130–1131.
35. Melamed, M. R., Flehinger, B. U., Zaman, M. B., *et al.*: Detection of true pathologic stage I lung cancer in a screening program and the effect on survival. *Cancer* **47**:1182–1187, 1981.
36. Taylor, W. F., Fontana, R. S., Uhlenhopp, M. A. *et al.*: Some results of screening for early lung cancer. *Cancer* **47**:1114–1120, 1981.
37. Simon, J. B.: Occult blood screening for colorectal carcinoma: A critical review. *Gastroenterology* **88**:820–837, 1985.
38. Gilbertsen, V. A., and Nelms, J. M.: The prevention of invasive cancer of the rectum. *Cancer* **41**:1137–1139, 1978.
39. Gilbertsen, V. A.: Proctosigmoidoscopy and polypectomy in reducing the incidence of rectal cancer. *Cancer* **34**:936–939, 1974.
40. Bolt, R. J.: Sigmoidoscopy in detection and diagnosis in the asymptomatic individual. *Cancer* **28**:230–232, 1971.
41. Winawer, S. J.: Detection and diagnosis of colorectal cancer. *Cancer* **51**:2519–2524, 1983.
42. Berlin, N. I.: Tumor markers in cancer prevention and detection. *Cancer* **47**:1151–1153, 1981.
43. Tests for occult blood. *Med. Lett.* **28**(705):5–6, 1986.
44. Greene, M. H., Clark, W. H., Tucker, M. A., *et al.*: Acquired precursors of cutaneous malignant melanoma. *N. Engl. J. Med.* **312**:91–97, 1985.
45. Fitzpatrick, T. B., Rhodes, A. R., and Sober, A. J.: Prevention of melanoma by recognition of its precursors. *N. Engl. J. Med.* **312**:115–116, 1985.
46. Arndt, K. A.: Precursors to malignant melanoma: Congenital and dysplastic nevi. *JAMA* **251**:1882–1883, 1984.
47. Friedman, R. J.: Early detection of malignant melanoma: The role of the physician examination and self examination of the skin. *Ca* **35**:130–151, 1985.
48. Consensus conference on precursors to malignant melanoma. *J. Dermatol. Surg. Oncol.* **11**:537–542, 1985.
49. Gusberg, S. B., and Milano, C.: Detection of endometrial cancer and its precursors. *Cancer* **47**:1173–1175, 1981.
50. Eddy, D. M.: The economics of cancer prevention and detection: Getting more for less. *Cancer* **47**:1200–1209, 1981.

17

Stroke

Joseph R. Berger and Roger E. Kelley

1. STROKE EPIDEMIOLOGY

Despite recent declines in the incidence of stroke, it still remains the third leading cause of death in the United States, ranking only behind heart disease and cancer. Stroke occurs in approximately 500,000 persons annually in the United States. Approximately 80% of the individuals experiencing a stroke will survive the initial ictus, though the prognosis is intimately related to the nature of the stroke (Table I).[1] The estimated prevalence of stroke survivors in the United States is two million. Of those surviving the ictus, 10% will have no disability; 40% will have a mild disability resulting in difficulties with ambulation, employment, and daily activities; 40% will have a marked disability and need special care; and 10% will require institutionalization.[2] Stroke victims constitute 16% of the patients in skilled-care nursing-home beds. The direct and indirect cost of stroke in the United States is estimated at $7 billion per year.

Nowhere in medicine is the expression ''an ounce of prevention is worth a pound of cure'' more appropriate than in the management of stroke and the stroke-prone patient. Despite extensive efforts to return vitality to ischemic brain tissue, the results have been far from rewarding. Therefore, a rational approach to stroke management must include early consideration and aggressive preventive treatment of the factors that increase stroke susceptibility.

1.1. Stroke Definition and Classification

The term *stroke* derives from a Middle English word meaning ''blow'' or ''sudden attack.'' It has been generically applied to cerebrovascular disease, often resulting in confusion regarding the specific etiology of a cerebrovascular insult. A logical approach to the prevention and management of stroke requires an adequate understanding of the pathogenesis of these disorders. A number of classifications have been devised to appropriately categorize stroke.[3] In a widely adopted scheme developed by the Harvard Stroke Registry, strokes are divided into thrombotic infarctions, embolic infarctions, lacunar infarctions, intraparenchymal hemorrhages, and subarachnoid hemorrhages.[4] Other clas-

Joseph R. Berger • Departments of Neurology and Internal Medicine, University of Miami School of Medicine, Miami, Florida 33101. *Roger E. Kelley* • Department of Neurology, University of Miami School of Medicine, Miami, Florida 33101.

Table I. Stroke Classification—Frequency and Mortality Rates[a]

	Frequency[b]	Mortality[c]
Atherosclerotic stroke	32%	15%
Lacunar infarction	18%	—
Embolic infarction	32%	16%
Hypertensive hemorrhage	11%	80%
Subarachnoid hemorrhage	7%	50%

[a]From Ref. 91.
[b]Frequency refers to the percentage of the total number of strokes.
[c]Mortality is based on the death rate in the first 30 days after the ictus.

sifications, such as that used in the Framingham study, combine thrombotic and lacunar strokes into a single group, atherothrombotic brain infarction, and list stroke from other causes and transient ischemic attack (TIA) as separate categories.[5] The latter classification represents results of a prospective study over 26 years. Undoubtedly, the routine adoption of computed tomographic (CT) imaging of the brain will improve diagnostic precision. The percentage of total numbers of strokes for each of the classes can be found in Table I.

Atherothrombotic cerebrovascular disease is typically characterized by a more variable evolution than is embolism or hemorrhage. TIAs precede the onset of thrombotic stroke in approximately 50% of cases.[6] Stroke occurs frequently during sleep—according to one major neurological textbook, in as many as 60% of cases. The neurological deficit may evolve over several hours, present in a "stuttering" fashion, or partially remit only to be completed some hours later. Headache may occur concomitantly with the thrombotic stroke in a minority of patients. Old age, hypertension, diabetes mellitus, and hyperlipidemia are risk factors for thrombotic disease.

In the Harvard Stroke Registry, cerebral embolism occurred as often as thrombotic stroke. It is characterized by the sudden appearance of the neurological deficit. Its onset has sometimes been referred to as "occurring as a bolt out of the blue." Embolic strokes tend to occur not only during the waking hours, but during periods of activity. They are occasionally preceded by transient neurological dysfunction, but not as often as occurs with thrombotic stroke. Embolic strokes are frequently seen in association with heart disease.[7,8]

Lacunar infarcts range in size from 0.5 mm to 15 mm. They have a predilection to occur in certain regions of the brain, such as the internal capsule, the thalamus, the frontal lobes, and the pons. They are typically multiple when observed at autopsy, but because of their small size may not be visualized by computed tomography of the brain. Their location dictates the nature of the neurological deficit observed. Pure motor hemiplegia is the most frequently recognized disorder resulting from a lacunar infarction. Other clinical pictures include pure hemisensory deficit, dysarthria and clumsy hand, contralateral hemiplegia and hemiataxia, and pseudobulbar palsy.[9] Generally, lacunar infarcts are seen in hypertensive individuals, but they are also seen in diabetics and otherwise normal individuals. These small infarcts are believed to arise as a result of disease of small penetrating vessels that often take their origin at right angles to large vessels.

Intraparenchymal hemorrhages generally occur in the setting of hypertension. They have a predilection for certain areas and therefore give rise to particular clinical pictures. The areas of predilection, their approximate frequency of occurrence, and the associated salient clinical features are noted in Table II. Among the other etiologies of intraparenchymal hemorrhage are ruptured arteriovenous malformations, hemorrhage into tumors, vasculitis, trauma, amyloid angiopathy, and coagulopathies. Intraparenchymal hemorrhage typically is rather sudden in onset, with a steady, progressive quality. It is characteristically accompanied by headache, and frequently consciousness is altered early in the course of the stroke owing to mass effect and resultant brain herniation.

Subarachnoid hemorrhage is characterized by the sudden appearance of an intense headache that is generally accompanied by meningismus as evidenced by nuchal rigidity. On rare occasions, it may be heralded by the onset of severe neck or back pain in the absence of headache. The most common nontraumatic etiology of subarachnoid bleeding is the rupture of an intracranial berry aneurysm. It accounts for 50–70% of spontaneous subarachnoid hemorrhage. Fifteen to twenty percent are due to secondary leakage of blood into the subarachnoid space from a primary intracerebral hemorrhage due to hypertensive or atherosclerotic vascular disease, and 6–12% represent rupture of an arteriovenous malformation.[10]

Berry aneurysms have a propensity to occur at various sites of the circle of Willis, and the resultant clinical picture will occasionally reflect the site of the lesion. The mortality of a subarachnoid hemorrhage is on the order of 45% in the first 30 days.[10] The

Table II. Location and Clinical Features of Intraparenchymal Hypertensive Hemorrhages[a]

Location	Finding
Putamen	1. Gradual weakening of contralateral arm and leg 2. Eyes deviate away from paretic side 3. Aphasia if in dominant hemisphere
Thalamus	1. Contralateral hemiparesis 2. Contralateral sensory deficit often exceeding degree of weakness 3. Forced downward eye deviation 4. Aphasia if in dominant hemisphere
Pons	1. Deep coma 2. Decerebrate rigidity 3. Small, reactive pupils 4. Abnormal reflex eye movements
Cerebellum	1. Vertigo 2. Paresis of conjugate gaze to the side of hemorrhage 3. Ipsilateral limb ataxia

[a]From Ref. 91.

two greatest complications resulting from a subarachnoid hemorrhage are rebleeding and vasospasm. Thirty percent of patients will have a recurrent hemorrhage in the first month, and this hemorrhage is particularly likely to recur between the fifth and ninth days.[11] Since the introduction of antifibrinolytic therapy, vasospasm is believed to be more often responsible for clinical deterioration in these patients than is recurrent hemorrhage.

1.2. Stroke Risk Factors

Arteriosclerosis is indisputably the most common cause of cerebrovascular disease. In that context, the risk factors for arteriosclerosis are also the risk factors that predispose one to cerebrovascular disease. A corollary to this axiom is the frequency with which coronary artery disease is found in patients with cerebrovascular disease, and vice versa. Coronary artery disease typically becomes symptomatic in men between the ages of 45 and 55, while symptoms of cerebrovascular disease do not occur until the succeeding decade.[12] Kannel *et al.* noted that the most reliable indicator of stroke proneness was evidence of cardiovascular disease manifested by electrocardiographic changes, angina pectoris, previous myocardial infarction, congestive heart failure, radiographic evidence of ventricular enlargement suggesting hypertension, and myocardial aneurysm.[13]

1.2.1. Aging

Appropriate management of the risk factors for arteriosclerosis can be expected to decrease the incidence of stroke. Unfortunately, some risk factors for arteriosclerosis, including age, male sex, and certain genetic traits, are irreversible. Aging alone appears to be the greatest risk for cerebrovascular disease. The prevalence of stroke rises rapidly after age 35 years and reaches 6% in persons 75 years and older.[14] Five percent of individuals aged 85 or older have strokes per year.[14] When the incidence of stroke is plotted logarithmically against age, the result is a straight line, with the incidence of stroke virtually doubling for every 5 years of age.[14]

1.2.2. Hypertension

There is a dramatic association of hypertension and stroke. Epidemiological surveys have demonstrated a decrease in stroke rate over the past 20 years that has been largely attributed to adequate means of hypertension control in the populations studied. The risk of stroke is directly proportional to the level of elevation of blood pressure.[15] In men with definite hypertension (blood pressure > 160/95 mm Hg) the relative risk for stroke is 4.0 relative to normotensives (blood pressure < 140/90 mm Hg), whereas in women the relative risk is 4.4.[16] Patients with borderline hypertension have approximately double the stroke risk compared to individuals with normal pressure. All measures of blood pressure, namely, pulse pressure, mean arterial pressure, systolic pressure, and diastolic pressure, are associated with increased stroke risk.[16] Systolic hypertension, even in isolation, is a strong predictor of stroke.[17] By promoting both arteriolosclerosis (hyaline and degenerative changes affecting the intima and media of small arterioles) and atherosclerosis (changes in large vessels), hypertension not only sets the stage for ischemic cerebral disease in the forms of thrombotic and lacunar infarction, but also predisposes to hypertensive hemorrhage. The latter was responsible for a much greater number of strokes in the past compared to the 11% current rate; however, the diagnosis was much less reliable in the pre-computed tomography era.[18]

1.2.3. Cardiac Disease

Patients with cardiac disease, whether clinically apparent or inapparent, have more than double the risk of stroke.[16] Coronary artery disease, congestive heart failure, left ventricular hypertrophy, and arrhythmias, particularly atrial fibrillation, are associated with risk of stroke. Furthermore, many stroke patients succumb to atherosclerotic cardiovascular disease. In light of the frequency of cardiac factors and the complexity of their management, a detailed discussion of this subject is included in this chapter (vide infra).

1.2.4. Cigarette Smoking

Though at one time cigarette smoking was considered to be a controversial risk factor for stroke, recent epidemiological studies from the Honolulu Heart Program have clearly established a relationship in men.[19] Compared to nonsmokers, cigarette smokers had two to three times the risk of thromboembolic or hemorrhagic stroke when controlled for other risk factors. Smoking cessation reduced the risk of stroke by more than half in this group. Cigarette smoking increases the risk of stroke by accelerating arteriosclerosis, increasing blood viscosity, and increasing platelet aggregability. It may also contribute to the ischemic insult as a result of associated hypoxemia.

1.2.5. Diabetes and Hyperlipidemia

Diabetes mellitus contributes independently to stroke risk, particularly ischemic brain disease, even after adjusting for its association with hypertension.[16] Casual blood sugars > 160 mg/dl are associated with a twofold increase in stroke.[16] With respect to hyperlipidemia, the risk of stroke correlates with total serum cholesterol. This association decreases after age 55.[20] The relationship of stroke risk to the various fractions of cholesterol is less well defined than with coronary artery disease, where high-density-lipoprotein cholesterol appears to exert a protective effect.[16] A strong significant negative association between levels of low-density-lipoprotein cholesterol and stroke in women was demonstrated in the Framingham study.[17] No significant protective effect of high-density-lipoprotein cholesterol or relationship to triglyceride was established in that study.[17]

1.2.6. Oral Contraceptives

Retrospective studies have detected a greater than fourfold increase in stroke in oral-contraceptive users compared to nonusers.[21] However, this finding remains controversial as most studies fail to reveal a substantial difference in incidence between healthy young men and women.[22,23] Data from Great Britain suggest a significant increased risk of fatal stroke from subarachnoid hemorrhage rather than from thromboembolism in oral-contraceptive users, particularly in smokers over the age of 35 years.[24]

1.2.7. Other Risk Factors

An elevated hematocrit appears to increase the risk of stroke. This factor may limit cerebral blood flow through stenotic arteries[25] or small penetrating vessels.[26] The association of elevated blood pressure and cigarette smoking with higher hematocrits may account to some degree for the increased risk. Similarly, obesity is related to systolic hypertension and impaired glucose tolerance, and the latter factors may be largely responsible for the association of obesity with stroke. Alcohol abuse has also been suggested as a risk factor for stroke.[16] Finally, several genetic diseases predispose to ischemic cerebrovascular disease. They include homocystinuria, Fabry's disease, and sickle cell anemia.

2. ASYMPTOMATIC CAROTID BRUITS

An asymptomatic carotid bruit is noted in up to 5% of the adult population in the United States.[27] It has generally been believed to be a risk factor for stroke. The Framingham study followed 245 patients with an asymptomatic carotid bruit over a 12-year period.[28] Sixteen strokes occurred in that time. Only five of these strokes were thromboembolic in nature and occurred on the side appropriate to the bruit. A high rate of symptomatic atherosclerotic cardiovascular disease was detected in this group of patients with a carotid bruit. A recent study by Chambers and Norris[29] prospectively followed 500 asymptomatic patients with cervical bruits for up to 4 years. An excess of cardiovascular events relative to cerebral ischemic events was also demonstrated in this group. The overall incidence of stroke at 1 year was 1.7%, and this risk was significantly greater in patients with severe carotid artery stenosis (>75%), progressing carotid artery stenosis, and coexistent heart disease.[29] The majority of patients who went on to have stroke had preceding TIAs. Because of the high risk of surgery in this condition compared to nonintervention, medical management in the context of properly conducted drug trials was recommended.[29]

In patients with asymptomatic carotid bruits undergoing surgical procedures, the incidence of postoperative stroke is not significantly different compared to an age-and-sex-matched control population of surgical patients.[30] The issue of the carotid bruit in the patient who is about to undergo cardiac surgery was not addressed in that article but has been the subject of several others.[31–34] The data regarding this matter are contradictory at present. Some cardiovascular surgeons feel that prophylactic carotid endarterectomy prior to cardiac surgery is necessary for patients with asymptomatic carotid disease.

3. TRANSIENT ISCHEMIC ATTACKS

TIAs are defined as focal neurological deficits resulting from ischemia that lasts no more than 24 hr. The vast majority of TIAs last no more than 2–15 min.[6] Approximately one-third of individuals with TIAs will subsequently develop a stroke within 5 years of follow-up.[35] These strokes most often occur in the first three months after the initial TIA.[35] Roughly one-half of strokes occur within 3 months of the TIA onset and two-thirds within 6 months.[16] The strokes are typically thromboembolic in nature. Ten percent of all strokes are preceded by TIAs,[4] with approximately 50% of thrombotic strokes preceded by TIAs.

The appropriate management of a TIA is keenly dependent on the part of the cerebral circulation that is affected (Table III). About 50% of TIAs occur in the posterior circulation (vertebrobasilar) and a similar number occur in the anterior circulation (carotid). The nature of the symptomatology allows a distinction between these two possibilities, though it is occasionally not entirely certain.

Probably no more than 15% of patients with TIAs are surgical candidates. Very few individuals with posterior circulation events are surgical candidates. The rare exceptions are the individuals with symptomatic subclavian artery obstruction proximal to the origin of the vertebral artery. Therefore, approximately 50% of patients with TIAs (i.e., those with posterior circulation events) are eliminated from surgical consideration immediately. The risk of arteriography and subsequent carotid endarterectomy needs to be carefully considered for the individual patient before surgical intervention is undertaken. There are no data from randomized, prospectively conducted studies to assist the physician in these difficult recommendations. A thorough discussion of the literature is beyond the scope of this chapter, but detailed review articles are available.[36,37]

The issue of surgery notwithstanding, the appropriate management of TIAs is a highly controversial matter and one that has become very individualized. Diagnostic measures in the management of TIAs are presented in Table IV. Anticoagulation with heparin acutely after the first TIA has been demonstrated to be of benefit in reducing the risk of recurrent TIAs and probably also the risk of subsequent stroke.[38] Sandok *et al.* recommend anticoagulation for patients who are not surgical candidates and who present

Table III. Symptoms and Signs Associated with Transient Ischemic Attacks[a]

Anterior circulation
1. Amaurosis fugax (absolutely diagnostic of anterior circulation event)
2. Hemiparesis or hemiplegia
3. Hemisensory loss
4. Hemianopsia
5. Aphasia
Posterior circulation[b]
1. Cortical blindness
2. Memory impairment
3. Diplopia
4. Vertigo
5. Dysarthria and dysphagia
6. Crossed motor deficits (ipsilateral face and contralateral body)
7. Crossed sensory deficits (ipsilateral face and contralateral body)
8. Ataxia

[a]From Ref. 91.

[b]With the exception of amaurosis fugax, the deficits observed with anterior-circulation TIAs may also occur with those in the posterior circulation. However, they are typically associated with other clinical features that suggest brain stem or cerebellar dysfunction.

Table IV. Relationship of Onset of Acute Myocardial Infarction and the Development of Cerebral Emboli[a]

Time	Emboli (%)
First week	11
Second week	33
Third week	16
Fourth week	24
Second month	6
Third month	8

[a]From Ref. 60.

within 2 months of their first TIA. Heparin is used initially followed by Coumadin for a period of 3 months.[38] In individuals presenting more than 2 months after their first TIA, antiplatelet therapy is recommended. The Canadian Cooperative Study clearly demonstrated that aspirin therapy was effective in reducing the risk of stroke and death in men with TIAs.[39] Unfortunately, in this and most other studies, aspirin proved ineffective in women. A combination of aspirin and dipyrimadole may be of benefit in these situations, but is as yet of unproven value. No data establish any superiority of anticoagulation therapy over antiplatelet therapy in the management of TIAs in men.

4. CARDIAC DISEASE AND STROKE

4.1. Atrial Fibrillation

Atrial fibrillation is associated with a predisposition to cerebral embolus, and the risk is directly related to the duration of the atrial fibrillation. The risk, based on data from the Framingham study,[40] is increased five- to sixfold for nonvalvular atrial fibrillation and is increased 17-fold when there is coexistent rheumatic heart disease. In addition, the risk for recurrent cerebral embolus appears to be greatest around the time of the initial event. According to one study,[41] the recurrence rate was 20% within 11 days of the initial cerebral embolus. This study stressed the urgency for initiating prophylactic therapy for preventing embolus as soon as possible.

There are several reasons for atrial fibrillation to be associated with an increased risk of cerebral embolus. First, it is often associated with rheumatic heart disease, a disorder that by itself increases the risk of both septic and nonseptic embolus. Furthermore, thrombus formation is commonly observed within the atrial appendage of the heart in patients with nonvalvular atrial fibrillation.[42] The detection of a source of cerebral embolus in an ischemic stroke patient remains one of the most reliable criteria for distinguishing embolic from thrombotic stroke.[43] On the other hand, it has been observed that patients with atrial fibrillation usually have risk factors for thrombotic stroke as well, and not all stroke patients with atrial fibrillation have cerebral embolus.[44]

Although atrial fibrillation is a significant marker for stroke risk and its importance directly correlates with increasing age,[45] considerable controversy still exists about proper prophylactic therapy for patients with atrial fibrillation. Most clinicians feel that the risk of stroke in patients with nonvalvular atrial fibrillation does not justify the risk of long-term anticoagulant therapy unless the patient has suffered symptoms of cerebral ischemia. On the other hand, it is certainly preferable to prevent a major stroke than to use a stroke as a post facto criterion for identifying someone who might have benefitted from preventive therapy. To further cloud the issue, there is no general agreement about the efficacy of anticoagulant therapy in preventing embolic stroke in patients with nonvalvular atrial fibrillation.[46] We and others[47] recommend the use of prophylactic anticoagulant therapy for patients experiencing focal neurological deficits attributable to emboli. However, in patients with acute embolic stroke, the immediate use of anticoagulant therapy risks converting an initially ischemic event into a hemorrhagic stroke.[48] The patient's age, presence of hypertension, size of the infarct, and level of compliance are all factors that must be taken into account when making a decision about the use of anticoagulant therapy.[49] A CT brain scan is mandatory in such circumstances to guarantee that there is no evidence of hemorrhage, which would contraindicate the use of anticoagulants.

4.2. Mitral Valve Prolapse

There continues to be considerable controversy about what role, if any, mitral valve prolapse plays in promoting cerebral ischemia. In one study 40% of patients with stroke under age 45 had mitral valve prolapse.[50] On the other hand, a number of stroke series, including those reporting on young patients,[51] have found no increase in the frequency of mitral valve prolapse.

There are a number of theoretical reasons to expect a higher frequency of cerebral ischemia in patients with mitral valve prolapse. Mitral valve prolapse may serve as a nidus for platelet–fibrin aggregation. Preliminary data suggest that this cardiac abnormality is associated with platelet hyperaggregability.[52] It is also associated with an increased risk of infective endocarditis,[53] which would be expected to result in an increased risk of septic cerebral embolus. Patients with mitral valve prolapse also have a predisposition to suffer atypical chest pain and sometimes end up undergoing coronarv angiography, which can be complicated by stroke.[54] In addition, there is a relatively high frequency of mitral valve prolapse in severe coronary artery disease.[55] Atrial fibrillation can be seen in association with mitral valve prolapse,[56] and there can be thrombus formation associated with prolapse of the mitral valve.[57] Mitral valve prolapse has been reported to occur in association with migraine,[58] and migraine can mimic TIA or there can actually be migrainous infarction.[59] Thus, it is not surprising that one population-based study reported that the prevalence rate for stroke in persons with mitral valve prolapse was four times higher than that for the non-mitral valve prolapse population.[60]

Up to 5% of stroke and TIA patients from large series have mitral valve prolapse.[61,62] This is actually lower than the 5–7% prevalence of mitral valve prolapse in the general population.[63,64] The discrepancy in the prevalence of mitral valve prolapse in different stroke series may be due to the variability in the ability to detect mitral valve prolapse. All series use echocardiography to detect mitral valve prolapse. Echocardiography may be normal in 10–20% of patients with proven mitral valve prolapse. In addition, interobserver concordance in diagnosing mitral valve prolapse by echocardiography varied between 52 and 80% in one series in which three board-certified cardiologists independently interpreted studies performed on patients with presumed mitral valve prolapse.[65]

It is generally acknowledged that mitral valve prolapse is an etiological factor of cerebral embolus. However, whether for young or old stroke patients, it should not be assumed that mitral valve prolapse is the primary mechanism of embolization until other possibilities are excluded. Associated factors such as coexistent aortic valve prolapse[66] or redundant mitral valves[67] may identify patients with mitral valve prolapse who are particularly susceptible to stroke.

For patients who do suffer cerebral ischemia in association with mitral valve prolapse, antiplatelet therapy is generally considered to be the therapy of choice.[68] If symptoms persist on antiplatelet therapy, then anticoagulant therapy may be necessary.

4.3. Rheumatic Heart Disease

Systemic embolism is a complication of rheumatic heart disease in 9–49% (average 15–20%) of patients.[69,70] Approximately 60% of these events are cerebral. It appears that mitral stenosis is the most common valvular abnormality associated with embolus, but embolic events have been reported in association with mitral insufficiency and aortic valve disease. There is a 17-fold increased risk of stroke when rheumatic heart disease coexists with atrial fibrillation.[40] It was initially reported that valvotomy was protective against embolism,[71] but later studies have not supported this view.[72] Effective anticoagulation appears to be the therapy of choice and has been reported to reduce the risk of recurrent embolization in rheumatic heart disease from 50% to 5–25%.[73]

4.4. Myocardial Infarction

Acute myocardial infarction is associated with cerebral embolus in 1.7–2.4% of patients.[73,74] This is presumably related to ventricular mural thrombus formation secondary to the infarct. Mural thrombus formation is most common when the infarct is large, involves the septum, and is associated with ventricular aneurysm formation and/or congestive heart failure.[70] According to one study,[75] approximately two-thirds of patients with cerebral emboli that complicated acute myocardial infarction developed symptoms within the first 3 weeks (Table IV).

Among patients with acute myocardial infarction, those with transmural anterior wall infarcts and early echocardiographic demonstration of apical dyskinesia or mural wall thrombus formation are at particularly high risk for cerebral embolus. By these criteria, approximately one-third of high-risk patients can be identified.[76] Of note, only 5–6% of patients with thrombi within ventricular aneurysm formation will suffer embolus.[77]

Anticoagulation appears to be beneficial for preventing cerebral embolus secondary to acute myocardial infarction, but because of its risks, it is not routinely recommended. It might be of value for short-term use, during the greatest risk of embolus, in high-risk patients. According to the Sixty Plus Reinfarction Study published in 1982,[78] anticoagulation reduced the number of intracranial events by 20% between the treated and untreated groups, but 20% of treated versus 2% of untreated patients developed intracranial hemorrhage with long-term anticoagulation.

4.5. Prosthetic Heart Valves

The introduction of prosthetic heart valves was associated with a significant risk of embolic complications, with prosthetic mitral valves posing greater risk than aortic valves. The early mitral ball valve, for example, was associated with an embolic rate of 17 per 100 patient-years despite the use of anticoagulation.[79] This rate has been significantly reduced with the use of newer, better-designed valves. The risk of embolus is directly related to the position of the valve, type of valve, use of anticoagulation, coexistent atrial fibrillation, left atrial enlargement, thrombus formation, and cardiomegaly.[76] For modern prosthetic aortic valves, in anticoagulated patients, the embolic risk has been estimated to be 4 per 100 patient-years for aortic valves.[80] There have been unsuccessful attempts to substitute antiplatelet therapy for anticoagulant therapy for prophylaxis against embolus in these settings.[76]

4.6. Cardiomyopathy

A number of cardiomyopathies of nonischemic origin can be associated with cerebral embolus. These entities promote heart chamber enlargement, which fosters thrombus formation. Cardiomyopathy should always be considered in young adults with stroke. Etiologies include viral infections, peripartum factors, amyloidosis, ethanol, Friedreich's ataxia, Refsum's disease, myotonic dystrophy, and Duchenne's dystrophy.[76]

5. INTRACRANIAL HEMORRHAGE

5.1. Congenital Berry Aneurysm

An aneurysm is a localized dilatation or outpouching of an artery, and the majority of intracerebral artery aneurysms (approximately 85%) are found at the base of the brain. In addition, there is a definite predilection for aneurysms to occur at vessel bifurcations. Most intracerebral aneurysms are assumed to develop from congenital defects in vessel walls. There has also been speculation that hemodynamic factors such as hypertension can promote enlargement and/or rupture of the aneurysm.

The typical presentation of a berry aneurysm is rupture with subarachnoid hemorrhage. Characteristic clinical features include severe headache, meningeal irritation, and focal neurological deficit. There will be demonstration of subarachnoid blood by CT in approximately 89% of instances,[81] but it is important to stress that a negative scan does not totally exclude a subarachnoid bleed. Lumbar puncture remains a primary diagnostic tool in the confirmation of aneurysmal rupture.

A large intracerebral aneurysm might be demonstrated on high-resolution CT brain scan, but confirmation generally requires cerebral angiography. However, CT techniques have potential to allow incidental detection of an unruptured aneurysm. These fortuitous findings have the potential to lead to prophylactic management. The natural history of unruptured aneurysms was the subject of a study of 65 patients with aneurysms documented by cerebral angiography.[82] This study found that none of the patients with an aneurysm smaller than 1 cm in diameter ruptured, in contrast to eight ruptured aneurysms

(38%) among patients with an aneurysm 1 cm or greater in diameter. Seven of the eight patients with ruptured aneurysms in this study died secondary to the event. Mean follow-up in this study was 8 years. This study supports a strategy of surgical clipping of large (> 1 cm), accessible intracerebral aneurysms to prevent rupture and, in all likelihood, death or severe disability.

The morbidity and mortality of aneurysmal rupture are greatest within the first 2 weeks of onset. Later complications usually are associated with rebleeding, vasospasm with secondary ischemic infarction, and the development of hydrocephalus.

It is generally accepted that surgical clipping of the aneurysm is the optimal therapy, especially if the patient is medically and neurologically stable, and the neurosurgeon has exceptional skill and experience. There is considerable controversy over optimal medical management prior to surgical clipping. Most studies report that antifibrinolytic therapy with either ϵ-aminocaproic acid or tranexemic acid, reduces the risk of rebleeding. Various therapies have been proposed to prevent vasospasm, and nimodipine appears to hold significant promise in this aspect of care.[83]

5.2. Arteriovenous Malformation

Arteriovenous malformations (AVMs) represent anomalous embryonal development in which there is a resultant tangle of arteries and veins. It is estimated that 0.14% of the population have an AMV, but the majority of these malformations remain clinically silent throughout life.[84] About 10% of patients with AVMs have a coexistent berry aneurysm.[84] The major neurological manifestations of AVMs are seizures and intracranial hemorrhage.

AVMs are usually detected by contrast-enhanced CT brain scan and are confirmed by cerebral angiography. Serious consequences, including death, occur in 28–50% of patients who have an intracranial bleed secondary to an AVM.[85] In addition, 7% of patients presenting with an intracranial hemorrhage will have a recurrence within 1 year and 1% of patients with AVMs who present with seizures have intracranial hemorrhage within 1 year.[86] This disturbing natural history has led to a search for therapies that may reduce the risk of intracranial hemorrhage.

The optimal therapy of an AVM is total surgical removal if this can be performed safely with minimal associated neurological sequelae. Attempts have been made to partially embolize nonsurgically accessible AVMs, but according to at least one report,[87] the recurrence rate for hemorrhage remained high. Conventional radiation therapy has been attempted, but has not provided an additional benefit.[86] One therapy that appears to hold promise consists of proton beam therapy[88] directed at the AVM. This treatment is designed to narrow the lumens of the vessels and to thicken the surrounding wall of the AVM. Proton beam therapy appears to reduce the risk of rebleeding, especially after the first 12 months following therapy. Improvement in neurological status was also reported.

6. CONCLUSION

Stroke implies the death of brain tissue. In light of the critical functions often subserved by small areas of the brain and the inability of the central nervous system to regenerate, the consequences of stroke are often disastrous. Despite intensive research efforts and the development of sophisticated diagnostic and investigative tools that have better defined the pathophysiology of stroke, therapy of ischemic brain disease has been largely unrewarding. Clearly, the most important role of the physician in managing ischemic cerebrovascular disease is to attempt to prevent it. This task requires the physician not only to identify patients who are at risk for stroke, but also to modify or eliminate their risk factors. Though the task may lack glamour, it is the critical issue in stroke management. Risk factors predisposing to stroke that can be affected by intervention include hypertension, cigarette smoking, diabetes mellitus, hyperlipidemia, and cardiac disease.

The greatest reversible risk factor for stroke is hypertension. The decline in the incidence of stroke in the United States parallels the development of the widespread use of effective antihypertensive therapy. Both diastolic and systolic hypertension are risk factors for stroke and require vigorous and continued therapy. Though there exists an identified risk of provoking or extending an area of brain infarction by overvigorous antihypertensive therapy,[89] the latter is not a major concern in the face of well-established, preexisting ischemic brain disease (stroke and TIA). Studies by Meyer and colleagues indicate that reducing blood pressure in hypertensive patients with prior stroke or prior TIA increases cerebral blood flow.[90] Other recommendations to the stroke-prone patient should include weight reduction, moderate daily physical activity, and cessation of smoking. Effective control of blood glucose in the diabetic patient and management of underlying cardiac disease, in particular, congestive heart failure, are also mandated.

These measures, however mundane, are the backbone of stroke prevention and can substantially reduce the risk of this debilitating and often fatal disorder.

REFERENCES

1. Sacco, R. L., Wolf, P. A., Kannel, W. B., and McNamara, P. M.: Survival and recurrence following stroke. *Stroke* **13**:290–295, 1982.
2. Cooper, B. S., and Rice, D. P.: The economic cost of illness revisted. *Soc. Sec. Bull.*, February 1986.
3. Capildeo, R., Haberman, S., and Rose, F. C.: The definition and classification of stroke. A new approach. *Q. J. Med.* **47**:177–196, 1978.
4. Mohr, J. P., Caplan, L. R., Melski, J. W., *et al.*: The Harvard Cooperative Stroke Registry. *Neurology* **28**:745–762, 1978.
5. Wolf, P. A., Kannel, W. B., and Verter, J.: Cerebrovascular diseases in the elderly: Epidemiology, in Albert, M. L. (ed.): *Clinical Neurology of Aging*. Oxford University Press, New York, 1984, p. 458.
6. Adams, R. D., and Victor, M.: *Principles of Neurology*. McGraw-Hill, New York, 1981, pp. 529–593.
7. Wolf, P. A., Kannel, W. B., McGee, D. L., *et al.*: Duration of atrial fibrillation and imminence of stroke: The Framingham study. *Stroke* **14**:664–667, 1983.
8. McAllen, P. M., and Marshall, J.: Cerebrovascular incidents after myocardial infarction. *J. Neurol. Neurosurg. Psychiatry* **40**:951–955, 1977.
9. Mohr, J. P.: Lacunes. *Stroke* **13**:3–11, 1982.
10. Locksley, H. B.: Natural history of subarachnoid hemorrhage, intracranial aneurysms and arteriovenous malformations, in Saks, A. L., Perret, G. E., Locksley, H. B., and Nishioka, H. (eds.): *Intracranial Aneurysms and Subarachnoid Hemorrhage*. Lippincott, Philadelphia, 1969, pp. 37–58.
11. Brust, J. C. M.: Subarachnoid hemorrhage, in Rowland, L. P. (ed.): *Merritt's Textbook of Neurology*, 7th ed. Lea & Febiger, Philadelphia, 1984, pp. 184–191.

12. Toole, J. F., and Cole, M.: Ischemic cerebrovascular disease, in Baker, A. B., and Baker, L. H. (eds.): *Clinical Neurology.* Harper & Row, Philadelphia, 1983, pp. 1–51.
13. Kannel, W. B., Blaisdell, F. W., Gifford, R., *et al.*: Risk factors in stroke due to cerebral infarction: A statement for physicians. *Stroke* **2**:423, 1971.
14. Kurtzke, J. F., and Kurland, L. T.: The epidemiology of neurologic disease, in Baker, A. B., and Baker, L. H. (eds.): *Clinical Neurology.* Harper & Row, Philadelphia, 1983, pp. 1–143.
15. Kannel, W. B., Wolf, P. A., Verter, J., *et al.*: Epidemiologic assessment of the role of blood pressure in stroke: The Framingham study. *JAMA* **214**:301–310, 1970.
16. Wolf, P. A., Kannel, W. B., and McGee, D. L.: Prevention of ischemic stroke: Risk factors, in Barnett, H. J. M., Mohr, J. P., Stein, B. M., and Yatsu, F. M. (eds.): *Stroke: Pathophysiology, Diagnosis and Management.* Churchill Livingstone, New York, 1986, pp. 967–988.
17. Wolf, P. A., Kannel, W. B., and Verter, J.: Current status of risk factors for stroke. *Neurol. Clin.* **1**:317–343, 1983.
18. Furlan, A. J., Whisnant, J. P., and Elveback, L. R.: The decreasing incidence of primary intracerebral hemorrhage: A population study. *Ann. Neurol.* **5**:367–373, 1979.
19. Abbott, R. D., Yin, Y., Reed, D. M., *et al.*: Risk of stroke in male cigarette smokers. *N. Engl. J. Med.* **315**:717–720, 1986.
20. Gordon, T., Castelli, W. P., Hjortland, M. C., *et al.*: High density lipoproteins as a protective factor against coronary heart disease: The Framingham study. *Am. J. Med.* **62**:707–713, 1977.
21. Collaborative Group for the Study of Stroke in Young Women: Oral contraception and increased risk of cerebral ischemia or thrombosis. *N. Engl. J. Med.* **288**:871–878, 1973.
22. Heyman, A., Arons, M., Quinn, M., *et al.*: The role of oral contraceptives in cerebral arterial occlusion. *Neurology* **19**:519–524, 1969.
23. Jennett, W. B., and Cross, J. N.: Influence of pregnancy and oral contraception on the incidence of strokes in women of childbearing age. *Lancet* **1**:1019–1023, 1967.
24. Royal College of General Practitioner's Oral Contraceptive Study: Further analysis of mortality in oral contraceptive users. *Lancet* **1**:541–546, 1981.
25. Grotta, J., Ackerman, R., Correia, J., *et al.*: Whole blood viscosity parameters and cerebral blood flow. *Stroke* **13**:296–301, 1982.
26. Toghi, H., Yamanouchi, H., Murakanu, M., *et al.*: Importance of hematocrit as a risk factor in cerebral infarction. *Stroke* **9**:369–374, 1978.
27. Wolf, P. A., Kannel, W. B., Sorlie, M. S., *et al.*: Asymptomatic carotid bruit and the risk of stroke. *JAMA* **248**:1442–1445, 1981.
28. Wolf, P. A.: Asymptomatic carotid bruit and risk of stroke: The Framingham study (abstract). *Stroke* **10**:96, 1979.
29. Chambers, B. R., and Norris, J. W.: Outcome in patients with asymptomatic neck bruits. *N. Engl. J. Med.* **315**:860–865, 1986.
30. Ropper, A. H., Wechsler, L. R., and Wilson, L. S.: Carotid bruit and the risk of stroke in elective surgery. *N. Engl. J. Med.* **307**:1388–1390, 1982.
31. Berhard, V. M., Johnson, W. D., and Evans, W. E.: Carotid artery stenosis: Association with surgery for coronary artery disease. *Arch. Surg.* **105**:837–840, 1972.
32. Mehigan, J. T., Buch, W. S., Pipkin, R. D., *et al.*: A planned approach to coexistent cerebrovascular disease in coronary artery bypass candidates. *Arch. Surg.* **112**:1403–1409, 1977.
33. Ennix, C. L., Lawrie, G. M., Morris, J., Jr., *et al.*: Improved results of carotid endarterectomy in patients with symptomatic coronary artery disease: An analysis of 1546 conservatic carotid operations. *Stroke* **10**:122–125, 1979.
34. Barnes, R., and Marazalek, P.: Asymptomatic carotid disease in the cardiovascular surgical patient: Is prophylactic endarterectomy necessary? *Stroke* **12**:497–500, 1981.
35. Whisnant, J. P., Matsumoto, N., and Elveback, L. R.: Transient cerebral ischemic attacks in a community: Rochester, Minnesota, 1955 through 1969. *Mayo Clin. Proc.* **48**:844–848, 1973.
36. Robertson, J. T.: Carotid endarterectomy. *Neurol. Clin.* **1**:119–129, 1983.
37. Murphey, F., and Miller, J. H.: Carotid insufficiency: Diagnosis and surgical treatment. *J. Neurosurg.* **16**:1–23, 1959.
38. Sandok, B. A., Furlan, A. J., Whisnant, J. P., *et al.*: Guidelines for the management of transient ischemic attacks. *Mayo Clin. Proc.* **53**:665–674, 1978.

39. Canadian Cooperative Stroke Study Group: A randomized trial of aspirin and sulfinpyrazone in threatened stroke. *N. Engl. J. Med.* **299**:53–59, 1978.
40. Wolf, P. A., Dawber, T. R., Thamer, H. E., Jr., and Kannel, W. B.: Epidemiological assessment of chronic atrial fibrillation and the risk of stroke: The Framingham study. *Neurology* **28**:973–977, 1978.
41. Hart, R. G., Coull, B. M., and Miller, V. T.: Anticoagulation and embolic infarction. *Neurology* **32**:274–275, 1982.
42. Adams, R. D.: Vascular diseases of the brain. *Annu. Rev. Med.* **4**:213–252, 1953.
43. Hakim, A. M., Rider-Cooke, A., and Melanson, D.: Sequential computerized tomographic appearance of strokes. *Stroke* **14**:893–897, 1983.
44. Britton, M., and Gustafson, C.: Non-rheumatic atrial fibrillation as a risk factor for stroke. *Stroke* **16**:182–188, 1985.
45. Wolf, P. A., Kannel, W. B., and Abbott, R. D.: Atrial fibrillation and stroke in the elderly, the Framingham study (abstract). *Stroke* **16**:138, 1985.
46. Ramirez-Lassepas, M., Quinones, M. R., and Nino, H. H.: Treatment of acute ischemic stroke. *Arch. Neurol.* **43**:386–390, 1986.
47. Yatsu, F. M., and Mohr, J. P.: Anticoagulation therapy for cardiogenic emboli to brain. *Neurology* **32**:274–275, 1982.
48. Kelley, R. E., Berger, J. R., Alter, M., and Kovacs, A. G.: Cerebral ischemia and atrial fibrillation: A prospective study. *Neurology* **4**:1285–1291, 1984.
49. Cerebral Embolism Study Group: Immediate anticoagulation of embolic stroke: Brain hemorrhage and management options. *Stroke* **15**:779–789, 1984.
50. Barnett, J. H. M., Boughner, D. R., Taylor, D. W., *et al.*: Further evidence relating mitral valve prolapse to cerebral ischemic events. *N. Engl. J. Med.* **302**:139–144, 1980.
51. Adams, H. P., Jr., Butler, M. J., Biller, J., and Toffol, G. J.: Nonhemorrhagic cerebral infarction in young adults. *Arch. Neurol.* **43**:793–796, 1986.
52. Scharf, R. E., Hennerici, M., Bluscheke, V., *et al.*: Cerebral ischemia in young patients. Is it associated with mitral valve prolapse and abnormal platelet activity *in vivo? Stroke* **13**:454–458, 1982.
53. Clemens, J. D., Horwitz, R. I., Jaffe, C. C., *et al.*: A controlled evaluation of the risk of bacterial endocarditis in persons with mitral valve prolapse. *N. Engl. J. Med.* **307**:776–781, 1982.
54. Dawson, D. M., and Fischer, G. G.: Neurologic complications of cardiac catheterization. *Neurology* **27**:496–497, 1977.
55. Verani, M. S., Carroll, R. J., and Falsetti, H. L.: Mitral valve prolapse in coronary artery disease. *Am. J. Cardiol.* **37**:1–11, 1976.
56. Schwartz, M. H., Teichholz, L. E., and Donoso, E.: Mitral valve prolapse. A review of associated arrhythmias. *Am. J. Med.* **62**:377–389, 1977.
57. Donaldson, R. M., Emanuel, R. W., and Earl, C. J.: The role of two-dimensional echocardiography in the detection of potentially embolic intracardiac masses in patients with cerebral ischemia. *J. Neurol. Neurosurg. Psychiatry* **44**:803–809, 1981.
58. Spence, J. D., Wong, D. G., Melendez, L. J., *et al.*: Increased prevalence of mitral valve prolapse in patients with migraine. *Can. Med. Assoc. J.* **131**:1457–1460, 1984.
59. Dorfman, L. J., Marshall, W. H., and Enzmann, D. R.: Cerebral infarction and migraine: Clinical and radiologic correlation. *Neurology* **29**:317–322, 1979.
60. Sandok, B. A., and Giuliani, E. R.: Cerebral ischemic events in patients with mitral valve prolapse. *Stroke* **13**:448–450, 1982.
61. Snyder, B. D., and Ramirez-Lassepas, M.: Cerebral infarction in young adults. Long-term prognosis. *Stroke* **11**:149–153, 1980.
62. Come, P. C., Riley, M. F., and Bivas, N. K.: Roles of echocardiography and arrhythmia monitoring in the evaluation of patients with suspected systemic embolism. *Ann. Neurol.* **13**:527–531, 1983.
63. Savage, D. D., Garrison, R. J., Devereux, R. B., *et al.*: Mitral valve prolapse in the general population. 1) Epidemiological features: The Framingham study. *Am. Heart J.* **106**:571–575, 1983.
64. Boughner, D. R., and Barnett, H. J. M.: The enigma of the risk of stroke in mitral valve prolapse. *Stroke* **16**:175–177, 1985.
65. Wann, L. S., Gross, C. M., Wakefield, R. J., *et al.*: Diagnostic precision of echocardiography in mitral valve prolapse. *Am. Heart J.* **109**:803–808, 1985.

66. Bartletta, G. A., Gagliardi, R., Benevenuti, L., *et al.:* Cerebral ischemic attacks as a complication of aortic and mitral valve prolapse. *Stroke* **16**:219–223, 1985.
67. Nishimura, R. A., McGoon, M. D., Shub, C., *et al.:* Echocardiographically documented mitral valve prolapse: Long-term follow-up of 237 patients. *N. Engl. J. Med.* **313**:1305–1309, 1985.
68. Barnett, H. J. M.: Embolism in mitral valve prolapse. *Annu. Rev. Med.* **33**:489–507, 1982.
69. Wood, P.: *Diseases of the Heart and Circulation,* 2nd ed. Eyre and Spottiswoode, London, 1956, p. 525.
70. Easton, J. D., and Sherman, D. G.: Management of cerebral embolism of cardiac origin. *Stroke* **11**:433–442, 1980.
71. Belcher, J. R., and Somerville, W.: Systemic embolization in relation to mitral valvuloplasty. *Br. Med. J.* **2**:1000–1003, 1955.
72. Wang, Y., Bland, E. F., and Scannel, J. G.: Evaluation of mitral commissuorotomy for the prevention of systemic embolism in mitral stenosis (abstract). *Circulation* **22**:829, 1960.
73. Thompson, P. L., and Robinson, J. S.: Stroke after acute myocardial infarction: Relation to infarct size. *Br. Med. J.* **2**:457–459, 1978.
74. Komrad, M. S., Coffey, C. E., Coffey, K. S., *et al.:* Myocardial infarction and stroke. *Neurology* **34**:1403–1409, 1984.
75. Bean, W. B.: Infarction of the heart. III. Clinical course and morphological findings. *Ann. Intern. Med.* **12**:71–94, 1938.
76. Hart, R. G., Sherman, D. G., Miller, V. T., *et al.:* Diagnosis and management of ischemic stroke. Part II—Selected controversies. *Curr. Prob. Cardiol.* **8**:7–80, 1983.
77. Reeder, G. S., Lengyel, M., Tajik, A. J., *et al.:* Mural thrombus in left ventricular aneurysm: Incidence, role of angiography and relation between anticoagulation and embolization. *Mayo Clin. Proc.* **56**:77–81, 1981.
78. Sixty Plus Reinfarction Study Research Group: Risks of long-term oral anticoagulant therapy in elderly patients after myocardial infarction. *Lancet* **1**:64–68, 1982.
79. McManus, Q., Grunkemeier, G., Thomas, D., *et al.:* The Starr–Edwards Model 6000 valve: A fifteen year follow-up of the first successful mitral prosthesis. *Circulation* **56**:623–625, 1977.
80. Edmunds, L. H.: Thromboembolic complications of current cardiac valvular prostheses. *Ann. Thorac. Surg.* **34**:96–106, 1982.
81. Adams, H. P., Jr., Kassell, N. F., Turner, J. C., *et al.:* CT and clinical correlations in recent aneurysmal subarachnoid hemorrhage: Preliminary report of Cooperative Aneurysm Study. *Neurology* **33**:981–988, 1983.
82. Wiebers, D. O., Whisnant, J. P., and O'Fallon, W. M.: The natural history of unruptured intracranial aneurysms. *N. Engl. J. Med.* **304**:696–698, 1981.
83. Allen, G. S., Ahn, H. S., Preziosi, T. J., *et al.:* Cerebral arterial spasm—A controlled trial of nimodipine in patients with subarachnoid hemorrhage. *N. Engl. J. Med.* **308**:619–624, 1983.
84. Mitchelson, W. S.: Natural history and pathophysiology of arteriovenous malformations. *Clin. Neurosurg.* **26**:307–318, 1979.
85. Stein, B. M., and Wolpert, S. M.: Arteriovenous malformations of the brain. II. Current concepts and treatment. *Arch. Neurol.* **37**:69–79, 1980.
86. Periet, G., and Nishioki, H.: Arteriovenous malformations, an analysis of 545 cases of craniocerebral arteriovenous malformations and fistuli reported to the cooperative study. *J. Neurosurg.* **25**:467–479, 1966.
87. Luesenhop, A. J., and Presper, J. H.: Surgical embolization of cerebral arteriovenous malformations through internal carotid and vertebral arteries. *J. Neurosurg.* **42**:443–451, 1975.
88. Kjellberg, R. N., Hanamura, T., Davis, K. R., *et al.:* Bragg-peak proton-beam therapy for arteriovenous malformations of the brain. *N. Engl. J. Med.* **309**:269–274, 1983.
89. Rosenfeld, W. E., Lippmann, S. M., Levin, I. H., and Scheinberg, P.: Hypotension—A cause for ischemic CVA (abstract). *Neurology* **33**(suppl 2):146, 1983.
90. Meyer, J. S., Sawada, T., Kitamura, A., *et al.:* Cerebral blood flow after control of hypertension in stroke. *Neurology* **18**:772–778, 1968.
91. Berger, J. R.: The diagnosis and management of cerebrovascular disorders, in Gardner, L. B. (ed.): *Acute Internal Medicine.* Elsevier, New York, 1986, pp. 417–429.

18

Osteoporosis

Eric Reiss

1. INTRODUCTION

1.1. Definition

Osteoporosis represents a decrease of bone mass that equally affects all elements of bone: the bone mass is small but normal in composition. Specifically, the proportion of organic and inorganic phases is normal, there are no defects in calcification, and the cellular architecture is not grossly distorted. This distinguishes osteoporosis from metabolic bone diseases that superficially resemble it, such as osteomalacia and osteitis fibrosa.

1.2. The Problem

Osteoporosis principally affects older women. It is the chief predisposing factor to fractures in the aged and poses an increasingly important health hazard as the population grows older. It has been estimated that the number of fractures of the femoral neck in the United States has increased from about 200,000 to 270,000 per year between 1970 and 1980, and this rate of change is likely to continue as the lifespan increases. The cost associated with treatment of these fractures rose from about $0.5 billion in 1970 to $1.2 billion in 1980 and could reach $5–10 billion by 2000.[1]

There is growing evidence that osteoporosis can be prevented, at least to a large extent. However, effective prevention often involves expenses and small, but definite, hazards. Although much has been learned in recent years, big gaps remain in our knowledge about how best to counsel individuals—let alone the population at large. The educated public's increasing awareness of osteoporosis as a genuine health problem has not been matched by the medical profession's appreciation of what can and cannot be accomplished by prevention. Some important issues involve nutrition—a subject on which everyone feels entitled to some opinion and which invites charlatanism.

1.3. Some New Ideas

New methods for assessing bone mass and its change with time have provided an essential tool for identifying subjects who are at a special risk for developing osteoporosis

Eric Reiss • Department of Medicine, University of Miami School of Medicine, Miami, Florida, 33101.
†Deceased.

and for determining the effectiveness of various prophylactic measures. Quantitative computed tomography correlates very well with bone mineral content by actual chemical analysis. It has the disadvantage of delivering several hundred mrads of radiation. Dual photon absorptiometry ("densitometry") correlates well with computed tomography at roughly one-hundredth the radiation dose and has emerged as the most frequently used clinical method for the study of osteoporosis.

New methods of prevention have been evaluated and old ones have been reassessed. As a result, the physician today has a substantial repertoire of approaches that permit individualization of regimens. Changes of calcium homeostasis with aging have been clearly delineated, but the relevance of these changes to osteoporosis remains problematic.

2. OSTEOPOROSIS IN CLINICAL PRACTICE

2.1. Diagnosis

Osteopenia is a nonspecific term describing an apparent decrease of bone density on roentgenograms. Radiographic assessment of bone mass is insensitive. It is also unreliable because it is affected by many uncontrollable technical variables. Although there are radiographic features that are characteristic of osteoporosis and others that suggest different bone diseases, the radiographic differentiation between various causes of osteopenia is often impossible.

Fortunately, the distinction between osteoporosis and other metabolic or neoplastic bone diseases is rarely complicated and requires only a thorough and systematic clinical evaluation. In osteoporosis, all clinical parameters, such as serum calcium, phosphorus, alkaline phosphatase, parathyroid hormone, and vitamin D metabolites, are grossly normal. If any abnormalities are uncovered, the diagnosis of osteoporosis is in question. An extensive workup is usually unnecessary. Multiple myeloma is the only disease that is easily mistaken for osteoporosis. When there is doubt, measurement of the sedimentation rate, serum and urine protein electrophoresis, and a bone marrow examination are in order.

2.2. Classification

Riggs and Melton have adduced new evidence supporting the distinction between the two principal forms of involutional osteoporosis—postmenopausal (type I) and senile (type II) osteoporosis.[2] Type I affects a relatively small subset of women within 10–15 years after the menopause. Bone loss is predominantly trabecular, so that vertebral fractures are the dominant clinical manifestation. Type II disease occurs in older subjects—65 and older. It involves cortical as well as trabecular bone, occurs in men as well as in women, and causes chiefly hip fractures.

The distinction between these types of abnormality is helpful in thinking about pathogenesis and prevention. In type I disease, excessive bone resorption owing to the loss of ovarian function is the main pathophysiological event. In type II disease, the problem is usually impaired bone formation. Bone biopsy in type II disease shows little cellular activity. Occasionally, the alterations of calcium homeostasis of aging compound the problem. These consist of decreasing efficiency of calcium absorption from the intestines due to a lessened efficiency of the synthesis of calcitriol (1,25-dihydroxyvitamin D) and a small but definite increase of serum parathyroid hormone.[3]

2.3. Risk Factors

The most important determinant of whether a person will develop clinically significant osteoporosis is the skeletal mass at maturity.[4] Heredity is the decisive factor influencing this variable. Blacks are genetically endowed with a large skeletal mass and are therefore relatively immune to osteoporosis except in very advanced age. Scandinavians appear to be especially susceptible to osteoporosis. Men are less at risk than women because of their larger skeletons; they also lose bone less rapidly than women when they grow old. Other genetic variables include diseases such as osteogenesis imperfecta at one extreme and, at the other, the occasional tendency for osteoporosis to occur more frequently in some families than in others in the absence of known disease.

A small body weight and a small muscle mass predispose to osteoporosis. This may well be the only condition in which being overweight has a protective influence!

Little is known about environmental factors that affect the peak adult bone mass. This mass increases well past the time when other tissues attain maturity.[4] Full skeletal maturation may not take place until age 30–35. It now seems possible or even likely that an abundant intake of calcium is essential for the attainment of maximal bone mass.[5] A diet deficient in calcium certainly decreases this mass and therefore predisposes to osteoporosis.

Women who experience menopause at an early age are very much at risk if they are untreated.[6] Premature loss of estrogenic function from any cause has a deleterious effect on bone. Amenorrheic athletes, for example, are at risk of excessive bone loss.[7] Drinking alcohol, smoking cigarettes, and being childless are predisposing factors. Breast feeding has an unexpected protective effect. Physical activity has the expected beneficial effect on bone.

Given this wide array of risk factors, one can identify women whose risk of becoming osteoporotic is greater than that of the population at large. They are the most important candidates for prophylactic regimens.

2.4. Screening

Ideally, all women should have a densitometric assessment of the spine in the perimenopausal period and periodically afterward. The objective is to identify women who enter the menopause with a low bone mass and are therefore at risk and to identify those who lose bone at an excessive rate. These are the women who require the most intensive intervention and the most careful follow-up.

Such widespread screening would involve a substantial cost and may therefore not be feasible. An alternative approach involves identifying those who are especially at risk based on the history and concentrating efforts on them. There is no consensus on this subject.

Densitometric assessment of many different parts of the skeleton is now possible. In the perimenopausal period, measurements of the spine are obviously of greatest interest. How frequently these should be done is uncertain, but yearly determinations for a few years in those at high risk should be considered.

3. PREVENTION

3.1. Calcium

An adequate intake of calcium is probably more important premenopausally than later since it may assure attainment of optimal skeletal mass. But what is adequate and what is optimal are unresolved questions.

Heaney *et al.* determined on the basis of very extensive and careful balance studies of 130 perimenopausal women that, on the average, zero calcium balance was attained at an intake of 1.24 g of calcium per day.[8] There is, of course, wide variation in the calcium intake required for the maintainance of balance. Furthermore, the capacity to adapt to marginal intakes decreases with age, so that older people may benefit from a larger intake. These considerations suggest that it is better to err on the side of a high calcium intake.

The assessment of bone mineral content by densitometry has yielded disappointing information about the efficacy of calcium supplements in the prevention of postmenopausal osteoporosis. A large intake of calcium does not by itself prevent postmenopausal loss of bone mass. The main reason for prescribing calcium supplements in midlife and beyond is to assure that calcium deficiency does not aggravate the normal aging of the skeleton.

The "average" American woman probably consumes no more than 500 mg of calcium daily. The recommended dietary allowance of calcium for adults is 800 mg daily—an amount that is likely to be much too low. Although there are no clear guidelines, most experts recommend an intake of calcium in the neighborhood of 1500 mg/day in the postmenopausal period. If this can be met by diet, all is well. Otherwise, the usual diet should be supplemented with 1000–1500 mg daily.

The only known hazard of calcium supplementation is hypercalciuria and the worsening of a preexisting tendency to form calcium-containing kidney stones. Calcium must be used cautiously in patients with a history of nephrolithiasis. In others, measurement of one 24-hr urine collection for calcium 4–6 weeks after starting calcium supplements is indicated. Any value in excess of 250 mg/24 hr or 4 mg/kg requires caution.

Calcium is available in many preparations—cheap and not so cheap. Many over-the-counter preparations without a trade name are perfectly satisfactory, but patients must be warned to read labels carefully: what matters is the amount of elemental calcium. The labels often give the amount of the actual compound—calcium carbonate or calcium lactate, and so forth. Calcium carbonate is a commonly used preparation: it contains only 40% calcium. Thus, 1200 mg of calcium carbonate provides only 480 mg of elemental calcium.

Recker has recently pointed out that calcium carbonate is poorly absorbed in subjects with achlorhydria. When calcium carbonate is given with meals, absorption is much improved—a good argument for counseling patients to take supplements with meals rather than between meals.[9]

3.2. Estrogens

The evidence that estrogens retard or abolish postmenopausal loss of bone is overwhelming.[10–12] Moreover, estrogens confer significant protection against fractures.[12] The references cited here are representative of a large number of convincing studies. In view of all these data, why are estrogens not universally recommended for postmenopausal white women?

Some women cannot tolerate estrogen therapy because of gastrointestinal or other side effects. Estrogens increase the probability of developing endometrial hyperplasia and cancer. The risk is small but definite.[13] Combining estrogens with progestins and thus allowing the endometrium to slough periodically is a good clinical practice. It probably lessens the risk of endometrial cancer, but many older women object to the periodic bleeding. Careful monitoring with examinations and endometrial biopsies can probably reduce the hazard to negligible, but accomplishing this requires time, effort, expense, and a high degree of physician understanding and responsibility.

The other potential dangers associated with estrogens are more elusive. The data on increased incidence of breast cancer are inconsistent and unconvincing. An increased as well as a decreased incidence of cardiovascular disease has been reported.[14,15] Estrogen-related hypertension has been reported but can be dealt with.

The potential dangers of estrogens have been given wide publicity, and many intelligent women hesitate to take estrogens in spite of strong indications for their use. Physicians must acquaint themselves with the relevant data in order to advise their patients honestly and effectively.

For practical purposes, there are few if any contraindications to the use of estrogens in women experiencing a premature menopause, spontaneously or surgically induced. Postmenopausal women at high risk, as defined earlier, are also candidates for estrogen replacement. For women with a good bone mass and who do not have major risk factors for osteoporosis, the use of estrogens in the postmenopausal period is not completely defined. If follow-up densitometry shows rapid bone loss, estrogens are clearly indicated. In others, the use of estrogens is probably optional, though a good case can be made for using estrogens unless there are strong contraindications. All women receiving estrogens require careful monitoring by periodic bone densitometry as well as gynecological surveillance.

3.3. Other Measures

3.3.1. Exercise

Physical stress on the skeleton tends to preserve bone mass. Immobilization and weightlessness (as experienced during flights in space) certainly promote rapid bone resorption. Whether active exercising is better than ordinary activity is less certain, but encouraging an active lifestyle contributes to a sense of well-being and may well be beneficial in many ways, including preservation of the skeleton.

3.3.2. Calcitonin and Other Approaches

Research on the prevention of osteoporosis has never been more active.[16] Although deficient secretion of calcitonin does not appear to be a factor in the genesis of osteoporosis,[17] calcitonin shows promise in preventing postmenopausal bone loss. At present use of calcitonin is not a practical approach because of its expense and the need for daily injections. Calcitonin administered by nasal snuff is now being evaluated.

Some anabolic steroids and dichlormethylene diphosphonate show promise in retarding or abolishing postmenopausal bone loss. Calcitriol may be of use in the elderly.[18] Other potentially useful agents are under active investigation. Sodium fluoride shows promise as a therapeutic agent in osteoporosis but has no place in prophylaxis.

REFERENCES

1. Linday, R., Dempster, D. W., Clemens, B. S., *et al.*: Incidence, cost, and risk factors of fracture of the proximal femur in the U.S.A., in Christiansen, C., Arnaud, C. D., Nordin, B. E. C., *et al.* (eds.): *Osteoporosis.* Proceedings of the Copenhagen International Symposium on Osteoporosis. Glostrup Hospital, Copenhagen, 1984, p. 311.
2. Riggs, B. L., and Melton, J. M., III: Evidence for two distinct syndromes of involutional osteoporosis. *Am. J. Med.* **75**:899–910, 1983.
3. Gallagher, J. C., Riggs, B. L., Eisman, J., *et al.*: Intestinal calcium absorption and serum vitamin D metabolites in normal subjects and osteoporotic patients. Effect of age and dietary calcium. *J. Clin. Invest.* **64**:729–736, 1979.
4. Heaney, R. P.: Risk factors in age-related bone loss and osteoporotic fracture, in Christiansen, C., Arnaud, C. D., Nordin, B. E. C., *et al.* (eds.): *Osteoporosis.* Proceedings of the Copenhagen International Symposium on Osteoporosis. Glostrup Hospital, Copenhagen, 1984, p. 245.
5. Heaney, R. P.: Calcium intake requirement and bone mass in the elderly. *J. Lab Clin. Med.* **100**:309–312, 1982.
6. Aloia, J. F., Cohn, S. H., Vaswani, A., *et al.*: Risk factors for postmenopausal osteoporosis. *Am. J. Med.* **78**:95–100, 1985.
7. Drinkwater, B. L., Nilson, K., Chestnut, C. H., III, *et al.*: Bone mineral content of amenorrheic and eumenorrheic athletes. *N. Engl. J. Med.* **311**:277–281, 1984.
8. Heaney, R. P., Recker, R. R., and Saville, P. D.: Calcium balance and calcium requirements in middle-aged women. *Am. J. Nutr.* **30**:1603–1611, 1977.
9. Recker, R. R.: Calcium absorption and achlorhydria. *N. Engl. J. Med.* **313**: 70–73, 1985.
10. Nachtigall, L. E., Nachtigall, R. H., Nachtigall, R. D., *et al.*: Estrogen replacement therapy. I. A 10-year prospective study in the relationship to osteoporosis. *Obstet. Gynecol.* **53**:277–280, 1979.
11. Lindsay, R., Hart, D. M., Forrest, C., *et al.*: Prevention of spinal osteoporosis in oophorectomised women. *Lancet* **2**:1151–1154, 1980.
12. Ettinger, B., Genant, H. K., Cann, C. E., *et al.*: Long-term estrogen replacement therapy prevents bone loss and fractures. *Ann. Intern. Med.* **102**:319–324, 1985.
13. Judd, H. L., Meldrum, D. R., Deftos, L. J., *et al.*: Estrogen replacement therapy: Indications and complications. *Ann. Intern. Med.* **98**:195–205, 1983.
14. Wilson, P. W. F., Garrison, R. J., and Castelli, W. P.: Postmenopausal estrogen use, cigarette smoking, and cardiovascular morbidity in women over 50. The Framingham study. *N. Engl. J. Med.* **313**:1038–1043, 1985.
15. Stampfer, M. J., Willett, W. C., Colditz, G. A., *et al.*: A prospective study of postmenopausal estrogen therapy and coronary heart disease. *N. Engl. J. Med.* **313**:1044–1049, 1985.
16. Christiansen, C., Arnaud, C. D., Nordin, B. E. C., *et al.*: *Osteoporosis.* Proceedings of the Copenhagen International Symposium on Osteoporosis. Glostrup Hospital, Copenhagen, 1984.

17. Tiegs, R. D., Body, J. J., Wahner, H. W., *et al.:* Calcitonin secretion in postmenopausal osteoporosis. *N. Engl. J. Med.* **312:**1097–1100, 1985.
18. Gallagher, J. C., Jerpbak, C. M., Jee, W. S. S., *et al.:* 1,25-dihydroxyvitamin D_3: Short- and long-term effects on bone and calcium metabolism in patients with postmenopausal osteoporosis. *Proc. Natl. Acad Sci. USA* **79:**3325–3329, 1982.

19

Preventable Visual Loss

Elizabeth Hodapp

1. INTRODUCTION

Ten million or so Americans have some visual disability, of whom perhaps half a million are legally blind with corrected vision of less than 20/200 in each eye. Another million or so have visual impairment such that despite wearing glasses they cannot read a newspaper.[1] Precise data regarding the prevalence and cause of visual problems do not exist. To attempt to generate such data, between 1979 and 1983 the National Eye Institute performed a study to determine whether it could obtain "estimates of the prevalence, by cause, of visual acuity impairment in persons 25 years of age or older."[2] The study concluded that such estimates could not be reliably obtained, largely because people were unwilling to be examined (P. F. Palmberg, personal communication).

Despite uncertainty as to their numbers, many people in this country do not see well. Any estimate of the economic impact of visual loss would be so speculative as to be useless. It has generally been accepted, without economic data to support the assertion, that blindness should be prevented. The particular details of preventive strategies and their cost/benefit ratios will probably be coming under additional scrutiny in the future.

This chapter deals with four preventable or treatable causes of visual loss and blindness that are within the purview of a primary-care physician. It does not include visual loss as part of syndromes, such as rubella or chromosome anomalies. Nor does it include those causes of poor vision, such as retrolental fibroplasia, that are well recognized by the physicians in a position to avoid them. The chapter, moreover, assumes that most patients will see an eye doctor if they perceive that they have something wrong specifically with their eyes or their vision. The conditions to be discussed are glaucoma, diabetic retinopathy, amblyopia, and ocular injuries.

2. GLAUCOMA

2.1. Definitions

Glaucoma refers to a group of conditions in which the intraocular pressure (IOP) is high enough to cause damage to the retinal ganglion cells that comprise the optic nerve.

Elizabeth Hodapp • Department of Ophthalmology, University of Miami School of Medicine, Miami, Florida 33101.

The level of IOP is determined by the relative rates of fluid formation and escape from the eye. Fluid is constantly secreted from the ciliary body located behind the iris and flows through the pupil into the anterior chamber. It exits the eye via the anterior chamber angle trabecular meshwork and enters the venous circulation in the sclera. Abnormal resistance to fluid egress at the level of the trabecular meshwork results in elevated pressure. Resistance may be of various sorts, and one of the most frequently used classifications of glaucoma separates the various forms of glaucoma by the presence or absence of a mechanical blockage of the trabecular meshwork. In open-angle glaucoma (Fig. 1), there is no mechanical blockage to the flow of fluid. The eye appears to be normal, but the pressure is elevated and there is a decreased rate of outflow. Angle closure glaucomas (Fig. 2), on the other hand, share the characteristic of a mechanical blockage to fluid flow. The iris is opposed to the trabecular meshwork and aqueous cannot escape from the eye. This type of glaucoma occurs most frequently in far-sighted eyes, which are shorter than average and have a relatively narrow space between the iris and trabecular mesh.

The intraocular pressure, which in normal individuals averages around 15–16 mm Hg, is usually 20–40 mm Hg in people with untreated open-angle glaucoma. Those with untreated angle closure may have a pressure as high as 60 or 70 mm Hg since the formation of aqueous humor continues until the intraocular pressure reaches ciliary body perfusion pressure.

Primary open-angle glaucoma—which accounts for perhaps 75% or 80% of all glaucomas—is a bilateral, insidious, blinding condition. The disease can usually be treated successfully with medication or surgery, and therefore early diagnosis is desirable. Primary angle closure glaucoma—perhaps 10% of glaucoma—may present either as an acute glaucoma or as a chronic glaucoma. The acute form is associated with pain and decreased vision and is usually recognized and treated promptly. The chronic form, for screening and prevention purposes, can be considered with primary open-angle glaucoma since the findings on all of the routinely used screening tests are similar. Secondary glaucomas make up the remainder of the cases, and this group includes corticosteroid-induced glaucoma, perhaps the most truly preventable glaucoma.

2.2. Epidemiology

Perhaps 70,000 people in America are legally blind because of glaucoma and about 5000–6000 individuals become legally blind every year as a result of the disease.[1]

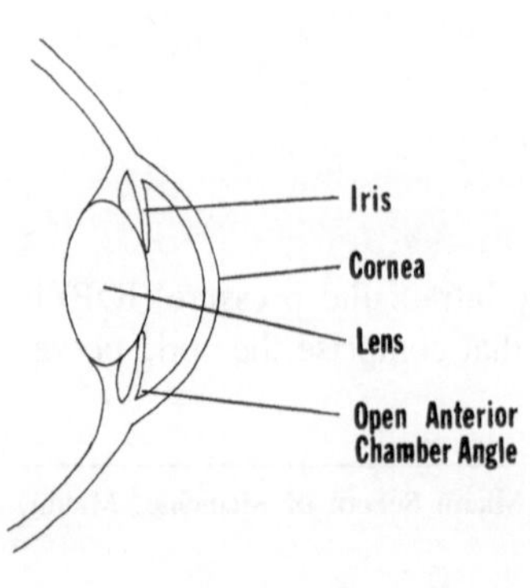

Figure 1. Ocular anatomy in open-angle glaucoma. There is no mechanical blockage to fluid flow from the site of formation behind the iris to the area of exit in the anterior chamber angle.

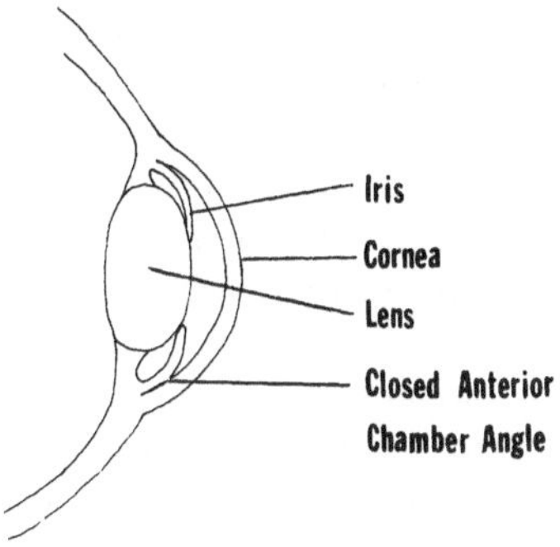

Figure 2. Angle closure glaucoma. The iris is mechanically obstructing the access of fluid to the anterior chamber angle.

Glaucomas as a whole become more frequent with increasing age, and the prevalence of the condition is felt to be somewhere around 1–2% of the population at age 65 and perhaps 3% of the population over the age of 65. It is familial in many cases, but over half of patients have no family history of glaucoma. Blacks appear to have a higher percentage of open-angle glaucoma as well as a higher rate of blindness from the disease. These increases appear to be independent of differences in health care between blacks and whites.[3]

2.3. *Pathophysiology*

The major site of glaucomatous damage is the optic disc. However, neither the way in which glaucomatous damage occurs nor the exact relationship of elevated pressure to disc damage is clear. Most people with glaucoma have pressures that are higher than average, but many people with high pressures do not have glaucoma, and some people with normal eye pressures have damage that appears to be glaucomatous. Various pathophysiological mechanisms can probably cause what we refer to as glaucoma, and although some are certainly related to pressure, perhaps others are not. In all forms of glaucoma there is retinal ganglion cell death, and with cell death the optic cup enlarges as the nerve tissue decreases. Associated with cell death, the visual field gradually deteriorates.

2.4. *Diagnosis and Screening*

There is no unequivocal clinical evidence that early treatment of glaucoma reduces the morbidity of the disease. Nonetheless it is a basic tenet of ophthalmologists that, especially in patients who have elevated intraocular pressure associated with glaucomatous damage, lowering the intraocular pressure slows or stops the progress of the disease. It is, moreover, a basic tenet that the earlier the diagnosis is made, the more likely it is that the patient will be able to maintain useful vision for his or her lifetime.

Because of these assumptions, a good deal of thought has been given to the most efficient way to identify patients with early glaucoma. For the purposes of discussion these will be divided into mass screening techniques and office screening techniques.

Mass glaucoma screening programs have been proposed as a method of identifying people at risk with glaucoma. Most such programs include only an intraocular pressure measurement, and all people with pressure exceeding a present level are referred for a follow-up complete examination. A major difficulty with intraocular pressure screening programs is the considerable overlap of intraocular pressure between glaucomatous and nonglaucomatous patients. Cutoff levels range from 21 to 25 mm Hg, with a common level being 22 mm Hg. At this level, approximately 10–20 normal individuals will be referred to an ophthalmologist for each patient who has glaucoma, and perhaps one of three individuals with manifest glaucomatous damage will have a pressure falling within the normal range at any given time of measurement. For this reason intraocular pressure screening is not a particularly efficient method for glaucoma detection.[4,5]

Office screening by the internist or family practitioner is preferable to mass intraocular pressure screening. The most useful single maneuver for glaucoma detection for the generalist to undertake is to encourage all of his/her patients to consult an ophthalmologist, not an optometrist, for glasses.[5] Ophthalmologists are trained to diagnose and treat all forms of ocular disease and routinely measure the intraocular pressure and examine the optic nerve. Optometrists are trained primarily in the recognition and correction of refractive problems.

The internist or family practioner can also, with very little expense of time and money, identify and refer people at particular risk to have glaucoma. The primary screening modalities are history and optic nerve examination. Tonometry is a third screening modality that may be considered despite the limitations mentioned.

The history allows identification of asymptomatic people who are at risk to have glaucoma. Anyone who has a family history of glaucoma should be seen regularly by an ophthalmologist. The ideal frequence of routine examination is unknown, but every 3 or 4 years prior to the age of 40, every 2 or 3 years between 40 and 55, and every year thereafter seems reasonable. Patients who have had facial trauma or ocular trauma, no matter how many years previously, should also be referred to an ophthalmologist because some such people develop glaucoma many years after injury.

Examination of the optic nerve through an undilated pupil is a useful screening method for the detection of abnormality, although not necessarily for the detection of complete normality. Patients with any of the following findings should be referred to an ophthalmologist:

1. Detectable asymmetry between the cups in the two eyes
2. A horizontal or vertical cup that occupies more than half the diameter of the disc (Figs. 3, 4)
3. Notching or irregularity of the cup (Fig. 5)
4. Peculiar appearance of the optic nerve (Fig. 6)

Examination through a dilated pupil is much easier than through an undilated pupil, although it is possible to precipitate angle closure glaucoma with dilation. Acute angle closure glaucoma is only rarely caused by mild dilation and can usually be treated well if diagnosed promptly. It is not, however, a desirable complication of an examination because eyes that have had acute angle closure glaucoma frequently develop a cataract some years sooner than their fellow eye. Also, cataract extraction in such patients causes more corneal complications than normally occur. Probably the safest course is to refer patients whose fundi cannot be seen through an undilated pupil for an ophthalmological

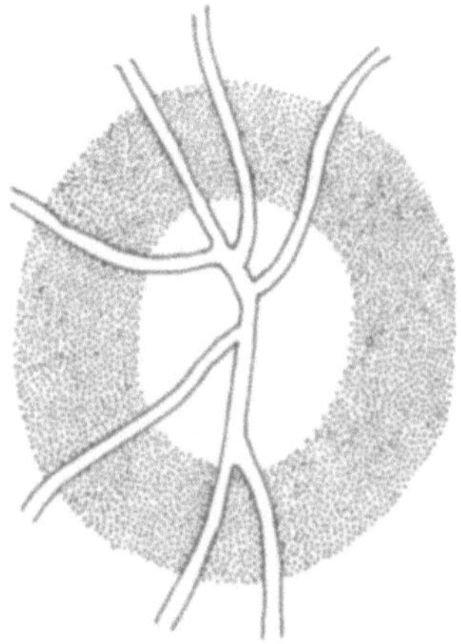

Figure 3. Normal optic nerve. The cup occupies less than half the horizontal or vertical diameter of the disc.

examination and to ask the ophthalmologist if the patient may be dilated in your office in the future. This may not always be practical, and depending on circumstances, it may be reasonable to dilate patients. A physician who routinely dilates and examines carefully his/her patient's fundi will probably identify several individuals with undiagnosed open-angle glaucoma for each person in whom angle closure is precipitated. Tropicamide, ½ %, one drop in each eye, should provide sufficient dilation for an adequate examination. Patients should be told to seek immediate ophthalmological care if their eyes hurt or if their vision is blurred following a dilated examination.

Office tonometry is a possible adjunct to a complete physical examination. There are two practical instruments for use in a general internist's office, the Schiotz tonometer and the hand-held applanation tonometer. The Schiotz tonometer is the less expensive; an instrument and ultraviolet sterilizer costs approximately $500. It is less accurate than the applanation tonometer and tends to give an inaccurately low reading in certain eyes, particularly those with near-sightedness. An applanation tonometer is highly accurate and

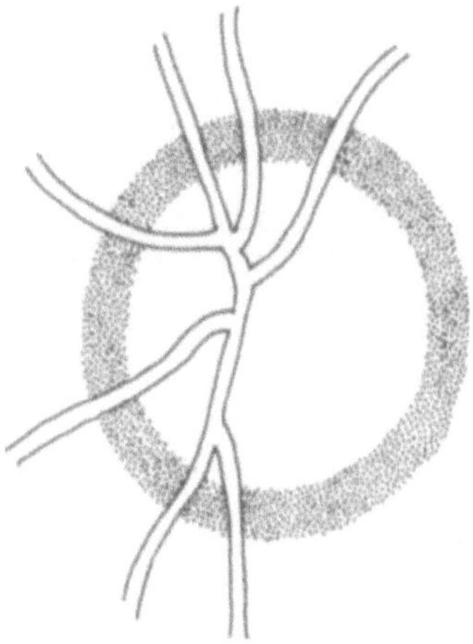

Figure 4. Suspicious optic nerve. The cup occupies substantially more than half the horizontal or vertical diameter of the disc. This could be a normal finding or could represent symmetrical acquired damage.

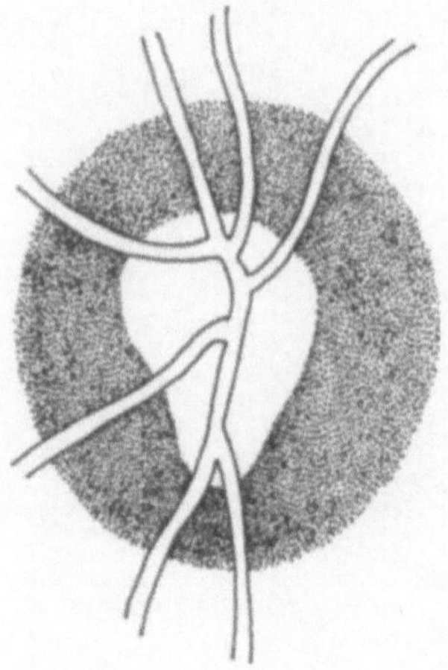

Figure 5. Abnormal optic nerve. The optic cup is notched toward the inferior rim of the disc.

costs approximately $750. The use of either of these tonometers requires a modest amount of training, but each instrument can be used accurately by a technician. A practitioner who chooses to perform tonometry should ask an ophthalmologist to teach him/her to use the instrument. Sterilization procedures between use are not difficult. Despite the overreferrals that will result, patients with a pressure above 22 mm Hg should be sent to an ophthalmologist. As noted earlier, all patients with abnormal nerves should be referred.

There is no information about the sensitivity or specificity of glaucoma screening performed as suggested here. Nonetheless, it seems reasonable and is unlikely to hurt patients in any way.

2.5. Corticosteroids and Glaucoma

One of the few preventable types of glaucoma is that associated with corticosteroid use. Topical corticosteroids delivered to the eye or skin as well as oral corticosteroids can cause an intraocular pressure rise that is indistinguishable from primary open-angle

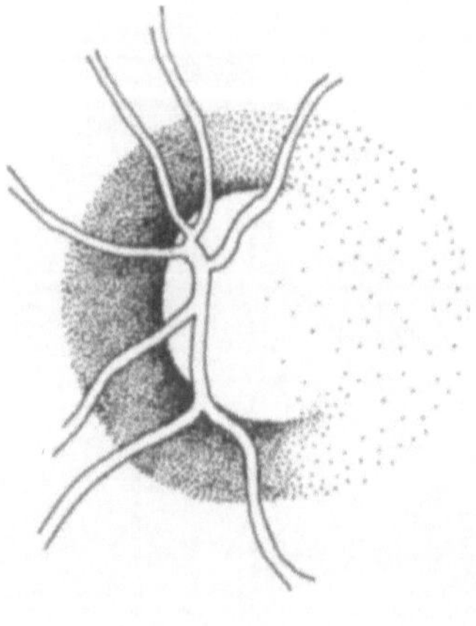

Figure 6. Suspicious optic nerve. The rim is not symmetrical all around, but one margin is sloped or flattened. This may occur normally or may be an acquired defect.

glaucoma in its effects. A marked pressure elevation following steroid use is more common in individuals with a family history of glaucoma than in the general population but it may occur in anyone. Nonophthalmologists should not prescribe corticosteroid eyedrops, and all patients who are being treated with oral or parenteral corticosteroids for more than a month should be followed in conjunction with an ophthalmologist. If topical corticosteroids are being applied to the face for more than a few weeks, such patients should also be referred for ophthalmological examination and follow-up. Topical corticosteroids applied to the skin away from the face have been reported to cause glaucoma only when used in substantial amounts for extended periods.

The pressure-raising effect of corticosteroids can occur at any stage in the use of the drugs, and such patients need to be followed for as long as they are being treated. Corticosteroid-induced glaucoma responds to ordinary glaucoma medications, so that if the steroids cannot be discontinued, a patient may nonetheless be helped by referral.

2.6. Costs

The cost of a history and fundus examination without a referral to an ophthalmologist is minimal, as physicians generally take histories and look in the eyes. Each referral to an ophthalmologist will probably cost at least $100, and one can probably expect at least 10 referrals per patient who is found to have glaucoma. Thus, case finding is expensive. Although it has not been proven that the early diagnosis of glaucoma decreases the economic impact of the disease, it seems worthwhile for the individual patient whose sight may be preserved.

3. DIABETIC RETINOPATHY

The incidence of diabetic retinopathy correlates directly with the duration of the disease. As the general medical care and thus the lifespan of diabetic patients improve, the problem of diabetic retinopathy increases. About 5000 patients become blind each year from diabetic retinopathy, and a total of perhaps 35,000 or so Americans are legally blind from the condition.[1] Many more have visual disability from the condition. Fortunately, panretinal photocoagulation has been well documented to decrease the incidence of substantial vision loss in both moderate and advanced retinopathy.[6,7] Treatment is easier and more successful if undertaken early, but retinopathy can at times be far advanced and at times associated with untreatable neovascular glaucoma by the time a patient notices symptoms. Internists doing direct fundoscopy can easily miss significant diabetic retinopathy.[8] Thus to prevent blindness from this condition early referral to an ophthalmologist is necessary.

It is currently recommended that any diabetic with a visual complaint be seen by an ophthalmologist. Any diabetic in whom any evidence of diabetic retinopathy is noted on fundus examination should be examined by an ophthalmologist. Patients with type 1 (juvenile-onset) diabetes should be seen by an ophthalmologist after 5 years and yearly thereafter; patients with type 2 diabetes should have a baseline examination at the time of diagnosis and an examination yearly thereafter.[9]

4. AMBLYOPIA

Amblyopia is a reduction in visual acuity related to inadequate visual experience during childhood. In order to develop good vision, the retina must receive a focused image so that the appropriate interneural connections can develop to allow clear vision. The most frequent treatable causes of amplyopia are crossed eyes and markedly unequal refractive errors. Amblyopia usually affects only one eye and does not cause legal blindness in the absence of a problem with the fellow eye. The frequency of significant amblyopia is not certain, but recent studies suggest that 1% or 2% of the population has vision in one eye below 20/40 (usual driving vision) in one eye, much of it presumably on the basis of ambyopia.[2]

Physicians who treat children should test visual acuity in their young patients before the age of 5. Children tend to peek, and the eye not being tested should be thoroughly and carefully covered. A letter, picture, number, or illiterate ''E'' chart at the end of a 20-ft hall with good light will suffice. Any child who has vision in either eye of less than 20/40 should be seen by an ophthalmologist. Not all causes of decreased vision in children can be successfully treated, but many children can be helped to develop reading and driving vision in an eye that would otherwise be of only limited use.

5. INJURY PREVENTION

Like amblyopia, ocular injuries rarely cause blindness, at least initially, because most injuries are unilateral. At least one million people are visually impaired in one or both eyes because of injuries.[1] Home injuries are more common than workplace injuries, perhaps because of enforcement of eye protection requirements by employers.[10] Not all accidents are preventable, but many eye injuries can be avoided by the wearing of appropriate protective eyewear. Carpentry injuries, home workshop injuries, sports injuries, and chemical injuries can often be avoided. As with other aspects of blindness prevention, the general rationale is that it is better to have two eyes than one. Moreover, virtually any eye injury, however minor, will end up costing more than a pair of protective lenses.[10]

Lens materials vary widely. Ordinary glass lenses are a very poor protection against trauma. The most appropriate material currently available is coated polycarbonate plastic. In a 2-mm central thickness such a lens is probably adequate for tennis, but a 3-mm central thickness mounted in a sports frame is probably a more appropriate recommendation for racket sports, as it is recommended for high-velocity sports such as racketball or squash. The 3-mm lenses in a sturdy frame with side shields or in the form of goggles is recommended for carpentry, power tool use, work with chemicals, and similar conditions with a high possibility of injury.[11]

Polycarbonate is also available in a one-piece, injection-molded wraparound lens/frame combination without correction, which can be used by people who do not require glasses or who wear contact lenses.[11]

Some prescription lenses are not available in polycarbonate, and for such patients a 3-mm CR-39 plastic lens in a sports frame is recommended.[11]

REFERENCES

1. National Society to Prevent Blindness: *Vision problems in the U.S.: Data analysis: Definitions, data sources, detailed data tables, analysis, interpretation.* National Society to Prevent Blindness, New York, 1980.
2. Kruger, D. E., Ederer, F., and NVAIS Project Team: *Report on the National Eye Institute's Visual Acuity Impairment Survey Pilot Study.* United States Government Printing Office, Washington, DC, 1984.
3. Leske, M. C., and Rosenthal, J.: Epidemiologic aspects of open-angle glaucoma. *Am. J. Epidemiol.* **109**:250–272, 1979.
4. Pollack, I. P.: The challenge of glaucoma screening. *Surv. Ophthalmol.* **4**:4–22, 1968.
5. Michaelson, I. C., and Berman, E. R. (eds.): *Causes and Prevention of Blindness.* Proceedings of the Jerusalem seminar on the prevention of blindness. Academic Press, New York/London, 1971.
6. The Diabetic Retinopathy Study Research Group: Preliminary report on effects of photocoagulation therapy. *Am. J. Ophthalmol.* **81**:383–396, 1976.
7. Early Treatment Diabetic Retinopathy Study Research Group: Photocoagulation for diabetic macular edema: Early treatment diabetic retinopathy study report number 1. *Arch. Ophthalmol.* **103**:1796–1806, 1985.
8. Sussman, E. J., Tsiaras, W. G., and Soper, K. A.: Diagnosis of diabetic eye disease. *JAMA* **247**:3231–3234, 1982.
9. Early Treatment Diabetic Retinopathy Study Research Group: Photocoagulation therapy for diabetic eye disease. *JAMA* **254**:3086, 1985.
10. Cohen, G. R., and Zaidman, G. W.: Work-related eye injuries. *Ann. Ophthalmol.* **18**:19–21, 1986.
11. Vinger, P. F.: The eye and sports medicine, in Duane, T. D. (ed.): *Clinical Ophthalmology,* Vol. 5. Harper & Row, Philadelphia, revised 1985.

20

Health Advice for International Travelers

Robert P. Smith, Jr., and James A. Wolff, Jr.

1. INTRODUCTION

Nearly 20 million Americans embark on international travel each year. Five million of these travelers visit undeveloped areas of the world with unfamiliar health hazards. Numerous vacationers participate in adventurous travel involving back-country treks, rafting trips, or natural-history tours that often result in exposure to food-, water-, or insect-borne infections. Unfortunately, many of these travelers are poorly prepared for the particular health risks common to these areas. For example, fewer than half of American travelers to malarious areas use appropriate malaria prophylaxis.[1] As a result, imported malaria and other infectious diseases of travelers have increased dramatically in the past decade.

Because of the growing public awareness of travel-related health problems, primary-care physicians and other health care providers are often asked to provide advice on appropriate immunizations, malaria prophylaxis, and other measures to protect the travelers' health. This chapter reviews the epidemiological data on travelers' illnesses and outlines the appropriate preventive strategies. Because travel between industrialized nations is rarely associated with unique health problems, our focus is on the traveler to developing countries, most of which are in the tropics.

2. EPIDEMIOLOGY OF TRAVEL-ASSOCIATED ILLNESS

The risk of illness during international travel depends on the itinerary, the nature of travel, and its duration. A tourist staying at a Caribbean resort is at relatively little risk of illness compared to a health care worker from the United States on a temporary assignment to a Haitian hospital. Similarly, businessmen attending a conference in a large city in

Robert P. Smith, Jr. • Department of Medicine, Dartmouth–Hitchcock Medical Center, Hanover, New Hampshire 03756. *James A. Wolff, Jr.* • Management Sciences for Health, Boston, Massachusetts 02130.

the developing world are at small risk of illness compared to back-country hikers in the same country.

Data on morbidity rates among tropical travelers are limited, but a high frequency of minor illness seems evident. One questionnaire study of U.S. travelers returning from short trips to the tropics demonstrated that 4% of travelers consulted a physician while abroad, and 0.5% were hospitalized.[2] Similar data from a Swiss study of 10,500 tropical travelers documented a 75% rate of illness during their brief (< 1 month) trip.[3] This was twice the rate of illness reported by a similar group of Swiss travelers to the United States and Canada. The commonly reported illnesses were minor ones, such as diarrhea, constipation, upper-respiratory infection, and skin ailments. However, 4% of these tropical travelers were confined to bed for at least a day, and 7% reported recurrent illness during the following year. Recent Finnish and British studies reveal similar results.[4,5]

Rates of more serious illness are also on the rise. For example, the Centers for Disease Control (CDC) reports that attack rates of *Plasmodium falciparum* malaria among U.S. tourists to East Africa increased from 20/100,000 travelers to 80/100,000 travelers between 1978 and 1983.[6] Other serious infections, such as hepatitis A, occur in unprotected travelers to Africa and South America at 500 times the expected rate in the United States. Amebiasis, typhoid fever, and schistosomiasis account for significant morbidity and occasional mortality in a small number of U.S. travelers to the tropics.[7]

A recent report on mortality in U.S. Peace Corps volunteers from 1962 to 1983 showed that accidental deaths outnumbered deaths from other causes by a ratio of 4:1.[8] One-third of all deaths among Peace Corps volunteers were attributable to motor vehicle accidents. The remainder of accidental deaths resulted from drownings, plane crashes, and a variety of other causes. Infectious diseases accounted for 25% of the mortality, with malaria leading the list. Surprisingly, the overall death rate abroad did not differ substantially from the expected death rate among U.S. citizens in the same age group, a finding that may reflect the health of the group chosen for Peace Corps work. Unlike most U.S. tourists, Peace Corps volunteers receive careful health preparations prior to their travel, and this effort appears to have decreased their morbidity from infectious diseases.[9]

3. HOW TO FIND HEALTH INFORMATION FOR TRAVELERS

The traveler's regular health provider is the usual source for pretravel advice and immunizations. A well-informed physician or nurse can best assess the needs of a particular traveler and then provide tailored recommendations. Unfortunately, most primary-care physicians are not well informed on the risks and benefits of the recommended and required immunizations, the need for malaria prophylaxis, or other precautions. Many patients receive bad advice; others seek advice from state health departments, which provide up-to-date public health information but are ignorant of the traveler's medical history.

Several sources of health information for travelers are available to physicians. The CDC publishes an excellent handbook, *Health Information for International Travel*, that is revised annually.[10] *The Morbidity and Mortality Weekly Report* provides a continuous update on these recommendations. State health departments usually can provide current immunization recommendations, and some medical centers have initiated specialized travelers' clinics which provide health advice and immunizations. Other organizations, such as the International Association for Medical Assistance to Travelers, provide health advice and names of English-speaking doctors in the countries on the tourists' itinerary. Office physicians with computer access may purchase a continuously updated software program that prints out medical requirements and recommendations by country.

4. PRETRIP EVALUATION

Physicians should encourage a pretrip office visit by their patients to review current medical problems, to assure an adequate supply of essential medications, and to counsel the patient regarding necessary immunizations, malaria prophylaxis, and other preventive measures. This visit should be planned at least 6 weeks prior to departure to tropical areas to allow adequate time for scheduling vaccinations.

Physicians should tailor their advice to persons with chronic disease to the particular individual's health status and the demands of the planned trip. Patients with severe cardiopulmonary disease, diabetes mellitus, and those on anticholinergic drugs are at increased risk of heat illness.[11] However, with judicious planning, these need not be reasons to avoid travel to hot climates. Insulin-dependent diabetics may need to modify their insulin regimen, taking into account changes in time zones and daily activities. The American Diabetes Association provides a pamphlet with specific suggestions.[12] Travelers with gastric achlorhydria, including patients on cimetidine or antacids, are at increased risk of serious enteric infection and may benefit from prophylactic antibiotics.[13] Splenectomized travelers to malarious areas should avoid mosquito exposure and be meticulous in taking antimalarial prophylaxis because they are at high risk of developing overwhelming parasitemia if infected.

Pregnant women planning tropical travel can safely take chloroquine, but they should avoid other antimalarials for prophylaxis. These women should not receive live viral vaccines or particular killed bacterial vaccines (cholera, typhoid) that can cause febrile reactions. Iodine-purified water should be avoided by pregnant women because it can cause congenital hypothyroidism in the newborn infant.[14] Boiled or chlorine-treated water should be used instead.

Most travelers to the tropics benefit from a review of common-sense precautions regarding food, water, and climate (Table I). A small medical kit (Table II) is often appropriate if extensive travel is planned, given the difficulty in obtaining familiar medications in certain countries. A handout summarizing the treatment of travelers' diarrhea (Table VII, VIII) is also appropriate.

More thorough preparations for prolonged travel (e.g., Peace Corps volunteers, foreign aid workers) should include a careful physical examination, dental examination, tuberculin skin test, and contingency plans for medical assistance abroad.

5. MEDICAL ASPECTS OF AIR TRAVEL

Jet travel poses a small risk to patients with severe cardiopulmonary disease because cabin pressures in high-altitude aircraft are similar to pressures at 5000–8000 ft above

Table I. Handout for Travelers to the Tropics[a]

1.	Avoid all untreated water, including ice.
	Safe water: boiled 10 minutes or treated with one of the following:
	Iodine tablets (1/quart, allow 30 min)
	2% Tincture of iodine (5 drops/qt, allow 30 min)
	Probably safe: sealed bottled water
2.	Carbonated soft drinks, beer, coffee, tea, undiluted fruit juice, and pasteurized milk are safe to drink.
3.	Avoid fresh leafy vegetables or raw vegetables unless known to be carefully washed in treated water. Eat only fruits you can peel or slice yourself.
4.	Avoid undercooked or "buffet style" meats, fish, shellfish. Eat well-cooked food served hot.
5.	Avoid dairy products in rural areas (milk, ice cream, soft cheese) unless known to be pasteurized.
6.	Use a diethyltoluamide-containing insect repellant when mosquitos are active.
7.	Swim with care. Inquire about undertow at ocean beaches and bilharzia (schistosomiasis) in freshwater lakes and streams.
8.	Avoid over-the-counter drugs unless you know what they are. Avoid drug injections for minor illness.
9.	Remember to take your malaria pills as prescribed.
10.	Check your health insurance policy to assure coverage abroad.

[a]Source: Smith.[46]

sealevel. Any travelers with severe cardiopulmonary disease or with homozygous sickle cell disease should have supplemental oxygen available by prior arrangement.[15] They should also be cautioned to avoid small, unpressurized aircraft.

As cabin pressure decreases, gas trapped in body cavities expands and can lead to various forms of barotrauma affecting the sinus cavities, ears, or abdomen. For this reason, air travel is contraindicated in patients who have had abdominal surgery within the previous 10 days.

Infants are particularly susceptible to otalgia during takeoff and landing. This can be prevented by giving the infant a bottle during these times. The constant sucking opens the eustachian tube and equalizes middle-ear pressures. Adults with sinus congestion should take an oral decongestant one-half hour prior to departure and use a nasal decongestant just before takeoff. Because "the bends" or decompression sickness can be precipitated by air travel too soon after a deep scuba dive, flying should be postponed for 12–24 hr after diving.

6. IMMUNIZATIONS

Immunizations against infectious diseases (i.e., cholera, yellow fever) are sometimes *required* for entry into foreign countries. The vaccinations required for each traveler can be checked by consulting the requirements listed annually in *Health Information for International Travel*.

Other immunizations, although not required, are *recommended* on the basis of risk of exposure. There is little argument about the benefit of an overdue tetanus–diphtheria booster, but the value of typhoid, poliomyelitis, cholera, and yellow fever vaccines varies with the proposed itinerary. All too often, appropriate immunizations are neglected be-

Table II. Traveler's Medical Kit[a]

Prescription items	
Antimalarial	Chloroquine phosphate (plus pyrimethamine–sulfadoxine if indicated)
Antibiotic	Trimethoprim–sulfamethoxizole (160 mg/800 mg) or tetracycline (500-mg tablets) for empirical treatment of severe diarrhea or urinary-tract infection
	Erythromycin (250-mg tablets) for severe respiratory or soft tissue infections
Antihistamine	Diphenhydramine (Benadryl) for systemic allergy (urticaria, etc.); can also be used as a soporific
Antimotion sickness	Meclizine (Antivert, 25 mg) or transdermal scopolamine for prevention of motion sickness
Antinausea remedy	Prochlorperazine (Compazine, 25-mg rectal suppositories) for severe nausea, vomiting
Antispasmodic	Loperamide (Imodium) for treatment of diarrhea and abdominal cramps with turista, should not be used for dysentery
For rapid ascent to high altitude	Acetazolamide (Diamox), 250-mg or 500-mg sustained-release b.i.d. 2 days prior to ascent and for 2–3 days after arrival at high altitude
Nonprescription items	
Aspirin or acetaminophen (Tylenol)	For treatment of minor arthralgias, febrile illness
Antibiotic ointment (Bacitracin, Neosporin, etc.)	For use on cuts and abrasions
Bismuth subsalicylate (Pepto-Bismol)	8-oz. liquid bottle for treatment of turista
Decongestant	Pseudephedrine preparation—a nasal spray decongestant may be helpful prior to air travel with a cold
0.5% Hydrocortisone skin cream (Cort-Aid)	For sunburn, insect bites, contact dermatitis
Sunscreen	(5% PABA as ingredient) and sunblocker (# 15 rating)
Iodine water purification tablets	Potable Aqua, Globaline, Coughlan's
Insect repellant	Containing diethyltoluamide
Glucose–electrolyte powder	Powdered mix for replacement of fluid losses
Povodone–Iodine liquid (Betadine)	For cleansing dirty cuts
Antifungal foot powder	Tinactin, Desitin
Moleskin	
Bandaids, sterile gauze and adhesive tape, ace bandage, and scissors	

[a]Source: Smith.[46]

Table III. Vaccinations Available for Protection of the Tropical Traveler[a]

Routine vaccinations that should be up-to-date for all travelers	
	Diphtheria–tetanus (booster every 10 years)
	Measles[b]
	Mumps[b]
	Rubella[b]
	Poliomyelitis[b] (booster every 5 years for those traveling to rural areas of developing countries)
Sometimes required for international travel	
	Cholera (valid for 6 months)
	Yellow fever[b] (valid for 10 years)
Often recommended for tropical travel to rural areas	
	Typhoid (booster every 3 years)
	Immunoglobulin for hepatitis A prophylaxis (renew every 3–6 months, depending on dose)
Vaccines for special circumstances	
	Rabies [human diploid cell vaccine (HDCV) booster every 2 years]
	Meningococcal
	Plague
	Hepatitis B
Discontinued or unavailable	
	Smallpox
	Typhus
	Japanese B encephalitis

[a]Source: Smith.[46]
[b]Live attenuated viral vaccine.

cause they are not a requirement for international travel. Table III summarizes the array of immunizations available for protection of the tropical traveler.

It is preferred to schedule vaccinations over several weeks to limit the side effects, which may be additive when multiple vaccinations are given on the same day. However, travelers commonly fail to leave enough time for orderly completion of their vaccinations before departure. In that case, immunizations can be given at separate sites, and up to three live vaccines or a live vaccine and a killed vaccine can be administered on the same day. Cholera and yellow-fever vaccinations should be given at least 3 weeks apart when possible, but they can be administered on the same day if necessary. Immune globulin should not be given prior to live attenuated vaccines as it may interfere with an effective immune response. If possible, immune globulin should be given no sooner than 14 days after live vaccines. Yellow-fever vaccine can be obtained only at a limited number of officially designated centers, which may give the vaccination only once or twice a month. For this reason, health providers should direct their patients to these sites well in advance of departure.

6.1. Routine Vaccinations

Travelers should update their routine vaccinations such as diphtheria–tetanus prior to departure. Individuals in a susceptible age group (birth date prior to 1956) without a history of measles or live measles vaccination should be immunized, as imported measles is a major impediment to the national goal of measles eradication. If there is no history of rubella or mumps immunity, a combined measles–mumps–rubella vaccine is recommended. Influenza and pneumothorax vaccinations should not be forgotten for prospective travelers who meet the usual indications for these vaccines.

Most U.S. adults have received complete immunizations to poliomyelitis with either the inactivated (Salk) or oral (Sabin) live vaccines. However, decreased immunity in adults is not unusual. As poliomyelitis is endemic (and epidemic) in most of the developing world, poliomyelitis boosters every 5 years are recommended for tropical travel, particularly if the trip includes close contact with local populations. Because of the remote risk of vaccine-acquired poliomyelitis (1/3,000,000) with oral vaccine, the inactivated (Salk) vaccine is preferable in previously unvaccinated or partially vaccinated adults. Oral poliomyelitis vaccine should not be given to pregnant women or to immunosuppressed patients or family members of these patients. These individuals should receive the inactivated vaccine. Travelers who are either unvaccinated or unsure of their vaccination status should follow the recommendations in Table IV.[16]

6.2. Vaccines Sometimes Required

6.2.1. Yellow Fever

Although seldom required for entry to equatorial countries, yellow-fever vaccine is recommended for all travelers to the endemic zone in Central and South America, Africa, and Trinidad, with the possible exception of brief travel restricted to large urban areas. Urban yellow fever has not occurred in decades in the Americas but is possible because of the presence of the vector mosquitos in cities. The highest-risk areas are lowland rainforests in continental South America and Panama and the forest–savannah interface in equatorial Africa.[17] The CDC provides weekly updates on areas of reported yellow fever, but substantial underreporting is likely. Yellow-fever vaccine is an effective, safe, attenuated, live-virus vaccine that confers immunity for at least 10 years. Mild reactions (sore arm, low-grade fever, headache) occur in 1–5% of those who receive the vaccine.

Table IV. Poliomyelitis Vaccination (Unknown Immunization Status or No Prior Vaccination)[a]

Time until departure	Vaccine criteria
< 1 month	One dose OPV[b]
> 1 month but < 2 months	Two doses IPV[c] 1. Now 2. 1 month later
2–7 months	Three doses IPV 1. Now 2. 1 month later 3. 1 month later
> 8 months	Full four doses IPV Primary series

[a]Modified from Mann *et al.*[16]
[b]OPV, oral poliomyelitis vaccine.
[c]IPV, inactivated poliomyelitis vaccine.

Although yellow-fever vaccine is well tolerated, it should not be given to infants less than 6 months old because they are at risk of vaccine-associated encephalitis, and the vaccine is contraindicated in patients with immune deficiencies and in pregnant women. Yellow-fever vaccine is grown in chick embryos and is also contraindicated in persons with egg allergy. In countries in which yellow fever is not endemic, the vaccination requirement for infants, pregnant women, and allergic individuals may be omitted if the traveler has a letter of explanation signed by a physician.

6.2.2. Cholera

The killed vaccine for cholera is not very effective and is usually advised only to satisfy immigration authorities. A single dose will suffice for this purpose. Although rarely required on entry to another country from the United States, it is often required when travelers cross between cholera-endemic countries. Travelers are at very low risk of contracting cholera (1/500,000) unless given to indiscrete dietary habits in the midst of an epidemic.[18] A British study estimated that five million dollars in vaccination costs would be required for each case of cholera prevented among travelers to cholera-endemic areas.[19] Complete cholera immunization (two doses in the primary series) might be considered for U.S. health care workers in a cholera-endemic area and for persons with gastric achlorhydria. The vaccine is not recommended in pregnancy or for children less than 6 months old.

6.3. Vaccines Often Recommended for Tropical Travel

6.3.1. Typhoid

Most cases of typhoid among U.S. travelers are acquired in India and Mexico.[20] Attack rates among European travelers range from 1/15000 cases per journey in parts of Asia and West Africa to 1/900,000 in Southern Europe.[7] Risks are highest in children, the elderly, or those with close contact with local populations. All travelers to areas off the usual tourist routes in the developing world are at risk of typhoid exposure through contaminated food and water, and vaccination is recommended. The current vaccine, though 70–90% effective, requires two immunizations a month apart for the primary series and a booster dose every 3 years. Local reactions to vaccination (a sore arm) and low-grade fever are common. A more effective and better-tolerated oral typhoid vaccine is currently under study.

6.3.2. Passive Immunization Against Hepatitis A

Immune globulin provides passive protection against hepatitis A for 3–6 months, depending on the dose administered. Hepatitis A is prevalent in most tropical and developing areas of the world as well as the Mediterranean littoral. A study of missionaries working abroad revealed a risk of symptomatic hepatitis A of 1–5/100 person-years of exposure.[21] Higher attack rates might be expected in groups of travelers whose exposure to contaminated food and water is greater. For the short-term traveler to Western-style hotels and resorts, the risk of hepatitis A is small and prophylaxis may be omitted. For prolonged residence (3 months or more) in countries with poor sanitation, hepatitis immune globulin injection may be warranted. For continuous protection, the injection must be repeated every 6 months. Travelers with extensive experience in developing countries may choose to check their immune status to hepatitis A. If serology is positive, immune globulin prophylaxis is unnecessary.

6.4. Vaccines for Special Circumstances

6.4.1. Rabies

Rabies is prevalent in domestic and wild animals in Africa, Latin America, and the Indian subcontinent. Peace Corps volunteers, anthropologists, biologists, and others planning prolonged residence in an endemic area should consider pretrip immunization with three doses of human diploid cell vaccine (HDCV). Although postexposure immunization is still required in the event of a bite, the pretrip vaccination provides some protection to the person with unsuspected exposure or who is unable to get immediate medical attention. It also simplifies postexposure management. Immunization, given by either intradermal or intramuscular route, requires a booster dose every 2 years. The HDCV vaccine, though expensive, is well tolerated and more effective than its predecessor, the duck embryo vaccine. However, serum sickness–like reactions have been reported in 5% of vaccines following booster doses of HDCV vaccine.[22] Antibody titers after preexposure vaccination are unnecessary. However, rabies immunization should be completed prior to chloroquine prophylaxis, which has been shown to interfere with the antibody response.[23] Physicians must alert all travelers to the developing world that any bite or scratch from an animal will require postexposure vaccination for treatment of rabies exposure.

6.4.2. Meningococcal Disease

Sub-Saharan Africa experiences annual (dry season) meningococcal epidemics, usually due to group A meningococcus. Visitors planning prolonged residence or involvement in health care in these countries may benefit from pretrip vaccination with meningococcal vaccine. Trekkers and other back-country visitors to India and Nepal should also consider vaccination with meningococcal vaccine because of recent reports of meningococcal outbreaks in these areas.

6.4.3. Plague

Plague vaccine is rarely indicated for travelers, with the exception of those planning prolonged residence in mountainous areas of rural Africa, Asia, or South America, when contact with wild rodents and their fleas is likely.

6.4.4. Hepatitis B

Hepatitis B prevalence is many times higher in South America, Africa, and Asia than it is in the United States. Therefore, all health care workers on assignment in these areas should be vaccinated against this virus. Since venereal transmission is possible, hepatitis B vaccine may be advisable in any nonimmune visitor anticipating immersion in local daily life. Travelers who are unable to complete the full three-dose series may benefit from two doses, which will provide 80–90% immunity.

6.5. *Discontinued or Unavailable Vaccines*

Smallpox vaccine is contraindicated to travelers due to global eradication of the disease (last case 1977) and the risk of vaccine-related illness. It is no longer required for entry into any country.

Reports of typhus acquired during travel are so rare that vaccine is no longer produced in the United States or Canada.

Travelers to the Far East occasionally inquire about protection against Japanese B encephalitis, an arboviral disease endemic to much of Asia, Nepal, and the western Pacific. Although vaccines are in use in Japan and China, they are currently available in the United States only on an experimental basis. Individuals with high risk of mosquito exposure in rural areas of the Far East (during June to October in temperate climates) can obtain the vaccine through limited distribution sites in the United States or at the U.S. Embassy in their destination country.

7. *MALARIA PROPHYLAXIS*

There has been a marked increase in travel-acquired malaria among Americans during the last decade. This is largely due to a resurgence of malaria in the developing world and to increased travel to these areas by unprotected tourists. Nearly 3000 U.S. citizens have acquired malaria while traveling abroad in the past decade.[24] The CDC's *Health Information for International Travel* provides extensive up-to-date information on malaria risk by locale and time of year. All travelers to malarious areas, even for a brief trip, should take antimalarial medication (Fig. 1).

Chloroquine remains the cornerstone of malaria prophylaxis. It is safe, cheap, well tolerated, and effective against most strains of malaria. Chloroquine is taken weekly (300 mg base or 500 mg chloroquine phosphate) for 1 or 2 weeks prior to entry into a malarious zone and is then continued during the stay and for 6 weeks after departure from the malarious area. Side effects (rash, hair loss) are rare. Retinopathy does not occur unless prophylaxis is continued for more than 5 years.[25,26] Hydroxychloroquine sulfate may be substituted for chloroquine if side effects occur (see Table V). Amodiaquine, another antimalarial, should no longer be used for prophylaxis because of recent reports of agranulocytosis associated with its use.[27]

Some areas of the world are host to strains of chloroquine-resistant *P. falciparum* malaria (see Table VI). Given the serious consequences of *P. falciparum* infection, a second antimalarial drug, pyrimethamine–sulfadoxine (Fansidar), in addition to chloroquine, had been recommended, until recently, for travelers to these areas. However, new information on the frequency of allergic Stevens–Johnson syndrome and fatal toxic epidermal necrolysis from Fansidar makes continued use of this agent for *P. falciparum* prophylaxis problematic. For many travelers the rate of fatal allergic reactions (1/10,000–20,000) is higher than their risk of developing *P. falciparum* malaria.[28] Therefore, the use

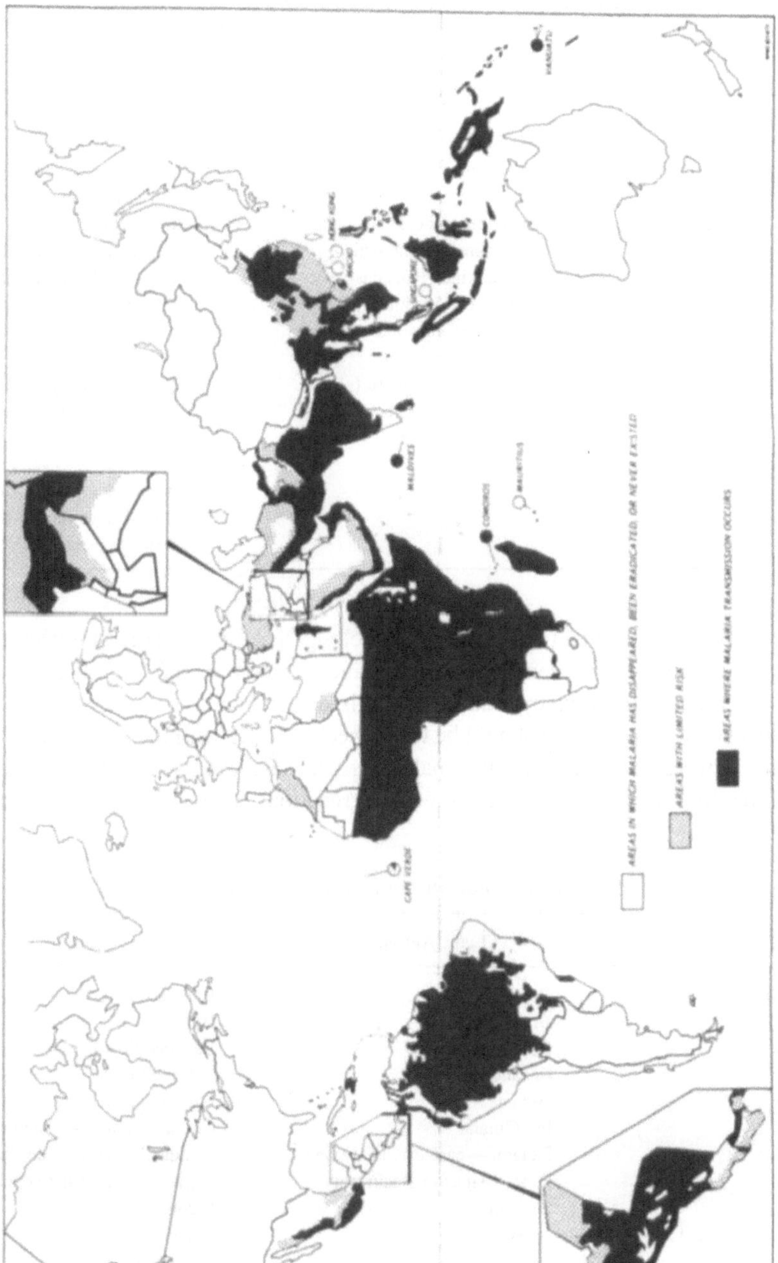

Figure 1. Epidemiological assessment of status of malaria, 1981. (Source: *Health Information for International Travel.*[47])

Table V. Malaria Chemoprophylaxis

Indication	Drug	Dose
1. All malarious areas, except those with chloroquine-resistant strains of *P. falciparum*	Chloroquine phosphate Alternates: Hydroxychloroquine Proguanil	Adult: 500 mg p.o. every week Pediatric: 8.3 mg/kg per week (not to exceed 500 mg total dose per week)
2. Areas with chloroquine-resistant *P. falciparum* if very high risk of malaria exposure is anticipated (greater than 3 weeks exposure anticipated)	Chloroquine phosphate plus pyrimethamine–sulfadoxine (Fansidar) (see text for caution with regard to Fansidar use)	Adult: As above plus 25 mg pyrimethamine and 500 mg sulfadoxine (1 tablet) every week
3. Terminal prophylaxis for individuals at heavy risk of malaria exposure	Primaquine phosphate (r/o G-6-PD deficiency first)	Adult: 26.3 mg/day for 14 days during last 2 weeks of chloroquine prophylaxis Pediatric: 0.5 mg/kg per day for 14 days (not to exceed 26.3 mg/day)

of Fansidar should be restricted to travelers with prolonged exposure (at least 3 weeks) in areas known to have high incidences of chloroquine-resistant *P. falciparum* infection. Alternative regimens using doxycycline prophylaxis or proguanil (Paludrine) are under study. If Fansidar is prescribed, it should be taken weekly along with the chloroquine and continued for 6 weeks after leaving the malarious area. Patients should be warned to discontinue the drug at the earliest sign of allergic reaction, such as skin rash or mouth

Table VI. Areas with Chloroquine-Resistant Malaria (1985)[a]

Africa	Latin America	Asia
Central African Republic	Bolivia	Bangladesh
Comoros	Brazil	Burma
Kenya	Colombia	Lao People's Democratic Republic
Madagascar	Ecuador	India—isolated areas
Malawi	Guyana	China—Southern China and areas bordering Lao People's Democratic Republic
Mozambique	Fr. Guiana	Indonesia
Rwanda	Panama—east of Canal zone	Malaysia
Tanzania	Peru—Amazon Basin only	Philippines
Uganda	Suriname	Papua New Guinea
Zaire (eastern provinces)	Venezuela	Solomon Islands
Zimbabwe		Thailand
		Vietnam

[a]Adapted from Centers for Disease Control.[10]

blisters. No traveler with a previous reaction to sulfa drugs should take Fansidar. Short-term (< 3 weeks) travelers to areas with high rates of chloroquine resistance may choose to take with them a treatment dose of Fansidar (three tablets) to use in the event of high fever if prompt medical evaluation is not possible. Some areas of the world (Thailand–Cambodia border) harbor chloroquine and Fansidar-resistant *P. falciparum* malaria. In these areas regimens of tetracycline, mefloquine, or quinine may be useful.

Individuals with intense exposure to malaria during a prolonged stay should consider the addition of primaquine (15 mg base/day for 14 days) at the end of their period of exposure. Primaquine eradicates latent *P. vivax* or *P. ovale* malaria parasites in the liver that are merely suppressed by chloroquine. Primaquine candidates should be screened for G-6-PD deficiency prior to its use. Terminal prophylaxis with primaquine is not necessary for short-term visitors to the tropics.

Malaria is a special risk to the mother and fetus during pregnancy, and all pregnant women are urged to take chloroquine prophylaxis during travel to malarious areas. Primaquine, however, should not be given until after delivery. Fansidar is not recommended for use during pregnancy because of potential pyrimethamine toxicity to the fetus. If a pregnant woman must travel to an area with resistant *P. falciparum* malaria, the small risk of pyrimethamine toxicity can be minimized by the addition of folinic acid supplements.[29]

In addition to chemoprophylaxis, travelers to malarious areas should use diethyltoluamide insect repellants when out at dawn or dusk and a mosquito net if sleeping in an unscreened dwelling.

8. COMMON-SENSE PRECAUTIONS WHILE TRAVELING

Many tropical travelers are unaware of simple health precautions. Physicians should briefly review these "rules of the road" at the pretrip office visit. In addition, a handout (Tables I, II) or a more detailed pamphlet such as *Health Hints for the Tropics*[30] can be provided.

8.1. Water

Tap water (including ice) in the developing world is often contaminated with enteric organisms despite testimonials to its safety by local authorities. It is best to avoid drinking water unless it is purified by 10 min of boiling or by chemical treatment. Water filters are unreliable. Iodine tablets (Potable Aqua, Globaline) or 2% tincture of iodine is more effective than chlorine (Halazone tablets) against protozoan cysts. Cold or turbid water will require longer treatment with iodide or chlorine than clear, warm water. Bottled water, if carbonated and sealed, is generally safe, as are carbonated soft drinks, beer, and undiluted fruit drinks.

8.2. Food

Although exotic cuisine is one of the delights of travel, the wise tourist will limit his intake of certain foods. Raw fruits and vegetables often harbor enteric parasites. Night soil is widely used, and untreated water is used to "freshen" produce. Therefore, fresh salads must be avoided, and only fruits that can be peeled by the traveler (i.e., bananas, oranges, mangoes) or washed in treated water should be eaten. Rare meats are a source of toxoplasmosis, trichinosis, and tapeworm and should therefore be avoided. Inadequately cooked pork is responsible for several possible enteric infections as well as hepatitis A. Dairy products may be unsafe in rural areas where milk is not pasteurized. They may lead to infections such as *Campylobacter* enteritis, brucellosis, or tuberculosis. Breads and canned foods are safe. In general, travelers should choose well-cooked foods served hot and ignore "buffet style" cold luncheons.

8.3. Climate

Physiological adaptation to a hot climate requires at least 2 weeks of acclimatization. Inadequate replacement of salt and water losses can lead to muscle cramps and heat exhaustion during strenuous physical exertion. Tourists should plan a gradual approach to physical activity, stay well hydrated, and salt their foods generously. Actual heat stroke is extremely rare among tourists, but the risk may be enhanced by medications with anticholinergic properties.

The effects of intense sunlight are also often underestimated. Individuals who will be regularly exposed to the sun during travel should use high-potency (#15–20) benzophenone sunscreens and lip balms, hats, and other protective clothing to assure a gradual tan. Sunscreens should be applied 0.5–1 hr prior to sun exposure and reapplied after swimming or sweating.

8.4. Altitude

Acute mountain sickness, a clinical syndrome due to incomplete adaptation to lower-atmospheric oxygen levels, is common among travelers arriving at elevations above 10,000 ft. It may occur as low as 8000 ft. Symptoms include headache, dyspnea on exertion, dizziness, nausea, and insomnia. These symptoms usually subside after 2–3 days at high altitude. Double-blind trials have demonstrated the effectiveness of acetazolamide (Diamox, 250 mg bid or 500 mg daily sustained release) in preventing acute mountain sickness. It should be given 2 days prior to arrival at high altitude and continued for 2–3 days after arrival.[31] It is not known yet whether acetazolamide can prevent the more serious and rare complications of altitude illness (pulmonary and cerebral edema) that afflict hikers and skiers at very high elevations, usually above 12,000 ft.

8.5. Traffic

Automobiles and their drivers are the greatest health hazard for the tropical traveler. Cars and drivers should be selected with care. As unlit vehicles and horse-drawn carts are common in the developing world, night driving is hazardous. Motorcycles are particularly dangerous—one-third of all motorcycles owned by Peace Corps volunteers are in an accident every year.[32]

8.6. Swimming

Undertow is a potential hazard on ocean beaches with good surf but no swimmers. Schistosomiasis is endemic in many freshwater ponds and streams in the tropics, so swimming or bathing sites should be chosen with care. Stagnant or slow-flowing streams near village washing and wading areas are particularly high-risk sites for contracting schistosomiasis. Inattention to these precautions recently led to an outbreak of acute schistosomiasis in a group of U.S. college students traveling in Kenya, with resulting myelitis in two of them.

8.7. Insects

In addition to malaria, mosquitos serve as vectors of a variety of viral and parasite diseases. Use of a diethyltoluamide-containing insect repellant is helpful. Light-colored, long-sleeved shirts and trousers should be worn at dawn and dusk, when most mosquito species are active. A mosquito net is advisable if the traveler is sleeping in an unscreened dwelling.

8.8. Animal Bites

Peace Corps statistics record a 10-fold increased incidence of animal bites in their volunteers over that expected in North America. Given the prevalence of rabies, contact with domestic animals should be limited to family pets and avoided completely if an animal appears ill. Animal bites should be washed carefully with soap and water and rabies prophylaxis obtained as soon as possible.

8.9. Medications

Potentially dangerous drugs such as chloramphenicol are sold over the counter in many developing countries. Travelers should not take medication blindly or at the suggestion of local pharmacists. They should also avoid injected drugs for mild illnesses, since the use of unsterile needles is frequent and could be the source of both hepatitis B virus and human T-cell lymphotrophic virus-III.

9. PREVENTION AND TREATMENT OF TRAVELER'S DIARRHEA

The bane of travelers from temperate zones to the tropics, traveler's diarrhea afflicts 30–50% of North Americans visiting the developing world. Enterotoxigenic *Escherichia coli* are the major cause of traveler's diarrhea, though other enteric pathogens, such as *Campylobacter, Shigella, Vibrio,* and rotavirus, may be important as well.[33]

"Turista" often begins during the first week of tropical travel and lasts 3–4 days. Abdominal cramps, nausea, and 3–15 watery bowel movements per day are typical. Dehydration is the major complication. Recurrent turista afflicts one-quarter of all travelers who remain in the tropics for more than 1 month. Although salad eaters and those adventurous enough to purchase meals from street vendors are at greatest risk, even fastidious individuals who follow the usual food and water precautions are susceptible.[34,35] Numerous regimens designed to avoid turista (e.g., yogurt) persist in travel folklore, but there are only two proven preventive approaches. The first, requiring 60 ml qid doses of bismuth subsalicylate (Pepto-Bismol), is cumbersome.[36] The second, the use of prophylactic doxycyline or trimethoprim–sulfamethoxazole (TM–SZ), puts travelers at risk of drug side effects (doxycyline: photosensitivity, vaginitis, *Candida* infection; TM–SZ: rash) and could potentiate infection by more troublesome organisms such as *Salmonella* or *Shigella*.[37,38] Resistance to tetracycline is prevalent among *E. coli* in some areas, and recent reports suggest that resistance to TM–SZ is also increasing. The effectiveness of these two drugs is thus limited.[39] Prophylactic antibiotic use should be restricted to travelers planning short stays for whom 1 or 2 days of diarrhea would pose a major problem and to other travelers with underlying illness that might be exacerbated by turista.

A preferable alternative for most travelers is to treat turista at its onset, with either bismuth subsalicylate (Pepto-Bismol), loperamide, or TM–SZ.[40–42] This will usually limit their illness to a day or 2 (Table VII). Maintaining adequate fluid intake is crucial. Travelers should carry a recipe for replacement of fluid losses, such as that advocated by the CDC (Table VIII). Electrolyte packets that can be reconstituted are available either over the counter or in pharmacies in most developing countries. Bowel antiperistalsis agents help control symptoms but do not shorten the duration of illness, and they may exacerbate incipient dysentery. Kaopectate is of no benefit. Iodohydroxy–chloroquine

Table VII. Medication for Prevention and Treatment of Traveler's Diarrhea[a]

I. Prevention of traveler's diarrhea	
Bismuth subsalicylate (Pepto-Bismol)	60 ml q.i.d.
Trimethoprim–sulfamethoxazole	160 mg TM/800 mg SZ (one double-strength tablet daily)
Doxycycline	200 mg once, then 100 mg every day (not on an empty stomach)
II. Treatment of traveler's diarrhea	
Fluid replacement (avoid dairy products)	
Bismuth subsalicylate	30 ml (1 oz) every 1/2 hour for a total of 8 doses (240 ml); may repeat on day 2
Trimethoprim–sulfamethoxazole	One double-strength tablet b.i.d. for 5 days
Trimethoprim	200 mg b.i.d. for 5 days (sulfa-allergic patient)
Loperamide (Imodium)[b]	4 mg; then 1 capsule (2 mg) after each loose movement up to 8 capsules within 24 hr
Dyphenoxylate HCI (with atropine sulfate—Lomotil)	Do not exceed 2 tablets q.i.d.

[a]Source: Smith.[46]
[b]For symptom relief only; do not use in dysentery.

Table VIII. Formula for Treatment of Diarrheal Disease[a]

Prepare 2 separate glasses of the following:	
Glass 1	
Orange, apple, or other fruit juice (rich in potassium)	8 oz
Honey or corn syrup (contains glucose necessary for absorption of essential salts)	1/4 teaspoon
Table salt (contains sodium and chloride)	1 pinch
Glass 2	
Water (carbonated or boiled)	8 oz
Baking soda (contains sodium bicarbonate)	1/4 teaspoon
Drink alternately from each glass until thirst is quenched. Supplement as desired with carbonated beverages, water, or tea made with boiled or carbonated water. Avoid solid foods and milk until recovery occurs. It is important that infants continue breast feeding and receive plain water while receiving these solutions.	

[a]Source: Centers for Disease Control.[10]

(Enterovioform), an over-the-counter remedy in many countries, should be avoided because it is ineffective and causes subacute myeloptic neuropathy.

Turista may recur repeatedly during long stays in the tropics, but travelers with persistent or recurrent diarrhea should be checked for other enteric pathogens. High fever, bloody diarrhea, and tenesmus (the dysentery syndrome) are not typical of turista and require immediate medical attention. True dysentery is fortunately uncommon among tourists to the tropics.

10. ASSESSING THE RETURNING TRAVELER

The asymptomatic traveler returning from a tour in the tropics seldom harbors latent infection. Routine studies are usually unnecessary, with the possible exception of a tuberculin skin test (PPD), a complete blood count with differential, and liver function tests.[43] The symptomatic returnee, however, warrants careful evaluation.[44,45]

REFERENCES

1. Reilly, P. C., Jr., Reilly, M. C., Catino, J., *et al.*: High-risk travel and malaria. *N. Engl. J. Med.* **296:**1536, 1977.
2. Kendrick, M. A.: Study of illness among Americans returning from international travel. *J. Infect. Dis.* **126:**684–685, 1972.
3. Steffen, R., Van Der Linde, F., and Meyer, H. E.: Risk of illness in 10,500 travelers to the tropics and 1300 to North America. *Schweiz. Med. Wochenschr.* **108:**1485–1494, 1978.
4. Peltola, H., Kryonseppa, H., and Holsa, P.: Trips to the South—a health hazard. *Scand. J. Infect. Dis.* **15:**375–381, 1983.

5. Reid, D., Dewar, R. D., Fallon, R. J., *et al.*: Infection and travel—The experience of package tourists and other travelers. *J. Infect. Dis.* **2**:365–370, 1980.
6. Lobel, H. O., Campbell, C. C., Schwartz, I. K., *et al.*: Recent trends in the importation of malaria caused by P. falciparum into the U.S. from Africa. *J. Infect. Dis.* **152**:613–617, 1985.
7. Steffen, R.: Typhoid vaccine, for whom? (letter). *Lancet* **1**:615–616, 1982.
8. Hargarten, S. W., and Baker, S. P.: Fatalities in the Peace Corps. *JAMA* **254**:1326–1329, 1985.
9. Banta, J. E., and Jungblut, E.: Health problems encountered by the Peace Corps overseas. *Am. J. Public Health* **56**:2121–2125, 1966.
10. Centers for Disease Control: Health information for international travel 1984. *Morbid. Mortal. Wkly. Rep.* **30**(suppl):1–28, 1984.
11. Kilbourne, E. M.: Risk factors for heat stroke. *JAMA* **247**:3332–3336, 1982.
12. American Diabetes Association: *Vacationing with Diabetes*. American Diabetic Association, New York.
13. Gianella, R. A., Broitmanm, S. A., and Zamcheck, N.: Influence of gastric acidity on bacterial and parasitic enteric infection. *Ann. Intern. Med.* **78**:271–276, 1973.
14. Galina, M. P., Avret, N. L., and Emhorn, A.: Iodides during pregnancy. *N. Engl. J. Med.* **267**:1124–1127, 1962.
15. Schwartz, J. S., Bencowitz, H. Z., and Moser, K. M.: Air travel hypoxemia with chronic obstructive pulmonary disease. *Ann. Intern. Med.* **100**:473–477, 1984.
16. Mann, J. M., Bernier, R. H., and Hurman, A. R.: Poliomyelitis vaccination for the international traveler. *Am. Fam. Physician* **26**:135–139, 1982.
17. Centers for Disease Control: Yellow fever vaccination. *Ann. Intern. Med.* **100**:540–542, 1984.
18. Snyder, J., and Blake, P. A.: Is cholera a problem for U.S. travelers? *JAMA* **247**:2268–2269, 1982.
19. Morger, H., Steffen, R., and Schar, M.: Epidemiology of cholera in travelers, and conclusions for vaccine recommendations. *Br. Med. J.* **286**:184–186, 1983.
20. Taylor, D. N., Pollard, R. A., and Blake, P. A.: Typhoid in the U.S. and the risk to the international traveler. *J. Infect. Dis.* **148**:599–602, 1983.
21. Kendrick, M.: Viral hepatitis in missionaries abroad. *J. Infect. Dis.* **129**:227–229, 1974.
22. Centers for Disease Control: Systemic allergic reactions following immunization with human diploid cell rabies vaccine. *Morbid. Mortal. Wkly. Rep.* **33**:185–187, 1984.
23. Pappaioanou, U., Fishbein, D., Dreeser, D. W., *et al.*: Antibody response to pre-exposure human diploid-cell rabies vaccines given concurrently with chloroquine. *N. Engl. J. Med.* **314**:280–284, 1986.
24. Centers for Disease Control: Imported malaria among travelers. *Morbid. Mortal. Wkly. Rep.* **33**:388–390, 1984.
25. Appleton, B., Wolfe, M. S., and Mishtowt, G. I.: Chloroquine as a malaria suppressive: Absence of visual effects. *Milit. Med.* **138**:225–226, 1973.
26. Editorial: Malaria prophylaxis for longterm visitors. *Br. Med. J.* **287**:1454–1455, 1983.
27. Hatton, C., Bunch, C., Peto, T., *et al.*: Frequency of severe neutropenia associated with amodiaquine prophylaxis against malaria. *Lancet* **1**:411–413, 1986.
28. Centers for Disease Control: Adverse reactions to Fansidar and updated recommendations for its use in the prevention of malaria. *Morbid. Mortal. Wkly. Rep.* **33**:713–714, 1985.
29. Editorial: Pyrimethamine combinations in pregnancy. *Lancet* **2**:1005–1007, 1983.
30. *Health Hints for the Tropics*, 8th ed. Supplement to *Tropical Medicine and Hygiene News*, The American Society of Tropical Medicine and Hygiene, Washington, D.C., 1980.
31. Larson, E., Roach, R. C., Schoene, R. B., *et al.*: Acute mountain sickness and acetazolamide; clinical efficiency and effect of ventilation. *JAMA* **248**:328–332, 1982.
32. Gangarosa, E. J., Kendrick, M. A., Lowenstein, M. S., *et al.*: Global travel and travelers' health. *Aviat. Space Environ. Med.* **51**:265–270, 1980.
33. Ericson, C. D., and Dupont, H. L.: Travelers' diarrhea: Recent developments, in *Current Topics in Infectious Diseases 6* (J. S. Remington and M. N. Swartz, eds.): McGraw-Hill, New York, 1985.
34. Tjoa, W. S., Du Pont, H. L., Sullivan, P., *et al.*: Location of food consumption and travelers' diarrhea. *Am. J. Epidemiol.* **106**:61–66, 1977.
35. Steffen, R., Van Der Linde, F., Gyr, K., and Scher, M.: Epidemiology of diarrhea in travelers. *JAMA* **249**:1176–1180, 1983.
36. DuPont, H. C., Sullivan, P., Evans, D. G., *et al.*: Prevention of travelers' diarrhea. Prophylactic administration of subsalicylate bismuth. *JAMA* **243**:237–241, 1980.

37. Sack, D. A., Kaminsky, D. C., Sack, R. B., *et al.*: Prophylactic doxycycline for travelers' diarrhea. *N. Engl. J. Med.* **298**:758–763, 1978.
38. Dupont, H. L., Galindo, E., Evans, D. G., *et al.*: Prevention of travelers' diarrhea with trimethoprim sulfamethoxazole and trimethoprim alone. *Gastroenterology* **84**:75–80, 1983.
39. Murray, B., Alvarado, T., Kim K.-H., *et al.*: Increasing resistance to trimethoprim–sulfa among isolated *E. coli* in developing countries. *J. Infect. Dis.* **152**:1107–1112, 1985.
40. Graham, D. Y., Estes, M., and Gentry, W.: Double-blind comparison of bismuth subsalicylate and placebo in the prevention and treatment of enteriotoxigenic *E. coli*-induced diarrhea in volunteers. *Gastroenterology* **85**:1017–1022, 1983.
41. DuPont, H. C., Reves, R. R., Galindo, E., *et al.*: Treatment of travelers' diarrhea with trimethoprim/sulfamethoxazole and with trimethoprim alone. *N. Engl. J. Med.* **307**:841–844, 1982.
42. Johnson, P. C., Ericcson, C. D., DuPont, H. L., *et al.*: Comparison of loperamide with bismuth subsalicylate for the treatment of acute travelers' diarrhea. *JAMA* **255**:751–760, 1986.
43. Effersoe, P.: Check-ups after tours of duty to the tropics. *Scand. J. Infect. Dis.* **9**:137–138, 1979.
44. Brown, K., and Phillips, S. M.: Tropical diseases of importance to the traveler. *Annu. Rev. Intern. Med.* **35**:59–84, 1984.
45. Wolfe, M. S.: Management of the returnee from exotic places. *J. Occup. Med.* **21**:691–695, 1979.
46. Smith, R.: Health advice for travelers, in Branch, W. T., Jr. (ed.): *Office Practice of Medicine*. Saunders, Philadelphia, 1987, 1264–1276.
47. Centers for Disease Control: *Health Information for International Travel. Morbid. Mortal. Wkly. Rep.*, August 1985. U.S. Dept. of Health and Human Services, HHS Pub. No. (CDC) 85-8280.

21

Occupational Medicine

Mark R. Cullen

1. INTRODUCTION

Although the evidence that chemical, physical, and biological factors at work play significant roles in the causation of medical disease has been recognized for over 285 years,[1] clinical attention to this area by all but a handful of industrial physicians has been minimal. Nonetheless, it is estimated that as many as half a million working people in the United States will acquire a work-related illness every year, many disabling and not a few lethal.[2] Furthermore, these illnesses will not be limited to a small number of unusual or high-risk workers like coal miners or lead smelters; virtually all occupations and work processes have attendant risks. Since the majority of adults—including women—now work outside the home,[3] the problems of recognition, treatment, and prevention of occupational disease will arise in virtually every type of medical practice.

While these realities impose a considerable burden for additional knowledge about an area traditionally ignored in medical education and training, there is an exciting reward to be gained: in no other area of clinical practice is the potential for truly preventive medicine so great. Not only can an early case of occupational disease generally be arrested or even reversed by removal of a patient from a noxious exposure or condition, but typically many present and future co-workers can be spared as well.

Unfortunately, in this opportunity lies a major if often unfulfilled responsibility. The role of governmental agencies and industrial hygienists and physicians in industry notwithstanding, the practicing physician remains the last safeguard of the workforce against these preventable and often tragic consequences of work. It can never be assumed that "someone else" is watching out for these possibilities or guaranteeing that such preventable disease will not occur, progress, or recur again in others. Thus, though the potential reward is high, so are the stakes.

Ironically, perhaps, while the role of the primary-care physician is so crucial, the potential for participation in the primary prevention of disease—i.e., limiting exposure to noxious substances and dangerous conditions at work—is small. Except when an actual disease occurs, neither the patient nor his/her doctor has very much control over the conditions of work itself, these being the province of plant managers and their industrial

Mark R. Cullen • Occupational Medicine Program, Yale University School of Medicine, New Haven, Connecticut 06510.

hygienists and industrial physicians, guided by existing (not entirely adequate) regulations. Therefore, the major emphasis in this chapter is on recognition of clinical manifestations of occupational disease and secondary strategies for prevention. This focus has been chosen because it is the act of recognition that will empower the physician to initiate change in the worker–patient and ultimately in the workplace itself. While it is true that detailed information about the work exposures and risks of even healthy patients should be an integral part of preventive health maintenance, the most crucial role for the physician outside the workplace itself is prompt recognition of working conditions that actually lead to disease.

2. GUIDE TO THIS CHAPTER

The field of occupational medicine, which includes both the bulk of clinical toxicology as well as principles of social medicine, vastly exceeds the scope of a single chapter in this text. Not only are there more than 10,000 toxic substances extant,[4] but their effects span all of the subspecialty domains within internal medicine as well as those of obstetrics, neurology, dermatology, and psychiatry. For this reason, much of what follows is devoted to the conceptual aspects and specialized skills and resources that are needed for an already skilled clinician to apply his or her prior knowledge to this new arena; discussion of some specific common occupational health problems will follow.

The chapter is divided into three sections. First, the basic principles of all occupational disease are outlined. In essence, this is an introduction to clinical toxicology.

Second, the special clinical skills needed to practice effectively are discussed. These include the occupational history, additional strategies for ascertaining what a patient has actually been exposed to, and approaches for parlaying this information into data regarding clinical findings and risks. A discussion of the concrete actions that practitioners can take when they suspect occupational disease, including workers' compensation and other legal/regulatory aspects of the field, follows.

Finally, the effects of work on the major organ systems are discussed. Since space is limited, only the most serious and prevalent disorders of proven occupational etiology are mentioned; preventive steps rather than treatment *per se* is emphasized. The focus is on organs, rather than chemicals, because the reader will far more readily recognize the effect clinically than the cause. Readers wishing to gain access to specific information about the effects of particular chemicals should consult the annotated reference list at the end of the chapter.

3. GENERAL PRINCIPLES OF OCCUPATIONAL DISEASE

1. Most occupational diseases lack distinctive clinical and pathological features. Many clinicians suppose, incorrectly, that the possibility that a given patient has an occupationally induced disorder will be suggested only after other, more usual, disorders are ruled out. Alternatively, they imagine (wrongly) that consultants such as radiologists and pathologists will "catch" these possibilities, shifting the burden of recognition away

from themselves. In reality, however, the majority of disturbances induced by chemicals and other working conditions are quite like, often identical to, disorders of other origins. For example, the typical patient with occupational asthma will behave clinically like any patient with extrinsic asthma; aplastic anemia caused by benzene is indistinguishable from that caused by drugs or viruses; asbestosis closely mimics so-called idiopathic pulmonary fibrosis.

Of course there are notable exceptions. For example, although silicosis closely resembles sarcoidosis on x-ray, lung biopsy will reveal its truly unique pathological characteristics. Similarly, inorganic mercury is known to cause a peculiar constellation of neurological, dermal, and salivary gland disturbances. But these cases are exceptions. In general, the historic relationship between the disease and biologically significant exposures—not the special features of the disease itself—will lead to correct diagnosis of a disease as occupationally caused. This implies, of course, that the primary clinician, not the specialist interpreting only part of the data, is most likely to recognize a disease as occupational.

This does not mean that occupational disorders cannot be differentiated—often with confidence—from other possible etiologies. In fact, it is the goal of this chapter to demonstrate how diagnosable they really are. But it does mean that without a high index of suspicion and collection of the prerequisite exposure information, the chance of making the correct and complete diagnosis is remote. Furthermore, this principle implies that the availability of a diagnostic category to explain an illness does not preclude the possibility that an occupational cause is responsible.

2. For occupational diseases of acute onset or periodic recurrence, the temporal relationship between exposure and symptoms is of diagnostic importance. Many of the most prominent effects of toxic exposures and dangerous conditions are abrupt in onset. Invariably, such clinical manifestations will occur shortly after the offending exposure. While this interval may be a few moments, as in the upper-airway irritation caused by acid fumes or ammonia, or several hours, as in the late asthmatic reaction to diisocyanates, or a few days, as in the acute renal failure caused by mercury fumes, the "incubation period" is invariably short and potentially clinically discernible. Rarely should prior or remote exposures be even relevant.

This cardinal feature of clinical toxicology has enormous diagnostic utility. For disorders that recur, like headaches or asthma or skin rashes, the pattern of illness in relationship to workshifts can easily be learned by history, just like the relationship of peptic ulcer symptoms to meals. Does the patient improve on weekends or holidays? Do the symptoms tend to recur at the same time of day, during or after work? Do the symptoms seem to occur only after use of certain substances or performance of certain tasks? If any of these is answered in the affirmative, the likelihood of an occupational disease is high.

For first occurrences, the focus in history should be on change in exposures preceding the illness. Since exposures that were previously well tolerated are unlikely to suddenly produce ill effects, the focus should center on unaccustomed, excessive, or accidental exposures. Has a new substance or operation been recently introduced? Did the ventilation malfunction? Has there been a leak or spill? Affirmative responses should prompt a detailed search for the cause, while negative answers suggest alternative etiological possibilities.

3. The lack of ongoing effects from a particular substance does not preclude the possibility of a delayed, latent chronic effect. Many toxic substances and hazardous conditions produce chronic damage to organ systems either by repeated insult to individual cells or subunits or by initiation or promotion of a tumor. Typically, these effects will not become clinically apparent until long after the onset of the process; indeed, the patient may already be long removed from the offending exposure by the time the effect becomes clinically apparent. This latency must be understood and accounted for by the clinician attempting to determine an environmental cause for a chronic illness or cancer. At a minimum, a careful review of prior exposures, often from 30 or 40 years before, may be required.

Unfortunately for both the victim and his/her physician, the toxins that cause such latent effects, often the most notorious and potentially lethal, may be free of any acute health effects whatsoever or may have acute effects entirely unrelated to the more serious chronic ones. Thus, the patient may have worked comfortably with the agent for a long time without any warning or awareness of the potential peril—most workers used such materials without precautions unless they were specifically instructed to do so. In fact, the absence of acute effects often led to gross mishandling of products containing cottonlike asbestos or emitting invisible radon daughters. Furthermore, since these substances seem quite harmless day to day, many workers do not even take particular note of the exposure and may not recall it very well, if at all, while other, more acutely irritating substances are well remembered.

The clinician, however, cannot afford to fall into the trap of assuming that exposures that did not bother a patient could not cause harm. Often knowledge of the import of these "historic" exposures can lead to valuable steps in the secondary prevention of bad outcomes. For example, it is now well recognized that surveillance of textile workers formerly exposed to benzidine-derived dyes can limit the risk of fatal bladder cancer[5]; similarly, intensive smoking cessation can reduce the lung cancer toll among the millions who have worked with asbestos.[6]

4. Many chronic occupational diseases have multifactorial origin. Although the growing body of data regarding the causation of disease should have sensitized most physicians to the possibility that a chronic disease can have more than one cause (e.g., coronary artery disease), many still approach diagnosis with the idea that either one cause will be found or none. This notion, which is really an extension of reasoning from acute and infectious disorders, is both wrong and detrimental to sound practice of preventive medicine. This is especially important in situations like lung cancer or chronic obstructive lung disease where one cause so often readily presents itself—cigarette smoking—sharply limiting inquiry into possible other causes. In fact, substantial data now exist demonstrating important additive, and sometimes synergistic, interactions between tobacco and respiratory toxins and carcinogens including asbestos,[7] radiation,[7] coal dust,[8] and grain.[9] In situations where both are contributing, failing to consider either is likely to limit important opportunities to reduce morbidity and mortality, for both the patient and those with whom he or she has worked.

Unfortunately, the science of causation of chronic disease remains quite primitive, so that many possible interactions are not yet appreciated, as those with tobacco are beginning to be. Nonetheless, there are already compelling reasons for considering a role for occupational factors in chronic disorders that might otherwise be singularly attributed to such risks as alcohol (liver and neurological disease), hypertension (stroke and chronic renal failure), diet (colon cancer), or genetics (asthma). It is almost certain that this list will expand exponentially as techniques improve for investigation of chronic diseases, by methods both epidemiological, i.e., studies of workers, and toxicological, i.e., studies with laboratory animals.

5. For both acute and chronic effects of toxins, the dose of exposure is a major determinant of risk or severity of disease (but not necessarily both). Although it will generally be difficult for the physician to directly assess the effective dose of toxins to which a patient is exposed, some basic understanding of the dose issue is essential, just as it is for effectively predicting and managing side effects of drugs. It may be particularly important in history taking, interacting with employers and industrial hygienists, and selecting therapeutic/preventive options.

An important first principle is that a toxin must enter the body to cause physiological harm; in the workplace the primary route is by inhalation, although skin is another portal for chemical and physical insults, while only rarely is the gastrointestinal (GI) tract a source. For chemicals, this means that the dose will be related to how much gets into the patient's breathing zone or on skin or clothing; thus welding, heating, or grinding a metal may pose risk, while bending or otherwise reshaping it will not.

Given that some exposure is truly occurring, toxins can be broadly divided into three types, depending on their mode of action. The first type—those that cause direct cellular injury—tend to cause a consistent pattern of effect, which increases with increasing dose. Examples include lead, mercury, silica, and carbon tetrachloride. In general, there is some "low" dose that is not harmful to virtually anyone. As levels rise, effects will eventually occur in almost everyone, although there will always be differences in the degree of effect, depending usually on undefinable host factors. Importantly too, the higher the level of exposure, the more severe will be the resultant disease.

Other substances act by idiosyncratic means, causing "allergic" types of problems such as asthma, allergic alveolitis, and dermatitis. As with drug reactions of this type, the dose of exposure primarily affects the proportion of exposed who may develop problems, not necessarily the severity in those affected. Furthermore, there may, for all intents and purposes, be no dose too low to produce illness in some exposed individuals. Obviously, host factors play an important role in who does and who does not get affected, although it is not often clear what the predisposing factors are (e.g., atopy is a proven risk in only a few settings!). Furthermore, once the "sensitization" process has occurred, extremely small exposures may trigger a response. Examples of culprits of this type are plastic accelerators (especially epoxies and polyurethanes), additives to cooling and cutting solutions, and the metals nickel, chromium, and beryllium.

Finally, there are the carcinogens like asbestos, radiation, and benzene. For these, the risk of developing cancer will in general rise proportionally with cumulative dose—no dose has been proven to be free of risk. Published epidemiological studies that demonstrate levels of risk, however, must be applied to individuals with an understanding of how the exposures compare. For example, a school teacher's risk of mesothelioma from schoolroom asbestos exposures cannot be assumed to be equal to that of an asbestos insulator; however, it will not be zero either. Similarly, even people living in the vicinity of a vinyl chloride plant have risk for the otherwise rare tumor angiosarcoma, but it is a far lower risk than for the chemical workers inside. Of course, for those who get the cancers, whatever their exposure, the severity of disease depends only on the stage of detection and treatment; dose has absolutely no bearing on outcome.

4. SPECIAL SKILLS FOR THE PRACTICE OF OCCUPATIONAL MEDICINE

4.1. Obtaining the Occupational History

Broadly speaking, the occupational history has two components. The first elicits from the patient the nature and extent of exposures he or she has had to toxic substances or dangerous working conditions. The second explores whether any of the patient's clinical problems or complaints bear a temporally logical relationship to these exposures. These components are analogous to, respectively, the dietary history and establishing a relationship between GI symptoms and meals or particular foods.

The first component—the job and exposure history—must be tailored to the constraints of the setting in which it is obtained. Not only will many patients not have access to information about substances with which they have worked or are working, but even if they did, the physician's lack of familiarity with work processes and time limitations makes it unfeasible to elicit everything. For this reason, the best approach initially is to get a brief summary of each job a patient has done—place of employment, dates, and job title—and to obtain a more detailed description of the present or most recent job. After this basic outline has been obtained, knowledge of present or past exposures to particular groups of harmful substances can be elicited in checklist style. The following is a brief list of "checkoffs" that might be included:

Mineral dusts, e.g., coal, silica, asbestos, talc, fiberglass
Metal fumes or dust, e.g., lead, mercury, arsenic
Organic solvents, e.g., benzene, trichlorethylene
Oils and coolants
Pesticides and fumigants
Noxious gases, e.g., chlorine, ammonia, carbon monoxide
Physical hazards, e.g., noise, radiation, repetitive trauma, heat, cold, vibration

The basic job and exposure history should take no more than a few minutes to record and can, ideally, be obtained by a simple questionnaire or by a nurse while other background data are recorded. This database can then serve as the framework for more detailed questioning if an occupational illness is suspected. A sample form for obtaining this basic information is shown in Fig. 1.

The second component of the history—the health and occupational history—should be adapted to the particular clinical problem or complaint under consideration. For patients with complaints of recent or recurrent onset, exploration of the temporal pattern in relationship to work, or particular aspects of work, is often rewarding. The special response to weekends and holidays should be explored specifically. An open-ended approach such as "Do you feel any of your symptoms might be related to exposures at work?" is provocative and may help you and the patient explore an unrecognized association. Another useful question is whether other co-workers seem to have similar complaints or symptoms, which allows the patient to express his/her impressions in lay "epidemiological" terms.

For the patient with a chronic health problem or cancer, however, this second part of the history must be entirely modified. The central diagnostic issue in this case is whether the patient has had a sufficient exposure, sufficiently long ago (to account for latency), to a substance known or suspected to cause his/her condition. To answer this, the physician needs to have in mind a list of etiological possibilities and carefully explore with the patient whether exposure occurred or may have occurred. Often, of course, both the lack of knowledge about working materials and the remoteness in time make this a challenge, requiring strategies for parlaying fragmentary information into a usable true exposure history. Both these tasks—ascertaining the possible causes and amplifying the patient's recollection into a specific environmental exposure history—are themselves special skills which will be discussed below.

4.2. Additional Sources of Exposure Information

The limitations of the occupational history—especially the job and exposure history—have already been alluded to. Explicitly, the major problems include the historic failure of employers to label substances by their chemical name (using instead either brand names or codes), the difficulty of assessing exposure dose, lack of knowledge about the potential exposures from nearby workers or operations, and failure to recall remote events. Physician lack of familiarity with the jobs and chemicals further compounds the difficulty.

For these reasons, the clinician must often obtain additional information about work exposures if suspicion of an occupational cause for an illness is high. While this imposes a time burden which can be cumbersome, the process often provides an opportunity to enhance understanding of a case beyond the mere names and dose range of toxic exposures and harmful processes; it also may provide the initial contact with individuals in a position to assist with patient management, procurement of necessary benefits, and, most important, institution of potentially necessary preventive changes in the workplace.

The following is a list of sources of additional exposure information. It must be emphasized at the outset that for usual ethical reasons it is imperative that the patient consent to any direct contact between the physician and employers, insurance carriers, unions, or other agencies—failure to discuss this with the patient could result in unforeseen repercussions which the physician may be powerless to alter.

1. *The Employer*. Large companies usually employ professionals who may be a source of detailed information about the workplace, including knowledge of previous related health problems in other workers. Smaller companies should, at a minimum, have forms, called material safety data sheets, which provide the name of the supplier of the product and sometimes further characterize its contents. Unfortunately, the health information is often both sparse and inaccurate—it should never be solely relied upon. On the other hand, more detailed data may be obtained by calling the named supplier.

2. *The Union*. Not all workers belong to unions and not all unions have expertise

Work and exposure history

A. Current employment

Questions 1–7 refer to your current or most recent job.

1. Job title ____________
2. Type of industry ____________
3. Name of employer ____________
4. Year job began ____________
   Still working?
   Yes ____ No ____ If no, year job ended ____________
5. Briefly describe this job, noting any part that you feel may be hazardous to your health.
   ____
   ____
6. Do you wear protective equipment for this job?
   Yes ____ No ____ If yes, check equipment used:
   Gloves ____ Air supply respirator ____
   Mask respirator ____ Coveralls or aprons ____
   Hearing protection ____ Safety glasses ____
7. In this job, are you exposed to any of the following?
   If yes, mark those to which you are exposed:
   Mineral dusts like coal, silica, or asbestos ____
   Metal dusts or fumes ____
   Oils or coolants ____
   Organic solvents or degreasers ____
   Noise
   Pesticides or fumigants ____
   Heat/cold
   Radiation ____
   Gases like chlorine, ammonia, carbon monoxide ____
   Vibration or repeated trauma ____

B. Employment history

It is important that we know all the jobs you have had for more than a few months. Job #1 is your current or most recent job. Beginning with the job before this one—Job #2—please fill in as much of the information requested as you can remember and continue to do so until all previous jobs have been listed. Include any military service you have had. If you need additional space, use the back of this form.

	Years (from–to)	Job title	Exposures
Job #2			
Job #3			
Job #4			
Job #5			
Job #6			
Job #7			
Job #8			
Wartime employment			

C. Other exposures

1. Does anyone in your household work at a job that you suspect involves exposures that may be brought home from work (e.g., asbestos fibers on clothes)?
   Yes No
2. Are there any industries in the area in which you live that may pollute your environment?
   Yes ____ No ____
3. Do you have any hobbies that expose you to chemicals, metals, or other substances?
   Yes ____ No ____

Figure 1. The occupational history. (Source: Rosenstock and Cullen,[19] p. 4.)

D. Health and occupational history
1. Is there any particular hazard or part of your job that you think relates to your problems?
   Yes _____ No _____
2. Do any of your co-workers have problems or complaints similar to yours?
   Yes _____ No _____
3. Are any of your symptoms brought on or made worse during or after work? If yes, which symptoms?
   ____
   ____
4. Are any of your symptoms much better on weekends or holidays? If yes, which symptoms?
   ____
   ____

Figure 1. (Continued)

regarding health and safety conditions of the workers they represent. Some unions are, however, very active in this area and may have considerable information regarding exposures and the health of other workers, as well as knowledge about options for job transfer and/or benefits if the patient cannot continue in his or her present status.

3. *Occupational Safety and Health Administration.* Since the Occupational Safety and Health Administration (OSHA) has primary responsibility for enforcing standards in the workplace, the local office may have some knowledge of exposures at your patient's place of work. They may also have data regarding exposure doses. If you are highly suspicious of a problem, a physician can file a complaint that may lead to an inspection of the facility. It must be remembered, however, that OSHA is not a medical evaluation unit and can only determine whether federal exposure guidelines are being met or not. Absence of an OSHA violation is not a guarantee that that environment could not be harmful, in view of the limitations of the regulatory process.

4. *State and Local Health Departments.* Many states now have units that can investigate suspect workplace health hazards; some actually perform on-site inspections. Other states have less direct capabilities but may assist in obtaining exposure data under new "right-to-know" laws. Similarly, local health officials may either have information or assist in obtaining it.

5. *Occupational Health Clinics and Programs.* Many medical centers now have established occupational health clinics, which may be invaluable sources of information about local plants or particular jobs. In addition, such clinics can often provide advice about particular toxins and approaches to patient evaluation and management. They can also be very useful in helping implement strategies for prevention. Lists of these programs can be found in the annotated bibliography at the end of the chapter (especially Refs. 9 and 10).

6. *Biological Monitoring.* Finally, when exposure information is incomplete, tests of biological fluids or other specimens for particular toxins of interest, e.g., heavy metals, may be feasible. Unfortunately, for many toxins, tests are either nonexistent, expensive, unreliable, or highly invasive. For this reason, biological monitoring should be strictly limited to situations where the use and meaning of the result will be clear-cut. Indiscriminate testing, as a substitute for a careful history or utilization of the above resources, is generally to be eschewed.

4.3. Translating Exposure Data into Clinical Terms

Even once a patient's exposure background has been clarified, it often remains difficult to decipher the data correlating exposure with clinical manifestations or risks. This is because such information is not covered in general clinical texts, while most occupational health literature is written in either toxicological or epidemiological, not clinical, terms. Several options exist:

1. *Texts.* Several useful texts now exist with which the reader should become familiar; these are described in the annotated bibliography at the end of this chapter.
2. *Computerized Literature Searches.* Several of the computerized database systems, available at most medical libraries, allow rapid access to current articles and texts. *Toxline* and *Medline* are particularly useful for finding materials on the effects of noxious agents.
3. *The National Institute for Occupational Safety and Health (NIOSH).* This federal agency, whose laboratories are located in Cincinnati, Ohio, has an extraordinary wealth of data regarding the effects of particular products and compounds. Staff will assist physicians investigating unusual cases or exposures.

4.4. Taking Action when Occupational Disease Is Suspected

Unfortunately for patient and doctor alike, the preventive steps that must be taken when occupational illness is diagnosed have implications far beyond the office or the patient's private life—they extend into the workplace where neither the physician nor the patient has direct control over the ostensible problem. Since this is true, effective practice requires knowledge of the steps needed to ensure the protection (and compliance) of the patient and the means for preventing other cases from potentially occurring.

4.5. Protecting the Patient

In general, treatment of any occupational illness requires removal from or reduction in exposure to the supposed causal conditions or toxins. Statement of a specific job restriction or exclusion in writing by the physician will, in general, accomplish this, but may also lead to other consequences such as dismissal or other disciplinary action, no matter how reasonable. For this reason, the following steps are essential:

1. The doctor's opinion should be discussed with the patient *before* anything is placed in writing.
2. The patient must be advised of the need to file for benefits under workman's compensation to protect his/her income and rights. In general, he/she should seek advice from a union or legal representative.
3. Regardless of workman's compensation rights, the patient must be warned that financial disruption may occur; the intervention of a social worker or other counselor may be advisable.
4. Most important, the physician must be aware that his/her opinion about the work-relatedness of an illness may by challenged by the employer, the insurance car-

riers, and/or their medical consultants. Accordingly, it is important that before an opinion is rendered, appropriate consultations are obtained if there is substantial doubt.

4.6. Protecting Present and Future Co-Workers

Of course, merely moving a patient from a noxious exposure leaves unchanged the underlying risk situation, transferring it instead to a different employee. Where the illness was caused, in large measure, by unique or unusual host factors, such as intercurrent disease, then subsequent workers are probably not at much risk. But in general, there will be continued potential or risk for disease unless working conditions themselves are changed. Unfortunately, unlike the comparable situation where a communicable disease is uncovered, no agency or authority can be relied on to assume responsibility for the "follow-up." The physician has several options for attempting to effect these preventive measures:

1. *Direct Approach to Management and/or Their Health and Safety Staff.* This is generally initiated by the act of notifying the employer about the patient's problems. Nonetheless, it is often worthwhile to inquire specifically about steps to prevent a reoccurrence in other workers, especially if the record suggests any degree of host susceptibility in the first case. Besides, there is often a tendency to disbelieve or dispute "bad" news, especially if the employer feels that no rules or standards have been violated (some consider the rules the limit of their responsibility).
2. *Approaching the Compensation Insurance Carrier.* The insurers may also dispute your view, but they do have direct liability for additional cases, hence a strong incentive to prevent them. Many insurance companies have experienced industrial hygienists who can further evaluate the environment and make recommendations. Ironically, a carrier's "risk appraisal" staff may take your comments very seriously, even while the "adjusters" are busy controverting your findings.
3. *Reporting to the State or Federal Occupational Health and Safety Administration.* OSHA has legislated responsibility to monitor workplace health and safety conditions. Unfortunately, their capacity is limited to enforcement of a set of rules which may or may not cover the situation that caused the patient's illness—they are *not* a health organization and cannot directly assess workplace disease or potential for it. A potential further drawback is that failure of OSHA to find a "violation" often further supports the view that nothing is wrong, even if it is.
4. *Requesting a NIOSH Health Hazard Evaluation.* NIOSH is obligated, under law, to investigate a suspicious workplace if requested to do so by an employer, union, or group of workers. These investigations may deal with health effects as well as measurement of environmental conditions. Unfortunately, NIOSH recommendations are not binding and may not lead to change. Information may be obtained from physicians in the Hazard Evaluation Unit at NIOSH offices in Cincinnati.
5. *Reporting to State and Local Health/Labor Departments.* Several states have independent capabilities to investigate adverse *health* conditions in a workplace, as well as power to dictate change. Even if they do not have such a structure, officials may help mediate change in a variety of ways.

6. *Referral to Regional or Local Occupational Health Clinics or Programs.* Although these professionals are "voluntary," they often have knowledge of effective means to bring about workplace change. A further advantage of such referral is that the clinics have the time, resources, and expertise to follow up on a case that may be beyond those of the individual practioner.

5. PRINCIPAL OCCUPATIONAL DISEASES AFFECTING THE MAJOR ORGANS

5.1. Lung Disease

Virtually all the major categories of lung disease, except vascular, have established environmental causes. Furthermore, occupational lung diseases are extremely prevalent. Although lethal varieties are now uncommon in the United States except for neoplasms, milder forms occur in virtually every workplace setting.

Acute conditions include *acute airway injury* (laryngotracheobronchitis, bronchiolitis, and pneumonitis) and *allergic alveolitis* (also known as hypersensitivity pneumonitis). The former generally occurs in accidental situations—fires, leaks, spills, or explosions—and is therefore difficult to manage in a preventive fashion. The most important culprits are noxious gases, including chlorine, phosgene, sulfur dioxide, nitrogen dioxide, and ammonia, often as part of combustion products, i.e., smoke. Allergic alveolitis, on the other hand, may present as repeated bouts of febrile respiratory illness, often with lung infiltrates, in individuals sensitized to molds and funguses contaminating virtually any animal or vegetable matter. Ventilation systems and humidifiers are potentially rich sources of these thermophilic organisms, as are birds, sewage, and silage. Early recognition and confirmation by finding serum IgG precipitins or typical findings on bronchoalveolar lavage (lymphocytosis, usually suppressor cells) or lung biopsy may allow interruption of an otherwise recurrent and ultimately scarring process by decontaminating the environment or removing the patient from it. Importantly, some resin systems, especially epoxies and polyurethanes (as in paint, for example) are now recognized as man-made causes.

The most important subacute or recurring disorder is *occupational asthma*—bronchospasm induced by sensitization to a single workplace agent. Patients typically present with cough or chest discomfort with a striking temporal pattern in relation to work shifts. Often there are no wheezes and no abnormalities whatsoever between episodes initially, so suspicion of asthma is crucial. Culprits include animal material (danders, shells), plastics, pharmaceuticals, some wood and metal dusts, and a wide range of organic chemicals. Early recognition is vital since the risk of progression to generalized asthma (i.e., reacting to all sorts of things) increases greatly with prolonged exposure to the causal agent; conversely, early removal usually leads to reversal to normal airway tone. Diagnosis hinges on the history; confirmation is by documentation of a reduction in flow rates temporally related to exposure, or by a prompt therapeutic response to removal. Serological tests for antibodies or similar studies remain largely experimental, as is specific inhalational challenge.

Chronic diseases include *industrial bronchitis, byssinosis, the pneumoconioses, and hypersensitivity disorders due to the metals beryllium and tungsten carbide.* Notably, panacinar emphysema is not well described in the occupational setting in the absence of either cigarette smoking or other risk factors (e.g., α_1-antitrypsin deficiency).

Industrial bronchitis is common in young workers exposed to mineral dusts, welding fumes, and irritants throughout the "dusty trades." Although significant obstruction uncommonly results, recurrent acute sinopulmonary infections are a source of morbidity. Reduction in exposure, through industrial hygiene or appropriate respiratory protective equipment, frequently results in diminution of cough and phlegm. Smoking, of course, is a major co-risk and should be discontinued.

Byssinosis is a more serious obstructive disease caused by some contaminant of the cotton boll; processors of unfinished cotton are at risk. Early clues include a characteristic tendency to bronchospasm early in the work week or progressive cough and phlegm production. Since both host and "mill" factors seem important, early symptoms and signs should prompt intervention to prevent an ultimately progressive, disabling disease.

The pneumoconioses include *silicosis, coal workers' pneumoconiosis* (CWP), and *asbestosis.* Each is due to heavy, usually long-term exposure to the respective dusts. Silicosis and, to a lesser extent, CWP are characterized by early radiographic changes (symmetrical small nodular infiltrates) and generally mild degrees of pulmonary fibrosis in "simple" or uncomplicated cases. The major complications are infection, often with mycobacteria, and progressive massive fibrosis, an uncommon but lethal progressive variant. Asbestosis, also a restricting disorder, is associated with a very high rate of pleural thickening and/or plaquing. Radiographic changes in the lungs themselves, primary irregular shadows in the bases, are often very subtle. The major complication is lung cancer, occurring in up to 25–50% of patients with lung scarring, especially in those who smoke.[10] Other cancers of the respiratory and GI tract also occur commonly and may be secondarily preventable. For all the pneumoconioses, it is felt that early removal from dust exposure and careful monitoring for complications are the mainstay of preventive care; co-workers must be evaluated as well.

Finally, two persistent hypersensitivity disorders due to inhaled metal may be devastating, even if recognized early. *Chronic beryllium disease* closely resembles sarcoidosis and seems to affect a small percentage of exposed workers, especially those who inhale fine fume. Suspicion should be high whenever sarcoid is considered because of the widespread use in electronics, aerospace, and metal processing of beryllium alloys and salts and the often prolonged latency between exposure and disease onset. *Hard-metal disease* is a virulent giant-cell alveolitis occurring in those who make and grind tungsten carbide (hard) tools. Cobalt is the suspect sensitizing agent; full recovery has been described after removal from exposure.

Lung cancer, mesothelioma. Respiratory tract malignancies are not rarely due to occupational factors. *Bronchogenic carcinoma* of all histological types is exceedingly common in asbestos-exposed workers, especially in those who smoke. Other major causes include radiation (especially alpha particles from underground mines), arsenic, nickel, chromium, polyaromatic hydrocarbons, and some alkylating agents; acrylonitrite, beryllium, cadmium, and vinyl chloride are suspect. Unfortunately, only primary preventive steps—eliminating exposure and tobacco use—have proven helpful; there is no evidence to support agressive surveillance or screening. *Malignant mesothelioma* of the pleura or peritonium is a rarer complication of asbestos work of long latency, averaging 30 years or more from first exposure. There is no known strategy for treatment or prevention in those who have been previously exposed.

5.2. Skin Disease

Dermatoses occur frequently in the industrial and service sector, causing extensive disability. Because they are visible, they are more likely to be recognized as work-related by patients. The major disease groups known to be associated with work include dermatitis, acne, traumatic lesions, and neoplasms.

Contact dermatitis is the most prevalent disorder. Most often the cause is irritation due to repetitive contact with such things as cutting oils, plating solutions, detergents, and organic solvents. *Allergic contact dermatitis* may be due to a wide range of metals (e.g., nickel, chromium, cobalt), as well as nitrogen and sulfur-containing organics often added as biocides or stablizers to industrial solutions and cleansers. Differentiation requires patch testing with nonirritating or standard dilutions of suspect culprits; diagnostic trials of removal and/or reexposure may be helpful.

Occupational acne may be due to oil exposures (e.g., in a machine operator), friction (e.g., the back of a driver), or internal exposure to alicyclic organochlorine compounds such as pesticides, polychlorinated biphenyls (PCBs), or dioxins. Acne caused by the latter group—called chloracne—is often quite striking in its distribution (e.g., nasal and ocular skin folds, groin) and resistant to usual therapies. Patients suspected of this require evaluation for chronic liver disease (see below) and peripheral neuropathy, which may be seen as well.

Skin cancers, except melanoma, the cause of which remains obscure, may be due to ultraviolet light, arsenic, ionizing radiation, and polyaromatic hydrocarbons found in mineral oils, tars, coal, and pitch. The major goal of recognition is enhanced surveillance for recurrences as well as the visceral malignancies that are caused by the same substances (except ultraviolet light)—especially lung cancer.

In addition to these effects, work conditions can affect the skin in numerous other ways, including discoloration (staining, pigmenting, or depigmenting), keratinization, or premature aging. Close inspection of the skin is also useful for determining patterns of extremity usage when evaluating muskuloskeletal disorders; occasionally skin signs are helpful in deciphering systemic intoxications, as in heavy-metal poisonings (e.g., arsenic, mercury).

5.3. Cardiovascular Disease

Although cardiovascular disease remains the leading cause of death in virtually all work groups, the effects of occupation remain largely undeciphered. It should be remembered, though, that known risk factors for atherosclerotic disease explain only about 50% of its occurrence[11]; environmental, physical, and stress factors are probably far more important than is presently realized.

Despite the lack of good data, certain cardiovascular sequelae of work are established. At least one chemical—the solvent carbon disulfide—causes premature atherosclerotic cardiovascular disease (ASCVD), leading to frequent coronary, cerebral, and peripheral ischemic events.[12] Asphyxiants, including carbon monoxide (CO) and the solvent methylene chloride (which is metabolized to CO), may cause *ischemia* in the absence of symptomatic coronary disease. Similarly, nitrites and nitrates used in the chemical and explosive industries may cause *coronary spasm* and sudden death.

Dysrhythmias, though usually due to intrinsic heart disease or metabolic disturbances, may be precipitated by a wide range of organic solvents, especially fluorocarbons such as freon; patients with unexplained rhythm disturbances should wear a Holter monitor during and after exposures to explore this.

Finally, a variety of heavy metals have cardiovascular effects. Lead and cadmium appear to elevate blood pressure, even in subtoxic doses. Arsenic, antimony, and cobalt may cause a cardiomyopathy with electrocardiographic changes and chamber dilatation; usually noncardiac effects dominate in heavily exposed individuals.

5.4. Musculoskeletal Disorders

It is hardly surprising that work contributes greatly to local problems of trunk and extremities, affecting secretaries and light assemblers almost as commonly as construction workers and truck drivers. Less predictable are the several systemic disorders, including scleroderma, acro-osteolysis, gout, plumbism, and fluorosis.

Regarding focal disorders—tenosynovitis, neural entrapment, arthritis, bursitis, and other enthesopathies—the range of possibilities and associations is exhaustive. Certain principles, however, apply broadly:

1. The presence of their risk factors, e.g., age or sex, should not discourage consideration of specific physical activities as causal.
2. Diagnosis should be based on detailed history and consistent physical examination of repeated trauma to the involved area. In general, the patient should be encouraged to literally "act out" his/her physical movements at work for the doctor.
3. Successful management and prevention require reduction of trauma, preferably by redesign of the work processes. While this is often feasible in principle, employers may be reluctant to do it, necessitating job transfer as an alternative, though far less desirable. The use of steroidal or nonsteroidal antiinflammatory agents to "cover" the problem without reducing the trauma is probably best avoided.

Of the systemic disorders, the *arthralgias of acute and chronic lead poisoning* are important to recognize because they may herald more fulminant GI or neurological involvement. Typically, blood lead levels are 40–80 μg/dl; other manifestations may or may not be present. Early removal of the patient from lead exposure may obviate severe morbidity. Diffuse muscle and joint involvement may also herald *chronic beryllium disease*, just as it does sarcoidosis.

Raynaud's phenomenon without other systemic effects may be caused by repetitive vibration, as in those who operate electric saws, jackhammers, and hand grinders. Digital blanching, often the earliest sign, requires immediate intervention lest this "vibration white finger" leads to permanent vascular insufficiency.

Scleroderma appears to occur too commonly in miners.[13] There is suspicion about solvent exposures as well, especially chlorinated ones. A similar disorder, dubbed *acro-osteolysis*, has been well described in workers heavily exposed to vinyl chloride monomer[14]; visceral scleroderma does not occur, but liver disease and a high rate of internal malignancies do; patients need diligent follow-up.

Gout is seen in late lead poisoning (at least 10 years after first exposure) and rarely in long-standing chronic beryllium disease. A history of prior exposure and associated pathology are key to recognition.

5.5. Gastrointestinal Disturbances

Although many common occupational diseases, including solvent and heavy metal intoxications, are associated with nonspecific GI complaints, most well-defined benign disorders of the GI tract have no established occupational causes. Study of these associations, however, is extremely limited so that patients with recurrent episodes of biliary, pancreatic, or peptic disease should be questioned about coincident chemical exposures.

Several patterns of nonmalignant hepatic injury are described. A variety of solvents and metals may cause *acute centrolubular necrosis* with elevations of serum alanine aminotransferace (ALT) (SGPT) and serum aspartate aminotransferase (AST) (SGOT), the latter usually lower than the former (as opposed to alcoholic injury). At least one organic chemical—methylene dianiline—has been established to cause *cholestatic hepatitis*. A prehepatic vascular lesion, *hepatoportal sclerosis*, with insidious portal hypertension, is seen after exposures to arsenicals and vinyl chloride monomer—unfortunately, the lesions may occur and progress without early symptoms or enzyme elevations, rendering early detection more difficult. *Granulomatous hepatitis* may be seen in chronic beryllium disease as well as in some occupationally acquired infections such as brucellosis.

Subacute or chronic active liver disease may occur if exposure to causal agents persists. In addition, the chlorinated alicyclic hydrocarbons, like pesticides, PCBs, and dioxins, can cause nonspecific, persistent dysfunction, usually associated with dermal chloracne. Whether any of these acute or subacute lesions may progress to outright cirrhosis, except after fulminant injury, is uncertain, but strong preventive steps, including removal from further exposure and discontinuance of alcohol, are surely prudent.

GI malignancies may also be environmental in origin. *Angiosarcoma of the liver*, often a sequela of hepatoportal sclerosis, is associated with exposure to thorium, arsenicals, or vinyl chloride in about 50% of cases.[15] *Hepatomas* may also result, although most cases are due to other causes. Asbestos dust seems to enhance the risk of carcinoma throughout the gut.[16] Routine colorectal screening, as recommended by the American Cancer Society, is probably warranted in those already exposed. More recently, other trades have been noted to have higher-than-average rates of colorectal cancer,[17] but these associations will require further study before surveillance strategies are clear.

5.6. Neurological Disease

The nervous system is highly susceptible to environmental insult. The clinical expression depends on the level and nature of the injury, as well as severity, before protective measures are initiated.

Acute encephalopathy, ranging from headache to coma, may result from solvents, asphyxiants, heavy metals (lead, mercury, manganese), and pesticides. Cases with recurrent mild attacks due to poor ventilation of solvents are extremely prevalent; usually mental symptoms predominate. Reduction in exposure is important because of the risk for development of *chronic organic brain syndrome* after many years, often heralded by depressive symptoms. Fortunately, the latter disorder tends to be nonprogressive after exposure stops, unlike idiopathic Alzheimer's disease.

Movement disorders may occur after CO poisoning as well as from exposures to manganese and certain narcotic derivatives. Unfortunately, techniques for early detection are still lacking.

Brain tumors, especially glioblastoma multiforme, seem to occur too frequently in workers exposed to various low-molecular-weight organic chemicals.[18] Unfortunately, neither specific chemical causes nor means for secondary prevention by clinicians are available.

Peripheral neuropathies, especially of the symmetrical axonal (as opposed to demyelinating) type, are seen after exposures to various chemicals including solvents (methyl butyl ketone, *n*-hexane, carbon disulfide, trichloroethylene), metals (lead, mercury, arsenic, thallium), plastics (acrylamide, dimethyl aminoproprionitrile), and pesticides. Early suspicion is imperative because electrophysiological studies become grossly abnormal only late in the course, when reversibility may be limited. Probably all patients with new-onset neuropathy should have toxic environmental causes strongly considered in the workup.

Focal peripheral neuropathy, like carpal tunnel syndrome, may be due to repetitive trauma. These lesions should be recognized by abnormal nerve conduction across the area of trauma (due to focal demyelination) and the corresponding history of asymmetrical compression or other stress to the region by occupational tasks.

5.7. Psychiatric Illness

The psychiatric consequences of work involve several interacting factors—chemical exposures, stress, and the various social systems in which work plays a crucial role. It is vital to recognize in this context that psychiatric symptoms may herald organic neurological or systemic disease and, conversely, somatic complaints referable to work exposures may be manifestations of a primarily psychological disorder.

Physical or chemical factors may cause psychiatric disorders in two settings. First, virtually all occupational injury or disease is complicated to some extent by psychological effects, ranging from mild "afterburn," where recovery is slightly delayed by persistence of initial symptoms until the victim adjusts and compensates, to more insidious and disabling *posttraumatic stress disorder,* in which the precipitating events are obsessively relived as the patient becomes more anxious and depressed. Sometimes the psychological nature of this disorder is obscured by fixation on physical symptoms resulting from even trivial exposure to conditions or chemicals that resemble the prior traumatic circumstances. Alternatively, certain neurotoxic chemicals—e.g., lead, mercury, arsenic, manganese, carbon disulfide—may cause affective disturbances before or without other accompanying signs. All patients with newly presenting manic or depressive illness should have an occupational history obtained to exclude a role for these reversible and potentially crippling poisons.

Because of the high prevalence of major and minor psychiatric disturbances in the population, it is not surprising that sometimes physical symptoms believed due to workplace substances are, in fact, initial signs of psychological distress. This is especially true when other work factors—e.g., fear of layoff, obsolescence of skills, or plant closing—are, in fact, important precipitants. Accordingly, patients with hard-to-substantiate complaints about chemicals at work should have these other aspects investigated early, before low-yield, expensive, exhaustive, and countertherapeutic workups are carried out. Well-studied strategies for primary and secondary prevention of such disruptions are, unfortunately, completely lacking.

5.8. Disorders of the Urinary Tract

Although many chemicals are nephrotoxic, the contribution of workplace exposures to well-recognized patterns of renal disease is only minimally characterized. Acute disturbances are better studied, but probably far rarer, than chronic.

Acute renal failure usually occurs under circumstances of accidental overexposure or extremely bad working conditions, uncommonly found in large industry today. Direct causes include heavy metals (especially mercury) and organic solvents (toluene is noteworthy). Tubular dysfunction may predominate with renal tubular acidosis or excessive clearance of phosphate, glucose, and organic acids, including uric acid. Acute renal failure may also be caused indirectly by exposures that induce abrupt hemolysis—e.g., arsine gas, strong oxidants—or rhabdomyolysis (e.g., carbon monoxide).

Chronic renal dysfunction has been convincingly demonstrated only for the heavy metals, especially lead, cadmium, and mercury. *Lead nephropathy* is noteworthy for its resemblance to hypertensive nephropathy—uric acid is often inappropriately elevated and gout (so-called saturnine gout) is relatively common. Removal from exposure is obligatory if ongoing; chelation may be of value. *Cadmium nephropathy* is pathologically nonspecific, but physiologically proximal tubular dysfunction precedes significant decrease in glomerular filtration. Exposure must stop if progression is to be halted. Mercury is unique in causing *membranous nephropathy,* often with significant proteinuria. The natural history remains uncertain.

There is speculation that exposure to organic solvents may cause *Goodpasture's syndrome* or other forms of *rapidly progressive glomerulonephritis*. The implication of this finding for prevention or treatment of these rare disorders is uncertain.

Bladder disease, especially epithelial *carcinoma,* is importantly tied to work. A wide range of dyes, especially benzidine and dyes derived from it, are potent bladder carcinogens. Exposed workers need vigilant ongoing surveillance with urine cytology and cystoscopy; newer screening and intervention strategies are being investigated.

5.9. Endocrine/Reproductive Disorders

Study of the effects of environmental conditions on endocrine function has been extremely limited. Thus far, three chemicals—lead, carbon disulfide, and polybrominated biphenyls—have been documented to depress thyroid function. Lead may also depress the hypothalamic pituitary axis as well as adrenal cortical hormone output. Testicular endocrine function, as opposed to spermatogenic, is relatively resistant to exogenous toxicity—only lead and estrogenic compounds have caused dysfunction after occupational exposures.

The role of the workplace in reproductive health has recently become an area of intense investigation; still there is only a little information to guide the practitioner. Patients usually seek medical attention because of infertility or, if pregnant, concern about some past, ongoing, or possible future risk to the fetus caused by workplace substances or conditions. Often risks of breast feeding are also at issue.

Infertility, at present, has only been studied in men; women are more difficult to study because of the absence of a simple measure of fertility. Some metals, solvents, pesticides, and plastics, as well as heat and radiation, are proven or suspected to reduce counts or quality of sperm. Except in azoospermic men, elimination of exposure results in gradual reversal over up to 18 months.

Advising pregnant workers regarding possible fetal risks is more challenging because of the inadequacy of the data and major social constraints—more than half of all reproductive-age women work outside the home and families depend on them for first and second incomes. If exposure has already occurred and is unlikely to be repeated, the only issue is whether there is enough information to predict that the risk is high enough to merit consideration of the only available therapeutic option. Table I lists the substances and conditions about which some data are available. Careful review of the history of exposure and biological monitoring of the mother are indicated to determine whether catastrophic fetal risk may have occurred. Noninvasive evaluation of the fetus may also be warranted. If risk is not judged to be high, optimistic support is crucial, since nothing but fear could be gained by a less clear-cut clinical decision.

If an exposure is ongoing, the options are several. If the toxin is on the list in Table I, the wisest course is to obtain transfer or reduction in exposure for the duration of the gestation. For less well-studied chemicals or situations of casual exposure (e.g., a clerical worker in an office at a factory using the toxin), slight job modifications are often satisfactory. In any event, the goal is to minimize the risk consistent with the financial and career needs of the patient. Unfortunately for prevention, no benefit system will remunerate a mother for income loss due to fetal risk.

Breast feeding is a different issue. Although there are psychological and physical advantages to breast feeding, these would surely be outweighed by the risk of intoxication of the fetus. Small (molecular weight under 200, including most metals) and lipophilic molecules (like pesticides and solvents) may be actively secreted, sometimes concentrated in breast milk. Since a highly satisfactory alternative exists for feeding the baby, this should be encouraged if there is any doubt, while the milk is being analyzed if the mother strongly prefers to breast feed.

5.10. Infectious Diseases

The recent epidemic of acquired immunodeficiency syndrome has forced a second look at the issue of occupational acquisition of infection. Not only health care workers, but laboratory and pharmaceutical workers, sanitation and waste treatment workers, meat

Table I. Agents Potentially Causing Adverse Reproductive Outcomes after Exposure in Pregnancy[a]

Established risk
Anesthetic gases
Diethylstilbestrol
Hepatitis B
Organic mercury
Lead
Polychlorinated biphenyls
Radiation
Suspected risk
Acrylonitrile
Arsenic
Cadmium
Carbon monoxide
Cytotoxic drugs
Dioxin
Ethylene oxide
Glycol ethers
Hexachlorophene
Inorganic mercury
Organic solvents
Organochlorine pesticides
Physical (including thermal) stress
Polybrominated biphenyls
Tellurium
Vinyl chloride
Vinylidene chloride
2,4,5-Trichlorophenol

[a]Source: Rosenstock and Cullen,[19] p. 112.

handlers, and others have opportunities for exposure to a broad range of organisms that should be considered in the workup of tuberculosis, hepatitis, cytomegalovirus infection, brucellosis, leptospirosis, and other conditions. In addition, outbreaks of histoplasmosis, legionnaires' disease, and sporotrichosis have frequently been traced to occupational settings. Since most of these occurrences are inherently preventable, early recognition of a possible workplace source is crucial.

5.11. Hematological Disorders

Workplace exposures may have an impact on hematological function in a variety of ways. Although an altered peripheral blood picture is often the presenting sign, prospective observation of workers exposed to relevant toxins suggests that significant injury may occur prior to observable changes in the complete blood count.

Hemolytic anemia may occur in a variety of settings. Workers heavily exposed to lead over a short period of time develop mild to moderately brisk hemolysis, often associated with GI and musculoskeletal symptoms. Arsine and stibine gases may cause acute red-cell membrane injury, with pigmenturia and acute renal failure. In workers with G-6-PD deficiency, a wide range of organic chemicals—oxidants—may similarly precipitate a hemolytic crisis.

Another dramatic effect of workplace toxins is *methemoglobinemia* with its attendant acrocyanosis. Causes include sodium nitrate as well as numerous related organic oxidants.

Hypoproliferative anemia, with injury occurring in the marrow, occurs in chronic lead and arsenic poisoning but is usually mild. The latter is often complicated by neutropenia. More serious marrow injuries, with hypoplastic red- and white-cell lines, may be caused by benzene, radiation, and organochlorine pesticides; the widely used ethylene glycol ethers are probable causes as well. These injuries, which may or may not be clinically apparent, may lead to serious outcomes, including *aplastic anemia* and *acute and chronic myeloproliferative* or *myelodysplastic disorders* including *acute nonlymphocytic leukemia.* Obviously, reduction of exposure is indicated whenever these toxic effects are noted.

Interestingly, occupational exposures have not been satisfactorily linked to lymphoproliferative disorders, although there is some evidence that benzene and radiation may induce certain *lymphomas* and *multiple myeloma.*

6. CONCLUSION

The need for all clinicians to incorporate skills in preventive occupational medicine is growing as workers, employers, and scientists increasingly recognize possible ill-health consequences of work. Practitioners are limited by (1) very minimal emphasis on this area in medical schools and training programs; (2) the lack of knowledge about the workplace; (3) the lack of a large, well-defined clinical database regarding most chemicals and most common disorders; and (4) the inaccessibility of the data that are available.

In this chapter, I have outlined the basic clinical principles and strategies for incorporating them into practice. The superficial survey of commonly seen occupational disorders is provided to indicate the breadth of possibilities. Given present information, the reader should consult the listed references to supplement this necessarily eclectic review.

ANNOTATED BIBLIOGRAPHY

1. Casarett, L. J., and Doull, J. (eds.): *Toxicology,* 2nd ed. Macmillan, New York, 1980.

This is the standard introductory toxicology text, exceedingly useful conceptually but limited in detail regarding specific toxins.

2. Clayton, G. D., and Clayton, F. E. (eds.): *Patty's Industrial Hygiene and Toxicology,* 3rd rev. ed., Vols. I, IIA, IIB, IIC, IIIA, IIIB. Wiley, New York, 1981.

This reference is a must for those in the field, the "Goodman and Gilman" of toxicology. Virtually any chemical can be conveniently researched here—a reasonably current review of the literature is provided, though clinical issues are not emphasized.

3. Finkel, A. J. (ed.): *Hamilton and Hardy's Industrial Toxicology,* 4th ed. John Wright PSG, Boston, 1983.

This is the "classic" text written by the great women of occupational medicine who saw it all, updated. Fabulous anecdotal clinical data.

4. Gosselin, R. E., Smith, R. P., and Hodge, H. C.: *Clinical Toxicology of Commercial Products,* 5th ed. Williams & Wilkins, Baltimore, 1984.

Once you get the knack of how to use it, a good way to determine or predict what a commercial product contains.

5. Levy, B. S., and Wegman, D. H. (eds.): *Occupational Health.* Little, Brown, Boston, 1983.

Excellent introductory text providing broad overview of the major issues and diseases. Less detail but more readable than standard texts.

6. Parmeggiani, L. (ed.): *Encyclopedia of Occupational Health and Safety,* 3rd rev. ed. International Labor Office, Geneva, 1983.

A truly encyclopedic work, these two volumes are the best source of information about jobs, trades, and industries, elucidating the major hazards in terms a clinician can understand.

7. Rom, W. N. (ed.): *Environmental and Occupational Medicine.* Little, Brown, Boston, 1983.

A relatively new, complete, and balanced general text of occupational medicine; clinical issues receive variable detail.

8. Zenz, C. (ed.): *Occupational Medicine, Principles and Practical Applications.* Year Book Medical Publishers, Chicago, 1975.

The former standard text; also large variability in the handling of different topics.

9. Rosenstock, L., and Cullen, M. R.: *Clinical Occupational Medicine.* Saunders, Philadelphia, 1986.

A new, inexpensive text exclusively oriented to practical issues in clinical management, presented in a "Washington manual" type format for easy reference; an extended version of this chapter.

10. Naviasky, L. M.: *A Directory of Independent Workers' Clinics.* Inform, Inc. (381 Park Avenue South, New York, NY 10016. 212-689-4040), 1986.

An inexpensive, nearly complete listing of independent occupational medicine clinics in the United States with information allowing easy and direct access to specialists around the country.

REFERENCES

1. Ramazzini, B.: *Diseases of Workers.* Translated by W. C. Wright from *De moribus artificum diatriba,* 1713. Hafner, New York, 1964.
2. Rosenstock, L.: Occupational medicine: Too long neglected. *Ann. Intern. Med.* **95:**774–776, 1981.
3. U.S. Dept. of Labor (Bureau of Labor Statistics): *Handbook of Labor Statistics,* Bulletin No. 2175. US Government Printing Office, Washington, DC, 1983.
4. Sax, N. I.: *Dangerous Properties of Industrial Materials.* Van Norstrand Reinhold, New York, 1979.
5. Schulte, P. A., Ringen, K., and Hemstreet, G. P.: Optimal management of asymptomatic workers at high risk of bladder cancer. *J. Occup. Med.* **28:**13–17, 1986.
6. Hammond, E. C., Selikoff, I. J., and Seidman, H.: Asbestos exposure, cigarette smoking and death rates. *Ann. NY Acad. Sci.* **330:**473–490, 1979.
7. Steenland, K., and Thun, M.: Interaction between tobacco smoking and occupational exposures in the causation of lung cancer. *J. Occup. Med.* **28:**110–18, 1986.
8. Seaton, A.: Coal and the lung. *Thorax* **38:**241–243, 1983.
9. Cotton, D. J., Graham, B. L., Li, K. Y. R., *et al.:* Effects of grain dust exposure and smoking on respiratory symptoms and lung function. *J. Occup. Med.* **25:**131–141, 1983.
10. Buchanan, W. D.: Asbestosis and primary intra-thoracic neoplasms. *Ann. NY Acad. Sci.* **132:**507–518, 1965.
11. Corday, E., and Corday, S. R.: Prevention of heart disease by control of risk factors: The time has come to face the facts. *Am. J. Cardiol.* **35:**330–333, 1975.
12. Hernberg, S., Nurminen, M., and Tolonen, M.: Excess mortality from coronary heart disease in viscose rayon workers exposed to carbon disulfide. *Scand. J. Work Environ. Health* **10:**93–99, 1973.
13. Rodnan, G. P., Benedek, T. G., Medsger, T. A., *et al.:* The association of progressive systemic sclerosis

(scleroderma) with coal miners' pneumoconiosis and other forms of silicosis. *Ann. Intern. Med.* **66**:323–334, 1967.
14. Dodson, V. N., Dinman, B. D., and Whitchouse, W. M.: Occupational acro osteolysis, *Arch. Environ. Health* **22**:83–91, 1971.
15. Vianna, N. J., Brady, J. A., and Cardamone, A.: Epidemiology of angiosarcoma of liver in New York state. *NY State J. Med.* **81**:895–899, 1981.
16. Levine, D. S.: Does asbestos exposure cause gastrointestinal cancer? *Dig. Dis. Sci.* **30**:1189–1198, 1985.
17. Swanson, G. M., Belle, S. H., and Burrows, R. W., Jr.: Colon cancer incidence among model makers and pattern makers in the automobile manufacturing industry: A continuing dilemma. *J. Occup. Med.* **27**:567–569, 1985.
18. Thomas, T. L., and Waxweiler, R. J.: Brain tumors and occupational risk factors: A review. *Scand. J. Work Environ. Health* **12**:1–15, 1986.
19. Rosenstock, L., and Cullen, M. R.: *Clinical Occupational Medicine*. Saunders, Philadelphia, 1986.

22

Nutrition

Eugene C. Corbett, Jr., and Daniel M. Becker

1. INTRODUCTION

The nutritional aspects of health and disease, although increasingly studied and publicized, remain incompletely understood. Nutritional science developed in the late 19th and early 20th centuries as dietary deficiency states were associated with specific diseases and biochemical findings. Vitamins were identified and the clinical consequences of caloric and protein deprivation were described. Following the recognition of essential nutrients, recommendations for daily allowances of these nutrients have been developed (Table I). Many complicated nutritional questions remain.

Although minimal nutritional standards for recognized nutrients can be established, it does not necessarily follow that larger quantities are better. Indeed, some vitamins are toxic in large doses, and the health problems of excess calories are all too prevalent. In industrialized nations where overt nutritional deficiency is rare and almost everyone can choose what and how much to eat, what is the ideal healthy diet? Can dietary discretion help to prevent the vascular disease and cancer that account for most of the mortality among older adults? While the links between dietary factors and chronic diseases are increasingly apparent, at the same time it is clear that nutritional variables are only part of the story. Genetic endowments may allow some to eat freely while severely curtailing the diet of others. In addition, behavior such as tobacco use may magnify a diet-associated risk factor (e.g., low vitamin A intake). The scientific investigation of these interactions is slow and cumbersome. It is difficult to move from an epidemiological association to a rigorous nutritional explanation of health or disease. Yet, in clinical settings it is now important to translate these evolving notions of diet and health into practical recommendations for preventive care. Indeed, physicians need to keep up with nutritionists, dietitians, and even the federal government in acknowledging the importance of diet in maintaining health (see Table II).[1]

Public interest in nutrition is high. Links between diet and disease, however tenuous, seem to capture the public imagination. Vitamin C for the common cold or to prevent cancer, vitamin E for aging, the Pritikin diet for vascular disease, megavitamins for behavioral disorders, and many other unproven or disproven nutritional treatments are

Eugene C. Corbett, Jr., and Daniel M. Becker • Department of Internal Medicine, University of Virginia School of Medicine, Charlottesville, Virginia 22908.

Table I. Recommended Daily Dietary Allowances (1980), Food and

	Age (years)	Weight kg	Weight lb	Height cm	Height in	Protein (g)	Fat-soluble vitamins: Vitamin A (μg RE)	Vitamin D (μg)	Vitamin E (mg aTE)
Infants	0.0–0.5	6	13	60	24	kg × 2.2	420	10	3
	0.5–1.0	9	20	71	28	kg × 2.0	400	10	4
Children	1–3	13	29	90	35	23	400	10	5
	4–6	20	44	112	44	30	500	10	6
	7–10	28	62	132	52	34	700	10	7
	11–14	45	99	157	62	45	1000	10	8
	15–18	66	145	176	69	56	1000	10	10
	19–22	70	154	177	70	56	1000	7.5	10
	23–50	70	154	178	70	56	1000	5	10
	51+	70	154	178	70	56	1000	5	10
Females	11–14	46	101	157	62	46	800	10	8
	15–18	55	120	163	64	46	800	10	8
	19–22	55	120	163	64	44	800	7.5	8
	23–50	55	120	163	64	44	800	5	8
	51+	55	120	163	64	44	800	5	8
Pregnant[b]						+30	+200	+5	+2
Lactating[b]						+20	+400	+5	+3

[a]RE, retinol equivalent; aTE, α-tocopherol equivalent; NE, niacin equivalent.
[b]Values are in addition to recommended daily allowance according to age.
[c]Dietary iron must be supplemented to meet nutritional needs.

widely and enthusiastically proclaimed. Yet amid a flourishing health food industry and rampant nutritional quackery, dietary common sense is taking hold. The extended debate about salt, fat, cholesterol, fiber, and sugar has convinced many that there are nutritional means of preserving and protecting health. The national interest in diet is an opportunity for wholesale prevention. Indeed, recent downward trends in cardiovascular mortality may be a consequence of a changing American diet. As perceptions of a healthy diet evolve, primary-care practitioners should continue to have a major role in interpreting nutritional science and promoting individual change. In doing so it will be necessary to point out to patients the limits as well as the benefits of preventive nutrition.

This chapter presents an overview of nutrition-related disease in the United States. Many of the important issues remain controversial. Topics with major public health implications are emphasized. In addition, aspects of food preparation and promotion, insofar as they relate to the concept of preventive nutrition, are discussed.

2. NUTRITION IN THE UNITED STATES

Estimating the prevalence of nutritional disease in the United States is difficult for many reasons: both dietary deficiency and excess can lead to disease; the relationships between diet and chronic disease remain poorly understood; measuring nutritional status requires biochemical, anthropometric, clinical, historical, and dietary assessments; the dietary history is difficult to determine and easily biased. Nevertheless, there have been determined efforts to collect nutritional information about the American people.

Nutrition Board, National Academy of Sciences—National Research Council[a]

Water-soluble vitamins							Minerals					
Vitamin C (mg)	Thiamine (mg)	Riboflavin (mg)	Niacin (mg NE)	Vitamin B_6 (mg)	Folacin (μg)	Vitamin B_{12} (μg)	Calcium (mg)	Phosphorus (mg)	Magnesium (mg)	Iron (mg)	Zinc (mg)	Iodine (μg)
35	0.3	0.4	6	0.3	30	0.5	360	240	50	10	3	40
35	0.5	0.6	8	0.6	45	1.5	540	360	70	15	5	50
45	0.7	0.8	9	0.9	100	2.0	800	800	150	15	10	70
45	0.9	1.0	11	1.3	200	2.5	800	800	200	10	10	90
45	1.2	1.4	16	1.6	300	3.0	800	800	250	10	10	120
50	1.4	1.6	18	1.8	400	3.0	1200	1200	350	18	15	150
60	1.4	1.7	18	2.0	400	3.0	1200	1200	400	18	15	150
60	1.5	1.7	19	2.2	400	3.0	800	800	350	10	15	150
60	1.4	1.6	18	2.2	400	3.0	800	800	350	10	15	150
60	1.2	1.4	16	2.2	400	3.0	800	800	350	10	15	150
50	1.1	1.3	15	1.8	400	3.0	1200	1200	300	18	15	150
60	1.1	1.3	14	2.0	400	3.0	1200	1200	300	18	15	150
60	1.1	1.3	14	2.0	400	3.0	800	800	300	18	15	150
60	1.0	1.2	13	2.0	400	3.0	800	800	300	18	15	150
60	1.0	1.2	13	2.0	400	3.0	800	800	300	30	15	150
+20	+0.4	+0.3	+2	+0.6	+400	+1.0	+400	+400	+150	[c]	+5	+25
+40	+0.5	+0.5	+5	+0.5	+100	+1.0	+400	+400	+150	[c]	+10	+50

2.1. Surveys

There are two major sources of information about food consumption and nutritional status: the Nationwide Food Consumption Survey (NFCS), sponsored by the U.S. Department of Agriculture (USDA), and the National Health and Nutrition Examination Survey (NHANES), conducted by the U.S. Department of Health and Human Services (HHS).[2,3] The NFCS and NHANES provide different but complementary data. The NFCS contains information about how food is consumed (when and where people eat, household food expenses) as well as dietary patterns. This information has been gathered over the past 40 years. HHS began a national health survey in the 1950s and added a nutritional component (the 10-state survey) in 1968. During 1971–1974 and 1976–1980 NHANES 1 and 2 studied a probability sample of the U.S. population aged 1–74. Unique to the NHANES programs is that the data are based on measured health indices collected in a standardized manner. These data include dietary information, results of dental and medical examination including anthropometric measures, and measurements of nutritionally important biochemical markers.

Nationwide Food Consumption Survey data from 1977–1978 show that 25% of money for food is spent for restaurant and takeout meals. The amount spent per household per day for food increases with income. Comparing before-tax household incomes of $5000 and $20,000 in 1977, $15.42 and $18.46, respectively, were spent per day for food. Lower-income families got more nutrient value per dollar spent compared to higher-income families. Among lower-income families, 9% reported insufficient food quantity.

In terms of dietary information, data from NHANES and NFCS are similar even though differences in study design make comparisons difficult. Nutrient intake data regarding total energy, protein, calcium, iron, vitamin A, vitamin C, thiamine, riboflavin,

Table II. Dietary Recommendations[a]

	Maintain ideal body weight	Reduce fat (% calories)	Reduce saturated fat	Increase polyunsaturated fat	Reduce cholesterol	Reduce simple sugar	Increase complex carbohydrates	Reduce sodium (g. NaCl equivalent)	Increase fiber	Other recommendations[b]
American Heart Association (1978)	Yes	Yes (30–35%)	Yes	Yes	Yes	Yes	Yes	Yes	No	1
Select Committee on Nutrition and Human Needs, U.S. Senate (1977)	Yes	Yes (27–33%)	Yes	Yes	Yes (250–350 mg)	Yes	Yes	Yes (<8 g)	Yes	1–6
U.S. Surgeon General (1979)	Yes	Yes	Yes	No	Yes	Yes	Yes	Yes	—	5,6
American Medical Association	Yes	High-risk groups	High-risk groups	High-risk groups	High-risk groups	Moderate	—	Yes (<12 g)	—	1,5,6
National Cancer Institute	Yes	Yes	—	No	—	—	—	—	Yes	1,5,6
Food and Nutrition Board, National Academy of Sciences	Yes	Adjust to caloric needs	No	No	No	If energy needs, low for diabetics	For diabetics	Yes (3–8 g)	As dictated by basic four food groups	1,5,6

[a]Source: McNutt.[1]

[b]Other recommendations: (1) moderate reduction of alcohol, (2) moderate reduction of additives, (3) moderate reduction of processed foods, (4) associate use of sugar with diabetes, (5) encourage exercise, (6) stress importance of food variety.

fat, and cholesterol are available. Information regarding folacin, vitamin B_6, and trace elements is limited in these surveys. Considerable day-to-day variation was noted. For example, there was a 20-fold range in daily intake for vitamin A and a fourfold range for energy intake. For many the energy intake was so low that only a sedentary lifestyle could be maintained. In terms of dietary intake, some of the nutrients seemed deficient. Iron and calcium intakes were low for many women. Intake of vitamin A, vitamin C, and protein was low for some population subgroups. There was no consistent relation between race, income, sex, or age with regard to inadequate intake. However, low income did not necessarily mean that the overall amount of food was less. Some nutrients were consumed excessively. Cholesterol and fat intake were high. In the NFCS study, fat accounted for 41% of the estimated energy intake. In NHANES 2 cholesterol intake averaged 405 mg/day for men and 266 mg/day for women. Both mean cholesterol intake and mean serum cholesterol values have decreased slightly since the 1960s.

Nutritional status is not defined simply by diet. Among the various dietary deficiencies noted in NHANES intake data, only iron deficiency had clearly associated biochemical and clinical findings (i.e., anemia). While these surveys show that malnutrition, in the form of nutrient deficiency, is very rare in the United States,[4] the data also point out the detrimental health effects of nutritional excess. There is evidence from NHANES and NFCS that relates obesity, dental caries, atherosclerosis, and hypertension to overeating and dietary misuse of fat, cholesterol, sugar, and sodium salt.

2.2. Nutritional Deficiency in Special Groups

Although in the United States and other industrialized nations nutritional deficiency states are rare, certain segments of the population are at higher risk to suffer from inadequate nutrition. Hospitalized patients, whether medical or surgical, frequently suffer protein and caloric malnutrition. The prevalance of malnutrition in general-medical patients is consistently more than 33%.[5] Some nutritional deficiency is acquired in the hospital, but in one study 22% of hospital patients were undernourished at the time of admission.[6] Various nutritional diseases, including protein, folate, and thiamine deficiency states, complicate chronic alcoholism. The elderly, whether at home, in the hospital, or in nursing homes, are particularly prone to poor nutrition.[7] The causes for this are multiple and include physical disability, poverty, social isolation, mental disorders, impaired appetite, inefficient mastication, intestinal malabsorption, and drug effects (including alcohol). While they suffer from chronic diseases that reduce both appetite and efficiency of eating, their nutrient needs are often increased by frequent acute illness.

3. NATURAL FOOD VERSUS PROCESSED FOOD

3.1. Organic Food

Although the United States has the most abundant and available food supply in the world, there is growing concern that it is unsafe. At issue is whether proper nutrition requires "health food" (natural, organic) as opposed to processed, refined, animal "junk food." This debate has assumed moralistic overtones: which foods are good and which bad?

It is difficult to define organic or natural food. Most foods are grown or raised, and in the chemical sense manufactured foods consist of organic compounds. Nevertheless, organic or natural foods are relatively free from fertilizers, pesticides, additives, and commercial processing. In this sense, such foods are pure but not necessarily better. Of necessity, production of organic foods is limited. In contrast, modern agriculture and food science manage to feed huge urban populations. As food is processed along the way from farm to store shelf, does it become less nutritious as well as less natural? How toxic are the various chemicals that increase productivity and retard spoilage?

Organic and natural foods can be compared to the foods that are generally available in stores and restaurants. Such comparisons should examine nutritional value, cost, and toxicity. It appears that an organic apple is as nutritious as a nonorganic apple, but it costs much more.[8]

The nutritional content of "fast foods" has been examined in detail. Perhaps surprisingly, examples of fast-food meals conform closely to modern dietary standards in terms of carbohydrate, fat, protein, vitamins, and minerals. Although the sodium content of fast-food meals is high, it is no higher than that of the traditional American meal purchased at a restaurant (steak, French fries, salad with dressing).[9]

3.2. Pesticides and Additives

Although it is relatively easy to defend the nutritional value of processed food, the question of toxicity from pesticide contaminants and food additives is more difficult to answer. Although hazards from pesticide residues are of concern, there are no known injuries or deaths related to their presence in foods.[10] It is difficult, if not impossible, to produce food absolutely free of pesticides. Pesticide residues are commonly found even in organic produce. There are certainly environmental and occupational risks associated with the pesticide industry, but their potential ill effects as food contaminants have been prevented by policies enforced by the Food and Drug Administration (FDA) and the USDA. There have been instances in which environmental and other industrial toxins (mercury, polybrominated biphenyls) have tragically contaminated the food chain.

A number of food additives concern the public.[11] These include nitrites, synthetic antioxidants, food colors, mold inhibitors, monosodium glutamate, diethylstilbestrol (DES), refined sugar, and salt. The latter two items can most easily be related to illness and will be discussed in another section. All additives are scrutinized by the FDA for reproductive, teratogenic, mutagenic, carcinogenic, and toxic effects. Many synthetic food dyes have been replaced by natural compounds, such as carotene, with inherent food value. Because of public feeling about "chemicals" in food, mold inhibitors (propionates and sorbates) and synthetic antioxidants (butylated hydroxyanisole and butylated hydroxytoluene) are used less frequently by food manufacturers. Natural antioxidants such as vitamins E and C may be useful instead of synthetic antioxidants. DES, used in the cattle industry to lower beef fat content, may carry a risk of carcinogenesis since it has been related to vaginal adenocarcinoma following *in utero* exposure. DES has been detected in trace quantities in beef liver but not in muscle; 100,000 tons of beef liver yield

12.3 g of DES, a dose that had no cancer risk in human studies. Antibiotics enter the food chain through their use in animal feeds. There is legitimate concern that these practices lead to increased antibiotic resistance in bacteria that are human pathogens.

Nitrites have received particular publicity. They are added to preserved foods to inhibit growth of *Clostridium botulinum* and are easily converted to nitrosamines. The latter are carcinogenic in laboratory animals at very low doses. Unfortunately, it is difficult to avoid nitrosamines. Although the FDA and the USDA are taking steps to limit nitrite content in cured meat, most nitrites reaching the stomach are derived from nitrates, found in many common vegetables including celery, spinach, lettuce, carrots, and beets. Dietary nitrites can be converted to nitrosamines by cooking (e.g., frying bacon) or by enzymes in saliva.

Food allergies can sometimes be explained by additives.[12] Sulfites (sodium and potassium sulfite or metabisulfite) are used as antioxidants in fresh fruits, fresh vegetables, and wines. They can cause urticaria or wheezing, usually in atopic individuals. Vegetable gums have been identified as allergents. Tartrazine yellow dye has been indicated as a cause of asthma and chronic urticaria. More commonly, food allergies with urticaria are due to foods such as shellfish, eggs, peanuts, strawberries, and tomatoes.

Concern over food additives includes their behavioral effects as well as their potential toxic, allergic, and carcinogenic properties. It has also been claimed that artificial food colorings, artificial flavorings, and foods that contain salicylates are the cause of hyperkinetic behavior and learning disabilities in children. Disturbed behavior in children has been blamed on foods with high sugar content. Furthermore, megavitamin treatment has been touted for various behavioral disorders in children and adults (see Section 3.4). Scientific investigations have failed to confirm any relationships between dietary factors and behavior.[13] However, studies in this area have been limited.

It should be mentioned that there are intrinsic hazards of food in addition to the risks added with modern farming and processing techniques.[14,15] Food poisoning due to microbiological contamination affects 10 million Americans per year. Potential toxins in commonly consumed foods include tannin in tea and coffee, goitrogens in broccoli and cabbage, and arsenic in shrimp. Although these substances do not reach toxic levels when consumed, they have not been studied in the same way as food additives. Traditional cooking methods also contribute to the dangers of food. Smoking and barbecuing meat add polycyclic hydrocarbon carcinogens to the food. Risks associated with vegetarian diets, megavitamins, and ''herbal'' remedies are discussed in the following sections.

3.3. Vegetarian Diets

In developed nations such as the United States, vegetarian diets are increasingly popular. Although such diets are generally quite healthy, there have been a few reports of nutrient deficiency resulting from strict vegetarianism (i.e., no eggs, fish, poultry, or milk products). Despite low vitamin B_{12} intake, most vegetarians have enhanced vitamin B_{12} absorptive capacity and do not become deficient. However, overt hematological and neurological signs can develop if low intake is coupled with subtle malabsorption.[16] Breast-fed infants of strict vegetarian mothers have been reported to develop vitamin B_{12} deficiency.[17] Milk-free vegetarian diets can lead to rickets in young children.[18] Trace metal deficiencies, particularly of zinc, can occur among vegetarians consuming diets high in phytate, an organic acid found in cereals. In the intestinal lumen phytate binds minerals and thereby reduces their absorption.[19]

3.4. Vitamin Misuse

Large doses of vitamins (see Table I for recommended daily allowances) are used at times in ill-conceived efforts to improve medical and psychological health. While the benefits of pharmacological doses of certain vitamins have not been proven, toxicity from overzealous vitamin use does occur.

3.4.1. Vitamin A

Acute vitamin A poisoning (single dose greater than 1,500,000 IU) causes increased intracranial pressure. Chronic poisoning (25,000–50,000 IU daily for months) features dermatological changes (hair loss, brittle nails, glossitis, dry skin), hepatosplenomegaly, fever, bone tenderness, increased intracranial pressure, and hypercalcemia. Vitamin A toxicity has been reported in young children taking large doses of vitamin A in quasi-medical attempts to control behavior or health.[20,21]

3.4.2. Vitamin D

Vitamin D is the nutrient most likely to cause toxicity. Its therapeutic index is low, and it is widely available as a food supplement and in vitamin preparations. Doses of 60,000 IU daily can lead to hypercalcemia, with weakness, volume depletion, ectopic calfication, gastrointestinal (GI) symptoms, headache, and hypertension. Vitamin D intoxication is often iatrogenic since it is used frequently in adult and pediatric practice.

3.4.3. Vitamin B_6 (Pyridoxine)

Recently, a sensory neuropathy (decreased pain, touch, pinprick temperature, vibration, and position senses) has followed use of large doses of pyridoxine for premenstrual symptoms or as part of a body-building program.[22] The neuropathy appeared after taking gram quantities on a daily basis (recommended daily allowance 2.0–2.2 mg/day). After the vitamin was stopped, significant but incomplete improvement gradually occurred.

3.4.4. Niacin (Nicotinic Acid)

Large doses of niacin, up to 3 g daily (recommended daily allowance 18 mg daily) have well-established efficacy in lowering serum cholesterol. Similar doses have dubious value in treating psychiatric conditions (''orthomolecular therapy''). These large doses routinely cause flushing, pruritus, and GI upset as a consequence of niacin-induced histamine release. There have been a few reports of acute hepatitis following regular use of high-dose niacin (0.75–4.5 g daily) for its alleged antipsychotic properties.[23,24]

3.4.5. Vitamin C

Scientific evidence notwithstanding, high-dose ascorbic acid, used commonly to prevent colds, has some potentially harmful side effects, including diarrhea, hemolysis in

G-6-PD-deficient patients, uricosuria, and hyperoxaluria.[25] The latter two metabolic changes create a theoretical risk of kidney stone formation. Breast-fed infants of mothers taking large doses of vitamin C can develop scurvy after being weaned.[25] Large amounts of vitamin C (as well as vitamin K) can reduce the anticoagulant effect of warfarin.

3.5. Herbal Remedies

Herbal teas are widely available. Their pharmacological properties can be potent and dangerous. Table III lists some plant products and their harmful effects.[15]

4. OBESITY

4.1. Epidemiology

The most prevelant nutritional disorder is overeating.[25] Obesity is defined by the National Center for Health Statistics as having triceps subscapular skinfold thickness greater than that of the 85th percentile of men or women aged 20–29. Overweight is defined similarly, but using body mass index (weight in kilograms divided by surface area in meters squared) rather than subcutaneous fat measurements. Severe obesity or severe overweight corresponds to the 95th percentile of the respective index. Although it is possible to be overweight but not obese (e.g., body builders), and vice versa, in most instances the two conditions coexist.

According to NHANES 2 data, between 1976 and 1980 34 million Americans were overweight, and among these 12.4 million were severely overweight.[26] This prevalence increases with age for black and white people of either sex. The highest prevalence of overweight occurs among black women: 30% at age 25; 60% at age 45. Poverty increases the frequency of this condition, and the association of obesity and poverty is particularly strong for women.

Table III. Pharmacological and Toxic Effects of Herbal Remedies

Pharmacological or toxic effect	Plant
Diuretic	Buchu, quack grass, dandelion, juniper berries, shave grass, horsetail
Cathartic	Buckthorn bark, senna, dock roots, aloe leaves
Anticholinergic or psychotogenic	Catnip, juniper, mandrake, snakeroot, hydrangea, jimson, wormwood, nutmeg
Aldosteronelike	Licorice root
Abortifacient	Devil's claw root, penny royal oil
Carcinogenic	Sassafras root
Estrogenic	Ginseng
Cyanogenetic glycosides	Leaves, seeds, or bark of apricot, cassava, cherry, choke cherry, peach, pear, apple, plum

4.2. Associated Diseases

There is ample clinical and epidemiological evidence that obesity is detrimental to health. Obesity-associated diseases, metabolic changes, and symptoms include diabetes mellitus, hyperlipidemia, hyperuricemia, gout, gallstones, kidney stones, fatty liver, nephrosis, hypertension, musculoskeletal disorders, hernia, pulmonary insufficiency, congestive heart failure, coronary artery disease, cerebrovascular disease, peripheral vascular disease, venous stasis, surgical and anesthetic complications, obstetrical complications, and various cancers (particularly uterine). Finally, significant psychosocial problems are related to obesity: poor self-image, social discrimination, increased psychoneurosis. Not unexpectedly, obesity adversely affects longevity. Data from the Framingham study suggest that overweight nonsmoking men had 30-year mortality rates 3.9 times higher than those of men of desirable weight.[27] To explain the underlying causes of this increased mortality, some of the more important diseases associated with obesity will be discussed in detail.

4.2.1. Coronary Artery Disease

Although obesity is associated with various risk factors for heart disease, including hypertension, diabetes mellitus, elevated total serum cholesterol, reduced high-density lipoprotein, and elevated triglycerides, the evidence that obesity or overweight is a risk factor for coronary artery disease is inconsistent.[28] Some epidemiological studies show no relationship, others a linear relationship (i.e., risk increases with obesity index), and others a U-shaped relationship (i.e., negative relationship at low weights but positive relationship with high weights). Autopsy studies of obese men have not consistently demonstrated increased coronary atherosclerosis. Cross-cultural studies are inconsistent. In Finland, fatter men have lower rates of cardiac death and myocardial infarction. As the rate of obesity in the U.S. population increases, there have been overall declines in mortality rates from myocardial infarction, cardiovascular disease, and stroke.

It is difficult to explain these negative results. They may be due to methodological problems in the various studies or poorly understood physiological factors. There are different types of obesity, and perhaps only abdominal obesity is a risk factor. Obesity may be protective due to dietary differences (more trace elements, increased alcohol intake), better stress adaptation, or endogenous factors (e.g., increased estrogen). Obesity may be a surrogate risk factor, concealing the atherogenic aspects of fattening diets or lack of exercise.

4.2.2. Hypertension

Although the association of hypertension and obesity has been known for years, it remains poorly understood.[29] As body mass increases with age, so does the arterial pressure. Industrialized populations steadily gain weight through the adult years, and the prevelance of hypertension increases accordingly. In primitive societies, weight is stable after full skeletal growth and the prevalence of hypertension does not increase with age. Data from the Framingham studies show that weight gain in young adult life predicts the later development of hypertension. Conversely, weight loss leads to reduction of blood pressure in large proportions of overweight hypertensive patients. Weight loss can also reduce blood pressure in normal patients, as shown in World War II studies during conditions of semistarvation. Weight loss without salt restriction will lower blood pressure, suggesting that the association of obesity and hypertension is not simply due to dietary salt.

4.2.3. Diabetes Mellitus

Non-insulin-dependent diabetes mellitus (NIDDM, or adult-onset diabetes mellitus) commonly affects obese elderly people. In 1916 Dr. Elliot Joslin wrote, "No pre-existent abnormal condition has occurred more frequently among my diabetic patients than has obesity.[30] Data from the 1976 National Health Information Survey confirm relationships between obesity, NIDDM, and age. For whites and blacks of both sexes, the reported frequency of diabetes increases with age and body mass index. The affected proportions of the surveyed population ranged from 0.5% among the least obese group aged 20–44 to 20.2% among black males older than 65 years in the most obese group (body mass index greater than 28.49 kg/m^2).[31]

The physiological factors underlying the development of diabetes in obese individuals include increased insulin resistance mediated at the cellular site of insulin action by decreased insulin receptors and postreceptor blockade; genetic predisposition; carbohydrate dietary composition; less exercise-induced glucose transport into cells; and impaired pancreatic beta-cell insulin production.

Given the host of morbid conditions associated with obesity and overweight, and the potential benefit of proper eating and exercise, obese patients should be targeted for preventive care. However, it is difficult for physicians or anyone else to meaningfully influence another person's dietary habits. This important subject will be discussed in Section 10.

5. LIPIDS

Dietary fat is important in the pathogenesis of atherosclerotic heart disease (ASHD) and perhaps in the development of certain cancers. This section discusses the various sources and types of dietary lipids, briefly defines the normal and abnormal constituents of serum lipids, and reviews the evidence that links fat to vascular disease. Although certain patterns of fat consumption have been associated with prostate, breast, and colon cancer, this topic is discussed in Chapter 16.

5.1. Definitions

Lipids are organic substances insoluble in water. Triglycerides are the major form of fat in food, blood, and fatty tissue. They serve as fuel and as sources of fatty acids necessary for the manufacture of cell membranes, phospholipids, and prostaglandins. Cholesterol is the primary sterol, needed for the synthesis of adrenal cortical hormones, sex hormones, and bile acids. Cholesterol is available both from the diet and by endogenous synthesis. Triglycerides and cholesterol are packaged with specific proteins, termed apoproteins, for plasma transport as lipoproteins. Genetic and acquired abnormalities in

Table IV. Lipid Classification

Lipoprotein	Pattern of associated hyperlipidemia	Major lipids	Apoproteins	Clinical effects
Chylomicrons	1, 5	Dietary triglycerides	AI, AIII, CI, CII, CIII	Eruptive xanthoma, pancreatitis
Very-low-density lipoprotein	2b, 4	Endogenous triglycerides	B, CI, CII, CIII, E	Eruptive xanthoma, pancreatitis, possible increased ASHD
Remnants	3	Cholesterol triglycerides	B, CIII, E	Tuberous xanthelasma, premature ASHD
Low-density lipoprotein	2a, 2b	Cholesterol	B	Tendon xanthelasma, premature ASHD
High-density lipoprotein		Cholesterol	AI, AII	Reduced ASHD risk

serum lipoproteins are associated with various diseases (see Table IV). By far the most important associated disease is ASHD. Both triglyceride and cholesterol elevations have been studied in this context, but the triglyceride data are inconclusive and will not be reviewed.

5.2. Lipids and Atherosclerosis

Epidemiological, clinical, and animal research supports the causal relationship between dietary fat and atherosclerosis.

5.2.1. Epidemiological Research

The association between elevated serum cholesterol and coronary artery disease has been a consistent finding in epidemiological studies throughout the world. This association precedes the clinical manifestations of the disease, holds for men and women, and becomes stronger as the serum cholesterol increases.

The Framingham study is the most frequently quoted investigation of ASHD risk factors.[32] Among the multiple interrelated host and environmental variables studied in this prospective evaluation of 2282 men and 2845 women, blood lipids were the strongest and most consistent risk factor. Cholesterol values between 250 mg/dl and 350 mg/dl represented the upper quartile of the study population. Elevations in this range increase the risk of ASHD two to five times. The risk associated with an elevated cholesterol increases steeply above a serum cholesterol of 210 mg/dl, even though this value is close to the population mean. This risk is age related and is strongest with patients younger than 65 years.

Estimates of fat intake correlated with average serum cholesterol values and ASHD in various cross-cultural studies. In countries such as Greece and Yugoslavia, where fat represents 30% of total calories, hypercholesterolemia and ASHD are three to five times less common than in the United States, where fat accounts for 40% of total calories.[33] In this cross-cultural study (the seven-countries study) differences in ASHD death rates between the various cohorts were related to differences in blood pressure, serum cholesterol, and dietary saturated (hydrogenated) fat. In a study from South Africa, poor blacks were shown to eat little animal fat, to have low serum cholesterol levels, and to suffer only rarely from ASHD.[34] Among vegetarian Seventh-Day Adventists the mortality rate from ASHD is one-third that of nonvegetarian Seventh-Day Adventists.[35] A cohort study of 1900 male employees of Western Electric Company (Chicago) followed prospectively for 20 years showed that dietary fat intake correlated with serum cholesterol and risk of ASHD.[36]

As it became clear that total serum cholesterol was related to risk of ASHD, various lipoproteins fractions were studied to determine their association with ASHD (see Table IV). The inverse correlation of high-density lipoprotein (HDL) and ASHD was noted more than 20 years ago.[37] Prospective data from the Framingham study confirmed that the higher the HDL levels, the lower the risk of ASHD.[38] In fact, these relatively recent Framingham data show that HDL levels are more powerful than other lipid indicators in predicting ASHD.

5.2.2. Clinical Research

The most obvious clinical phenomenon relating cholesterol and ASHD is the extraordinary risk associated with familial hypercholesterolemia (type IIA). The striking elevations of serum cholesterol in this disease are due to genetic defects in the production of the low-density lipoprotein (LDL) cellular receptor. Patients who are homozygous for this defect develop ASHD in childhood, and myocardial infarction has been reported as early as 18 months.[39] Heterozygotes develop ASHD in the third or fourth decade. By age 60 approximately 85% have had a myocardial infarction.[39]

A multicenter randomized clinical trial (Lipid Research Council Coronary Prevention Trial) tested the benefit of lowered cholesterol in reducing ASHD among men with type II hypercholesterolemia.[40] Approximately 4000 men were randomized. Treated and control groups followed low-cholesterol diets, but the treated patients also took cholestyramine. After approximately 7 years, treated patients had lower total serum cholesterol and LDL as well as 24% less ASHD deaths and 19% less nonfatal myocardial infarctions.

Clinical studies have examined the role of apoproteins in ASHD. Low levels of apoprotein A and high levels of apoprotein B have been reported in survivors of myocardial infarction.[41] Apoprotein B is the major apoprotein of LDL, and apoprotein A-I is the major apoprotein of HDL. The ratio of apoprotein A-I to apoprotein B is low in survivors of myocardial infarction compared to healthy sex-and-age-matched controls.[41] Furthermore, this ratio discriminated between normolipemic myocardial infarction survivors and controls. In this study serum HDL levels were also significantly lower in the myocardial infarction group.

Although high levels of HDL seem protective for ASHD and low levels appear to be a risk factor, patients with congenital HDL deficiency do not necessarily have precocious ASHD. The frequency of ASHD is not increased in patients with Tangier disease, in which HDL cholesterol is about 8% of normal.[42] However, two sisters with premature

ASHD were shown to have severe deficiencies of HDL, apoprotein A-I, and apoprotein C-III.[42]

5.2.3. *Animal Studies*

Many animal studies have shown that high-cholesterol diets raise serum cholesterol and lead to atherosclerosis. In addition, stopping the high-cholesterol feedings will then reverse the atherosclerotic process. Rhesus monkeys fed a high-fat, high-cholesterol diet developed coronary disease in 12 months. Control monkeys fed on the same atherogenic diet were then switched to low-cholesterol diets, and 12 months later these animals had evidence of regression of ASHD.[43]

5.3. *Determinants of Serum Cholesterol*

The determinants of serum cholesterol are incompletely understood.[39] Genetic, dietary, and lifestyle factors have been recognized. Cholesterol levels increase with aging, and stress can temporarily cause an increase in lipoprotein production and hence serum cholesterol.

5.3.1. *Genetics*

Familial hypercholesterolemia (type II-A) affects 1 in 500 people in the general population and 1 in 20 people with abnormally elevated serum cholesterol. Familial combined hyperlipidemia, leading to elevations in cholesterol, triglycerides, or both (types II-A, II-B, 4), accounts for about 10% of cholesterol elevation. The majority (approximately 85%) of people with elevated cholesterol have so-called polygenic hypercholesterolemia, determined by unknown genetic and environmental interactions. Diet is important regardless of the genetic predisposition.

5.3.2. *Diet*

As mentioned, estimates of fat intake correlate with serum cholesterol in cross-cultural studies. Saturated fat intake correlates with serum cholesterol, whereas monounsaturated fat and polyunsaturated fat intake does not. Saturated fats are generally solid in consistency (e.g., lard) and derived from animal sources. Red meat is the most important dietary source of saturated fat. Unsaturated fats are generally liquid (e.g., corn oil, safflower oil) and derived from plant sources. Cholesterol is found in all animal tissue, with particularly high levels in liver and eggs. The effects of cholesterol intake on serum cholesterol levels are quite variable. Genetic differences between individuals, dietary saturated and polyunsaturated fats, and the baseline serum cholesterol all influence the relationship between dietary and serum cholesterol. For example, among vegetarians no relationship was noted between dietary or egg cholesterol intakes and plasma lipid levels. However, comparing low-fat vegetarians (fat 23–33% of total energy intake) to high-fat vegetarians (35–48% energy intake), the former had 11% lower mean serum cholesterol and 14% higher high-density serum cholesterol.[44] Aside from dietary fat, there may be a connection between carbohydrate intake and serum cholesterol. This relationship is discussed in Section 6, "Sugar."

Serum cholesterol has been shown to vary with diet in studies where genetic variables have been controlled. Men of Japanese ancestry living in Japan, Hawaii, and California have progressively increasing intakes of total fat with parallel increases in serum cholesterol (181.1 mg/dl, 218.3 mg/dl, and 228.2 mg/dl, respectively).[45] Although from country to country the relationship between diet and serum cholesterol seems clear, within populations it is harder to demonstrate that diet determines serum cholesterol.[46,47] Thus in the Framingham data, there was no clear relationship between individual diet and serum cholesterol.

In controlled situations with human subjects, such as in metabolic wards, there is a strong correlation between serum and dietary lipids.[46] Although restricted diet in a metabolic ward will consistently lower serum cholesterol, the reduction is not uniform between individuals, and those with initially high levels will remain with relatively high levels after dieting.[46]

5.3.3. High-Density Lipoprotein

HDL cholesterol levels may be increased by regular vigorous exercise, moderate alcohol consumption, caloric restriction with weight loss, and cessation of smoking. The data determining these effects are limited, but exercise is consistently associated with higher HDL levels. Furthermore, there is a dose effect, with marathon runners having higher values than joggers, who have higher values than inactive men.[48]

5.4. Fish Oils

There is growing evidence that high fish consumption is a protective factor against ASHD.[49] Eskimos eat 400 g of fish daily and have a low prevalence of ASHD. High fish consumption in Japan may also explain the low rate of ASHD there. Within Japan, areas of higher fish consumption have lower ASHD rates. A 20-year cohort study of 852 Dutch men showed that fish consumption correlated inversely with the incidence of ASHD.[50] There was a dose effect in this study: the more fish eaten, the lower the risk of ASHD death. As little as two fish dishes per week seemed to provide protection.

Dietary and physiological research has added to the plausibility of these fish tales. In limited studies of normolipemic and hyperlipemic subjects, fish oil diets have been shown to lower cholesterol and triglyceride levels impressively.[51] *In vitro* studies of monocyte and neutrophil function following increases in dietary fish oils showed decreased cyclooxygenase-related inflammatory effects.[52] This change reflects the competitive inhibition by eicosapentaenoic and docosahexaenoic acids of arachidonic acid utilization by cyclooxygenase. As a result there are less leukotriene B-4-mediated inflammatory effects. In terms of atherogenesis, fish oil-related antiinflammation may alter the process by which monocytes adhere to damaged arterial endothelium.

6. SUGAR

The use of sugar as a nutrient is a relatively recent phenomenon in the dietary history of humans. Although it has been known about for centuries (Pliny the elder referred to it as "a kind of honey made from reeds"), its cheaper production in the 19th and 20th centuries has allowed it to become widely and abundantly available.[53] Between 1900 and 1980, the world sugar production increased from 8 to 93 million tons.

In the United States since 1900, the consumption of carbohydrate in the form of starch has decreased nearly 50% while that of sugar has increased by 25%.[53] The estimated annual amount of per capita sugar consumption in 1909 was 75 lb compared to 102 lb now, and the trend appears to be continuing upward.[53]

Sugar contributes to excessive weight gain because of its attractive taste and widespread availability. In addition, it contributes to other health problems, including dental caries and diabetes mellitus. It may also be a factor in the development of atherosclerosis.

6.1. *Dietary Sugar*

Dietary sugars include mono- and disaccharides. The primary disaccharides in foods include sucrose, the common table sugar derived from plant sources, and the milk sugar lactose, the only sugar from an animal source. Simple sugars or monosaccharides include galactose (from lactose), dextrose (D-glucose), and fructose (primarily from fruits). Glucose, the form of sugar utilized in human biological systems, forms the basic substrate for human metabolic functions. It is derived from ingested mono- and disaccharides as well as from the polysaccharides of plant (starch) and animal (glycogen) sources.

Sugars constitute approximately 25% of the calories in the typical American diet.[54] Three-fourths of this amount comes from processed or refined sugars compared to one-quarter from natural fruit sources such as fruit and honey. In comparison, starches (polysaccharides) provide another 25% of the typical American caloric intake, while fat (42%) and protein (12%) account for the remaining dietary intake. In less developed societies refined sugars are not as widely available, and starches provide the predominant form of dietary carbohydrates. For example, in some areas of Africa 80% of the total caloric intake is from nonrefined vegetable sources of carbohydrate; the remainder is from protein and fat foods.[55,56]

6.2. *Sugar and Diabetes*

The increased consumption of sugar in the United States in the 20th century has been paralleled by an increasing prevalence of diabetes. For example, in 1959, the prevalence of diabetes was 8.7 cases per 1000 population compared to 16.2 in 1968 and 24.7 in 1979.[57] Although it is not clear whether sugar is involved directly in the etiology of diabetes mellitus, excess caloric intake in the form of simple sugars adds to the metabolic burden of the diabetic. For both insulin-dependent diabetes and non-insulin-dependent diabetes, insulin and glucose responses to processed carbohydrates (e.g., white bread, refined sugar) are high compared to caloric equivalents of whole-grain breads and vegetables. For diabetics with impaired insulin secretion or increased insulin resistance, diets low in sugars and high in complex carbohydrates decrease insulin demand and help to improve glucose tolerance.[58–60]

6.3. *Sugar and Dental Caries*

Dietary sugar is clearly involved in the development of dental caries and pyorrhea.[61] Eating sugar lowers the pH of the oral cavity and thereby allows the proliferation of acid-dependent, plaque-producing bacteria. The acid environment and the increased plaque enhance enamel destruction and subsequent dental infection. Dental caries are generally not found in cultures that do not use simple sugars in the diet. Use of fluoride in drinking water has helped stem the 20th-century epidemic of tooth decay. However, conservative dietary use of refined sugar and dental hygiene remain the mainstays of prevention in tooth and gum disease.

6.4. Obesity

It is easy to gain weight with high sugar consumption. Relatively small amounts of digested sugar represent large amounts of stored energy. Thus, 1 lb of body weight, equivalent to 3500 kcal of energy, would be provided by 1.75 lb of sugar. It would be difficult to utilize this amount of metabolic fuel. For example, walking or jogging 5 mph for 1 hr uses a mere 420–600 kcal.[62]

Sugar not only tastes good, but it is easily digested and thus large quantities can be consumed. Compared to fats and proteins, carbohydrate digestion is more rapid and is associated with less satiety.[59] Similarly, simple sugars provide less satiety than complex carbohydrates. Thus, on a high-carbohydrate, high-sugar diet, it is relatively easy to eat more food and therefore store more calories. The psychological appeal of sweet foods, the nutritional efficiency of refined carbohydrate diets, and the ubiquity of sugar in the American diet together help to explain why obesity is at present the major nutritional disease in the United States.

6.5. Fruits, Vegetables, Grains

The presence of fiber in the diet modifies some of the metabolic disadvantages of simple sugar. For example, comparing caloric equivalents of apple juice and whole apple, the latter induces a flatter insulin response and a lower glycemic index (a measure of incremental blood glucose following a meal) while providing greater satiety.[59] The fiber content of "sugar substitutes" (fruits, vegetables, grains) has other potential advantages associated with higher-fiber diets. These advantages are discussed in Section 7, "Fiber." In addition, experiments involving the isocaloric substitution of starch for sugar have demonstrated that serum cholesterol and triglyceride levels are lowered as much as 20% following the reduction of dietary simple sugar.[63] These observations may help to explain the relationship between diabetes and atherosclerosis. Dietary use of complex carbohydrates in lieu of simple sugars also has the important advantage of providing minerals and vitamins as well as calories.

7. FIBER

Prior to the mid-1960s, fiber was not considered an important nutrient. Nutritional textbooks at that time suggested that fiber was a relatively inert portion of dietary intake, and thus its connection to nutrition or to diseases was minimized. However, since then, interest in fiber has grown considerably because of evidence that it is an active ingredient in a variety of gastrointestinal and metabolic functions.

7.1. Definitions

Fiber refers to six plant cell wall constituents (gum, mucilage, pectin, hemicellulose, lignin, cellulose) that are generally resistant to human digestive mechanisms. Gum, mucilage, pectin, and some hemicellulose are digested by colonic bacteria in the colon. Lignin, cellulose, and a variable amount of hemicellulose are passed unaltered in the stool.

Crude fiber refers to the portion of fiber that remains after dissolution of fiber in dilute acid and alkali mediums. However, this term is not nutritionally relevant, and it is not useful in a clinical discussion.

Bran, a commonly used term, refers to the form of fiber that passes through the human gut unaltered by human or bacterial degradation. It is usually made up of variable amounts of cellulose, hemicellulose, and lignin.

7.2. Physiological Effects

7.2.1. Water-Holding Capacity

All fiber types have considerable hydrophilic activity, resulting in a greater water content of small intestinal contents and colonic feces. This activity is greatest with the soluble gel-forming gums, pectins, and mucilages and least with the insoluble celluloses, hemicelluloses, and lignins. However, since the latter forms are primarily passed unaltered in the stool, the formation of stool bulk is primarily a function of this undigested fiber. Because of their resistance to digestive and bacterial degredation, the more coarse preparations of bran have been shown to be the most effective stool softeners.[64] The majority of the increase in stool weight with bran supplementation is related to its water-holding capacity.

7.2.2. Transit Time and Stool Weight

A highly refined diet, with the least dietary fiber content, results in smaller, more firm, heavier stools, which take longer to transit through the GI tract. The presence of fiber increases stool bulk and diminishes bowel transit time.[65] Burkitt's studies indicate a two- to threefold difference in the average intestinal transit time between rural African villagers, with high-fiber unrefined diets, and British citizens, with typically refined western diets (35 hr versus 80 hr with 300 g of stool versus 100 g, respectively). For the westerner this results in increased contact time of the stool with the colonic mucosa. This increased contact time is postulated to be a mechanism in the pathogenesis of colon cancer in industrialized societies (see Chapter 16).

Although the increase in stool weight from the addition of fiber to the diet is heavily related to water content, it is also a function of increased bacterial mass and increased weight from the fiber content itself.

As opposed to enhanced colonic transit, gastric emptying appears to be delayed by the presence of dietary fiber. This effect has been noted to be quantitatively similar to the pharmacological effect of 30 mg of propantheline.[66] Delayed gastric emptying is associated with slower absorption of certain nutrients (e.g., sugar) as well as certain drugs (e.g., acetaminophen).

Higher-fiber diets increase the subjective sense of satiety after eating.[59] Thus, to feel "full" on a refined low-fiber diet, one must eat more. This phenomenon implies a role for fiber in the behavioral pattern underlying obesity.

7.2.3. Cation Exchange

Fiber enhances the excretion of various cations such as calcium, magnesium, zinc, and iron.[67] It is thus theoretically possible that increasing fiber in the diet might lead to cation deficiency. However, no clinically significant cation loss syndromes have been noted in populations with extremely high-fiber diets. Nor has cation loss been seen in individuals known to change from low to high dietary fiber. This cation-binding property however, raises the possibility of a carcinogenic cation-binding mechanism whereby fiber-containing diets might decrease the carcinogenic potential of western diets. It has been shown, for example, that the addition of wheat bran to the diet diminishes considerably the mutagenic activity of stools from patients with colon carcinoma.[68]

7.2.4. Adsorption and Excretion of Nutrients

The addition of fiber to diets has been shown to result in an increase in fecal excretion of bile acids, bile salts, nitrogen, fatty acids, and overall calories.[64]

Fecal energy loss occurs in the range of 20–95 kcal/day with dietary fiber supplementation in the form of bran biscuits.[69] A comparison of low-, middle-, and high-fiber diets showed a stool caloric excretion of 83, 127, and 210 kcal/day, respectively.[70] In a more recent study, the use of high-fiber intake in the form of fruits and vegetables led to a similar increase in fecal calorie excretion compared to a fiber-poor diet.[71] A similar phenomenon seems to be true with nitrogen and fat excretion. For example, addition of 15 g of citrus pectin to the controlled diets of experimental subjects increased fecal fat excretion by 44%.[72] Similarly, the addition of 10–15 g of dietary fiber in the form of bran biscuits resulted in a 30–50% increase in fecal nitrogen.[69] Although the clinical relevance of these phenomena is open to speculation, it is likely that high-fiber diets diminish caloric absorption compared to an isocaloric refined diet and therefore help to prevent obesity.

7.3. Fiber and Disease

The various fiber-related physiological changes reviewed here provide background for a consideration of the relationship of dietary fiber to disease. The following discussion highlights the currently considered role of dietary fiber in diverticulosis coli and constipation, colon carcinoma, diabetes mellitus, and atherosclerosis.

7.3.1. Diverticulosis Coli and Constipation

Presumably, diverticulosis results from sustained high intraluminal pressures, while high-fiber diets allow fecal passage at lower pressures.[73,74] Until 1971, however, diverticular disease had been treated with highly refined diets. In 1971 Painter showed that high-fiber diets enhance fecal passage and relieve symptoms of diverticulitis.[75] This salutary effect of dietary fiber has been observed in many studies since then, including a randomized trial in 1977.[76] Fiber may reverse the disease as well as improve symptoms. In a study of 40 patients with diverticulosis given 24 g of bran daily for 6 months, three patients no longer had demonstrable diverticula upon follow-up barium enema studies.[74]

Perhaps more important is the question of the role of dietary fiber in the prevention of diverticular disease. Epidemiological studies of diverticular disease demonstrate an inverse relationship between the development of diverticula in the colon and the fiber content of the diet.[77] Thus, African villagers (high-fiber diet) have very little diverticulosis compared to urban African populations (less dietary fiber).[78] As diets in Western industrialized nations have become more and more refined in the 20th century, the prevalence of colonic diverticulosis has also increased.[79,80] Japanese immigrants to Hawaii develop diverticulosis as they assume a western diet.[81] Vegetarians have less diverticulosis than nonvegetarian matched controls.[82] In another case-control study, fiber intake in patients with diverticular disease was half that of controls without diverticulosis.[83]

Although it appears that a fiber-rich diet is effective in the prevention as well as treatment of diverticular disease, further clinical trials are needed to clarify the dose and type of dietary fiber, the length of treatment, and the extent of disease reversal.

7.3.2. Cancer of the Colon

In 1971, Burkitt pointed out the lower incidence of colon cancer in African societies (3.5–5.5 per 100,000) compared to the population in Connecticut (51.8), New York (45.3), and Scotland (51.5).[84] Burkitt related these differences to variations of fiber in the diet. He noted much higher amounts of fiber in the diets of African villagers compared to the highly refined low-fiber diets of the average western diet.[84,65] In a more detailed and recent study of urban Denmark and rural Finland, between which there is a threefold difference in carcinoma of the colon incidence (14.2 per 100,000 versus 42.1 per 100,000), investigators observed that the low-incidence area was associated with both a high intake of nonstarch polysaccharides (i.e., dietary fiber) and an increase in stool bulk compared to the high-incidence areas.[85]

Burkitt's African data may be confounded by genetic differences between the urban and rural populations. However, blacks entering the United States from low-risk-colon-cancer areas develop incidence rates of colon cancer similar to those of the general U.S. population.[84] A similar change from low to high incidence has been shown for immigrants from Japan to the San Francisco/Oakland Bay area.[86]

While the epidemiological data linking colon cancer rates to patterns of dietary fiber are imposing, the mechanism for this relationship remains to be determined.

7.3.3. Diabetes

The glycemic effects of various foods are affected by their fiber content. For example, nondiabetic human experimental subjects have different insulin and glycemic responses to caloric equivalents of whole apples, crushed apples, and apple juice.[59] Insulin levels and glucose peaks were higher for apple juice compared to whole apple. Similar results have been shown by adding various types of fiber to a 10-g glucose load.[87] Thus, dietary fiber somehow moderates meal-associated blood glucose changes.

As might be expected, studies with diabetic patients have shown that increasing dietary fiber can improve glucose intolerance. For example, the medication needs of a group of diabetics (type I and type II) assigned to standard American Diabetic Association (ADA) diets or 15-g crude fiber diets were examined during a 2-week study.[88] In the high-fiber diet 75% of the calories were carbohydrate-derived compared to 43% for the ADA diet. Among insulin-requiring diabetics on the high-fiber diet, four of nine were able to stop insulin and the remainder required smaller dosages. Furthermore, the high-fiber diet allowed five of five subjects taking sulfonylureas to discontinue their medication. In another study that compared 3-g and 20-g crude-fiber diets for eight insulin-requiring diabetics, average daily glucose fell from 164 mg% to 120 mg% as the diet changed from low to high fiber.[89] At the same time there were more hypoglycemic reactions during the high-fiber phase, suggesting reduced insulin needs.

As mentioned in Section 6, "Sugar," epidemiological studies have shown that the prevalence of diabetes in a culture is directly related to sugar consumption by the population. As sugar consumption increases, dietary fiber decreases, and thus diabetes and dietary fiber have been inversely related in population studies. Thus, among hunter–gatherers (Bushmen, Hottentots, aborigines), diabetes does not exist.[90] Diabetes seems to be more common in urban than in rural Bantu in South Africa. Furthermore, comparisons of different racial and cultural groups in Africa show distinct differences with regard to glucose and insulin levels than urban whites.[56,90] In a study of a more homogeneous population in an industrialized society, Trowell examined death rates from diabetes in England during a World War II forced shift to a higher-fiber flour.[91] During 1941–1956, diabetic death rates fell more than 50% for men and women.

These various sources of epidemiological evidence suggest that diabetes becomes more common as a society shifts to a processed diet.[92] It is possible that this phenomenon is not casual but rather a reflection of genetic, cultural, or socioeconomic relationships.

7.3.4. Atherosclerosis

Various forms of dietary fiber have been shown to influence serum lipid levels. Depending on the amount and type of fiber, serum cholesterol can be lowered 20–100%.[93] For example, oat and bean fiber, in the range of 60 g/day, lowers cholesterol in hypercholesterolemic men by approximately 20%.[94] In this regard, soluble fiber, such as pectin or guar gum, is more effective than insoluble fiber, such as lignin or cellulose. The mechanism of this lipid-lowering effect is not known. It may involve fiber-induced fecal excretion of bile acids or enhanced metabolic degradation of lipoproteins.

In relatively small studies, high-fiber diets correlate inversely with atherosclerotic endpoints. In a cohort study of 871 middle-aged men in Zutphen, the Netherlands, mortality from coronary heart disease was four times higher for men in the lowest quintile of dietary fiber compared to those in the highest quintile.[95] It should be noted that this inverse relationship disappeared with an analysis that employed multiple logistic regression. Another relatively small cohort study from England showed an inverse relationship between dietary fiber and coronary disease.[96] These data are suggestive but limited, and the fiber–atherosclerosis hypothesis needs further investigation.

8. SALT

Salt, most commonly used for human consumption as sodium chloride, is important in the pathogenesis of hypertension. It is therefore included in the list of nutrients contributing to major diseases of our time.

8.1. Physiology

Sodium, primarily with the anion chloride, is the primary extracellular cation, essential to the maintainance of the osmotic equilibrium and the extracellular volume of the body. It forms approximately 0.15% of the body by weight. Sodium is absorbed only through the gastrointestinal tract, and it is excreted through the renal, integumentary, and gastrointestinal organs. Renal excretion accounts for approximately 90% of sodium loss under normal circumstances. Under conditions of heightened sweating, vomiting, or diarrhea, considerable amounts of sodium are lost via these routes. On the other hand, under conditions of restricted salt intake, renal and integumentary excretion of sodium approaches zero. The homeostatic control of sodium excretion is primarily under the influence of the renin–angiotensin–aldosterone system. In addition, natriuretic peptides in the atria and vascular tree recently have been shown to have a major role in blood volume and pressure regulation.[97]

8.2. Diet and Sodium

The normal human is capable of adapting to a very wide range of sodium intake, from less than 500 mg/day of sodium, to more than 25 g/day. Among various cultures there is a wide range of dietary salt use. In some nonindustrialized societies there is minimal sodium in the diet, whereas in some Oriental cultures large amounts of sodium are used to store and prepare food for eating.[98,99] In the NHANES I health and nutrition survey the average sodium chloride intake for various groups ranged from 3.8 to 7.5 g/day.[99] A 1957 study of employees at a large single workplace used urinary sodium measurements to infer daily intakes of 4–24 g (mean 10 gm).[101] A more recent review suggests similar daily salt intakes with approximately 20% of sodium chloride from meat, fish, and poultry foods; 15% from milk and milk products; and 50% from the salt added by the consumer as seasoning and flavoring.

Virtually all foodstuffs contain some amount of sodium, but there is a wide range of salt content. Fresh vegetables contain the least amount of sodium, whereas processed foods contain considerably more sodium. For example, 3½ oz of fresh peas contains 2 mg of sodium, and a similar amount of canned peas contains 236 mg. Meat sources are generally higher in salt than vegetable sources. Naturally occurring sources of sodium include dairy products, fish, poultry, and eggs. Soft water contains more sodium than naturally occurring hard water. A wide variety of food preservatives contain sodium, including monosodium glutamate, sodium sulfate, and the sodium nitrate and nitrites. Cooking fats originating from animal sources contain more salt than those from vegetable sources, the former being the kind most widely used in fast-food restaurants and commercial cooking.

8.3. Sodium Requirements

Based on observations in ambulatory settings over an extended period of time, Dahl estimates the average daily sodium requirement to be at most 40–185 mg.[102] In metabolic wards subjects on salt-free diets suffer no ill effects.[103,104] Some populations exist with virtually no salt (less than 10 mg of sodium per person per day) in their diets.[105–107]

While physiological adaptions to low sodium intakes are well tolerated, some individuals develop hypertension in response to excessive dietary sodium.

8.4. Sodium and Hypertension

The role of salt in the pathogenesis of hypertension has long been the focus of clinical, epidemiological, and experimental study (useful reviews in Refs. 98, 99, 104, 108).

8.4.1. Experimental Research

Dahl *et al.* demonstrated a cause-and-effect relationship between salt intake and hypertension in the rat.[109] By inbreeding techniques they developed two distinct populations of hypertensive (salt-sensitive) and nonhypertensive (salt-resistant) rats. In the salt-sensitive rats, they demonstrated a linear relationship between sodium intake and blood pressure. At higher levels of sodium intake and subsequent hypertension, increases in mortality and morbidity were seen. Hypertension was more likely if the high-salt diet was started early in life. In some cases hypertension persisted despite deletion of dietary salt.

The hypertensive effect of sodium may be mediated at the cellular level. In hypertensive individuals, red-blood-cell and white-blood-cell intracellular sodium is increased, and these levels reflect overall sodium balance.[110] Some studies have shown similar increases among normotensive relatives of hypertensive patients.

The hypertensive effect of sodium is in part a result of its role in maintaining extracellular volume. Increased salt intake will expand the extracellular space, and since extracellular volume is an important determinant of blood pressure, hypertension can result from volume expansion. Thus, Murray *et al.* were able to demonstrate a linear relationship between ingested sodium (over a range of 200 mg to 30 g) and cardiac output, stroke volume, body weight, and blood pressure.[111]

8.4.2. Epidemiological Research

In various cultures dietary sodium correlates with the prevalence of hypertension. At the lower end of the salt-use spectrum, studies in Uganda [105] and New Guinea[107] document salt intakes of less than 1 g daily and a corresponding absence of hypertension, hypertension-related diseases, and age-related increases in blood pressure. At the other end of the spectrum, one finds an average intake of 27 g of salt per day in certain areas of Japan, where there are also high prevalences of hypertension and hypertension-related diseases. Thus, in Japan cerebral vascular disease related to hypertension is the most important cause of death, and this is seen among young as well as old people.[112] Dahl and others document this relationship in other settings, showing that the frequency of hypertension in a population increases linearly with salt intake.[99,104] In a study of 1124 individuals in a single workplace, blood pressure correlated with self-described salt use. Only 1 of 101 who added no salt to the diet was hypertensive, whereas 38 of 522 who occasionally added salt and 58 of 501 who always added salt were hypertensive.[101]

An increased prevalence of hypertension in conjunction with an increase in dietary salt has been observed in genetically similar populations who migrate from rural areas to the city. This has been observed among the Zulu in Africa,[113] in New Guinea,[114] and in Polynesia.[115]

8.4.3. Clinical Research

As early as 1920, Allen documented that hypertension could be treated by salt restriction.[103,116] In 1950, on a metabolic ward, Dole *et al.* showed that a rice–fruit diet (less than 500 mg/day of sodium) reduced the blood pressure of six hypertensive patients.[117] A return of hypertension was effected when 2.5 g of sodium was added back to the daily diet. In another metabolic ward study these researchers documented hypertension in five patients on a 10-g salt diet, normalization of the blood pressure on ½ g of salt per day, and recurrence of hypertension when a similar 10-g amount was reinstituted in the diet.[118] Similar lowering of blood pressure in hypertensive individuals has been documented by others when diets containing less than 1 g of sodium per day are successfully followed.[119–121] More recent clinical trials have also shown the hypotensive effect of sodium restriction.[122–124] One of these, a double-blind, randomized, crossover trial using sodium tablets versus placebo, showed a 6.1% lowering of blood pressure for the low-salt (placebo) group.[125]

Estimates of the proportion of the population sensitive to the hypertensive effects of sodium suggest an even distribution of sodium-sensitive and -nonsensitive hypertensive individuals.[99,104,123] Thus, if half of the hypertensive population responded to sodium restriction, a considerable reduction in the prevalence of hypertension and hypertension-mediated vascular disease would follow.

9. VITAMINS AND TRACE MINERALS

9.1. Vitamins

Vitamins are a group of organic substances that, except for vitamin D, need to be obtained from the diet or through bacterial production (e.g., vitamin K). They are usually required in small amounts and have variable amounts of storage in the body. The fat-soluble vitamins, A, D, E, and K, are generally stored in larger amounts than the water-soluble vitamins, B and C, and therefore are less often associated with the deficiency states but more often associated with toxicity states. Vitamins function as cofactors and coenzymes in various metabolic systems. Overt vitamin deficiency states are now extremely rare in the general population in the United States. However, there is growing interest in the relationships between vitamins A and C and cancer, and between vitamin C and the common cold. Randomized clinical trials have disproved the latter connection, and there is little epidemiological evidence to support the theory that vitamin C can prevent cancer. The role of vitamin A in the development of cancer requires further discussion.

Vitamin A is necessary for the functioning of light-sensitive pigments of the retina. The amount of vitamin A needed for this is in the range of 500–600 μg of retinol per day, an amount more than adequately provided in a marginal American diet. A more controversial role for vitamin A involves the development of various cancers. There appears to be an inverse relationship between the amount of dietary vitamin A and its carotene precursors and the risk of cancers of the lung, larnyx, bladder, esophagus, stomach, and prostate.[126]

9.1.1. Dietary Sources and Requirements of Vitamin A

Vitamin A has both animal and plant sources in the diet. The fat-soluble forms are found primarily in dairy products, but meats are also good sources of vitamin A. The richest sources of the water-soluble vitamin A precursors, the carotenoids (e.g., beta carotene) are the darker-green and yellow vegetables, apricots, cherries, watermelon, and cantaloupe. Grains are also a relatively good source of vitamin A.

Vitamin A toxicity is seen with excessive intake of the fat-soluble forms of the vitamin, but not with the water-soluble caretenoid forms. There is a large variation in the serum and liver levels of vitamin A in Americans. Approximately 15% are around or below the lower limit of normal. Furthermore, NHANES data show that vitamin A intake is marginal for many people.[3] Thus there is a relatively large group of people who may suffer chronic mild vitamin A deficiency, and this dietary state may represent exposure to a cancer risk factor.

9.1.2. Cancer and Vitamin A

Vitamin A is essential to epithelial cell growth and differentiation, a function that underlies its possible role in neoplastic development. Mild deficiency of vitamin A leads to a metaplastic follicular hyperkeratinization in humans. *In vitro* experiments have shown an enhancement effect on tumor development in epithileal tissue in vitamin A-deficient cultures as well as a protective effect of vitamin A added to chemically carcinogenic media. Similar results have been observed in experimental animals under conditions of vitamin A deficiency and carcinogen-induced tumor development.[127]

Epidemiological studies in humans have consistently demonstrated an inverse relationship between the incidence of long carcinoma and the intake of dietary forms of vitamin A. There also appears to be an inverse relationship between serum levels of vitamin A and the development of cancer in general and lung cancer in particular.[128]

The consistency of these findings in both experimental and epidemiological investigations demands further study. The actual mechanism of this relationship remains to be elucidated.

9.2. Minerals, Elements, Electrolytes

Although 15 minerals, elements, and electrolytes are known to be essential in the human diet (calcium, phosphorus, magnesium, iron, zinc, iodine, copper, manganese, fluoride, chromium, selenium, molybdenum, sodium, potassium, chloride), only a few are important in the context of this chapter. Although trace elements have been implicated in the pathogenesis of some important diseases (selenium and cancer, chromium and diabetes), these relationships are controversial and beyond the scope of this discussion. Sodium, calcium, iodine, and iron are most commonly associated with disease. Sodium was discussed earlier. Iodine deficiency is an important cause of thyroid disease in developing countries, but iodine-deficiency goiter has been virtually eradicated in the United States and other developed countries through the widespread use of iodized table salt. Dietary calcium has been related to osteoporosis and hypertension. The former disease is discussed in Chapter 18. The relationship of calcium to hypertension requires further discussion, as does the subject of iron deficiency anemia.

9.2.1. Calcium and Hypertension

A number of studies have pointed to a relationship between dietary calcium and hypertension. NHANES 1 data indicate that low calcium intake is associated with hypertension.[129] It has also been shown that 1–2 g of supplemental calcium, the amount in a quart of milk, will lower blood pressure in hypertensive individuals.[130] However, in double-blind, crossover, placebo-controlled trials of patients with essential hypertension, supplemental calcium significantly lowered blood pressure in only half the patients.[131]

The physiological connection between calcium and hypertension is not understood. Serum levels of ionized calcium may be determinants of renin production.[132] Increased intracellular calcium may mediate the increased vascular tone of essential hypertension, and this effect may be altered by changes in dietary calcium.

Further research is necessary before specific dietary recommendations for calcium can be made to hypertensives. However, since many of these patients follow low-fat diets and therefore avoid dairy foods, their dietary calcium intake may be marginal and calcium supplementation may be in order.

9.2.2. Iron

Several nutritional surveys, including both HANES 1 and 2, have shown that dietary iron deficiency is quite common in the United States. Young children, women of child-bearing age, and the elderly are particularly affected. Lower socioeconomic status increases the likelihood of iron deficiency anemia. Table V lists the iron requirements for men, women, and children.[133] Menstruating or pregnant women have two to four times the iron needs of men or nonmenstruating women. Fortunately, iron replacement during pregnancy and lactation is almost universally recommended. Although dietary iron dimin-

Table V. Iron Requirements[a]

	Dietary intake (mg/day)	Absorbed iron (mg/day)
Men and nonmenstruating women	5–10	0.5–1
Menstruating women	7–20	0.7–2
Pregnant women	20–48	2–4.8
Adolescents	10–20	1–2
Children	4–10	0.4–1
Infants	5–15	0.5–1.5

[a]Source: Ref. 133.

ishes as eating patterns change with aging, average daily iron intake is adequate for most elderly Americans when adjusted according to caloric intake and biological needs.[134]

10. DIETARY CHANGE

The preceding discussion makes it clear that some dietary changes would lead to better health. Table II presents recommendations from various expert groups. These dietary goals focus on total calories, sugar, fat, fiber, and salt. In terms of preventive nutrition, these recommendations are important for all patients, not just those with diabetes, cardiovascular disease, hypertension, or obesity. Since dietary change is probably easier earlier in life, it makes more sense to intervene during adolescence and early adulthood than to struggle with a problem such as obesity in middle age. Although it is relatively easy to point out to patients which dietary changes might be important, it is much more difficult to change eating behavior and then document a benefit. The following discussion on the dietary management of obesity, hypertension, and hyperlipidemia illustrates these problems. The general subject of diet and cancer is discussed in Chapter 16.

10.1. Obesity and Weight Loss

Americans are anxious to lose weight. Approximately $10 billion is spent annually for weight reduction treatments.[135] However, most attempts to lose and maintain weight fail, and this failure is as common in a physician's practice as it is for the unsupervised dieter. In various clinical studies from 1966 to 1977, only about 20% of patients lost more than 9 kg, with an average weight loss of only 5.4 kg.[131] To succeed, weight loss programs must be able to help people change their eating and exercise patterns, and to do this psychological factors must be addressed.[136] A comprehensive approach is necessary, and this type of broad-based effort is beyond the reach of most primary-care practitioners. It is important for physicians to accept the limits of simple dietary advice and to rely on dietitians, nutritionists, nurses, psychologists, and community groups (e.g., Weight Watchers) to help with dietary management.

Some of the results of comprehensive outpatient obesity management programs are encouraging. Among all patients treated in a nurse-and-dietitian-managed obesity clinic at the University of Virginia, 39% remained actively involved after enrollment, and these active participants maintained an average of 21.4 kg weight loss over 12 months.[135]

However well managed and comprehensive, weight reduction programs serve a selected population. They are not generally available, and most obese patients lack the financial or personal resources to remain continuously involved in programs that insist on committed participants. Therefore, nondietary treatment options for morbid obesity are sometimes necessary, and several surgical approaches have been developed. Intestinal bypass is fraught with complications (chronic liver disease, arthritis) and should no longer be recommended. Gastric bypass procedures can achieve weight loss without the serious side effects of intestinal bypass. Long-term follow-up of such patients is limited, but in one recent study of 123 operated patients, 59% achieved long-term (19–47 months) weight loss greater than 30% of the excess weight. At the same time job status as a marker of personal function was stable or improved in 95%, and use of insulin and hypertensive medications decreased, a reflection of the benefits of weight loss on diabetes and hypertension.[137] Gastric restriction is still in a developmental stage. It is anticipated that simpler techniques (e.g., endoscopic) will soon be available.

10.2. Hypertension and Salt Restriction

Although blood pressure can be reduced by weight loss and salt restriction, this effect is difficult to maintain. Furthermore, even though in clinical trials sodium restriction reduces blood pressure, it does not work for every patient.[131] Some hypertensive patients—the elderly, those with low renin, and those with higher blood pressures—respond better to salt restriction. Monitoring urinary sodium will help the physician to follow salt restriction efforts by his patients. Patients should be taught that salt restriction becomes easier over several months as taste preferences change. To make it more convenient to reduce salt intake, more low-salt processed foods are being marketed.

10.3. Vascular Disease and Lipid Restriction

Although dietary restriction of cholesterol is generally advocated, no clinical trials have proven that dietary intervention prevents or reduces coronary disease.[138] In a recent ambitious effort to intervene with regard to multiple risk factors (reduction of dietary cholesterol, cessation of smoking, control of hypertension) in high-risk men, there was no reduction in mortality from coronary disease in the "special-intervention" group compared to the group that received "usual care."[139] However, other nonexperimental approaches do attribute part of the recent decline in the ischemic heart disease mortality rate to lifestyle changes such as lower-cholesterol diets and smoking cessation. Between 1968 and 1976, mortality from coronary disease declined by 21%, and this decline seems to have continued from 1976 to 1980.[140] Goldman and Cook estimate that about one-third of this decline is due to reduction in dietary cholesterol.[100]

As discussed in Chapter 11, coronary disease can be anticipated in certain patients. Regardless of evidence from clinical trials, it makes sense for physicians to modify risk factors once they have been recognized, whether by treating hypertension, helping patients to stop smoking, or recommending diet change. Dietary modifications aimed at reducing serum cholesterol (e.g., less red meat, more fish and poultry, less refined sugar, more grains and vegetables) are not difficult in a culinary sense, allow coincident salt and caloric restrictions, create no extra costs or risks, and perhaps most important, involve the patient in health promotion.

11. SUMMARY

This chapter summarizes a large body of evidence that links modern diet with modern disease. The strength of this evidence is variable: very convincing with regard to lipids and cardiovascular disease as well as for sodium and hypertension; more tentative for the various disorders associated with low-fiber, highly processed diets and for some of the illnesses associated with marginal vitamin intake. What seems clear is that nutrition-related disease in the United States is more often a question of too much than too little. Patients advised to eat less salt, less fat, and less sugar would end up eating foods with higher fiber, vitamin, and trace metal content. Such dietary advice seems prudent. Primary-care physicians now have the opportunity to practice preventive nutrition with all their patients. As the epidemiological and clinical evidence accrues, it will be possible to combine selective as well as general dietary changes with other risk factor modifications to intervene earlier in the natural history of chronic diseases.

REFERENCES

1. McNutt, K.: Dietary advice to the public: 1957 to 1980. *Nutr. Rev.* **38**:353–360, 1980.
2. Swan, P. B.: Food consumption by individuals in the United States: Two major surveys. *Annu. Rev. Nutr.* **3**:413–432, 1983.
3. Simopoulos, A. P.: Overview of nutritional status in the United States. *Prog. Clin. Biol. Res.* **67**:237–247, 1981.
4. Graham, G. G.: Poverty, hunger, malnutrition, prematurity, and infant mortality in the United States. *Pediatrics* **75**:117–125, 1985.
5. Bistrian, B. R., Blackburn, G. L., Vitale, J., *et al.*: Prevalence of malnutrition in general medical patients. *JAMA* **235**:1567–1570, 1976.
6. Albion, N., Asplund, K., and Bjermer, L.: Nutritional status of medical patients on emergency admission to hospital. *Acta Med. Scand.* **212**:151–156, 1982.
7. Exton-Smith, A. N.: Malnutrition in the elderly. *Proc. Roy. Soc. Med.* **70**:615–619, 1977.
8. Jukes, T. H.: Organic food. *CRC Crit. Rev. Food Sci. Nutr.* **9**:395–418, 1977.
9. Appledorf, H.: Nutritional analysis of foods from fast food chains. *Food Technol.* **28**:50–55, 1974.
10. Jukes, T. H.: How safe is our food supply? *Arch. Intern. Med.* **138**:772–774, 1978.
11. Jukes, T. H.: Current concepts in nutrition: Food additives. *N. Engl. J. Med.* **297**:427–430, 1977.
12. Mathews, K. P.: Urticaria and angioedema. *J. Allergy Clin. Immunol.* **72**:1–14, 1983.
13. Wender, E. H.: Diet and hyperkinesis, in Ellenbogen, L. (ed.): *Controversies in Nutrition.* Churchill Livingstone, New York, 1981, pp. 125–138.
14. Jukes, T. H.: Organic foods and food additives, in Ellenbogen, L. (ed.): *Controversies in Nutrition.* Churchill Livingstone, New York, 1981, pp. 139–158.
15. Toxic reactions to plant products sold in health food stores. *Med. Lett.* **21**:29–30, 1979.
16. Carmel, R.: Nutritional vitamin B-12 deficiency: Possible contributory role of subtle vitamin B-12 malabsorption. *Ann. Intern. Med.* **88**:647–649, 1978.
17. Higginbottom, M. C., Sweetman, L., and Nyhan, W. L.: A syndrome of methylmalonic aciduria, homocystinuria, megaloblastic anemia, and neurologic abnormalities in a vitamin B12-deficient breast-fed infant of a strict vegetarian. *N. Engl. J. Med.* **299**:317–320, 1978.
18. Dwyer, J. T., Dietz, W. M., Huss, G., *et al.*: Risk of nutritional rickets among vegetarian children. *Am. J. Dis. Child.* **133**:134–140, 1979.
19. Harland, B. T., and Peterson, M.: Nutritional Status of lacto-ovo vegetarian Trappist monks. *J. Am. Diet. Assoc.* **72**:259–265, 1978.
20. Shaywitz, B. A., Siegel, N. J., and Pearson, M. A.: Megavitamins for minimal brain dysfunction: A potentially dangerous therapy. *JAMA* **238**:1749–1750, 1977.
21. Lippe, B., Hensen, L., Mendoza, G., *et al.*: Chronic vitamin A intoxication. *Am. J. Dis. Child.* **135**:634–636, 1981.
22. Schaimburg, H., Kaplan, J., Windebank, A., *et al.*: Sensory neuropathy from pyridoxine abuse. *N. Engl. J. Med.* **309**:445–448, 1983.
23. Sugar, A. A., and Clark, C. G.: Jaundice following the administration of niacin. *JAMA* **228**:202–203, 1974.

24. Patterson, D. J., Dew, E. W., Gyorkey, F., *et al.:* Niacin hepatitis. *South. Med. J.* **76:**239–240, 1983.
25. Toxic effects of vitamin overdosage. *Med. Lett.* **26:**73–74, 1984.
26. VanItallie, T. B.: Health implications of overweight and obesity in the United States. *Ann. Intern. Med.* **103**(6 pt 2):983–988, 1985.
27. Garrison, R. J., and Castelli, W. P.: Weight and thirty year mortality in the Framingham study. *Ann. Intern. Med.* **103**(6 pt 2):1006–1009, 1985.
28. Barrett-Connor, E. L.: Obesity, atherosclerosis, and coronary artery disease. *Ann. Intern. Med.* **103**(6 pt 2):1010–1019, 1985.
29. Dusten, H. P.: Obesity and hypertension. *Ann. Intern. Med.* **103**(6 pt 2):1047–1049, 1985.
30. Cooppan, R., and Flood, T. M.: Obesity and diabetes, in Marble, A., Kroll, L. P., Bradley, R. F., *et al.* (eds.): *Joslin's Diabetes Mellitus.* Lea & Febiger, Philadelphia, 1985, p. 373.
31. Bonham, G. S., and Brock, D. B.: The relationship of diabetes with race, sex, and obesity. *Am. J. Clin. Nutr.* **41:**776–783, 1985.
32. Kannel, W. B., Castelli, W. P., Gordon, T., *et al.:* Serum cholesterol, lipoproteins, and the risk of coronary heart disease: The Framingham study. *Ann. Intern. Med.* **74:**1–12, 1971.
33. The diet and all-causes death rate in the seven countries study. *Lancet* **1:**58–61, 1981.
34. Bronte-Stewart, A., Keys, A., Brock, J. P., *et al.:* Serum cholesterol, diet, and coronary heart disease: An inter-racial survey in the cape peninsula. *Lancet* **2:**1103–1107, 1955.
35. Phillips, R. L., Lemon, F. R., Beeson, V. L., *et al.:* Coronary heart disease mortality among Seventh Day Adventists with differing dietary habits. *Am. J. Clin. Nutr.* **31:**5191–5198, 1978.
36. Shekelle, R. B., Shryock, A. M., Paul, O., *et al.:* Diet, serum cholesterol, and death from coronary heart disease: The Western Electric study. *N. Engl. J. Med.* **304:**65–70, 1981.
37. Gofman, J. W., Young, W., and Tandy, R. L.: Ischemic heart disease, atherosclerosis, and longevity. *Circulation* **34:**679–696, 1966.
38. Gordon, T., Castellki, W., and Hjortland, M. C.: High density lipoprotein as a protective factor against coronary heart disease: The Framingham study. *Am. J. Med.* **62:**707–714, 1977.
39. Brown, M. S., and Goldstein, J. L.: The hyperlipoproteinemias and other disorders of lipid metabolism, in Peterdorf, R. G., Adams, R. D., Braunwald, E., *et al.* (eds.): *Harrison's Principles of Internal Medicine.* McGraw-Hill, New York, 1983, pp. 547–558.
40. The lipid research clinics coronary prevention trial results: Reduction in incidence of coronary heart disease. *JAMA* **251:**351–361, 1984.
41. Avugaro, P., Cazzolato, G., Bittolo Bon, G., *et al.:* Are apolipoproteins better discriminators than lipids for atherosclerosis? *Lancet* **1:**901–903, 1979.
42. Norum, R. A., Lakier, J. B., Goldstein, S., *et al.:* Familial deficiency of apolipoproteins A-I and C-III and precocious coronary artery disease. *N. Engl. J. Med.* **306:**1513–1519, 1982.
43. Armstrong, M. L., Warner, E. D., and Conner, W. S.: Regression of coronary atheromatosis in rhesus monkeys. *Circ. Res.* **27:**59–67, 1970.
44. Liebman, M., and Bazarre, T. L.: Plasma lipids of vegetarian and nonvegetarian males: Effects of egg consumption. *Am. J. Clin. Nutr.* **38:**612–619, 1983.
45. Kato, H., Tillotson, J., Nichaman, M. Z., *et al.:* Epidemiologic studies of coronary heart disease and stroke in Japanese men living in Japan, Hawaii, and California: Serum lipid and diet. *Am. J. Epidemiol.* **97:**372–384, 1973.
46. Levy, R. I., and Feinleib, M.: Risk factors for coronary artery disease and their management, in Braunwald, E. (ed.): *Heart Disease.* Saunders, Philadelphia, 1984, pp. 1205–1234.
47. Kuller, L. H.: Epidemiology of cardiovascular diseases: Current perspectives. *Am. J. Epidemiol.* **104:**425–456, 1976.
48. Hartug, G. M., Foreyt, J. P., Mitchell, R. S., *et al.:* Relation of diet to high density lipoprotein cholesterol in middle aged marathon runners, joggers, and inactive men. *N. Engl. J. Med.* **302:**357–361, 1980.
49. Herold, P. M., and Kinsella, J. E.: Fish oil consumption and decreased risk of cardiovascular disease: A comparison of findings from animal and human feeding trials. *Am. J. Clin. Nutr.* **43:**566–598, 1986.
50. Kromhout, D., Bosschieter, E. B., and Coulander, C. L.: The inverse relation between fish consumption and 20 year mortality from coronary heart disease. *N. Engl. J. Med.* **312:**1205–1209, 1985.
51. Phillipson, B. E., Rothrock, D. W., Connor, W. E., *et al.:* Reduction of plasma lipids, lipoproteins, and apoproteins by dietary fish oils in patients with hypertriglyceridemia. *N. Engl. J. Med.* **312:**1210–1216, 1985.

52. Lee, T. H., Hoover, R. L., Williams, J. D., *et al.*: Effect of dietary enrichment with eicosapentaenoic and docosahexaenoic acids on in vitro neutrophil and monocyte leukotriene generation and neutrophil function. *N. Engl. J. Med.* **312:**1217–1219, 1985.
53. Sipple, H. L., and McNutt, K. W.: *Sugars in Nutrition.* Academic Press, New York, 1974, pp. 3–9, 93–107.
54. Garrison, R. H., and Somer, E.: *Nutrition Desk Reference.* Keats, New Caanan, CT, 1985, p. 5.
55. *Dietary Goals for the United States,* 2nd ed. Select Commission on Nutrition and Human Needs, US Senate. US Government Printing Office, Washington, DC, 1977, p. 5.
56. Rubenstein, A. H., Seftel, H. C., Miller, K., *et al.*: Metabolic response to oral glucose in healthy South African White, Indian and African subjects. *Br. Med. J.* **1:**748–751, 1969.
57. National Center for Health Statistics: Diabetes in America. PHS, NIH Pub. No. 85–1468. USDHHS, Washington, DC, August 1985.
58. Jenkins, D. J. A., Wolever, T. M. S., Jenkins, A. L., *et al.*: Low glycemic response to traditionally processed wheat and rye products. *Am. J. Clin. Nutr.* **43:**516–520, 1986.
59. Haber, G. B., Heaton, K. W., and Murphy, D.: Depletion and disruption of dietary fiber; effects on satiety, plasma glucose and serum insulin. *Lancet* **2:**679–682, 1977.
60. Anderson, J. W., Midgley, W. R., and Wedman, B. W.: Fiber and diabetes. *Diabetes Care* **2:**369–379, 1979.
61. Leske, G. S., Ripa, L. W., Leske, M. C., *et al.*: Dental public health, in Last, J. M. (Ed.): *Public Health and Preventive Medicine.* Appleton, Century Crofts, Norwalk, CT, 1986, pp. 1473–1513.
62. Williams, S. R.: *Nutrition and Diet Therapy.* Mosby, St. Louis, 1985.
63. Reiser, S., Hallfrisch, J., Michaelis, D. E., *et al.*: Isocaloric exchange of dietary starch and sucrose in humans; effects on levels of fasting blood lipids. *Am. J. Clin. Nutr.* **32:**1659–1669, 1979.
64. Eastwood, M. A., Brydon, W. G., and Tadesse, K.: Effects of fiber on colon function, in Spiller, G. A., and Kay, R. M. (eds.): *Medical Aspects of Dietary Fiber.* Plenum Press, New York, 1980, pp. 1–26.
65. Burkitt, D. P., Walker, A. R. P., and Printer, N. S.: Effect of dietary fiber on stools and transit times, and its role in the causation of disease. *Lancet* **2:**1408–1411, 1972.
66. Holt, S., Heading, R. C., Carter, D. C., *et al.*: Effect of gel, fibre or gastric emptying on absorption of glucose and paracetamol. *Lancet* **1:**636–639, 1979.
67. James, W. P. T.: Dietary fiber and mineral absorption, in Spiller, G. A., and Kay, R. M. (eds.): *Medical Aspects of Dietary Fiber.* Plenum Press, New York, 1980, pp. 39–59.
68. Land, P. C., and Bruce, W. R.: Fecal mutagens: A possible relationship with colorectal cancer. *Sci. Proc. Am. Assoc. Cancer Res.* **19:**167, 1978.
69. Southgate, D. A. T., Branch, W. J., Hill, M. J., *et al.*: Metabolic responses to dietary supplements of bran. *Metabolism* **25:**1129–1135, 1976.
70. Southgate, D. A. T., and Durnin, J. V. G. A.: An experimental reassessment of the factors used in the calculation of the energy value of human diets. *Br. J. Nutr.* **24:**517–535, 1970.
71. Kelsay, J. L., Behall, K. M., and Prather, E. S.: Effect of fiber from fruits and vegetables on metabolic responses of human subjects. *Am. J. Clin. Nutr.* **31:**1149–1153, 1978.
72. Kay, R. M., and Truswell, A. S.: Effect of citrus pectin or blood lipids and fecal steroid excretion in man. *Am. J. Clin. Nutr.* **30:**171–175, 1977.
73. Painter, N. S., Truelove, S. C., Ardran, G. M., *et al.*: Segmentation and localization of intraluminal pressures in the human colon with special reference to the pathogenesis of colon diverticula. *Gastroenterology* **49:**169–177, 1965.
74. Broadribb, A. J. M., and Humphreys, D. M.: Diverticular disease: Three studies—Treatment with bran (part II). *Br. Med. J.* **1:**425–428, 1976.
75. Painter, N. S.: Treatment of diverticular disease (abstract). *Br. Med. J.* **2:**156, 1971.
76. Broadribb, A. J. M.: Treatment of symptomatic diverticular disease with a high fiber diet. *Lancet* **1:**664–666, 1977.
77. Almy, T. P., and Howell, D. A.: Diverticular disease of the colon. *N. Engl. J. Med.* **302:**324–331, 1980.
78. Segal, I., Solomon, A., and Hunt, J. A.: Emergence of diverticular disease in the urban South African Black. *Gastroenterology* **72:**215–219, 1977.
79. Painter, N. S., and Burkitt, D. P.: Diverticular disease of the colon: A deficiency disease of Western civilization. *Br. Med. J.* **2:**450–454, 1971.

80. Heller, S. N., and Hackler, L. R.: Changes in the crude fiber content of the American diet. *Am. J. Clin. Nutr.* **31**:1510–1514, 1978.
81. Stemmerman, G. N., and Yatani, R.: Diverticulosis and polyps of the large intestine: A necropsy study of Hawaii–Japanese. *CA* **31**:1260–1270, 1973.
82. Gear, J. S. S., Ware, A., Fursdon, P., *et al.*: Svmptomless diverticular disease and intake of dietary fiber. *Lancet* **1**:511–514, 1979.
83. Broadribb, A. J. M., and Humphries, D. M.: Diverticular disease: Three studies—Relation to other disorders and fiber intake (part I). *Br. Med. J.* **1**:424–425, 1976.
84. Burkitt, D. P.: Epidemiology of cancer of the colon and rectum. *Cancer* **28**:3–13, 1971.
85. Jensen, O. M., MacLennan, R., and Wahrendorf, J.: Diet, bowel function, fecal characteristics, and large bowel cancer in Denmark and Finland. *Nutr. Cancer* **4**:5–22, 1982.
86. Haenszel, W., and Kurihara, M.: Studies of Japanese migrants. I. Mortality from cancer and other diseases among Japanese in the United States. *J. Natl. Cancer Inst.* **40**:43–68, 1968.
87. Jenkins, D. J. A.: Dietary fiber and carbohydrate metabolism, in Spiller, G. A., and Kay, R. M. (eds.): *Medical Aspects of Dietary Fiber.* Plenum Press, New York, 1980, pp. 175–192.
88. Kichm, T. G., Anderson, J. W., and Ward, K.: Beneficial effects of a high carbohydrate, high fiber diet on hyperglycemic diabetic men. *Am. J. Clin. Nutr.* **29**:895–899, 1976.
89. Mirinda, P. M., and Horwitz, D. L.: High fiber diets in the treatment of diabetes mellitus. *Ann. Intern. Med.* **88**:482–486, 1978.
90. Jackson, W. P. U.: Diabetes mellitus in different countries and different races: Prevalence and major features. *Acta Diabetol. Lat.* **7**:361–401, 1970.
91. Trowell, H.: Diabetes mellitus death rates in England and Wales 1920–1970 and food supplies. *Lancet* **2**:998–1002, 1974.
92. Trowell, H. C.: Dietary fiber hypothesis of the etiology of diabetes mellitus. *Diabetes* **24**:762–765, 1975.
93. Anderson, J. W., and Chen, W. L.: Plant fiber—Carbohydrate and lipid metabolism. Am. J. Clin. Nutr. **32**:346–363, 1979.
94. Anderson, J. W., Chen, W., Story, L., *et al.*: Hypocholesterolemic effects of soluble-fiber rich foods for hypercholesterolemic men (abstract). *Am. J. Clin. Nutr.* **37**:699, 1983.
95. Kromhout, D., Bosschieter, E. B., and Coulander, C. D. L.: Dietary fiber and 10 year mortality from coronary heart disease, cancer, and all causes, the Zutphen study. *Lancet* **2**:518–522, 1982.
96. Morris, J. N., Marr, J. C. N., and Clayton, D. G.: Diet and heart: A postscript. *Br. Med. J.* **2**:1307–1314, 1977.
97. Needleman, P., and Greenwald, J. E.: Atriopeptin: A cardiac hormone intimately involved in fluid, electrolyte, and blood pressure homeostasis. *N. Engl. J. Med.* **314**:828–834, 1986.
98. Fries, E. D.: Salt, volume and the prevention of hypertension. *Circulation* **53**:589–595, 1976.
99. Fregly, M. J.: Attempts to estimate sodium intake in humans, in Horan, M. J., Blaustein, M., and Dunbar, J. B. (eds.): *National Institute of Health Workshop on Nutrition and Hypertension.* Biomedical Information Corp, New York, 1985, pp. 93–112.
100. Goldman, L., and Cook, E. F.: The deline in ischemic heart disease mortality rates: An analysis of the comparative effects of medical interventions and changes in lifestyle. *Ann. Intern. Med.* **101**:825–836, 1984.
101. Dahl, L. K., and Love, R. A.: Etiological role of sodium chloride intake in essential hypertension in humans. *JAMA* **164**:397–400, 1957.
102. Dahl, L. K.: Salt intake and salt need. *N. Engl. J. Med.* **258**:1152–1205, 1958.
103. Allen, F. M.: Treatment of arterial hypertension. *Med. Clin. North Am.* **6**:475–481, 1922.
104. Dahl, L. K.: Salt and hypertension. *Am. J. Clin. Nutr.* **25**:231–244, 1972.
105. Shaper, A. G.: Cardiovascular disease in the tropics. III. Blood pressure and hypertension. *Br. Med. J.* **3**:805–807, 1972.
106. Oliver, W. J., Cohen, E. L., and Neel, J. V.: Blood pressure, sodium intake and sodium related hormones in the Yanomamo indians, a "no-salt" culture. *Circulation* **52**:146–151, 1975.
107. Sinnett, P. F., and Whyte, H. M.: Epidemiological studies in a total highland population, Tukisenta, New Guinea. *J. Chronic Dis.* **26**:265–290, 1973.
108. Meneely, G. R., and Battarbee, H. D.: Sodium and potassium. *Nutr. Rev.* **34**:225–235, 1976.
109. Dahl, L. K., Knudsen, K. D., Heine, M. A., *et al.*: Effects of chronic excess salt ingestion, modification of experimental hypertension in the rat by variations in the diet. *Circ. Res.* **22**:11–18, 1968.

110. Hilton, P. J.: Cellular sodium transport in essential hypertension. *N. Engl. J. Med.* **314**:222–229, 1986.
111. Murray, R. H., Luft, F. C., Bloch, R., *et al.*: Blood pressures responses to extremes of sodium intake in normal man. *Proc. Soc. Exp. Biol. Med.* **159**:432–436, 1978.
112. Sasaki, N.: The relationship of salt intake to hypertension in the Japanese. *Geriatrics* **19**:735–744, 1964.
113. Scotch, N. A.: A preliminary report on the relation of sociocultural factors to hypertension among the Zulu. *Ann. NY Acad. Sci.* **84**:1000–1009, 1960.
114. Maddocks, I.: Blood pressure in melanesians. *Med. J. Aust.* **1**:1123–1126, 1967.
115. Prior, I., Evans, J., Harvey, H., *et al.*: Sodium intake and blood pressure in two polynesian populations. *N. Engl. J. Med.* **279**:515–520, 1968.
116. Allen, F. M.: Arterial hypertension. *JAMA* **74**:652–655, 1920.
117. Dole, V. P., Dahl, L. K., Cotzias, G. C., *et al.*: Dietary treatment of hypertension: Clinical and metabolic studies of patients on the rice-fruit diet. *J. Clin. Invest.* **29**:1189–1206, 1950.
118. Dole, V. P., Dahl, L. K., Cotzias, G., *et al.*: Dietary treatment of hypertension (part II). Sodium depletion as related to the therapeutic effect. *J. Clin. Invest.* **30**:584–595, 1951.
119. McDonough, J., and Wilhelm, C. M.: The effect of excess salt intake on human blood pressure. *Am. J. Dig. Dis.* **21**:180–181, 1964.
120. Watkin, D., Froeb, H., Hatch, F., *et al.*: Effects of diet in essential hypertension. Results with unmodified Kempner rice diet in fifty hospitalized patients (part II). *Am. J. Med.* **9**:441–493, 1950.
121. Parijs, J., Joossens, J., Van Der Linden, L., *et al.*: Moderate sodium restriction and diuretics in the treatment of hypertension. *Am. Heart J.* **85**:22–34, 1973.
122. Morgan, T., Gillies, A., Morgan, G., *et al.*: Hypertension treated by salt restriction. *Lancet* **1**:227–230, 1978.
123. Sullivan, J., Ratts, T., Taylor, J., *et al.*: Hemodynamic effects of dietary sodium in man. *Hypertension* **2**:506–514, 1980.
124. Beard, T., Gray, W., Cooke, H., *et al.*: Randomized controlled trial of a no-added-sodium diet for mild hypertension. *Lancet* **2**:455–458, 1982.
125. MacGregor, G., Best, F., Cam, J., *et al.*: Double-blind randomized crossover trial of moderate sodium restriction in essential hypertension. *Lancet* **1**:351–355, 1982.
126. Committee on Diet, Nutrition and Cancer, Assembly of Life Sciences: *Diet, Nutrition and Cancer.* National Research Council, National Academy Press, Washington, DC, 1982.
127. Sporn, M. B., and Newton, D. L.: Chemoprevention of cancer with retinoids. *Fed. Proc.* **38**:2528–2534, 1979.
128. Kummet, T., Moon, T. E., and Meyskens, F. L.: Vitamin A: Evidence for its preventive role in human cancer. *Nutr. Cancer* **5**:96–106, 1983.
129. McCarron, D. A., Morris, C. D., Henry, H. J., *et al.*: Nutrient intake and blood pressure in the United States. *Science* **224**:1392–1398, 1984.
130. McCarron, D. A., and Morris, C. D.: Calcium and hypertension, evidence for a protective action of the cation, in *NIH Workshop on Nutrition and Hypertension.* Biomed Information Corp., New York, 1985, pp. 167–186.
131. Kaplan, N. M.: Non-drug treatment of hypertension. *Ann. Intern. Med.* **102**:359–373, 1985.
132. Resnick, L. M., Laragh, J. H., Sealey, J. E., *et al.*: Divalent cations in essential hypertension. Relations between serum ionized calcium, magnesium and plasma renin activity. *N. Engl. J. Med.* **309**:888–891, 1983.
133. Committee on Iron Deficiency, Council on Foods and Nutrition, American Medical Association: Iron deficiency in the United States. *JAMA* **203**:119–124, 1968.
134. Lynch, S. R., Finch, C. A., Monsen, E. R., *et al.*: Iron status of elderly Americans. *Am. J. Clin. Nutr.* **36**:1032–1045, 1982.
135. Atkinson, R. L., Russ, C. S., Ciavarella, P. A., *et al.*: A comprehensive approach to outpatient obesity management. *J. Am. Diet. Assoc.* **84**:439–444, 1984.
136. Brownell, K. D.: The psychology and physiology of obesity: Implications for screening and treatment. *J. Am. Diet. Assoc.* **84**:406–413, 1984.
137. Thompson, K., Fletcher, S., O'Malley, M. S., *et al.*: Long term outcomes of morbidly obese patients treated with gastrogastrostomy. *J. Gen. Intern. Med.* **1**:85–89, 1986.
138. Levy, R. I., and Feinlieb, M.: Risk factors for coronary artery disease and their management, in Braunwald, E. (ed.): *Heart Disease.* Saunders, Philadelphia, 1984, pp. 1209–1234.

139. Multiple Risk Factor Intervention Trial: Risk factor changes and mortality results. *JAMA* **248:**1465–1477, 1982.
140. Stern, M. P.: The recent decline in ischemic heart disease. *Ann. Intern. Med.* **91:**630–640, 1979.

23

Smoking

Edward J. Trapido

Cigarette smoking is the chief preventable cause of mortality in the United States. It is estimated that the annual excess mortality attributable to smoking in the United States exceeds 500,000. The bulk of these deaths are due to coronary heart disease, cancer, and chronic obstructive lung disease.[1–3] In addition, smoking has been linked to gastrointestinal diseases,[4] nonmalignant diseases of the mouth,[5–7] and respiratory disease in children.[8–10] In 1986, more people will die of smoking-related diseases than died in World War I, World War II, Korea, and the Vietnam War.

1. PREVALENCE

It has been estimated that nearly one-third of Americans are smokers.[11,12] This estimate is strikingly consistent among sex and racial groups. Although it appears that men have higher rates than women, the National Center for Health Statistics has shown a consistently declining prevalence in men, at all ages. However, in women, the decline is not apparent at all age groups, with the most recent survey actually showing a rise in prevalence since 1980 in women under age 35, and a tapering off of the decline in women aged 35–64. It is interesting to note that the per capita consumption of cigarettes was greatest in the mid-1970s and has been declining more recently.[13]

Even more striking is the high prevalence of cigarette usage among high-school students. In 1985, 68.6% of high-school students in a National Institute on Drug Abuse survey[14] reported ever having smoked, with 30.1% having smoked within the previous month and 19.5% smoking daily. Whereas this rate had been higher in males between 1975 and 1979, after this time the rate in females exceeded that in males (see Fig. 1).

It should be noted that there has been a general decline in these rates since 1977. Of note is that 22.7% of students who intended to complete college had smoked at least once in the month before the survey, whereas 37.9% of those students who did not intend to go to or complete college smoked. Finally, students in the Northeast were 1.5 times more likely to be smokers than students in the West. Most of the initial use of cigarettes took place before high school. It is alarming that daily smoking had begun for 14% before 10th

Edward J. Trapido • Department of Oncology, University of Miami School of Medicine, Miami, Florida 33101.

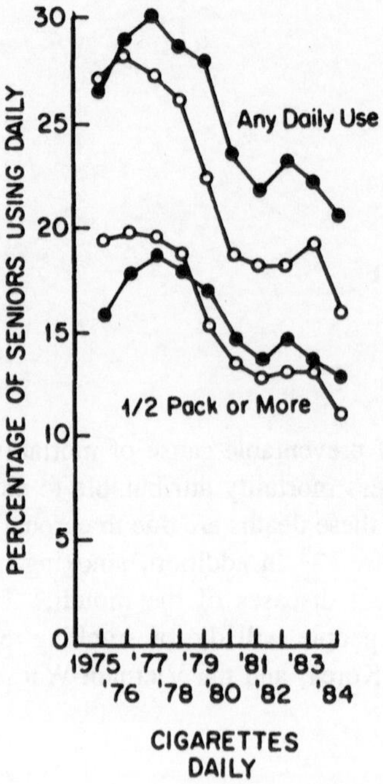

Figure 1. Trends in 30-day prevalence of daily use of cigarettes. (○) Male; (●) female.

grade, with only 8% more students starting in high school. Thus, in spite of the presumed awareness of the hazardous effects of smoking, teenagers, as well as women, continue to smoke at an alarming rate.

2. LUNG CANCER

Lung cancer is the leading cause of cancer deaths in men and women. For men, lung cancer has long been known to be the leading killer. In women, the death rate began to overtake the mortality rate from breast cancer in 1985.[15] Lung cancer is the most commonly diagnosed site in men (incidence), but is the third most common in women.[16] The

Table I. Age-Adjusted Lung and Bronchus Cancer Incidence (Rates × 100,000, 1983)

White men	79.3
White women	33.5
Black men	125.3
Black women	33.9

incidence rate of lung and bronchus cancer from the Surveillance, Epidemiology and End Results (SEER) Program[17] is presented in Table I.

The incidence rates and mortality rates show that survival from lung cancer is poor. The 5-year survival from lung cancer is 10% in blacks and 13% in whites, for all stages; even when localized at diagnosis, survival rates are 33% and 42%, respectively.[18] In part, this is because about 1,000,000 lung cancer cells are already present by the time a lesion is visible on x-ray (it is estimated that a visible lung tumor has been developed for 9–10 years before it is seen). Roughly, 75% of staged cases presented at stage III in SEER, among both whites and blacks.[17]

There can now be little doubt about the causation of lung cancer by cigarette smoking. It is estimated that between 80 and 85% of all lung cancer deaths are attributable to smoking,[19] with greater percentages in men (85%)[20] than in women (75%). The impact of smoking on male mortality was seen before that among women, which is usually attributed to the relatively recent increase in the prevalence of smoking among women, beginning after World War II. Rates of lung cancer have been shown to rise with increasing amount smoked, as shown in Table II.

Increasing risk has also been seen with increasing duration of smoking,[1] total pack years of use, and increasing years since first use.[33] Cessation of smoking appears to be accompanied by a drop in risk,[28,35] as shown in Table III.

The risk of lung cancer in smokers approaches that of nonsmokers after about 15 years since cessation, with varying degrees of decrease in risk after shorter periods. However, it appears that the magnitude of the decrease is dependent on the extent of prior inhalation, amount smoked, age at initiation of smoking, inhalation practices, and the reasons for smoking cessation.[1]

The adverse effects of tobacco use on risk of lung cancer exist for those who smoke cigars and pipes, but the association is not as strong as for cigarettes. This lesser effect has been linked to the lack of inhalation of tobacco smoke in pipe and cigar smokers, and thus a lower total intake of tobacco. In general, pipe smokers show a higher risk of lung cancer than cigar smokers,[1] with some studies[26,33] showing evidence of a dose–response relationship between cigar and/or pipe smoking and lung cancer mortality. Risks of dying from lung cancer more than doubled with either eight or more cigars smoked per day, or 20 or more pipefuls smoked per day. It has been suggested that this lesser effect from pipe or cigar smoking is probably due not to the cigarette paper or tobacco additives,[43] but to the fact that the smoke from cigarettes is less alkaline than that from cigars or pipes.

3. PATHOLOGICAL CHANGES

During smoking, the lung is exposed to a variety of compounds, including tar, nicotine, carbon monoxide, and other substances that act as initiators, promoters, cocarcinogens, or complete carcinogens. The mucous membranes are recipients of these irritating substances, and the cilia are paralyzed. As the mucosal cells continue to accumulate these deposits, they may become hyperplastic and ultimately anaplastic.

In addition to these changes, studies indicate that there is a greater likelihood of smokers to develop premalignant changes in the bronchial epithelium than nonsmokers.[2]

Table II. Lung Cancer Mortality Ratios for Men and Women, by Current Number of Cigarettes Smoked per Day[a]

Population	Men: Cigarettes smoked per day	Men: Mortality ratios	Women: Cigarettes smoked per day	Women: Mortality ratios
ACS 25-state study	Nonsmoker	1.00	Nonsmoker	1.00
	1–9	4.62	1–9	1.30
	10–19	8.62	10–19	2.40
	20–39	14.69	20–39	4.90
	40+	18.71	40+	7.50
British physicians study	Nonsmoker	1.00	Nonsmoker	1.00
	1–14	7.80	1–14	1.28
	15–24	12.70	15–24	6.41
	25+	25.10	25+	29.71
Swedish study	Nonsmoker	1.00	Nonsmoker	1.00
	1–7	2.30	1–7	1.80
	8–15	8.80	8–15	11.30
	16+	13.70	16+	—
Japanese study, all ages	Nonsmoker	1.00	Nonsmoker	1.0
	1–19	3.49	<20	1.90
	20–39	5.69	20–29	4.20
	40+	6.45		
U.S. veterans study	Nonsmoker	1.00		
	1–9	3.89		
	10–20	9.63		
	21–39	16.70		
	≥40	23.70		
ACS 9-state study	Nonsmoker	1.00		
	1–9	8.00		
	10–20	10.50		
	20+	23.40		
Canadian veterans	Nonsmoker	1.00		
	1–9	9.50		
	10–20	15.80		
	20+	17.30		
California men in 9 occupations	Nonsmoker	1.00		
	About ½ pk	3.72		
	About 1 pk	9.05		
	About 1½ pk	9.56		

[a]Source: Refs. 21–42.

As the number of cigarettes smoked increases, loss of cilia, basal cell hyperplasia, and the presence of atypical cells increase. Similarly, several studies have shown that smokers' sputum is more likely to show atypical epithelial cells than nonsmokers' sputum.[44,45] Cigarette smoke paralyzes the ciliary cleaning mechanism of the respiratory system for about 10 min. Long-term smokers have bronchi with impaired cleaning mechanism. The long-term smoker's only mechanism to clear the lungs is coughing. The higher irritation causes more mucous production, often causing obstruction (C. Tate, personal communication, Feb. 5, 1986).

Table III. Lung Cancer Mortality Rates in Ex-Cigarette Smokers, by Number of Years Stopped Smoking[a]

Study	Years stopped smoking	Mortality ratio	
British physicians	1–4	16.0	
	5–9	5.9	
	10–14	5.3	
	15+	2.0	
	Current smokers	14.0	
U.S. veterans[b]	1–4	18.83	
	5–9	7.73	
	10–14	4.71	
	15–19	4.81	
	20+	2.10	
	Current smokers	11.28	
Japanese men	1–4	4.65	
	5–9	2.50	
	10+	1.35	
	Current smokers	3.76	
		Number of cigarettes smoked per day	
		1–19	20+
ACS 25-state study (men 50–69)	<1	7.20	29.13
	1–4	4.60	12.00
	5–9	1.00	7.20
	10+	0.40	1.06
	Current smokers	6.47	13.67

[a]Source: Refs. 21–28, 30–35.
[b]Includes data only for ex-cigarette smokers who stopped for other than physicians' orders.

4. CORONARY HEART DISEASE

Although lung cancer and its association with smoking receive a great share of the medical and political attention, even more deaths per year from cardiovascular disease than from lung cancer are attributable to tobacco. It has been estimated that 20–30% or more of coronary heart disease (CHD) mortality, amounting to about 120,000 deaths per year, is attributable to smoking. In addition, a proportion of stroke, peripheral vascular disease, and atherosclerosis deaths are attributable to smoking.

In the 1983 Report of the Surgeon General,[2] it was concluded that cigarette smoking was the most important mutable risk factor for CHD in the United States. The relationships between the incidence of CHD and various measures of cigarette use are presented in Table IV. These data represent the results of several cohorts participating in the National Cooperative Pooling Project.

In all five studies, the incidence of CHD was lower in nonsmokers than in smokers

Table IV. Analysis of the Incidence of Coronary Heart Disease by Smoking Behavior[a]

Smoking behavior	Standardized incidence ratio by study group[b]					
	Pool 5	ALB	CH–GAS	CH–WE	FRAM	TECUM
All	100	100	100	100	100	100
Nonsmokers	58	55	48	59	67	(53)
Never smoked	54	45	(53)	44	77	(60)
Past smoker	63	67	56	89	(46)	(50)
<½ pack/day	55	(67)		(43)	78	(43)
Cigar and pipe only	71	78	(58)	98	57	(61)
Cigarette smokers						
About ½ pack/day	104	(52)	(64)	139	106	(151)
About 1 pack/day	120	108	125	128	119	117
>1 pack/day	183	200	190	162	174	151
Risk ratio						
≥1 pack/day						
Nonsmokers	2.5	2.7	3.3	2.4	2.2	( )[c]
95% confidence interval						
Low	2.1	1.8	2.1	1.6	1.5	( )
High	3.1	4.3	6.2	3.7	3.4	( )
Risk ratio						
>1 pack/day						
Nonsmokers	3.2	3.7	4.0	2.8	2.6	( )
95% confidence interval						
Low	2.6	2.4	2.5	1.2	1.8	( )
High	4.2	6.1	8.4	5.5	4.5	( )
Number of men at risk	8,282	1,796	1,258	1,926	2,162	1,140
Person-years of experience	70,970	17,240	11,017	16,072	19,756	6,885
Number of first events	644	154	123	140	178	49

[a]Source: Pooling Project Research Group.[46]

[b]ALB, Albany Cardiovascular Health Center Study; CH–GAS, Chicago Peoples Gas Company Study; CH–WE, Chicago Western Electric Company Study; FRAM, Framingham Heart Disease Epidemiology Study; TECUM, Tecumseh Health Study.

[c]( ), based on fewer than 10 first events.

and lowest in individuals who had never smoked. Smokers who had smoked only pipes and cigars had higher rates of CHD than nonsmokers, although the former group's rates were still one-half to one-third lower than those of cigarette smokers. The risk ratio, i.e., the risk of CHD among smokers compared to the risk among nonsmokers, of CHD associated with smoking at least one pack per day was 2.5 with a 95% confidence interval of 2.1–3.1 and was 3.2 with a 95% confidence interval of 2.6–4.2 for smoking more than a single pack. The risk was greatest in heavy smokers, in all age groups (Table V).

Although the excess incidence attributable to smoking more than a single pack per day increased with age, the risk ratio declines, since the baseline risk of CHD, i.e., the denominator of the risk ratio, rises with age. Table V shows also that although there was a lower risk of CHD for cigar and pipe smokers compared to those who smoked more than one pack of cigarettes per day, the risk associated with cigar and pipe smoking was not significantly different from that of the nonsmoking or light-smoking group.

Table V. Average Annual Risk of First Major Coronary Event, National Collaborative Pooling Project[a]

Smoking pattern	Age at risk 40–44	45–49	50–54	55–59	60–64	40–64
	Average annual risk (per 1000 man-years)[b]					SIR[e]
All	3.1	6.4	8.0	22.6	19.9	100
Nonsmoker	(1.5)	3.0	3.6	7.3	15.5	58
Never smoked	(1.9)	(0.7)	(2.5)	8.7	11.4	54
Past smoker	(0.9)	5.5	4.3	6.1	15.5	63
<½ pack/day	(1.7)	(4.7)	(5.9)	(6.4)	(7.5)	55
Cigar and pipe only	(2.1)	(2.2)	(2.1)	12.1	19.5	71
Cigarette smokers						
About ½ pack/day	(3.1)	(5.0)	(6.2)	15.5	24.3	104
About 1 pack/day	3.9	8.4	10.3	13.8	22.0	120
>1 pack/day	4.9	12.2	17.4	22.5	26.8	183
Risk ratio						
> pack/day:nonsmokers	( )[c]	4.1	4.8	3.1	1.7	3.2[d]
	Number of first events					SIR
All	34	113	158	194	145	644
Never smoked	3	2	8	21	21	55
Past smoker	1	11	10	13	18	53
<½ pack/day	1	4	6	6	4	21
Cigar and pipe only	2	4	5	26	33	60
About ½ pack/day	3	7	9	19	15	53
About 1 pack/day	14	49	64	61	42	230
>1 pack/day	10	36	56	48	22	172

[a]Source: Pooling Project Research Group.[46]
[b]See footnote to Table IV for names of the five study groups.
[c]( ), based on fewer than 10 first events.
[d]Approximate 95% confidence interval: 2.6–4.2.
[e]SIR, Standardized incidence ratio.

CHD rates are lower in women than in men, with young and middle-aged women having only about 20% the CHD that men have. Not surprisingly, this is thought to be due to the lower prevalence of cigarette use among women. In addition, the 1983 report of the Surgeon General[2] suggests that female smokers tend to smoke fewer cigarettes than men daily, and to inhale less deeply. In fact, after adjustment for these differences in smoking habits, increments in death rates from CHD associated with cigarette smoking are similar in men and women.

Cigarettes have been found to be a causal factor in the etiology of myocardial infarction (MI).[47–49] In addition, oral-contraceptive users who smoke are at a substantially increased risk (risk ratio of about 10) of myocardial infarction, compared to nonsmoking oral-contraceptive users. The risk of nonfatal MI, a strong determinant of subsequent fatal coronary heart disesase,[50] has also been shown to be increased in oral-contraceptive users who smoke, with the relative risk in the heaviest smokers and oral-contraceptive users reaching a risk ratio as high as 39.[51] In addition, it appears that women who have risk factors that put them at a higher risk of MI, including elevated total serum cholesterol levels, decreased high-density-lipoprotein cholesterol levels, hypertension, diabetes mellitus, angina pectoris, blood group A, tendency to type A behavior, or family history of MI, are at further increased risk of MI if they smoke.[52] It is thought that cigarette smoking increases the likelihood of thrombosis, since the association between cigarette use and angina pectoris is much weaker than that of smoking and MI occurrence.[52–56] Since oral contraceptive use increases the risk of thromboembolic disease, it has been suggested that the reason the risk of MI is so greatly increased among smokers who use oral contraceptives may relate to the joint association with thromboembolism.[52]

There is also an association between MI and smoking among men.[57,58] Risk increases with number of cigarettes smoked,[59–63] with overall relative risk of MI associated with smoking being about 3. As with women, the effect of smoking on CHD is not confounded by other major risk factors,[46, 64–68] but there may be an interaction between smoking and other risk factors. This may be because cigarette smoking affects a number

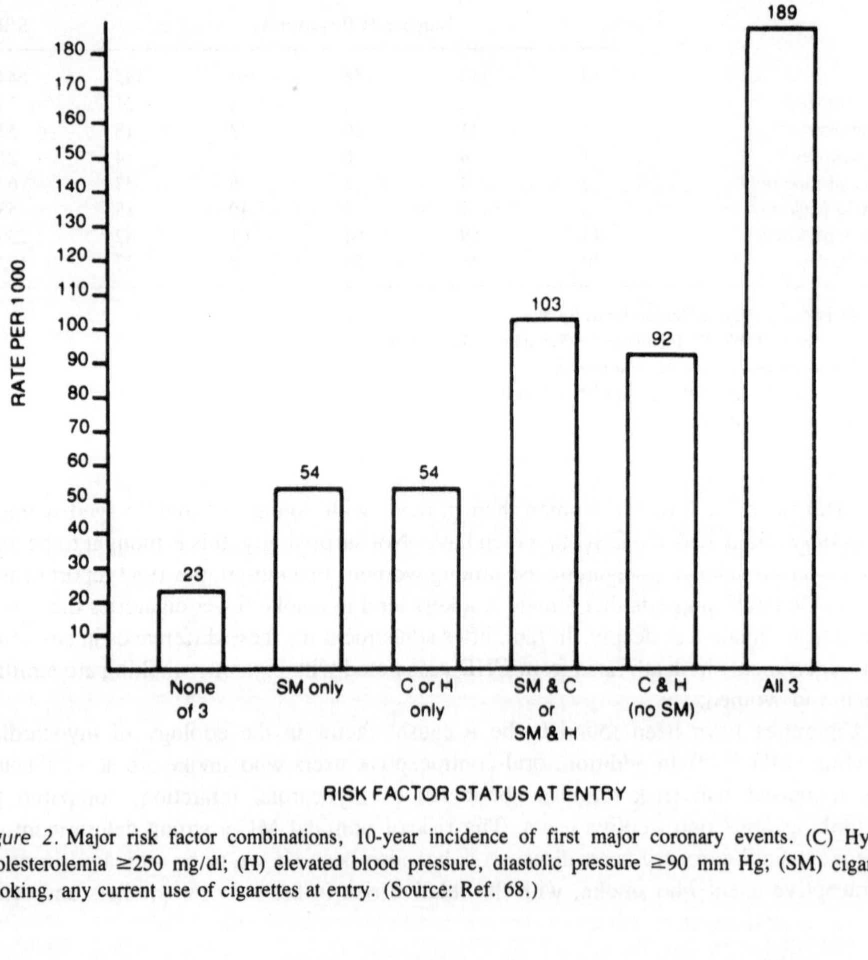

Figure 2. Major risk factor combinations, 10-year incidence of first major coronary events. (C) Hypercholesterolemia ≥250 mg/dl; (H) elevated blood pressure, diastolic pressure ≥90 mm Hg; (SM) cigarette smoking, any current use of cigarettes at entry. (Source: Ref. 68.)

of other factors, such as high-density lipoproteins, blood pressure, and serum cholesterol, as illustrated in Fig. 2.

A number of cohort studies have examined the association between CHD mortality, and smoking, in both men and women. The results of these studies, presented in Table VI, show that the risk of dying from CHD among smokers is probably about 50% higher than for nonsmokers.

These studies also found that death rates from CHD among smokers, compared to nonsmokers, decrease with increasing age, owing to the rapid increase of CHD mortality with age. Second, the studies found that the risk of dying of CHD is related to a variety of measures of cigarette use, including number of cigarettes smoked, [22,28,29,33–38,69,71,72,74–78,82] with heaviest smokers showing relative risks of about 2; inhalation characteristics,[22,28,29,74,75] with deep inhalers having relative risks of about 1.8 compared to nonsmokers; and age at initiation of smoking,[22,33,35,69,78,82] with smokers who began smoking at a young age having the most elevated risks. Although the risk of coronary heart disease is lower in lighter smokers than in heavier smokers, the evidence does not suggest a threshold effect. There is no evidence to suggest that any level of cigarette smoking is safe with regard to CHD risk.[2]

5. CEREBROVASCULAR DISEASE

After CHD and cancer, cerebrovascular disease is the most common killer in the United States, accounting for 7.7% of deaths.[16] About 500,000 individuals are newly diagnosed with some form of cerebrovascular disease per year, with approximately 200,000 deaths per year. The prospective study in Framingham, Massachusetts[54,66] estimated that there is a 5% chance of having a stroke by age 50. Stroke incidence rises sharply with age, especially after age 45.

The relationship between smoking and stroke incidence is felt to depend on the type of stroke or specific clinical manifestation of cerebrovascular disease. Smoking appears to

Table VI. Mortality Ratios from Prospective Studies of Coronary Heart Disease[a]

Study	Mortality ratio
Dorn	1.6 (men)
Hammond	1.7 (men)
Hirayama	1.7 (men), 1.8 (women)
Hammond	1.9–2.6 (men)
Best	1.6 (men)
Doll	1.6 (men)
Cederlof	1.7 (men), 1.3 (women)
Paffenbarger	1.6 (men)
Swiss physicians	1.3–2.2 (women)

[a]Source: Refs. 22,28,29,33,35,36,38,69–81.

be more strongly related to stroke before age 55, and more to nonfatal strokes than fatal strokes.

However, the association is not a simple and clear one. Some studies have found a positive association with smoking, with risk ratios of 1.2–1.5,[33,35] whereas others [72,83,84] have not. The relationship between cigarette smoking and stroke incidence or mortality is, at its weakest, barely suggestive of a positive association, and few studies have found dose–response relationships. The results of some of the studies are presented in Tables VII and VIII.

However, relationships between oral-contraceptive use, smoking, and stroke may be stronger, as illustrated by the results of a study[86] that found a relative risk of 21.9 among women who both smoked and used oral contraceptives compared to nonsmoking women who did not use the pill.

The relationship between transient ischemic attacks and cigarette smoking is unclear, since both positive[87] and negative[88] associations have been reported. However, the association with subarachnoid hemorrhage appears to be stronger, as shown in a number of studies.[89–91]

Since the incidence of stroke in young women is low, there are few studies on the interaction of smoking and oral-contraceptive use on stroke risk. However, a number of studies suggest that cigarette smoking acts independently and interactively with oral contraceptive use, heaviest users of both being at substantially elevated risk.[90,92–94]

6. *LARYNGEAL CANCER*

Cigarette smoking is considered to be the major cause of cancer of the larynx in the United States. About 1% of all cancer deaths are from laryngeal cancer, amounting to 3750 deaths in 1985 and 11,500 cases. Mortality is higher in men than in women. Among women, nonwhites experience higher rates than whites, and for nearly all of the last three decades, nonwhite men have had higher mortality rates than white men. Generally,

Table VII. Results of Stroke Incidence Studies

Study	Type[a]	Date	Disease[b]	Relationship between stroke and smoking[c]	Approximate relative risk
Hiroshima	P	1958–1964	CI	None	—
Washington	P	1961–1971	Stroke	None	0.9
			CI	None	0.8–1.1
Framingham	P	1949–1973	ABI	Yes, not sig	1.1–2.7 (men)
Manitoba	R	1970–1971	CI	Yes, sig?	2.4
Rural Japan	P	1964–1970	Stroke	Yes, not sig	1.9–2.7
Harvard	P	1916–1966	Nonfatal CI	Yes, sig	1.6
Walnut Creek	P	1969–1976	SAH	Yes, sig	5.7
Queen Square	R	1965–1978	Aneurysm	Yes, sig?	3.8

[a]P, prospective; R, retrospective.
[b]CI, cerebral infarction; ABI, atherothrombotic brain infarction; SAH, subarachnoid hemorrhage.
[c]? Denotes doubt about the study design.

Table VIII. Results of Stroke Mortality Studies[a]

Name	Type[b]	Date	Relationship between stroke and smoking	Approximate mortality ratio
Longshoremen	P	1951–1969	None	1.1
Washington	P, R	1952–1971	None	0.9
Harvard	P	1916–1966	Yes	2.1
Dorn	P	1954–1962	Yes	1.3–1.9
British physicians (10 year)	P	1951–1961	None	1.2
British physicians (20 year)	P[c]	1951–1971	Yes	1.1–1.5
American Cancer Society	P	1959–1965	Yes	1.3–2.8

[a]Source: Ref. 85.
[b]P, prospective; R, retrospective.
[c]Based on cerebral thrombosis only.

mortality rises consistently after age 40, although in nonwhite men, the rate peaks and falls after age 70.[1] Table IX shows the relative risk of laryngeal cancer associated with smoking.

As shown, there is a positive association between smoking and laryngeal cancer, with risks being at least doubled among smokers. Several studies have shown a dose–response relationship between the number of cigarettes smoked per day and the risk of dying from laryngeal cancer. As with lung cancer, there does not appear to be a threshold below which no increased risk is observed among smokers, and risks rise with increasing amount smoked.[105] Cohort studies have similarly shown relative risks that are elevated

Table IX. Selected Mortality Ratios for Cancer of the Larynx[a]

Study	Population size	Number of deaths	Nonsmokers	Cigarette smokers	Comments
ACS 9-state study	188,000 men	24	—	—	All larynx cancer deaths occurred in smokers
British physicians	34,000 men	38	1.00	13.00	Includes cancer of larynx and other upper-respiratory sites
U.S. veterans	290,000 men	116	1.00	11.49	
ACS 25-state study	358,000 men	67	1.00	6.52	Includes buccal, pharyngeal, and laryngeal cancers
	483,000 women	11	1.00	3.25	
California men in 9 occupations	68,000 men	11	—	>2.90	All larynx cancer deaths occurred in smokers[b]
Japanese study	122,000 men	38	1.00	13.59	
	142,800 women	6	1.00	6.52	

[a]Source: Refs. 95–104.
[b]Ratio derived by comparing smokers of half a pack with all other smokers.

with smoking,[1] with comparable dose–response relationships. A positive association is also seen when exposure has been related to the tar and nicotine content of the cigarettes that are smoked, the degree of inhalation, or the age at first smoking.[106,107]

Other findings add to the idea that this association is a causal one. Studies among Mormons and Seventh-Day Adventists, both of whom have a low percentage of smokers, suggest that the incidence of laryngeal cancer is markedly lower than in populations with higher prevalences of smoking.[108–112] Also, mortality among women has increased over the past 20 years, similar to lung cancer, consistent with the rise in female smoking over time. Laryngeal cancer has been found to be more common in alcoholics than non-alcoholics.[113–115] This risk appears to be synergistic with smoking use. It is estimated, in fact, that 80–90% of all head and neck tumors are attributable to use of both alcohol and tobacco.[116] Thus, if there were an increase in alcohol use by women, over the period of time that smoking increased, the joint effects of smoking and alcohol might be more directly responsible for the rise in female laryngeal cancer mortality rates than from smoking alone.

Finally, although the relationships between other forms of tobacco use and laryngeal cancer have received little attention, the few studies that have focused on cigar and pipe use (e.g., Refs. 22,28,33,74) have found that these smokers have mortality rates from laryngeal cancer similar to those of cigarette smokers.

7. ORAL CANCER

Cigarette smoking and alcohol use are major factors in the etiology of cancer of the oral cavity. Cancers of the oral cavity consist of cancers of the lip, tongue, major and minor salivary glands, floor of the mouth, and nasopharynx and hypopharynx. In 1986, there will be an estimated 29,500 cases and 9400 deaths[117] diagnosed in the United States. The male-to-female ratio of cases is about 3:1, although this varies to a high as 9:1 in different geographical regions of the United States. Cancer of the lip is uncommon, with 4600 cases expected in this country in 1986. Cancer of the lip also appears to be associated with smoking.[116]

The incidence of cancers of the buccal cavity and pharynx has remained relatively stable over the past 35 years, except among nonwhite men, for whom rates have doubled over this period. Men consistently have a higher rate than women. Among men, whites have higher rates than blacks, whereas among women, the reverse is true, although differences in the latter rates are small. Death rates are low until age 40 and then rise steeply in both sexes.

Both cohort and case-control studies have shown an adverse effect of smoking on incidence and/or mortality from cancer of the oral cavity (Table X). The average relative risks from these studies are difficult to determine, since some studies group the various oral sites together, and some do not. However, the relative risks associated with smoking appear higher in men than in women and higher for pharyngeal cancers than for those of the buccal cavity.[2]

In addition, a recent report from China reported that in men, 93% of pharyngeal cancer was related to smoking.[118] A dose–response relationship between number of

Table X. Mortality Ratios for Cancer of the Oral Cavity[a]

Study	Population size	Number of deaths	Nonsmokers	Cigarette smokers
ACS 9-state study	188,000 men	55	1.00	5.06
British physicians	34,000 men	38	1.00	13.00
U.S. veterans	290,000	61	1.00	4.22
			1.00	14.05
ACS 25-state study	358,000 men	167	1.00	6.52
	483,000 women	65	1.00	3.25
California men in 9 occupations	68,000 men	19	1.00	2.76
Japanese study	122,200 men	43	1.00	2.88 men
	142,800 women	11	1.00	1.22 women
Swedish study	55,000 men and women	15	NA[b]	NA[b]

[a]Source: Ref. 2.
[b]Ratio not available.

cigarettes smoked per day and risk of dying of oral cancer has been observed in several studies,[26,33,75,107,119] with individuals smoking more than one pack per day having greater than 5 times the risk of death from oral cancer than that of nonsmokers.

In populations who do not tend to smoke, the occurrence of cancers of the oral cavity and pharynx is low. Both Mormons and Seventh-Day Adventists have lower-than-expected rates of cancer of the gum, mouth, tongue, and pharynx.[108–112] Evidence from a number of studies suggests that whatever form of tobacco is smoked is associated with an increased risk of cancer of these sites associated with smoking.

Oral cancer occurs with greater frequency among individuals who both smoke and drink. Whether the synergistic effect is multiplicative[120] or additive[121] remains to be determined. However, a recent study of oral squamous cell carcinoma found that the joint exposure increased risk from 15 to 27.5 times, whereas either one, alone, increased the risk only 2.5 times.[122]

8. ESOPHAGEAL CANCER

Cancer of the esophagus is not a common cancer in the United States, with an estimated 9300 cases and 8800 deaths estimated for 1986.[16] There is a predominance of men with the disease, and the mortality rate is about 3.5 times higher for men than for women. Esophageal cancer is more common in blacks than in whites.[117] That cancer of the esophagus has some "environmental" etiology is suggested by the marked differences in regional rates.[123] Cancer of the esophagus has been fairly stable over time among whites, but among nonwhites has risen in women, with a sharp rise in men over the last 30 years. A number of studies have looked at the role of smoking and esophageal cancer, and although they find a variation in the amount of disease attributable to smoking, they consistently find a positive association between cigarette smoking and mortality from esophageal cancer. Mortality ratios range from 1.3 to 11.1 among smokers. In four of the largest cohort studies, a dose–response relationship was observed.

Since the esophagus is not directly exposed to smoke, instead receiving the condensates of smoke either after being swallowed, or through ciliary action of the lung, or from coughing, variations in the degree of inhalation (from pipes and cigars) would not be expected to change the amount of smoke reaching the esophagus. Increased risk is found for all forms of use, but little differences exist by mode of smoking. In studies looking at this issue, rates of cancer of the esophagus were similar in persons smoking cigars, cigarettes, and pipes, but all were greater than the rates in nonsmokers. Alcohol and cigarette use seem to have a synergistic effect on rates of esophageal cancer.[1]

9. BLADDER CANCER

There are approximately 40,500 new cases of bladder cancer in the United States each year and 10,600 deaths.[16] The incidence of bladder cancer among males is roughly three times that of females. The age-adjusted mortality for bladder cancer has fallen slightly among nonwhite and white men over the past 30 years. Among women, the drop has been more dramatic.[1] Most cancers of the bladder are transitional or squamous cell, and many are not discovered until they have spread beyond the local stage.[17] The 5-year survival rates are substantially higher in whites than in nonwhites. The proportion of bladder cancer deaths attributable to smoking ranges between 40 and 60% in men and 25 and 35% in women.[1,124,125]

Many studies have found a positive association between smoking and bladder cancer.[1,126–130] Compared to nonsmokers, smokers experience about 2–4 times the risk of bladder cancer. Cole *et al.*[125] found that risk of bladder cancer rose with more cigarettes smoked and with greater degrees of inhalation. Other case-control studies,[131] as well as cohort studies,[29,35,42] have shown dose–response relationships. The cohort studies have generally shown a doubling of risk of dying from bladder cancer among smokers, compared to nonsmokers. Like other smoking-related cancers, cancer of the bladder occurs less often than expected among Mormons and Seventh-Day Adventists.[108–110,112]

The evidence supporting a positive relationship between cigarette smoking and bladder cancer is clearly not as strong as for cancers of the lung, larynx, oral cavity, or esophagus, and it is likely that other factors (such as occupational exposures) are playing a major role in the etiology of this disease.

10. OTHER CANCERS

Smoking is associated with cancer of the uterine cervix,[132–135] kidney, stomach, liver, biliary passages,[2] and pancreas.[127,133,136] However, the strength of these associations is not as strong as for the other sites. Recent studies relating cigarette smoking to cancer of the breast[137,138] are contradictory, and evidence of a positive association with vulvar cancer[139] and skin cancer[140] and a negative association with endometrial cancer[141] not supported by Tyler *et al.*,[142] suggest the need for further studies.

11. CHRONIC LUNG DISEASES

In 1983, there were about 62,000 deaths from chronic lung disease (composed largely of asthma, emphysema, and chronic bronchitis). About 80–90% of these have been attributed to smoking. In fact, in population-based studies conducted in the United States cigarette smoking is usually the only predictor for development of chronic obstructive lung disease.[3] Cigarettes produce both acute and chronic effects on the mucosa of the nasopharynx, tongue, vocal cords, bronchioles, cilia, mucous glands, alveolar macrophages, and collagen, as described previously.

Within a few years after initiation of smoking, the small airways (<2 mm in diameter) begin to become inflamed. This inflammation is a response to the irritants found in smoke and is often followed by ulceration and squamous metaplasia. A later manifestation of this is hypertrophy of smooth muscle, goblet cell hyperplasia, and peribronchiolar fibrosis. The prevalence of these conditions is greater in older people and in heavy smokers.[143] This inflammation is often a precursor to lobular emphysema. Respiratory bronchiolitis is among the most noticeable differences between smokers and nonsmokers.

Both cohort and case-control studies show an increase in death from chronic obstructive lung disease in smokers, compared to nonsmokers, with relative risks even greater than those observed for lung cancer, ranging from 2 to 24. The death rate from chronic obstructive lung disease is higher in men than women, probably reflecting the sex differential in smoking exposure cited earlier.

There is a marked dose–response effect relating tobacco to mortality from chronic obstructive lung disease, whether measured by number of cigarettes, years of smoking, or degree of inhalation.[4] Pipe and cigar smokers are also at elevated risk, but not as high as cigarette smokers are. Like the findings for lung cancer, populations where cigarette smoking is uncommon (Seventh-Day Adventists, Mormons, Old Order Amish) have lower lung disease rates than otherwise would be expected. However, immigrant studies suggest that ethnic background is not a major determinant of chronic obstructive lung disease.

12. THE ECONOMICS OF SMOKING

The costs related to smoking have been calculated from the direct costs of illness, disability, and early death for all related diseases and estimation of the proportion of disease that is attributable to smoking. Direct costs include expenses for hospital and home nursing care, services of professionals and paraprofessionals, drugs, medical research and training, facility construction, and public health expenditures. Indirect costs are those relating to loss of a worker due to disease, disability, or death. The combination of direct and indirect costs results in the total underlying costs of tobacco-related illness.[144]

In 1980, the costs of smoking-attributable disease in the United States were estimated to be $42.2 billion dollars, of which $16.1 billion were direct costs, $19.2 billion were indirect mortality costs, and $6.9 billion were indirect morbidity costs, based on 1980 dollars.[145]

The Office of Technology Assessment (OTA) estimated that the 1985 cost of treating smoking-related diseases ranged between $12 billion and $35 billion dollars, with a middle range estimated to be $22 billion dollars. Loss of productivity was estimated to result in a cost of between $27 billion and $61 billion dollars, with a middle estimate of $43 billion dollars. Thus the total smoking-related costs amounted in 1985 to between $39 billion and $96 billion, with a middle estimate of $65 billion dollars, or about $2.17 per pack of cigarettes.[146] Lewit, as modified by the OTA,[146] calculated that the direct health care costs for the period from 1964 to 1983 were $338.6 billion dollars in direct health care costs and $712 billion dollars in indirect costs.

The health care expenditures vary by disease entity and are a function of the proportion of the disease attributed to smoking. Roughly 30% of cancer deaths have been attributed to smoking,[43] as mentioned previously. Between 11%[146,147] and 30%[2] of cardiovascular and cerebrovascular disease deaths have been attributed to smoking; for respiratory disease deaths, 20%[144] to 90%[4]; for digestive disease deaths 8%,[147] to 39%,[148] with smaller percentages of deaths from injuries and perinatal deaths attributed to smoking.

From a public health standpoint, the crude mortality and years of life lost may well be the crucial aspect of assessing the impact of smoking. For the three major categories of smoking-related disease (cancer, cardio- and cerebrovascular disease, and chronic lung diseases), there are about 16 years lost per death per person (calculated using the average number of years of life remaining for smokers and nonsmokers), amounting to 4,896,000 years of lost life for the 314,000 deaths occurring each year from these disease categories.

Thus, if broken down by disease categories, about $6.9 billion dollars is spent on tobacco-related cancers, $8 billion for circulatory system illnesses, and $6.7 billion for diseases of the respiratory system. In addition, the cost of smoking-related lost productivity is estimated to be $18.9 billion for cancer, $17.4 billion for circulatory diseases, and $7.1 billion for diseases of the respiratory system. The result of these additions are about $25.8 billion for cancer, $25.4 billion for diseases of the circulatory system, and $13.8 billion for respiratory diseases.[146]

13. SMOKING CESSATION

Since smoking is the single largest preventable cause of premature death and disability in the United States, the best single way to prevent these losses is to prevent and/or decrease cigarette smoking.[1] For the major mortality categories of cardiovascular disease, cancer, and cerebrovascular disease, the length of time since cessation appears to be critical in lowering a smoker's risk. The reduced prevalence of smoking among some age- and sex-specific groups, as well as some occupational groups, suggests that large numbers of smokers have or would like to quit.[19] It is interesting to note that although smoking is still very prevalent among nurses, physicians and dentists have reduced their prevalences of smoking.[149]

Physicians can have a substantial impact on the smoking practices of their patients. Over 70% of Americans visit their physician at least once per year.[3] After a single physician recommendation to a patient without known smoking-related disease, one study found a (1–5%) drop in smoking prevalence.[150] Another study found that 98% of primary-care physicians encouraged their patients to stop smoking, and 45% were at least partly successful.[151] In a clinical trial in England, the smoking prevalence among enrollees dropped by 31% after a 15-min physician–patient session, and an additional 20% changed from cigarette use to use of pipes or cigars.[152] Finally, another intervention trial found that nearly twice as many individuals receiving "special attention" stopped cigarette use, compared to those who did not receive such attention.[2,3,153] Of those who quit, more than half continued to refrain from smoking for at least 5 years.

To encourage people to quit smoking, it may be useful to explore why they smoke. The following factors may act alone or in combination: (1) Cigarette smokers report an increased *sense of stimulation* or sharpening of their intellectual capacities when they smoke. (2) Cigarette smokers enjoy or rely on physically *handling the cigarette.* (3) Smokers find pleasure in smoking, and smoking *produces a relaxed feeling.* (4) Cigarette smoking offers a way of *reducing tension,* stress, and fear. (5) Smokers are *physiologically addicted* and often *crave* a cigarette. (6) Some smokers smoke by *habit,* apparently not necessarily even realizing that they want a cigarette.[154] Programs that attempt to foster smoking cessation should take into account the probable causes/behavioral manifestations of the individual's habit. For example, substitution of cigarettes with other activities (such as exercise) may not help the 30% of smokers for whom smoking is an immediate response to a stressful situation.[155]

It has been estimated that more than 90% of smokers have tried to quit at least once.[106] Between 1978 and 1980, roughly 1,800,000 smokers quit their habit; 60% of these were women. Since the initial Surgeon General's Report on Smoking, the prevalence of smoking fell by 13%, from 50% in men, and by 4%, from 29% in women. Smoking seems to have generally declined in both men and women, except for girls aged 17–18 years, in recent years.[1,14,156,157] Pinney[156] found that women who continue smoking are more likely to use low-tar and nicotine cigarettes than are men.

Most smokers try to quit on their own, without involvement in a formal program.[1] The reasons for wanting to quit are varied, and studies suggest they may emanate from the individual's health concerns, family or peer pressure, fear of adverse health consequences for the individual's family, concern for cleanliness or social acceptance, and cost of cigarettes.[3,106,158]

In addition to a smoker trying to quit totally on his/her own (which has been reported to be successful up to 63.5% of the time)[159] self-help aids, such as mass media, have reported successful cessation proportions of up to 50%. More formalized programs, such as smoking-cessation classes, often use a variety of behavior modification techniques, such as systematic desensitization or contracting. The success rates of these programs vary depending on the type and content of the program, cost and site of program, and degree of motivation.[19] In most programs, success is expected to be initially high among those who complete the entire program, but successful cessation drops off by as much as two-thirds with a year.[160] The cessation success rate of nicotine-containing gum has not been conclusively determined, although early indications are that the gum is useful. In addition, the use of the gum requires a prescription, and hence requires patient–physician interaction, which has been demonstrated to be effective in increasing cessation.[161]

It is not unlikely that reported cessation percentages are somewhat inaccurate, since those who do not succeed in quitting during a cessation program may quit in a subsequent program. Presumably those individuals were likely to have been highly motivated. Conversely, intitial quitting is not the same as continued cessation, resulting in overestimates of cessation percentages. For example, information from the MRFIT trial shows that smoking may recur even after periods of long cessation.[153]

In addition to smoking cessation, smoking prevention programs have become more widely accepted.[162] These programs have focused on children and adolescents and have been incorporated into health education curricula. Prevention programs have switched from emphasizing the evils of smoking to emphasizing the child's ability to control his/her own body, and hence his/her own health. Curricula usually teach social or psychological reasons for why smoking is started. Few comparative evaluations of the effectiveness of various programs have been published.

14. COMMUNITY RESPONSE TO SMOKING

In recent years, national and local legislative groups, as well as professional organizations, have taken a pronounced role in antismoking campaigns. Many states have passed legislation that prohibits smoking in specific public locations or creates either specified nonsmoking or smoking areas. Some states have passed cigarette sales taxes, which are designated to be spent on cancer control activities or on other smoking-related diseases (Idaho, Nebraska, New Jersey, Pennsylvania, Minnesota, New Mexico). The American Medical Association has supported the elimination of federal price support for growing tobacco, the use of rotating warning labels on cigarettes, financial incentives by insurance companies to nonsmokers, the expansion of education programs targeted at adolescents and teenagers, the prohibition of cigarette vending machines, and most important, the elimination of any form of advertising of tobacco via legislation prohibiting such advertising.[163,164] Some insurance companies have developed new premium rate tables for nonsmokers, and one company no longer wants to insure smokers.[165]

15. PASSIVE SMOKING

It has been estimated that three-fourths of Americans are exposed to passive (also referred to as involuntary) smoking. Involuntary smoking refers to exposure of nonsmokers to tobacco combustion products in the indoor environment.[106] There has been increasing public concern and pressure over the hazards associated with involuntary exposure to smoke, leading to the enactment of legislation, as described earlier.

Tobacco smoke in the environment comes both from the exhaled breath of people smoking and from "sidestream" smoke from the end of a burning cigarette. Many of the same compounds are found in both types of smoke. Sidestream smoke has higher concentrations of carbon monoxide, tar, nicotine, benzo(a)pyrene, and other dangerous gas and particulate phase constituents. Since there is dilution into ambient air of this smoke, sidestream smokers receive different quantities and types of noxious substances than smokers. In part, this depends on the amount of smoke, volume of the room, and type and amount of ventilation.[1]

The relationship between passive smoking and chronic diseases is difficult to assess, because exposure is difficult to quantitate, i.e., amount of exposure, length of time exposed. Even in studies of spouses of smokers, misclassification may occur since nonsmoking spouses may themselves be former smokers, and current marital exposure to smoke may not reflect prior exposure to the same or a different spouse. Also, exposure in the workplace may provide prolonged exposure to smoke. Another difficulty is that the latency period associated with the development of chronic diseases is long, and current exposure to passive smoke may not be relevant. Finally, since smoking is known to have interacting effects with some occupational carcinogens, the effect of passive smoking may be confounded by such exposure.[1] Thus, the issue of long-term hazards associated with passive smoking is not nearly resolved.

It is, however, becoming increasingly evident that hazardous components of smoke are absorbed by nonsmokers. Elevations of carbon monoxide, nicotine concentration, and nicotine-to-creatinine ratios have been found in blood, urine, and saliva in individuals exposed to passive smoke.[166–169] Acute reactions, including complaints of headache, cough, and nasal and eye irritations,[142] have been reported to be in excess among those passively exposed to smoke.

The effects of passive smoking are observed in children, adult nonsmokers, and particular subgroups of individuals who have difficulty with respiration, such as asthmatics. Among children less than 2 years old, there appears to be an increased risk of bronchitis and pneumonia in families where the parents smoke. When both parents smoke, the risk is highest; when only one smokes, the risk is intermediate between that of nonsmoking parents and that when both parents smoke.[170] Older children appear to also have this increased risk.[171] Two studies have found that children of nonsmoking mothers were substantially less likely to be hospitalized for pneumonia or bronchitis than children of maternal smokers.[165] Other studies suggest that there are notable reductions in forced expiratory volume (FEV) in the first 7 years in children of smokers,[172] including a dose–response relationship between FEV reduction and number of smokers in the home.[165] Wheezing and asthma,[173,174], middle-ear infections, decreased height, and sudden infant death syndrome[175–177] are also more common in children of smokers than in children of nonsmokers.

In adults, passive smoking is associated with both short-term and long-term effects. The short-term effects include those conditions previously stated to occur in children, as well as aggravation of allergic attacks. Besides pulmonary problems, cardiovascular effects and cancer are associated with passive smoke exposure. Passive smoking decreases the time for symptoms of angina to begin after exercise.[178]

The most studied association between passive smoking and chronic disease is on lung cancer. Hirayama found the nonsmoking wives of smokers had twice the risk of developing lung cancer as wives of nonsmokers.[179] Trichopolous *et al.*[180] found a significantly elevated lung cancer risk among women whose husbands smoked. Garfinkel found an increased risk also, although it was not significantly elevated.[181] A study by Correa *et al.*[182] found that men who were exposed in their youth to both parents smoking had more than a 65% increase in lung cancer risk compared to those whose parents did not smoke; those having one parent smoking had an intermediate risk. This study also found that the risk of lung cancer among *nonsmoking* spouses was elevated if the smoking spouse was a heavy smoker, but the risk for a *smoking* spouse did not increase if his/her spouse was a heavy smoker. In summary, the strength of this association appears fairly strong and suggestive of a dose–response effect.

REFERENCES

1. *Report of the Surgeon General. The Health Consequences of Smoking. Cancer.* USDHHS (PHS) Office of Smoking and Health, Rockville, MD, 1982.
2. *Report of the Surgeon General. The Health Consequences of Smoking. Cardiovascular Disease.* USDHHS (PHS) Office of Smoking and Health, Rockville, MD, 1983.
3. *Report of the Surgeon General. The Health Consequences of Smoking. Chronic Obstructive Lung Disease.* USDHHS (PHS) Office of Smoking and Health, Rockville, MD, 1984.
4. Kikendall, J. W., Evaul, J., and Johnson, L. F.: Effect of cigarette smoking on gastrointestinal physiology and non-neoplastic digestive disease. *J. Clin. Gastroenterol.* **6**:65–79, 1984.
5. Bastiaan, R. J., and Waite, I. M.: Effects of tobacco smoking on plaque development and gingivitis. *J. Periodontol.* **42**:259–263, 1971.
6. Sheiham, A.: Periodontal disease and oral cleanliness in tobacco smokers. *J. Periodontol.* **42**:259–263, 1971.
7. Ismail, A. I., Burt, B. A., and Eklund, S. A.: Epidemiologic patterns of smoking and periodontal disease in the United States. *J. Am. Dent. Assoc.* **106**: 617–621, 1983.
8. Liard, R., Perdrizet, S., and Reinert, P.: Wheezy bronchitis in infants and parents' smoking habits. *Lancet* **1**:334–335, 1982.
9. Fergusson, D. M., Horwood, L. J., Shannon, F. T., and Taylor, B.: Parental smoking and lower repiratory illness in the first three years of life. *J. Epidemiol. Commun. Health* **35**:180–184, 1981.
10. Colley, J. R. T., Douglas, J. W. B., and Reid, D. D.: Respiratory disease in young adults: Influence of early childhood lower respiratory tract illness, social class, air pollution, and smoking. *Br. Med. J.* **3**:195–198, 1973.
11. Lusto, J.: Reducing the health consequences of smoking. A progress report. *Public Health Rep.* **98**:34–39, 1983.
12. Remington, P. L., Forman, M. R., Gentry, E. M., Marks, J. S., Hagelin, G. C., and Trowbridge, F. L.: Current smoking trends in the United States. *JAMA* **253**:2975–2978, 1985.
13. *The Tax Burden on Tobacco. 1983.* The Tobacco Institute, Washington, D.C., 1984.
14. Johnston, L., O'Malley, P. M., and Bachman, J. G.: Use of licit and illicit drugs by America's high school students 1975–1984. USPHHS, ADAMHA, Publ. no. (ADM) 85-1394, Rockville, MD, 1985.
15. DeVita, V.: *Update: Annual Cancer Statistics Update.* National Institutes of Health, Bethesda, Maryland, 1985.
16. Silverberg, E., and Lubera, J.: Cancer statistics 1986. *Ca* **36**:9–25, 1986.
17. *1985 Annual Cancer Statistics Review.* National Cancer Advisory Board, USDHHS (NCI), Rockville, MD, 1985.
18. *1984 Annual Cancer Statistics Review.* National Cancer Advisory Board, USDHHS (NCI), Rockville, MD, 1984.
19. Fielding, J. E.: Smoking: Health effects and control. *N. Engl. J. Med.* **313**(8):491–498; **313**(9):555–561, 1985.
20. *Cancer Facts and Figures, 1985.* American Cancer Society, New York, 1985.
21. Hammond, E. C.: Evidence on the effects of giving up cigarette smoking. *Am. J. Public Health* **55**(5):682–691, 1965.
22. Hammond, E. C.: Smoking in relation to the death rates of one million men and women, in Haenszel, W. (ed.): *Epidemiological Approaches to the Study of Cancer and Other Chronic Diseases.* NCI Mono 19 USDHEW (PHS), Rockville, MD, 1966, pp. 127–204.
23. Hammond, E. C., Garfinkel, L., Seidman, H., and Lew, E. A.: "Tar" and nicotine content of cigarette smoke in relation to death rates. *Environ. Res* **12**(3):263–274, 1976.
24. Doll, R., and Hill, A. B.: The mortality of doctors in relation to their smoking habits; a preliminary report. *Br. Med. J.* **1**:1451–1455, 1954.

25. Doll, R., and Hill, A. B.: Lung cancer and other causes of death in relation to smoking. A second report on the mortality of British doctors. *Br. Med. J.* **2**:1071–1081, 1956.
26. Doll, R., and Hill, A. B.: Mortality in relation to smoking: 10 years' observations of British doctors (Part 1). *Br. Med. J.* **1**:1399–1410, 1964.
27. Doll, R., and Hill, A. B.: Mortality in relation to smoking. Concluded. *Br. Med. J.* **1**:1462–1467, 1964.
28. Doll, R., and Peto, R.: Mortality in relation to smoking: 20 years' observations on male British doctors. *Br. Med. J.* **2**:1525–1536, 1976.
29. Cederlof, R., Friberg, L., Hrubec, Z., and Lorich, U.:*The Relationship of Smoking and Some Social Covariables to Mortality and Cancer Morbidity. A Ten Year Follow-up in a Probabity Sample of 55,000 Subjects, Age 18–69,* Pt 1,2. The Karolinska Institute, Stockholm, 1975, pp. 1–91.
30. Hirayama, T.: *Smoking in Relation to the Death Rates of 265,118 Men and Women in Japan.* National Cancer Center, Tokyo, 1967.
31. Hirayama, T.: Smoking in relation to the death rates of 265,118 men and women in Japan. A report on 5 years of follow-up. ACS 14th Science Writers Seminar, Clearwater Beach, FL, March 24–29, 1972.
32. Dorn, H. F.: The mortality of smokers and nonsmokers, in *Proceedings of the Social Statistics Section of the American Statistical Association, December 27–30, 1958.* American Statistical Association, Washington, DC, 1959, pp. 34–71.
33. Kahn, H. A.: The Dorn study of smoking and mortality among U.S. veterans, in Haenszel, W. (ed.): *Epidemiological Approaches to the Study of Cancer and Other Chronic Diseases.* NCI Mono. No. 19, USDHEW (NCI), Rockville, MD, 1966, pp. 1–125.
34. Rogot, E.: *Smoking and General Mortality among U.S. Veterans 1954–1969.* USDHEW (NHLBI) DHEW publ. no. (NIH) 74-554, Rockville, MO, 1974.
35. Rogot, E., and Murray, J. L.: Smoking and causes of death among U.S. veterans. 16 years of observations. *Public Health Rep.* **95**(3):213–222, 1980.
36. Hammond, E. C., and Horn, D.: Smoking and death rates—Report on forty-four months of follow-up on 187,783 men. I. Total mortality. *JAMA* **166**(10):1159–1172, 1958.
37. Hammond, E. C., and Horn, D.: Smoking and death rates—Report on forty-four months of follow-up on 187,783 men. II. Death rates by cause. *JAMA* **166**(11):1294–1308, 1958.
38. Best, E. W. R.: *A Canadian Study of Smoking and Health.* Department of National Health and Welfare, Ottawa, 1966, pp. 1–137.
39. Best, E. R. W., Josie, G. H., and Walker, C. B.: A Canadian study of mortality in relation to smoking habits. A preliminary report. *Can. J. Public Health* **52**:99–106, 1961.
40. Hammond, E. C., and Seidman, H.: Smoking and cancer in the United States. *Prev. Med.* **9**(2):169–173, 1980.
41. Dunn, J. E., Linden, G., and Breslow, L.: Lung cancer mortality experience of men in certain occupations in California. *Am. J. Public Health* **50**(10):1475–1487, 1960.
42. Weir, J. M., and Dunn, J. E.: Smoking and mortality, A prospective study. *Cancer* **25**(1):105–112, 1970.
43. Doll, R., and Peto, R.: *The Causes of Cancer.* Oxford University Press, Oxford, 1981.
44. Maltoni, C., Carretti, D., Canepari, C., and Ghetti, G.: Incidenza della metaplasia squamosa dellepitelio respirtorio in rapporto al fumo di sigaretta. *Cancro* **21**(4):349–356, 1968.
45. Nasiell, M.: *The Epithelial Picture in the Bronchial Mucosa in Chronic Inflammatory and Neoplastic Lung Disease and Its Relation to Smoking. A Comparative Histologic and Sputum Cytology Study.* Cytology Laboratory, Department of Pathology at Sabbatsberg Hospital, Karolinska Institute, Stockholm, 1968, pp. 1–72.
46. Pooling Project Research Group: Relationship of blood pressure, serum cholesterol, smoking habit, relative weight and ECG abnoralities to incidence of major coronary events: Final report of the pooling project. *J. Chronic Dis. 31*(4):201–206, 1978.
47. Mann, J. I., Doll, R., Thorogood, M., *et al.:* Risk factors for myocardial infarction in young women. *Br. J. Prev. Soc. Med.***30**:94–100, 1976.
48. Slone, D., Shapiro, S., Rosenberg, L., *et al.:* Relation of cigarette smoking to myocardial infarction in young women. *N. Engl. J. Med.***298**:1273–1276, 1978.
49. Rosenberg, L., Shapiro, S., Kaufman, D. W., *et al.:* Cigarette smoking in relation to the risk of myocardial infarction in young women. *Int. J. Epidemiol.* **9**:57–63, 1980.
50. Hennekens, C. H., and Buring, J. E.: Smoking and coronary heart disease in women. (editorial). *JAMA* **253**(20):3003–3004, 1985.

51. Rosenberg, L., Miller, D. R., Kaufman, D. W., *et al.*: Myocardial infarction in women under 50 years of age. *JAMA* **250**:2801–2806, 1983.
52. Rosenberg, L., Kaufman, D. W., Helmrich, S. P., Miller, D. L., Stolley, P. D., and Shapiro, S.: Myocardial infarction and cigarette smoking in women under 50 years of age. *JAMA* **253**:2965–2969, 1985.
53. Shapiro, S., Weinblatt, E., Frank, C. W., *et al.*: Incidence of coronary heart disease in a population insured for medical care (HIP): Myocardial infarction, angina pectoris, and possible myocardial infarction. *Am. J. Public Health* **59**(suppl 6):1–101, 1969.
54. Kannel, W. B., Castelli, W. P., and McNamara, P. M.: Cigarette smoking and risk of coronary heart disease: Epidemiologic clues to pathogensis: The Framingham study, in Wynder, E. L., and Hofmann, D. (eds.): *Toward A Less Harmful Cigarette.* NCI Mono. 28 , Bethesda, MD, 1968, pp. 9–20.
55. Oliver, M. F.: Ischaemic heart disease in young women. *Br. Med. J.* **4**:253–259, 1974.
56. Bengtsson, C.: Ishaemic heart disease in women: A study based on a randomized population sample of women and women with myocardial infarction in Goteberg, Sweden. *Acta Med. Scand.* **5** (suppl):1–128, 1973.
57. Carlson, L. A., and Bottiger, L.E.: Ischaemic heart disease in relation to fasting values of plasma triglycerides and cholesterol. Stockholm prospective study. *Lancet* **1**:865–870, 1972.
58. Carlson, L. A., Bottiger, L. E., and Ahfeldt, P-E.: Risk factors for myocardial infarction in the Stockholm prospective study. A 14 year follow-up focusing on the role of plasma triglycerides and cholesterol. *Acta Med. Scand.* **206**(5):351–360, 1979.
59. Hamman, R. F., Barancik, J. I., and Lilienfeld, A. M.: Patterns of mortality in the older order Amish. I. Background and major causes of death. *Am. J. Epidemiol.* **114**(6):845–861, 1981.
60. Holme, I., Helgeland, A., Hjermann, I., Leren, P., and Lund-Larson, P. G.: Four and two thirds years incidence of coronary heart disease in middle-aged men: The Oslo study. *Am. J. Epidemiol.* **112**(1):149–160, 1980.
61. Natvig, H., Borchgrevink, C. F., Dedichen, J., Owren, P. A., Schiotz, E. H., and Westlund, K.: A controlled trial on the effect of linoleic acid on incidence of coronary heart disease. The Norweigian vegetable oil experiment of 1965–1966. *Scand. J. Clin. Lab. Invest.* **22**(suppl 105):1–20, 1968.
62. Schroll, M., and Hagerup, L. M.: Risk factors of myocardial infarction and death in men aged 50 at entry. A ten-year prospective study from the Glostrup population studies. *Dan. Med. Bull.* **24**(6):252–255, 1977.
63. Wilhemsen, L., Bengtsson, C., Elmfeldt, D., Vedin, A., Wilhelmsson, C., Tibblin, G., Lindqvist, O., and Wedel, H.: Multiple risk prediction of myocardial infarction in women as compared to men. *Br. Heart J.* **39**(11):1179–1185, 1977.
64. Hopkins, P. N., and Williams, R. R.: A survey of 246 suggested coronary heart disease risk factors. *Atherosclerosis* **40**(1):1–52, 1981.
65. Inter Society Commission for Heart Disease Resources: Primary prevention of the atherosclerotic diseases. *Circulation* **42**(6):555–595, 1970.
66. Kannel, W. B.: Some lessons in cardiovascular epidemiology from Framingham. *Am. J. Cardiol.* **37**(2):269–282, 1976.
67. Levy, R. I., and Feinleib, M.: Risk factors for coronary artery disease and their management, in Braunwald, E. (ed.): *Heart Disease: A Textbook of Cardiovascular Medicine,* Vol. 2. Saunders, Philadelphia, 1980.
68. Stamler, J., and Epstein, F. H.: Coronary heart disease: Risk factors as guides to preventive action. *Prev. Med.* **1**(1–2):27–48, 1972.
69. Dorn, H. F.: Tobacco consumption and mortality from cancer and other diseases. *Public Health Rep.* **74**(7):581–593, 1959.
70. Hammond, E. C., and Garfinkel, L.: Coronary heart disease, stroke, and aortic aneurism. Factors in the etiology. *Arch. Environ. Health* **19**(2):167–182, 1969.
71. Salonen, J. T.: Oral contraceptives, smoking, and risk of myocardial infarction in young women. A longitudinal population study in eastern Finland. *Acta Med. Scand.* **212**(3):141–144, 1980.
72. Paffenbarger, R. S., Jr., Brand, R. J., Scholtz. R. I., and Jung, D. L.: Energy expenditure, cigarette smoking, and blood pressure level as related to death from specific diseases. *Am. J. Epidemiol.* **108**(1):12–18, 1978.
73. Gillium, R. F., and Paffenbarger, R. S., Jr.: Chronic disease in former college students. XVII. So-

ciocultural mobility as a precursor of coronary heart disease and hypertension. *Am. J. Epidemiol.* **108**(4):289–298, 1978.
74. Doll, R., Gray, R., Hafner, B., and Peto, R.: Mortality in relation to smoking: 22 years observations on female British doctors. *Br. Med. J.* **280**:967–971, 1980.
75. Doll, R., and Hill, A. B.: Mortality of British doctors in relation to smoking: Observations on coronary thrombosis, in Haenszel, W. (ed.): *Epidemiologic Approaches to the Study of Cancer and Other Chronic Diseases.* NCI Mono. 19, USDHEW (PHS), Rockville, MD, 1966, pp. 205–268.
76. Strobel, M., and Gsell, O.: Mortalitat in Bezeihung Zum Tabakrauchen. 9 Jahre Beobachtungen Bei Arzten in der Schweiz. (Mortality in relation to tobacco smoking. Nine years of observation in Swiss physicians.) *Helv. Med. Acta* **32**(6):547–592, 1965.
77. Gsell, O., Abelin, T., and Wieltchnig, E.: Rauchen und Mortlitat der Schweizer Arzte: Resultata nach 18 Jahriger Beobachtung. (Smoking and mortality of Swiss physicians: Results after 18 years of observation). *Bull. Schweiz. Akad. Med. Wissenschaft.* **35**(1–3):71–82, 1979.
78. Hiramyama, T.: Smoking and cadiovascular disease—An epidemiological study. *Korei Igaku* **13**(3):86–91, 1975.
79. Hiramyama, T.: An epidemiological study on smoking and ischaemic heart disease. *Gen. Clin. J.* **27**(2):265–274, 1978.
80. Hiramyama, T.: Smoking and arteriosclerosis—An epidemiological study. *Saishin Igaku* **36**(4):798–809, 1981.
81. Hirayama, T., and Hamano, Y.: Smoking and mortality from major causes of death. *Eisei No Shibyo* **28**(4):3–18, 1981.
82. Hrubec, Z., and Zukel, W. J.: Epidemiology of coronary heart disease among young army males of World War II. *Am. Heart J.* **87**(6):722–730, 1974.
83. Kagan, A., Popper, J. S., Rhoads, G. G., Takeya, Y., Kato, H., Goode, G. B., and Marmot. M.: Epidemiologic studies of coronary heart disease and stroke in Japanese men living in Japan, Hawaii, and California. Prevalence of stroke, in Scheinberg, P. (ed.): *Cerebrovascular Diseases.* Raven, New York, 1976.
84. Wolf, P. A., Dawber, T. R., Thomas, H. E., and Kannel, W. B.: Epidemiologic assessment of chronic atrial fibrillation and risk of stroke. The Framingham study. *Neurology* **28**(10):973–977, 1978.
85. Haberman, S., Capildeo, R., and Rose, F. C.: Smoking: A risk factor for stroke, in Greenhalgh, W. (ed.): *Smoking and Arterial Disease.* Pitman Press, Bath, Great Britain, 1981.
86. Wolf, P. A., Dawber, T. R., and Kannel, W. B.: Heart disease as a precursor of stroke, in Schoenberg, D. S. (ed.): *Neurological Epidemiology: Principles and Clinical Applications. Advances in Neurology,* Vol 19. Raven, New York, 1978.
87. Rhoads, G. G., Popper, J. S., Kagan, A., and Yano, K.: Incidence of transient cerebral ischaemic attack in Hawaii Japanese men. The Honolulu heart study. *Stroke* **11**(1):21–26, 1980.
88. Ostfield, A. M., Shekelle, R. B., and Klawans, H. L.: Transient ischaemic attacks and risk of stroke in an elderly poor population. *Am. J. Public Health* **64**(5):450–458, 1974.
89. Bell, B. A., and Symon, L.: Smoking and subarachnoid hemorrhage. *Br. Med. J.* **1**:577–582, 1979.
90. Petitti, D. B., and Wingerd, J.: Use of oral contraceptives, cigarette smoking, and risk of subarachnoid hemorrhage. *Lancet* **2**:234–236, 1978.
91. Petitti, D. B., Wingerd, J., Pelligren, F., and Ramcharan, S.: Risk of vascular disease in women, smoking, oral contraceptives, noncontraceptive estrogens, and other factors. *JAMA* **242**(11):1150–1154, 1979.
92. Collaborative Group for the Study of Stroke in Young Women: Oral contraceptives and stroke in young women, Associated risk factors. *JAMA* **231**(7):718–722, 1975.
93. Collaborative Group for the Study of Stroke in Young Women: Oral contraception and increased risk of cerebral ischaemia or thrombosis. *N. Engl. J. Med.* **288**(17):871–878, 1973.
94. Royal College of General Practitioners: Oral contraceptive study. Mortality among oral contraceptive users. *Lancet* **2**:727–731, 1977.
95. Schrek, R., Baker, A., Ballard, G. P., and Dolgoff, S.: Tobacco smoking as an etiologic factor in disease. I. Cancer. *Cancer Res.* **10**:49–58, 1960.
96. Valko, P.: Smoking and occurrence of malignant tumors of the larxnx. *Ceskoslovenska Otolaryngol.* **1**:102–105, 1952.

97. Saffioti, U.: Experimental respiratory tract carcinogenesis and its relation to inhalation exposures, in Hanna, M.G., Nettesheim, P., Gilbert, J. R., *et al.* (eds.): *Inhalation Carcinogenesis.* Proceedings of a Biology Division, Oak Ridge National Conference, Gatlinberg, TN. AEC, EDC Symposium Series, 1970, pp. 27–54.
98. Bradshaw, E., and Schonland, M.: Oesophageal and lung cancers in natal African males in relation to socio-economic factors. An analysis of 484 interviews. *Br. J. Cancer* **23**(2):275–284, 1969.
99. Wynder, E. L., Bross, I. J., and Day, E.: A study of environmental factors in cancer of the laranyx. *Cancer* **9**(1):86–110, 1956.
100. Schwartz, D., Denoix, P-F., and Anguera, G.: Research on the localizations of cancer associated with tobacco and alcoholic factors in man. *Sem. Hop. Paris* **33**(62/7):3630–3645, 1957.
101. Wynder, E. L., Kmet, J., Dungal, N., and Segi, M.: An epidemiological investigation of gastric cancer. *Cancer* **16**(11):1461–1496, 1963.
102. Dutta-Choudhuri, R., Roy, H., and Sen-Gupta, B. K.: Cancer of the laraynx and hypopharaynx. A clinicopathological study with special reference to aetiology. *J. Indian Med. Assoc.* **32**(9):352–362, 1959.
103. Staszewski, J.: Tobacco smoking and its relation to cancer of the mouth, tonsils, and laranyx. *Nowotwory* **10**(2):121–132, 1960.
104. Svoboda, V.: An analysis of some possible epidemiologic factors involved in cancer of the larynx. *Neoplasma* **15**(6):677–684, 1968.
105. Wynder, E. L., and Hoffman, D.: Tobacco and tobacco smoke. *Semin. Oncol* **3**(1):5–15, 1976.
106. *Report of the Surgeon General. Smoking and Health.* USDHEW (PHS) Office of Smoking and Health, Rockville, MD, 1979.
107. *Report of the Surgeon General. The Health Consequences of Smoking.* USDHEW (HSM) Health Services and Mental Health Administration, Rockville, MD, 1971.
108. Engstrom, J. E.: Cancer mortality among Mormons in California during 1968–1975. *J. Natl. Cancer Inst.* **65**(5):1073–1082, 1980.
109. Lyon, J. L., Gardner, J. W., and West, D. W.: Cancer incidence in Mormons and non-Mormons in Utah during 1967–1975. *J. Natl. Cancer Inst.* **65**(5):1055–1061, 1980.
110. Lyon, J. L., Gardner, J. W., and West, D. W.: Cancer risk and life-style: Cancer among Mormons from 1967–1975, in Cairns, J., Lyon, J. L., and Skolnick, M. (eds.): *Cancer Incidence in Defined Populations.* Banbury Report No. 4. Cold Spring Harbor Laboratory, Cold Spring Harbor, NY, 1980, pp. 3–30.
111. Phillips, R. L., Kuzma, J. W., and Lotz, T. M.: Cancer mortality among comparable members versus nonmembers of the Seventh Day Adventist Church, in Cairns, J., Lyon, J. L., and Skolnick, M. (eds.): *Cancer Incidence in Defined Populations.* Banbury Report No. 4. Cold Spring Harbor Laboratory, Cold Spring Harbor, NY, 1980, pp. 93–108.
112. West, D. W.: An assessment of cancer risk factors in Latter-day Saints and non-Latter-day Saints in Utah, in Cairns, J., Lyon, J. L., and Skolnick, M. (eds.): *Cancer Incidence in Defined Populations.* Banbury Report No. 4. Cold Spring Harbor Laboratory, Cold Spring Harbor, NY, 1980, pp. 31–49.
113. Monson, R. R., and Lyons, J. L.: Proportional mortality among alcoholics. *Cancer* **36**(3):1077–1079, 1975.
114. Pell, S., and ĎAlonzo, C. A.: A five year mortality study of alcoholics. *J. Occup. Med.* **15**(2):120–125, 1973.
115. Schmidt, W., and DeLint, J.: Causes of deaths in alcoholics. *Q. J. Stud. Alcohol* **93**(1):171–185, 1972.
116. Chow, J. W.: Head and neck cancers 1. Who's at risk and why. *Diagnosis* **6**(10):106–108, 111–112, 1984.
117. *Surveillance, Epidemiology, End Results. Incidence and Mortality Data. 1973–1977.* USDHHS (NIH) Publ. no. 81–2330, Rockville, MD, 1981.
118. Shimizu, M.: Oral cancer of Tokyo—Peculiarity, TMN classification, histopathological type and relation between smoking and prevention. *Shikai Tenbo* **62**(4):717–730, 1983.
119. Hirayama, T.: Changing patterns of cancer in Japan with special reference to the decrease in stomach cancer mortality, in Hiatt, H. H., Watson, J. D., and Winsten, J. A. (eds.): *Origins of Human Cancer.* Book A: *Incidence of Cancer in Humans.* Cold Spring Harbor Conference on Cell Proliferation, Vol 4. Cold Spring Harbor Laboratory, Cold Spring Harbor, NY, 1977.
120. US Department of Health and Human Services (DeLuca, J. R., ed.): *Fourth Special Report to the U.S. Congress on Alcohol and Health.* USDHHS, PHS, ADAMHA, NIAAA. DHHS Publ. No. (ADM) 81–1080, Rockville, MD, 1981.

121. McCoy, D. G., Hecht, S. S., and Wynder, E. L.: The roles of tobacco, alcohol, and diet in the etiology of upper alimentary and respiratory tract cancers. *Prev. Med.* **9**(5):622–629, 1980.
122. Hoffman, L., and Heher, W.: Squamous cell carcinomas of the oral cavity. *Deutsche Med. Wochenschr.* **108**(30):1150–1152, 1983.
123. Page, H. S., and Asire, A. J.: *Cancer Rates and Risks.* USPHHS Publ. No. (NIH) 85–691, Rockville, MD, 1985.
124. Wigle, D. T., Mao, Y., and Grace, M.: Relative importance of smoking as a risk factor for selective cancers. *Can. J. Public Health* **71**:269–275, 1980.
125. Cole, P., Monson, R. R., Haning, H., and Friedell, G. H.: Smoking and cancer of the lower urinary tract. *N. Engl. J. Med.* **284**(3):129–134, 1971.
126. Hartge, P., Hoover, R., and Kantor, A.: Bladder cancer risk and pipes, cigars and smokeless tobacco. *CA* **55**(4):901–906, 1985.
127. Whittemore, A. S., Paffenbarger, R. S., Anderson, K., *et al.*: Early precursors of site-specific cancers in college men and women. *J. Natl. Cancer Inst.* **74**(1):43–61, 1985.
128. Morrison, A. S.: Advances in the etiology of urothelial cancer. *Urol. Clin. North Am.* **11**(4):557–566, 1984.
129. Vineis, P., Ciccone, G., Ghisetti, V., *et al.*: Cigarette smoking and bladder cancer in females. *Ca Lett.* **26**(1):61–66, 1985.
130. Howe, G. R., Burch, J. D., Miller, A. B., *et al.*: Tobacco use, occupation, coffee, various nutrients, and bladder cancer. *J. Natl. Cancer Inst.* **64**(4):701–713, 1980.
131. Hoover, R., and Cole, P.: Population trends in cigarette smoking and bladder cancer. *Am. J. Epidemiol.* **94**:409–491, 1971.
132. Lyon, J. L., Gardner, J. W., West, D. W., Stanish, W. M., and Hebertson, R. M.: Smoking and carcinoma-*in-situ* of the uterine cervix. *Am. J. Public Health* **73**:558–562, 1983.
133. Trevathan, E., Layde, P., Webster, L. A., *et al.*: Cigarette smoking and dysplasia and carcinoma *in situ* of the uterine cervix. *JAMA* **250**:499–502, 1983.
134. Greenberg, E. R., Vessey, M., McPherson, K., *et al.*: Cigarette smoking and cancer of the uterine cervix. *Br. J. Cancer* **51**(1):139–141, 1985.
135. LaVecchia, C., Franceschi, S., DeCarli, A., *et al.*: Cigarette smoking and the risk of cervical neoplasia. *Am. J. Epidemiol.* **123**(1):22–29, 1986.
136. Gordis, L., and Gold, E. B.: Epidemiology of pancreatic cancer. *World J. Surg.* **8**(6):808–821, 1984.
137. Schechter, M. T., Miller, A. B., and Howe, G. R.: Cigarette smoking and breast cancer: A case-control study of screening program participants. *Am. J. Epidemiol.* **121**(4):479–487, 1985.
138. Brinton, L. A., Schairer, C., Stanford, J. L., and Hoover, R. N.: Cigarette smoking and breast cancer. *Am. J. Epidemiol.* **123**(4):614–622, 1986.
139. Mabuchi, K., Bross, D. S., and Kessler, I. I.: Epidemiology of cancer of the vulva. A case-control study. *Cancer* **55**(8):1843–1848, 1985.
140. Aubry, F., and MacGibbon, B.: Risk factors of squamous cell carcinoma of the skin. A case control study in the Montreal region. *Cancer* **55**(4):909–911, 1985.
141. Lesko, S. M., Rosenberg, L., Kaufman, D. W., *et al.*: Cigarette smoking and the risk of endometrial cancer. *N. Engl. J. Med.* **313**(10):593–596, 1985.
142. Tyler, C. W., Webster, L. A., Ory, H. W., *et al.*: Endometrial cancer: How does cigarette smoking influence the risk of women under 55 years of age having this tumor? *Am. J. Obstet. Gynecol.* **151**(7):899–905, 1985.
143. Jackson, F. N., and Holle, R. H.: Smoking: Perspectives 1985. *Prim. Care* **12**(2):197–216, 1985.
144. Rice, D. P., and Hodgson, T. A.: Economic costs of smoking: An analysis of data for the United States. Draft of paper presented at Allied Social Science Association Annual Meetings, San Francisco, Dec. 25, 1983.
145. Shultz, J. M.: Perspectives on the economic magnitude of cigarette smoking. *NY State J. Med.* **85**(7):302–306, 1985.
146. *Smoking Related Deaths and Financial Costs.* Health Program Office, Office of Technology Assessment, Washington, D.C., September 1985.
147. Schultz, J. M.: *Smoking Attributable Mortality, Morbidity, and Economic Costs. Methodology and Guide to Computer Software.* Center for Nonsmoking and Health, Minneapolis, 1985.

148. Ravenholt, R. T.: Addictive mortality in the U.S., 1980: Tobacco, alcohol and other statistics. *Pop. Dev. Rev.* **10**(4):697–724, 1984.
149. Engstrom, J. E.: Trends in mortality among California physicians after giving up smoking. 1950–79. *Br. Med. J.* **286**:1101–1105, 1983.
150. Russell, M. A., Wildson, C., Taylor, C., and Baker, C. D.: Effects of general practitioners advice against smoking. *Br. Med. J.* **2**:231–235, 1979.
151. Battista, R. N.: Adult cancer prevention in primary care: Patterns of practice in Quebec. *Am. J. Public Health* **73**:1036–1039, 1983.
152. Rose, G., Hamilton, P. J. S., Colwell, L., and Shipley, M. J.: A randomized controlled trial of antismoking advice: 10 year results. *J. Epidemiol. Commun. Health* **36**:102–108, 1982.
153. Ockene, J. K., Hymnowitz, N., Sexton, M., and Brotke, S. K.: Comparison of patterns of smoking behavior change among smokers in the Multiple Risk Intervention Trial (MRFIT). *Prev. Med.* **11**:621–628, 1982.
154. Horn, D., and Waingrow, S.: Some dimensions of a model for smoking behavior change. *Am. J. Public Health* **56**:21–26, 1966.
155. Christen, A. G., and Cooper, K. H.: *Strategic Withdrawal from Cigarette Smoking*. American Cancer Society, New York, 1979.
156. Pinney, J. M.: Speech delivered to the American Lung Association of Maryland, Baltimore, May 5, 1981. As cited in *Cancer Prevention Research Summary—Tobacco*. USDHHS, NIH Publ. No. 84–2614, Rockville, MD, 1984.
157. National Institute of Education: *Teenage Smoking: Intermediate and Long Term Patterns*. US Govt. Printing Office, Washington, DC, 1979.
158. Schwartz, J. L.: Myths and realities of smoking cessation. *NY State J. Med.* **83**:1355–1357, 1983.
159. Schachter, S.: Don't sell habit breakers short. *Psychol. Today* **283**:457, 1982.
160. Leventhal, H., and Cleary, P. D.: The smoking problem: A review of the research and theory in behavioral risk modification. *Psychiatry Bull.* **88**:370–405, 1980.
161. Rimer, B. K., Strecher, V. J., Kentz, M. K., and Engstrom, P. L.: A survey of physicians views and practices on patient education for smoking cessation. *Prev. Med.* **15**(1):92–98, 1986.
162. Glynn, T.: National Cancer Institute, Hispanic Cancer Control Conference, April 17, 1986.
163. Board of Trustees, AMA: Media advertising for tobacco products. *JAMA* **255**(8):1033, 1986.
164. Lindberg, G. D., and Knoll, E.: Tobacco: For consenting adults in private only (editiorial). *JAMA* **255**(8):151–153, 1986.
165. Fielding, J. E.: Smoking: Health effects and control, in Last, J. M., Chin, J., Fielding, J. E., Frank, A. L., Lashof, J. C., and Wallace, R. B. (eds.): Maxcy Rosenau: *Public Health and Preventive Medicine*. Appleton Century Crofts, Norwalk, CT, 1986.
166. Sterling, T. D., Dimich, H., and Kobayashi, D.: Indoor byproduct levels of tobacco smoke: A critical review of the literature. *J. Air Pollut. Control Assoc.* **32**:250–259, 1982.
167. Seppanen, A.: Smoking in closed space and its effect on carboxyhemoglobin saturation in smoking and nonsmoking subjects. *Ann. Clin. Res.* **9**:281–283, 1977.
168. Feyerbend, C., Higginbottam, T., and Russsell, M. A.: Nicotine concentrations in urine and saliva of smokers and nonsmokers. *Br. J. Med.* **284**:1002–1004, 1982.
169. Greenberg, R. A., Haley, N. J., Etzel, R. A., and Loda, F. A.: Measuring the exposure of infants to tobaccos smoke: Nicotine and cotinine in urine and saliva. *N. Engl. J. Med.* **310**:1075–1078, 1984.
170. Fergussen, D. M., Horwood, L. J., Shannon, F. T., and Taylor, B.: Parental smoking and lower respiratory illness in the first 3 years of life. *J. Epidemiol. Commun. Health* **25**:180–184, 1981.
171. Colley, J. R., Douglas, J. W., and Reid, D. D.: Respiratory disease in young adults: Influence of early childhood lower respiratory tract illness, social class, air pollution and smoking. *Br. Med. J.* **3**:195–198, 1973.
172. Tager, I. B., Weiss, S. T., Munoz, A., *et al.*: Longitudinal study of the effects of maternal smoking on pulmonary function. *N. Engl. J. Med.* **309**:699–703, 1980.
173. Bonham, G. S., and Wilson, R. W.: Children's health in families with cigarette smokers. *Am. J. Public Health* **71**:290–293, 1981.
174. O'Connell, E. J., and Logan, G. B.: Parental smoking in childhood asthma. *Ann. Allergy* **32**:142–145, 1974.

175. Kraemer, M. J., Richardson, M. A., Weiss, N. S., *et al.*: Risk factors for persistent middle ear infections: Otitis media, catarrh, cigarette smoke exposure and atopy. *JAMA* **249:**1022–1025, 1983.
176. Rona, R. J;, Florey, C. V., Ckarle, G. C., and Chinn, S.: Parental smoking at home and height of children. *Br. Med. J.* **283:**1363, 1981.
177. Bergman, A. B., and Weisner, L. A.: Relationship of passive cigarette smoking to sudden infant death syndrome. *Pediatrics* **58:**665–668, 1976.
178. Aronow, W. S.: Effect of passive smoking on angina pectoris. *N. Engl. J. Med.* **299:**21–24, 1981.
179. Hirayama, T.: Nonsmoking wives of heavy smokers have a higher rate of lung cancer. A study from Japan. *Br. Med. J.* **282:**183–185, 1981.
180. Trichopoulos, D., Kalandi, L., Sparros, L., and MacMahon, B.: Lung cancer and passive smoking. *Int. J. Cancer* **27:**1–4, 1981.
181. Garfinkel, L : Time trends in lung cancer mortality among nonsmokers and a note on passive smoking. *J. Natl. Cancer Inst.* **66**(6):1061–1066, 1981.
182. Correa, P., Pickle, L. W., Fontham, E., *et al.*: Passive smoking and lung cancer. *Lancet* **2:**595–597, 1983.

24

Mental Disorders

Mary P. Harward and Julia E. Connelly

1. INTRODUCTION

Primary-care practice includes the diagnosis and treatment of both medical and mental disorders. However, primary-care practitioners infrequently diagnose mental disorders.[1,2] Such "missed diagnoses" may be due to several factors: lack of education about detection and treatment of mental disorders; the constraints on time in a busy office practice that preclude indepth psychiatric interviews with every patient; and the difficulty of distinguishing symptoms of mental disorders amid physical complaints. Just as with medical illnesses, preventing the complications of mental disorders begins with early and accurate diagnosis. This chapter outlines the means of improving the detection of mental disorders by discussing (1) the role of prevention in mental disorders; (2) the epidemiology of mental disorders in the community and in the medical office; (3) the groups at risk for mental disorders; and (4) the symptoms (anxiety and depression) associated with the major mental disorders seen in office practices.

2. PREVENTION OF MENTAL DISORDERS

Prevention of mental disorders is not as well defined as prevention of infectious diseases, nor is screening for mental disorders as clear cut as screening for breast or colon carcinoma. The prevention of mental disorders is complicated by their multifactorial etiologies, e.g., life stress, genetic factors, and neurochemical alterations. Even though it is difficult to alter all these factors in order to prevent a mental disorder before it occurs, the course of a mental disorder can be influenced by early identification and intervention. At this time, diagnosis can be made only after the symptoms of the mental disorder are present. Major mental disorders cannot be diagnosed while the individual is asymptomatic except in mental disorders with a clearly defined etiology, such as asymptomatic neurosyphilis. In 1980, the Canadian Task Force on the Periodic Health Examination reviewed the indications for periodic screening for major affective disorders and suicide risk factors. Because no diagnostic method is available for the detection of these problems

Mary P. Harward • Department of Internal Medicine, Northwestern University School of Medicine, Chicago, Illinois 60611. *Julia E. Connelly* • Department of Internal Medicine, University of Virginia School of Medicine, Charlottesville, Virginia 22908.

while the patient remains asymptomatic, screening was not recommended.[3] Even though genetic and biochemical abnormalities are present in some mental disorders, screening tests for the asymptomatic detection of these disorders are not available. The study of the neurochemical changes present with such disorders as schizophrenia, major depression, and some anxiety disorders is an advancing field of psychiatric research, and future developments may make screening tests available.

Questionnaires designed to detect mental disorders before symptoms are obvious include the General Health Questionnaire,[4] the Hamilton Rating Scale,[5] and the Beck Depression Scale.[6] These instruments are available to practitioners and are beginning to be used in the primary-care office.[7] This, too, is an area of active research, and specific recommendations regarding the utility of these questionnaires in office practice may be forthcoming.

Early detection and interventions can shorten the duration of a mental disorder once the symptoms are present. For example, treatment of a major depression with antidepressants can elevate the mood within 2–3 weeks, allowing the patient to return to his or her usual activities. Early treatment can also be effective in preventing the complications of mental disorders. The complications of mental disorders include the progression of untreated psychiatric symptoms to a more dysfunctional state, disruption of the family of the ill person, recurrence of episodic illness as in bipolar disorder, death through suicide, and the overutilization of medical services.

Patients with untreated mental disorders will frequently have associated somatic complaints, particularly when depression and anxiety disorders are present. Failure of the physician to recognize and treat the underlying depression or anxiety can lead to multiple return visits for evaluation of complaints such as chest pain, fatigue, or shortness of breath. Diagnostic tests, with high costs and potential risks, may be ordered to evaluate the somatic complaints.

Patients with clearly diagnosed mental disorders may also receive inadequate medical care. The frequency of undiagnosed physical disorders has been shown to be high in medical outpatients referred for psychiatric evaluation.[8] Patients with chronic mental disorders are at risk for developing the medical illnesses common to their sex and age group. The primary-care physician treating a patient with primary symptoms of a mental disorder nevertheless should be diligent in performing the periodic health examination as indicated. The recommendations for the periodic health examination are described in Chapter 26.

3. EPIDEMIOLOGY OF MENTAL DISORDERS

Mental disorders are prevalent both in the community and in the primary-care-practitioner's office. Knowledge about the range of mental disorders in these two populations may help the practitioner to target his or her preventive efforts regarding mental disorders.

Data on mental illness in the community have recently become available from a preliminary report of the Epidemiology Catchment Area Program (ECA Program), an ongoing survey of mental disorders in the community conducted by the National Institute of Mental Health.[9] Overall, 19% of the community population surveyed had experienced the symptoms suggestive of a mental disorder according to the criteria of the American Psychiatric Association's *Diagnostic and Statistical Manual,* 3rd edition (DSM-III) within the preceding 6 months. Preliminary data from three communities show that alcohol abuse and dependence, anxiety (including phobias), major depressive episode, and dysthymia are the most prevalent mental disorders.[10]

The ECA Program also revealed that 67% of people with a DSM-III-defined mental disorder visited a health care professional during the 6-month period. Only 10% of such individuals had made a mental health–related visit to a mental health specialist.[11] The primary-care practitioner appears to be the major health care provider for these psychologically distressed patients.

It is difficult to estimate the prevalence of mental disorders among primary-care patients because of the difficulty in defining a "mental disorder." If any form of psychological distress is included, the prevalence may be as high as 80%.[12] If strict research diagnostic criteria are applied, the prevalence is 27%.[13] Both figures identify mental distress and disorder as common problems. The National Ambulatory Care Survey (NACS) of 1980–1981 lists the principal reason for the visit and the principal diagnosis of office visits to general and family practitioners.[14] These data may be difficult to interpret since both patients and physicians may underrecognize the symptoms of mental disorders or attribute them to physical causes. The NACS listed mental disorders as the principal diagnosis in 2.6% of office visits. Psychotherapy or therapeutic listening was provided in 2.5% of the office visits.

4. IDENTIFYING THE GROUPS AT RISK FOR MENTAL DISORDERS

Several groups of individuals are at increased risk of developing mental disorders. Such groups include (1) persons experiencing significant life stress; (2) persons with a family history of mental disorders such as depression, schizophrenia, and alcoholism; and (3) persons with an acute or chronic medical illness.

4.1. Life Stress

An association between life stressors and the onset of mental disorders such as depression,[15] bipolar disorder,[16] and schizophrenia[17] has been suggested. Suicide is often accompanied by a number of life stresses.[18] Indeed, life stress has also been shown to be a precipitant for illness in general. Using the Social Readjustment Scale, Holmes and Rahe observed that individuals who have high scores for "changes in life events" were at relatively higher risk for developing mental and physical illness within the following 6-month–2-year period than were individuals with lower scores.[19] Interestingly, life changes such as marriage which are generally thought of as pleasurable or positive can be stressful, and this stress may at times have a negative influence on one's overall health. The Social Readjustment Scale quantitatively defines the significance of a life change.

The primary-care physician can help patients recognize the causes of their stress and offer suggestions for adaptation to the stress. The physician must first be aware of the situation causing the stressful reaction. One study in a university medical clinic revealed that house officers failed to recognize 76% of the stressful life events experienced by their patients.[2] This observation may be attributed in part to the predominant emphasis on the biomedical model of disease during medical education.

The biomedical model defines ''normality'' in chemical, physical, and physiological terms. Diseases measured by alterations in chemical or physiological functions are considered deviations from this normal state. The etiology of the disease is usually defined by diagnostic tests. This narrow focus commonly results in failure to diagnose the actual problem and the cause of the symptoms—the psychosocial stressor or the unexpressed emotional response. Yet, such ''psychophysiological'' reactions are commonly seen in general practice. For example, the adolescent boy may develop abdominal pain every day at school in response to his parent's threatened divorce, or a middle-aged woman who is depressed may complain of multiple aches and pains.

An approach that integrates the biological, social, and psychological symptoms has been proposed by Engel. This ''new medical model''—the biopsychosocial model—incorporates the psychosocial environment of the patient with the biomedical aspects of the disease.[20] Unexpressed emotional responses that accompany social factors such as loss, conflict, and frustrated expectations are sometimes expressed through physical complaints. McWhinney has proposed a system of classifying the social phenomena that may produce psychological and physical symptoms (see Table I).[21] Attention to the social, psychological, and physical complaints helps interpret the patient's behavior and symptoms and allows the physician to design a treatment plan that addresses many pertinent issues.

4.2. Family History

In addition to the individuals experiencing life stress, those with a family history of mental disorders are at increased risk of mental distress. Part of this distress may result

Table I. Taxonomy of Social Factors in Illness and Patient Behavior[a]

1. Loss—(a) Personal loss—loss of a loved one through death or desertion. (b) Loss of things—imposed loss of home, cherished possession, or job.
2. Conflict—(a) Interpersonal—conflict within family, with neighbors, or at work, where hostility is recognized. (b) Intrapersonal—role conflict or conflicting demands on the patient (as in a working mother).
3. Change—(a) Development—where time of life is the major problem (as adolescence, menopause, or senescence). (b) Geographical—where a move to an unfamiliar environment is the major problem (as in immigration).
4. Maladjustment—(a) Interpersonal—problems between people with no overt conflict (as in failure to achieve a satisfactory sexual relation without hostility between partners). (b) Personal—failure to adjust to the environment (home or job) in the absence of the above-mentioned loss, conflict, or change.
5. Stress—(a) Acute—unexpected event not covered under loss, conflict, or change (for example, the sudden illness of a family member or friend). (b) Chronic—long-term situation not included in loss, conflict, or change (for instance, the presence of a handicapped child in the family).
6. Isolation—not due to any recent loss, change, or conflict (as in an elderly widow).
7. Failure or frustrated expectations—when the patient's goals in life are not fulfilled and when there is no evidence of an intervening event covered by loss, conflict, or change (e.g., failure at school or failure to achieve occupational promotion).

[a]Source: McWhinney.[21]

from the disruption of living with a family member with a mental disorder such as depression or alcoholism. In addition, there is a genetic predisposition to mental disorder. A family history of alcoholism carries an increased risk of both alcoholism and depression. First-degree relatives of patients with major depressive disorder have a 9% (males) or 14% (females) chance of developing depression. For bipolar disorder (manic–depressive illness), the risk is 15–21% for developing some form of affective illness. Children of two schizophrenic parents have a 40% chance of developing schizophrenia. The risk if one parent is schizophrenic is 10–15%, and the risk of a sibling of an affected child developing schizophrenia is 2–3%, similar to the incidence in the general population. Anxiety and the somatoform disorders also tend to occur in families, but exact data on risk are not available.[22]

4.3. Acute and Chronic Medical Illness

A final group of individuals at risk of mental disorders are those with acute and chronic physical illness. The diagnosis of any illness with or without a significant physical disability carries with it a psychological burden. This burden may include such reactions as anger over the loss of good health, depression over the loss of physical function, or anxiety over the uncertainty of prognosis. This may alter the patient's ability to function at work or within the family.

The patient's reaction to the distress of a chronic illness can have a marked effect on the ultimate recovery and rehabilitation of the patient and on the associated psychological consequences. Patients will have different ways of coping with illness. The coping skills will reflect the personality style of the patient. By recognizing the individual's coping abilities, the physician may be able to prevent further complications from the distress of the illness and the development of a mental disorder such as depression or anxiety.

Kahana and Bibring outline several different personality styles frequently encountered in primary care and their means of coping with illness.[23] For example, the compulsive personality can be very orderly, conscientious, controlling, and even obstinate. Becoming ill represents a "loss of control" and is often followed by an attempt to regain control. If this patient is given sufficient information about his illness and the opportunity to gain some control through participation in his medical care, angry outbursts and noncompliance can be diminished.

Among individuals with physical complaints are those with a reason other than their symptom for visiting a primary-care practitioner. There are many "hidden reasons" that patients visit doctors, including psychological, social, and informational reasons.[24] Connelly and Mushlin have shown that 45% of patients requesting a "checkup" have psychosocial problems, with or without other problems, as the reason for the request. In addition, 50% of the patients seen for a "checkup" had symptoms that fulfilled the DSM-III criteria for a major mental disorder.[25]

5. DISORDERS ASSOCIATED WITH DEPRESSION

Depression and its symptoms are among the most frequent mental disorders seen in the primary-care office. Using the nomenclature of the DSM-III, the disorders of depression include adjustment reaction with depressed mood, dysthymic disorder, major depressive episode, cyclothymic disorder, and bipolar disorder.[26] Bereavement and unresolved grief reactions are special categories that may include depression. From a preventive standpoint, recognition of the depression allows further evaluation and treatment before complications occur.

Knowledge of the risk factors for depression can aid in the recognition. Life events such as loss of a job can predictably be accompanied by a depressed mood. Life-cycle changes such as aging, retirement, or the disruption of family ties when grown children leave home or marry may precipitate depression. The postpartum period and the menopausal period may be a particularly risky period for women to experience depression.

The patient who presents with multiple somatic complaints, appetite disturbance with associated weight fluctuation (either gain or loss), loss of enjoyment of pleasurable activities, decreased libido, sleep disturbance, or lack of energy should be suspected of having a depressed mood. The patient is not likely to volunteer that he or she is depressed. Asking the patient directly, "How have your spirits been lately" or routinely questioning all patients about sleep, sexual function, daily interests, appetite, and energy may provide the answer.

Some medical problems are associated with a depressed mood. Such medical disorders include Cushing's syndrome, hypothyroidism, hypercalcemia, hyperparathyroidism, vitamin B_{12} deficiency, viral infection (hepatitis, infectious mononucleosis), rheumatoid arthritis, systemic lupus erythematosus, pancreatic carcinoma, temporal lobe epilepsy, senile dementia of the Alzheimer's type, frontal-lobe tumor, subdural hematoma, multiple sclerosis, cerebrovascular disease, drug withdrawal, and alcoholism. Many drugs may also cause a depression (see Table II). The history and physical examination coupled with judicious use of laboratory and diagnostic tests will aid the physician in separating the primary depression from the secondary depression due to medical illness. Evaluating the patient for primary depression while considering the possibility of an underlying medical disorder is important. Frequently, the physician initiates an extensive, costly, and risky diagnostic evaluation searching for a "medical" problem without simultaneously addressing the question of depression. When nothing measurable is found (as dictated by the medical model), the patient is assumed to have a "mental" problem. Continuing to assess the patient for signs and symptoms of depression while waiting for the thyroid function tests or complete blood count is fundamentally important.

Once the physician has identified that the patient does have a depressed mood, determination of the duration of the symptoms, the degree of social and occupational

Table II. Drugs That Can Cause a Depressed Mood

Alcohol	Cimetidine
Amphetamines (on withdrawal)	Contraceptives, oral
Anticonvulsants	Corticosteroids
Antihypertensives (beta blockers, clonidine, methyldopa, reserpine, spironolactone)	Disulfiram
	Isoniazid
	Nonsteroidal antiinflammatory agents
Barbiturates	Thyroid hormones
Benzodiazepines	

dysfunction, and the presence of vegetative signs will aid in determining the appropriate therapeutic intervention.

The DSM-III criteria for an adjustment reaction with a depressed mood include a maladaptive response to a stressor that has occurred in the previous 3 months.[26] The patient is unable to carry out his or her usual family or job responsibilities owing to the depressed mood. Therapeutic listening often helps establish a supportive relationship with the patient that permits discussion of the emotional reaction to the stressor. The role of the physician is not to pass judgment or give advice, but to serve as a mediator and clarifier, allowing the patient to arrive at a possible solution.

Dysthymic disorder can be diagnosed when a depressed mood has been present for 2 years. The presence and severity of the depression usually impair the day-to-day life of the patient.[26] This may be the most difficult disorder for the primary physician to treat, although a supportive role can be offered by the physician. The risk of major depressive episode and suicide gestures is high in this group.

A major depressive episode is characterized by the same depressed mood as seen in adjustment reaction or dysthymic disorder. Additionally, the major depression is accompanied by vegetative symptoms of depression that are listed in Table III.[26]

Bereavement follows the loss or death of a loved one and is an expected reaction to this loss. Grief does not include the loss of self-esteem and the sense of worthlessness common in depression; however, a significant number of bereaved develop a major depression. The primary-care physician may be called on to assist his or her patient in the grief process. Holmes and Rahe identified the loss of a spouse as the most stressful life event on the Social Readjustment Scale.[19] Assistance early in the bereavement may prevent future development of a major depression.

Grief work can be done easily in the physician's office. Frequent, short visits are most beneficial for both the physician and patient. Usually, a limited number of visits (six to eight) are arranged. During the first visit, the physician needs to assess the patient's symptoms and differentiate between normal grief and a major depression (see above). It is

Table III. Symptoms of a Major Depressive Episode[a]

Poor appetite; increased appetite
Insomnia; hypersomnia
Psychomotor agitation–retardation
Loss of interest in usual activities or decrease in sexual drive
Loss of energy; fatigue
Feelings of worthlessness; excessive or inappropriate guilt
Diminished ability to think or concentrate
Recurrent thoughts of death, suicidal ideation, wishes to be dead; suicide attempt

[a]Adapted from DSM-III.[26] At least four of the above must have been present nearly every day for at least 2 weeks.

useful to remember, though, that signs and symptoms of a major depression are a part of bereavement and may exist for up to a year after the death.

During the grief work, the physician aids the patient in loosening the bonds held to the deceased, forming new relationships, and readjusting to the environment without the deceased.[27] If these goals are not accomplished, the grieving patient may develop a major depression that requires further treatment.

All medications should be used judiciously during this period. Anxiety, depression, and sleep disturbances are to be expected and need not be treated unless they become persistent or extremely dysfunctional. At most, a mild sedative–hypnotic agent may be prescribed for short-term use at bedtime if a sleep disturbance is prominent.

Once a loss has occurred, the physician should note the date of its occurence in the patient's chart since anniversary reactions are common. Also, the age of the deceased should be noted. Some patients experience anxiety or somatic symptoms when they reach the age at which a parent died. The anniversary reaction can occur on any significant date, such as birthdays, marriage anniversaries, or holidays, in addition to the date of death or when the patient reaches the age of the deceased. At the time of the anniversary, the patient may only be aware of a general feeling of anxiety or depression that may take the form of numerous somatic complaints. The patient may even adopt some of the symptoms present in the deceased before death. Awareness of the psychophysiological connection will allow the physician to discuss the feelings of grief with the patient instead of merely embarking on an extensive "medical" evaluation.

A major depression can be effectively treated with resultant reduction of morbidity (low self-esteem, low energy level, and anhedonia) and mortality (suicide). Since the discovery of amitryptyline and imipramine in the 1950s, antidepressants have been found to alter the natural history of major depression by elevating the depressed mood and shortening the length of the illness. Discussion of drug therapy and selection of patients for drug therapy is beyond the scope of this chapter, but the reader is referred to the discussion by DePaulo.[28]

Counseling is an effective adjunctive therapy for depression. Such counseling does not always require a mental health specialist and can be done by a trained primary-care practitioner with weekly to biweekly office visits of 20–30-min duration. The counseling can allow the patient to discuss the depressed mood and the associated social and occupational impairment, to plan for the recovery period of the depression and a return to normal functioning, and to discuss the stresses that may have precipitated the depression.

The patient who does require a referral to a psychiatrist is one who is actively suicidal (see below), who has psychotic symptoms in addition to depression, who does not respond to antidepressant therapy after 4–6 weeks of treatment with an adequate dose, who may require electroconvulsive therapy because of medical illnesses that complicate the use of antidepressants, or who is so severely depressed that eating and self-care are neglected. Also, a psychiatric consultation can be helpful if there is doubt about the diagnosis of a major depression.

Manic symptoms are present in cyclothymic disorder and bipolar disorder. Mania causes an elevated, often irritable, mood with accompanying symptoms of increased activity, talkativeness, flight of ideas or thought racing, grandiosity, decreased sleep, distractibility, and involvement in potentially damaging activities, such as buying sprees, sexual indiscretions, reckless driving, or foolish business investments.[26] In bipolar disorder, manic episodes typically alternate with depressive episodes. To diagnose bipolar disorder, though, a history of depression is not needed, only the presence of a manic episode.

A cyclothymic disorder has similar criteria as a bipolar disorder, but not to the same extent. The manic episodes are referred to as "hypomanic."

Lithium is the treatment of choice for bipolar disorder and is particularly efficacious in preventing recurrence of the illness. Typically, patients with bipolar disorder have cycles of mania and depression. Lithium helps to stabilize the mood and decrease the severity of the mania and depression if not totally prevent the recurrence. The first episode of mania nearly always requires psychiatric hospitalization because of the poor judgment of the patient and the possibility of physical, social, or financial ruin during the manic state. The primary-care practitioner will have difficulty managing a patient with manic episodes without psychiatric consultation.

The possibility of suicide should always be considered in any patient with a depression whether it is simple sadness or a major depression. Patients experiencing a manic episode are always at risk of self-destruction because of their poor judgment. Approximately 20,000–50,000 suicides are successfully committed annually. The number of estimated suicide gestures is probably 10 times that of successful suicides. The impact of suicide can be dramatically seen when expressed in terms of years of potential life lost (YPLL). This reflects the young age at which many suicides occur. In 1983, suicide accounted for 631,990 YPLL and was the fifth leading cause of YPLL in the United States. The YPLL due to suicide were highest among white men.[29]

Suicide can be prevented through early detection of suicidal thoughts and appropriate protection of the patient from self-destructive acts. The management of suicidal behavior is not confined to the psychiatrist. The primary-care physician may be the only caregiver for many suicidal patients. Just as one needs to question for the presence of depression, the patient should be directly asked about suicidal thoughts. Many primary physicians are uncomfortable doing this, fearing that this may plant the idea of suicide in a nonsuicidal patient. This is simply not true. The question needs to be asked in a nonthreatening way, allowing the patient to respond affirmatively without fearing repercussions from the physician. The physician might ask: "Have you ever felt so depressed that you have thought about harming or killing yourself?" If the patient responds yes, specific inquiries need to be made about previous suicide plans, specific current plans and feasibility of those plans, feelings of hopelessness, future orientation, presence of significant psychosocial stress, presence of major depression, and social support. The patient with previous suicide attempts, a well-conceived, practical plan, no social supports, recent diagnosis of a major depression, and lack of future orientation is at risk of imminent suicide. Additional features that are associated with a high suicide rate are listed in Table IV.

All suicidal patients do not require hospitalization. Patients with a characterological disorder with many suicide gestures may actually become more dysfunctional when hospitalized. Repeated hospitalization may reinforce the behavior of repeated suicide threats. Some patients may have suicidal thoughts but low likelihood of acting on them, and these patients can be managed as outpatients with continued participation by the primary physician. The assessment of suicide risk may be difficult for the primary-care practitioner, and consultation with a psychiatrist will be helpful. If the patient is actively suicidal, an immediate referral of the patient to a psychiatrist is mandatory. If a psychia-

Table IV. Risk Factors for Suicide

Male sex[a]	Family history of suicide attempts
Single or widowed	"Anniversary reaction"
Social isolation	Chronic or terminal illness
Unemployment	Recent surgery
Urban residence	Chronic pain
White (within United States)	Depression
Recent loss	Psychosis
History of previous suicide attempt	Alcoholism or other substance abuse
History of impulsive behavior	Organic brain syndrome

[a]Women attempt suicide more often than men, but men commit suicide successfully more often.

trist is not available, the primary physician could consider admission to the medical ward with close observation of the patient while consultation is obtained. Above all, the patient must be protected from himself. Suicidal threats should be treated as an emergency. If the patient absolutely refuses psychiatric referral or hospital admission, involuntary commitment should be considered. Commitment laws vary between states, and the physician should be familiar with the procedure in his or her area.

6. DISORDERS ASSOCIATED WITH ANXIETY

Anxiety is another frequent mood disturbance seen by the primary physician. Again, the purpose of the physician is to differentiate the anxious mood that is an appropriate response to a stressful or threatening situation from the phobic disorder or generalized anxiety disorder that will require specific pharamacological therapy for prevention of further dysfunction. Common anxiety disorders, according to DSM-III nomenclature, include adjustment reaction with anxious mood, agoraphobia, panic disorder, generalized anxiety disorder, and posttraumatic stress disorder.[26]

Normal anxiety is a common response to any threatening or stressful event. Anxiety often accompanies symptoms and is frequently the main reason the patient sought medical care. Recognition and discussion of the etiology of the anxiety may alleviate or reduce it.

An adjustment reaction can also involve an anxious mood. The patient may become quite dysfunctional but may respond to therapeutic listening. Agoraphobia has classically been considered "fear of the marketplace." The term has been generalized to include fear of public places from which escape might be difficult (crowds, bridges, or public transportation). This fear leads the patient to a reclusive life with marked constriction of any normal activity. Agoraphobia may or may not be accompanied by panic attacks. Panic attacks are discrete episodes manifested by dyspnea, palpitations, chest pain, choking or smothering sensations, dizziness, feeling of unreality, paresthesias, hot and cold flashes, sweating, faintness, trembling, and fear of dying or going crazy. The diagnosis of panic disorder requires that at least three panic attacks must occur within a 3-week period. The panic attacks are not precipitated by a life-threatening situation.[26] These symptoms are also typical of many medical disorders, such as asthma, alcohol withdrawal, atherosclerotic coronary vascular disease, arrhythmias, or endocrine disorders. Frequently, the patient with anxiety symptoms will come to a primary-care practitioner requesting medical evaluation. A panic disorder should always be included in the differential diagnosis of anxiety. As emphasized earlier, a careful history is necessary to make these diagnoses.

For panic disorder, therapy with imipramine or alprazolam may prevent future attacks and can be so dramatic as to turn a recluse into an active, social person.[30] This therapy can easily be initiated by the primary-care physician. If the diagnosis is questionable or the patent does not respond as expected to the therapy, then psychiatric referral may be helpful.

Generalized anxiety disorder requires at least three of the four categories of symptoms listed in Table V to be present for at least a month.[26] Therapy includes anxiolytic agents (benzodiazepines) and counseling. For a discussion for the treatment of anxiety, the reader is referred to Baile.[31]

Another category of mental disorders that frequently present with anxiety and symptoms are the somatoform disorders. Patients with a somatoform disorder adopt "illness as a way of life."[32] The patient's whole existence centers around his or her bodily complaints. These people are high utilizers of the medical system and will be seen in every physician's practice. Because these patients talk only in terms of their bodily complaints and never mention their emotions, the physician also focuses on medical diagnoses. The patient is at risk of undergoing many unnecessary diagnostic tests. This is both costly and potentially harmful to the patient.

The inability to express emotions is termed "alexithymia" and is characteristic of patients with a somatoform illness. When asked to describe their feelings during a stressful event, such as a funeral, the patient will describe physical feelings such as headaches, chest pain, or abdominal pain rather than emotions such as sadness or anger. The emotions are expressed through the body.

Somatoform disorders include hypochondriasis, somatization disorder, psychogenic pain disorder, and conversion disorder. The main feature of hypochondriasis is an unrealistic intepretation of physical symptoms with preoccupation of fear of a serious disease.

Table V. Symptoms of Generalized Anxiety Disorder[a]

1. Motor tension: shakiness, jitteriness, jumpiness, trembling, tension, muscle aches, fatigability, inability to relax, eyelid twitch, furrowed brow, strained face, fidgeting, restlessness, easy startle.
2. Autonomic hyperactivity: sweating, heart pounding or racing, cold, clammy hands, dry mouth, dizziness, light-headedness, paresthesias, upset stomach, hot or cold spells, frequent urination, diarrhea, discomfort in the pit of the stomach, lump in the throat, flushing, pallor, high resting pulse and respiratory rate.
3. Apprehensive expectation: anxiety, worry, fear, rumination, anticipation of misfortune to self or others.
4. Vigilance and scanning: hyperattentiveness resulting in distractibility, difficulty in concentrating, insomnia, feeling "on edge," irritability, impatience.

[a]Adapted from DSM-III.[26]

Multiple system complaints of several years' duration are found in somatization disorder. Pain is the predominant symptom in psychogenic pain disorder. The pain is not in an anatomical distribution, and psychological factors are thought to play an important role. Conversion disorder occurs with the involuntary loss of physical functioning due to psychological factors.[26]

Although specific diagnosis of the type of somatoform disorder is helpful, a few general principles of treatment do apply. The patient should be seen on a regular basis for brief appointments, regardless of whether he is experiencing symptoms. This may be as often as 15 min weekly. The patient needs to understand that the appointment should be kept even if he is feeling fine. Let the patient know that he will always be ill and therefore require a physician's attention. It will not be productive to try to convince the patient that "nothing is wrong." The patient needs to be allowed to have his illness without pejorative judgment. The stresses of the job, home, and family should be discussed since they are probably the cause of the disorder. Trying to convince the patient that these stresses are related to their physical complaints may not be beneficial. The doctor should not feel obligated to make a diagnosis or expect the patient to ever feel fine. Diagnostic tests and therapeutic remedies should be ordered with restraint. These are some of the most difficult and challenging patients to take care of, requiring all the clinical and counseling skills of the physician. These patients are just as likely to develop coronary artery disease or malignancy as anyone else with similar risk factors. It can be quite difficult to determine when a new complaint is related to the somatoform disorder or the development of a new pathophysiological process.

Most of the somatoform disorders will be handled solely by the primary-care practitioner, mainly because of the refusal of the patient to believe that there is a psychological component to his complaints. Referral to a psvchiatrist is difficult. Conversion disorder, though, will require psychotherapy, and rapid referral to a psychiatrist may facilitate recovery of the patient with few complications.

REFERENCES

1. Brody, D. S.: Physician recognition of behavioral, psychological, and social aspects of medical care. *Arch. Intern. Med.* **140:**1286–1289, 1980.
2. Thompson, T. L., Stoudmire, A., Mitchell, W. D., *et al.:* Underrecognition of patients' psychosocial distress in a university hospital medical clinic. *Am. J. Psychiatry* **140:**158–161, 1983.
3. Report of the Task Force on the Periodic Health Examination. *Can. Med. Assoc. J.*, **121:**1193–1254, 1974.
4. Johnstone, A., and Goldberg, D.: Psychiatric screening in general practice. *Lancet* **1:**605–608, 1976.
5. Hamilton, M.: A rating scale for depression. *J. Neurol. Neurosurg. Psychiatry* **23:**56–62, 1960.
6. Beck, A. T.: *Depression: Clinical, Experimental, and Theoretical Aspects.* Hoeber, New York, 1967.
7. Rucker, L., Frye, E. B., and Cygan, R. W.: Feasibility and usefulness of depression screening in medical outpatients. *Arch. Intern. Med.* **146:**729–731, 1986.
8. Koranyi, E. K.: Morbidity and rate of undiagnosed physical illnesses in a psychiatric clinic population. *Arch. Gen. Psychiatry* **36:**414–419, 1978.
9. Regier, D. A., Meyers, J. K., Kramer, M., *et al.:* The NIMH epidemiologic catchment area program. Historical context, major objectives, and study population characteristics. *Arch. Gen. Psychiatry* **41:**934–941, 1984.
10. Meyers, J. K., Weissman, M. M., Tischler, G. L., *et al.:* Six-month prevalence of psychiatric disorders in three communities. 1980 to 1982. *Arch Gen. Psychiatry* **41:**959–967, 1984.

11. Shapiro, S., Skinner, E. A., and Kessler, L. G.: Utilization of health and mental health services. *Arch. Gen. Psychiatry* **41**:971–978, 1984.
12. Stoeckle, J. D., Zola, I. K., and Davidson, G. E.: The quality and significance of psychological distress in medical practice. *J. Chronic Dis.* **17**:959–976, 1966.
13. Hoeper, E. W., Nycz, G. R., Cleary, P. D., *et al.*: Estimated prevalence of RDC mental disorder in primary medical care. *Int. J. Mental Health* **8**:6–15, 1979.
14. National Center for Health Statistics, Cypress, B. K.: *Patterns of Ambulatory Care in General and Family Practice, the National Ambulatory and Medical Care Survey, United States, January 1980–December 1981*. Vital and Health Statistics. Series 13, No. 73. DHHS Pub. No. (83) 1734. Public Health Service. US Government Printing Office, Washington, DC, 1983.
15. Warheit, G. J.: Life events, coping, stress, and depression symptomatology. *Am. J. Psychiatry* **136**:502–507, 1979.
16. Dunner, D. L., Patrick, V., and Fieve, R. R.: Life events at the onset of bipolar affective illness. *Am. J. Psychiatry* **136**:508–511, 1979.
17. Brown, G. W., and Berley, J. L. T.: Crises and life changes and the onset of schizophrenia. *J. Health Social Behav.* **9**:203–214, 1968.
18. Paykel, E. S.: Suicide attempts and recent life events. *Arch. Gen. Psychiatry* **32**:327–333, 1978.
19. Holmes, T. H., and Rahe, R. H.: The Social Readjustment Rating scale. *J. Psychosom Res.* **11**:213–218, 1967.
20. Engel, G. L.: The need for a new medical model. A challenge for biomedicine. *Science* **196**:129–136, 1977.
21. McWhinney, I. R.: Beyond diagnosis. An approach to the integration of behavioral science and clinical medicine. *N. Engl. J. Med.* **287**:384–387, 1972.
22. Rainer, J. D.: Genetics and psychiatry, in Kaplan, H. I., and Sadoch, B. J. (eds.): *Comprehensive Textbook of Psychiatry*, 4th ed. Williams & Wilkins, Baltimore, 1985, pp. 36–41.
23. Kahana, R. J., and Bibring, G. L.: Personality types in medical management, in Zibring, N. (ed.): *Psychiatry and Medical Practice in a General Hospital*. International Universities Press, New York, 1964.
24. Barsky, A.: Hidden reasons some patients visit doctors. *Ann. Intern. Med.* **94**:492–498, 1981.
25. Connelly, J. E., and Mushlin, A. I.: The reasons patients request "checkups": Implications for office practice. *J. Gen. Intern. Med.* **1**:163–165, 1986.
26. American Psychiatric Association: *Diagnostic and Statistical Manual of Mental Disorders*, 3rd ed. APA, Washington, DC, 1980.
27. Lindemann, E.: The symptomatology and management of acute grief. *Am. J. Psychiatry* **101**:141–149, 1944.
28. DePaulo, J. R.: Affective disorders, in Barker, L. R., Burton, J. R., and Zieve, P. D. (eds.): *Principles of Ambulatory Medicine*, 2nd ed. Williams & Wilkins, Baltimore, 1986, pp. 183–195.
29. Centers for Disease Control: Premature mortality due to suicide and homicide—United States, 1983. *Morbid. Mortal. Wkly. Rep.* **35**:357–361, 1986.
30. Sheehan, D. V.: Monoamine oxidase inhibitors and alprazolam in the treatment of panic disorder and agoraphobia. *Psychiatr. Clin. North Am.* **8**:49–62, 1985.
31. Baile, W. F.: The anxious patient, in Barker, L. R., Burton, J. R., and Zieve, P. D. (eds.): *Principles of Ambulatory Medicine*, 2nd ed. Williams & Wilkins, Baltimore, 1986, pp. 156–175.
32. Ford, C. V.: *Somatizing Disorders. Illness as a Way of Life*. Elsevier, New York, 1983.

25

Alcoholism and Drug Abuse

Randolph J. Canterbury

1. EPIDEMIOLOGY

1.1. Alcoholism

One of the greatest public health problems in the United States today is alcoholism and drug abuse. Alcoholism alone is responsible for more morbidity than all the cancers and respiratory diseases combined. The lifetime incidence of alcoholism has been estimated at approximately 10% for men and 3% for women. There is a strong familial trend for the disease evidenced by the two times or greater risk for the identical twin of an alcoholic to share the disease as compared to a fraternal twin. Adoption studies demonstrate a fourfold increase in the incidence of alcoholism in children of alcoholic biological parents adopted at birth as compared to adopted children of nonalcoholic biological parents.[1,2] Not only is the disease a major one today, but its prevalence appears to be increasing. It is estimated that the consumption of alcohol in the United States has increased by 30% during the last 20 years resulting, in the current mean consumption per year by Americans over the age of 14 of 2.75 gallons of absolute ethanol.[3]

1.2. Drug Abuse

There have also been increasing trends in the abuse of other drugs in this country during the past few years. It is estimated that over 16 million Americans use marijuana each month, and approximately 10% of high-school seniors are said to be daily users of the drug. A strong statistical association exists between marijuana use and the abuse of more serious drugs.

Over the past 10 years cocaine abuse has become a major problem. One of the most expensive drugs abused, cocaine has been associated with an increasing number of emergency room mentions in the data from that Drug Abuse Warning Network system. This is a system that reviews emergency room records for mentions of drug use associated with the visit. The number of mentions for the 6-month period January–June 1982 was 2353, as compared to the 6-month period July–December 1984, when there were 5146 men-

Randolph J. Canterbury • Departments of Behavioral Medicine and Psychiatry and Internal Medicine, University of Virginia School of Medicine, Charlottesville, Virginia 22908.

tions.[4] There are no metropolitan areas where cocaine abuse has been reported to be decreasing. It is estimated that over 33 million Americans have tried cocaine and there are between one and two million current users. The abuse of this drug has commonly resulted in the arrest and conviction of many business and professional people for whom abuse of this costly drug has become a routine part of their lifestyle.

Although the overall rate of narcotic abuse may be falling, heroin addiction is still considered by many to be one of the most serious drug abuse problems in the United States. The drug is extremely addicting both psychologically and physically, and it has often been associated with crime because of the expense of the drug and its addictive potential. Current estimates indicate that approximately one-half million Americans are addicted to heroin. This is a drug that is more associated with large metropolitan areas and ports of entry than many other drugs of abuse.

The group at risk for substance abuse is nearly the entire population, although some groups appear more vulnerable. Certain factors that tend to predict future abuse behavior have been identified. For example, those people who adopt substance abuse behaviors early in life (especially near puberty) are more likely to sustain ingrained patterns of substance abuse. Men are still the more common substance abusers, but women are rapidly increasing their abuse patterns. Lower socioeconomic class more strongly correlates with substance abuse; however, it is common across all class boundaries (and cocaine abuse is more common in the upper classes). Parental modeling is another factor that increases the likelihood of substance abuse in offspring. That is, families in which substance abuse is an accepted mechanism for coping with stress tend to imply approval to their children. Peer modeling is also a powerful motivator toward substance abuse in adolescents, and social gatherings are also associated with increased substance abuse in the college age population and in adults.

2. ASSOCIATED PSYCHIATRIC ILLNESS

From the psychiatric perspective alcoholism and drug abuse are often associated with dysphoric mood states and with thought disorders. In fact, it is not uncommon to find patients with affective disorders or anxiety disorders who self-medicate with alcohol or other depressant drugs in order to be able to concentrate or to sleep better. As many as one-half of patients applying for methadone maintenance programs have been diagnosed with significant depression. If the abusive pattern has not become imprinted, the substance abuse may subside when the primary psychiatric disorder is treated. Unfortunately, the abused substances themselves may alter sleep patterns and adversely affect the patient's mood and self-esteem, resulting in an exacerbation of the dysphoria, and a sustained pattern of abuse may begin. This process tends to be cybernetic.

Chronic substance abuse may also result in psychiatric symptoms that mimic primary psychiatric illnesses. Cocaine abuse is often associated with other psychiatric illnesses. Diagnostic interviews on cocaine abusers have led to the diagnoses of depressive disorders in as many as 30% of the patients. Others have had bipolar disorder or attention deficit disorder. The immediate withdrawal period from cocaine often results in depressive symptomatology, and the complete syndrome of major depression is not infrequent.

Alcoholics commonly have alterations in sleep architecture that clinically resemble those of major affective disorders. Psychic and somatic anxiety are commonly associated with alcoholism and may be mistaken for a primary anxiety disorder. It is not uncommon for alcoholics to develop a depressed mood, isolation, and suspiciousness to a paranoid degree, and alcohol withdrawal delirium has been at times misdiagnosed as a primary thought disorder (such as schizophrenia) when an adequate history was not obtained.

3. ASSOCIATED MEDICAL ILLNESS

Alcoholism is related to a number of other diseases of various organ systems. Cancer (especially of the head, neck, and esophagus), chronic lung disease, hypertension, cardiac arrhythmias, cardiomyopathy, peptic ulcer disease, pancreatitis, gastritis, malabsorption syndromes, alcoholic hepatitis, and Laënnec's cirrhosis are common alcohol-related disorders. In addition, diseases of the central and peripheral nervous systems are frequently associated with prolonged alcohol abuse (delirium tremens, alcohol amnestic syndrome, Wernicke's encephalopathy, cerebral atrophy, cerebellar degeneration, central pontine myelinolysis, and polyneuritis). Fetal alcohol syndrome occurs commonly in infants born to mothers who drink 150 g or more of alcohol a day during gestation and is increasing in frequency as the incidence of alcoholism increases among women of childbearing age. Trauma of all kinds is commonly associated with alcohol abuse. A study by the National Institute of Medicine[5] indicated that alcoholism reduces the life expectancy of its victims in the United States by an average of 12 years.

Individuals who abuse drugs by intravenous injection are at relatively high risk for developing infectious endocarditis, phlebitis, hepatitis, and acquired immunodeficiency syndrome. Those who "snort" cocaine are at risk for serious mucosal damage. Seizures are not uncommon in illicit drug abusers. Recently there have been a number of syndromes associated with the use of various types of "designer drugs." One of these is a severe form of Parkinson's syndrome associated with the injection of 1-methyl-4-phenyl-1,2,3,6-tetrahydropyridine (MPTP), an occasional contaminant of synthetic opioids prepared illicitly by chemists.[6] The MPTP-induced form of Parkinson's syndrome is irreversible and appears to worsen with time.

4. SOCIAL COSTS

4.1. Economic Implications

According to the study by the National Institute of Medicine,[5] alcoholism costs this country 60 billion dollars a year. The Metropolitan Life Insurance Company estimates that alcoholism creates a direct cost to industry of 85 billion dollars per year. In particular, alcoholics are heavy users of the medical care system. Twenty percent of our national expenditure for hospital care is alcohol related. Twelve percent of the total health care budget for adults is related directly or indirectly to alcohol abuse. As many as one-third of all hospitalized adult patients have problems related to alcoholism; however, fewer than a third of these are so designated in the discharge diagnoses and only 1 in 10 of those identified is actually referred for alcoholism treatment. More than 200,000 Americans die each year from alcoholism, i.e., 1 out of every 10 deaths.

A significant problem with substance abuse exists in the American workplace. This results in a tremendous loss of productivity associated with injuries to self and others (four times non-substance abusers), illness, absenteeism (16 times non-substance abusers), breakage, poor workmanship, and theft. Workers who are substance abusers have five times the workman's compensation claims of their counterparts who do not abuse substances. Forty-seven percent of all industrial injuries and 40% of industrial fatalities are related to alcohol abuse. It is estimated that between 3% and 7% of the employed population use some form of illicit drug on a daily basis, and between 5% and 10% of the workforce is alcoholic. This high rate of impairment leads to a loss of productivity and contributes heavily to the annual cost of substance abuse.

4.2. ASSOCIATED VIOLENCE

Approximately two-thirds of all domestic violence is alcohol related, and one-third of all cases of child abuse are alcohol related. Between 50% and 80% of all traffic fatalities, two-thirds of all drownings, two-thirds of all homicides, 40% of all rapes, and at least a third of all suicides are related to alcohol abuse.[7]

5. RECOGNITION OF ALCOHOLISM

Despite these impressive statistics, a large national survey has demonstrated that fewer than 20% of all persons perceive alcoholism as a health problem.[5] Physicians and nurses apparently do not have a good understanding of the significance of alcoholism as a health problem. Histories of drug and alcohol use taken by health care providers in general hospitals are notoriously inaccurate and incomplete. Patients in these facilities tend to minimize their drinking behavior, and their doctors and nurses collude with them in these deceptive alcohol histories. Physicians often do not identify a patient's alcoholism as a medical problem even when they know it exists. And as mentioned earlier, only about 1 in 10 patients with identified and designated alcoholism is referred for treatment. This form of denial on the part of the health care professionals represents their own ignorance about the gravity of this problem and may relate to their denial about their own drinking habits. Also, physicians do not like to identify problems for which they think no effective treatment exists, and most physicians are not aware of the success that substance abuse treatment enjoys today.

The diagnosis of substance abuse disorders historically has been difficult and inconsistent because there has been little agreement on the definitions of these disorders and their diagnostic criteria. How much does a person have to drink in order to be diagnosed as having alcoholism? With what frequency does one have to drink? How much family difficulty has to result from substance abuse? How much social or occupational dysfunction must be present? These are all questions that professionals have debated for many years. The American Psychiatric Associations's Diagnostic and Statistical Manual, third edition,[8] gives specific diagnostic criteria for various substance abuse disorders. These criteria may be easily applied in the clinical setting for consistent diagnosis of patients who give reliable histories. In essence, any individual who suffers any significant physiological, psychological, social, legal, or occupational dysfunction because of the use of a substance and continues to use that substance can be classified in one of the substance abuse diagnostic categories.

Unknown to many physicians is the fact that screening for substance abuse is easy, cheap, and available. It is rarely employed as a part of health maintenance, however. It is crucial that substance abuse be detected early in order to increase the likelihood of successful treatment. Treatment must be initiated while the patient still has a substantial support system and before his/her denial reaches a prohibitive level. Therefore, physicians must be aware of the proportions of the problem and be alert to the diagnosis, especially since the disease masquerades under the guises of many other illnesses.

What are some simple and inexpensive indicators of drug abuse in office patients? There are several screening instruments that can help identify which patients in an office practice are most likely abusing drugs. One of these is the Addiction Assessment Form.[9] This is a test that gives indications about the abuse of various drugs and alcohol through a very detailed and specific drug history. This instrument relies on self-report, and most substance abusers have a large amount of denial about the severity of their illness. It is also important to know some of the drug-seeking behavior patterns of addicted people. The physician must be aware that many substance abusers come to the office complaining of pain and requesting narcotics for treatment. These patients often "doctor shop," moving to another unsuspecting physician when a doctor recognizes their pattern. Requesting "diet pills" is not an unusual mechanism for acquiring amphetamines or other sympathomimetic amines. Sedative/hypnotic abusers may complain of anxiety or insomnia in order to acquire their drug of choice. These patients often come to the physician's office toward the end of a busy day when detailed questions about their requests are less likely to be asked, and they tend to avoid intake appointments when they are scheduled. There are many more indicators of excessive alcohol consumption, and the focus will be on these.

The blood alcohol level (BAL) may be of some use in making the diagnosis of alcohol abuse or dependence. It is often said that a BAL of 0.1 g/dl during an office visit is diagnostic of alcoholism. Any random BAL of 0.3 g% would also be diagnostic because of the alcohol tolerance such a high level implies. On the other end of the spectrum, a BAL of zero is of no significance in the diagnosis, because an alcoholic may have periods of time when he does not drink. Whitfield[10] has evaluated and rated various aspects of the history, physical examination, laboratory evaluation, and diagnoses that are suggestive of alcoholism. These are summarized in Table I. In particular, over 75% of patients who admit to having blackouts (periods of time for which memory is lost) while drinking have alcoholism. If a family member complains of the patient's drinking behavior, this is associated with alcoholism in over 75% of cases. If a patient admits that alcohol is interfering with his health, occupational functioning, or social functioning, he has alcoholism by definition. Patients who say that they are unable to stop drinking for any period of time and those who say that they have stopped drinking for a period of time are very likely to have alcoholism.

On the physical examination, those patients who have the odor of alcohol on their breath, bilateral parotid gland enlargement, spider nevi or angiomata, or have trem-

Table I. Medical, Psychiatric, Legal, and Other Findings Suggestive or Highly Suggestive of Alcoholism

Presenting complaint or history

Blackouts with drinking[a]
Family violence[b]
Child abuse[b]
First seizure in an adult[b]
Prison record[b]
Job performance problem[b]
Spouse/other complaints of patient's drinking[b]
DWI (driving while intoxicated) record[b]

Drug-use history

Alcohol use interfering with health, job, or social function[c]
Patient says, ''I can stop drinking anytime,'' or the equivalent, or patient gets evasive or angry or talks glibly while drinking history is taken[a]
Patient states that he has stopped drinking completely for any length of time[a]
Word ''drinker'' said in rounds or report[a]
Heavy alcohol use (more than 3 drinks/day or more than 5 drinks at an occasion for a 154-lb person)[b]

Physical examination

Odor of beverage alcohol on breath[a]
Parotid gland enlargement, bilateral[a]
Spider nevi or angiomata[a]
Tremulousness, hallucinosis, and/or 1 or 2 seizures[a]
Cigarette stains on fingers[b]
Small testicles[b]
Unexplained bruises[b]
Many scars, tattoos[b]
Edematous, ''puffy'' face (may be subtle)[a]

Laboratory abnormalities

Blood alcohol level greater than 300 mg%[a]
Blood alcohol level greater than 100 mg%[a]
Blood alcohol level positive, any amount[b]
High serum osmolality (about 70% due to alcohol)[a]
High serum ammonia[a]
High amylase[b]
Abnormal liver function tests[b]
SGOT elevated on admission, normal by discharge[a]
Gamma glutamyl transferase (GGT) elevation[a]

X-ray film findings

Pancreatic calcifications[a]
Multiple rib fractures[a]

Associated diagnosis

Pancreatitis, acute or chronic (40–95%)[a]
Hepatitis, alcoholic[c]
Cirrhosis (85%)[a]
Portal hypertension[a]
Fatty liver[b]
Gastritis[b]
Refractory hypertension[b]
Wernicke–Korsakoff syndrome[a]
Cerebellar degeneration[b]
Peripheral neuropathy[b]
Aspiration pneumonia[b]
Frequent automobile or other accidents[a]
Drownings[b]
Freezing or cold injury[a]
Burns, esp. 3rd degree[b]
Attempted suicide[b]
Leaves hospital against medical advice[b]

[a]Seventy-five or more are percent alcoholic.
[b]Fifty percent or more are alcoholic.
[c]Diagnostic of alcoholism.

ulousness, hallucinosis, and/or one to two seizures are very likely to have alcoholism (again a 75% chance). From the laboratory perspective a BAL of 0.3 g% is diagnostic and 0.1 g% is highly suggestive of alcoholism. High serum osmolality is also suggestive (about 70% of such elevations are due to ethanol). Elevations of serum ammonia, serum glutamate–oxalacetate transaminase, or γ-glutamyl transferase are highly suggestive. Radiographs demonstrating pancreatic calcifications or multiple rib fractures are also commonly seen in patients who have alcoholism.

Acute or chronic pancreatitis, cirrhosis, portal hypertension, Wernicke–Korsakoff syndrome, frequent automobile accidents, and freezing or cold injuries are all highly suggestive of alcoholism.

In addition to the above indicators of alcoholism, a study recently reported by Ryback *et al.*[11] demonstrated the effectiveness of an algorithm, derived from multiple discriminant analysis of several routine chemical and hematological tests, in screening for alcoholism. Applying this method 100% of alcoholic patients in the medical wards of a hospital and 94% of those in an alcoholism treatment program were correctly identified as alcoholic. Equally as important as the sensitivity of this algorithm is the fact that 100% of the medical control group were correctly identified as nonalcoholic.

Beyond these observations and tests that may be made as part of the primary health care of patients, a simple, rapid, and inexpensive screening procedure has been available since 1971—the Michigan Alcoholism Screening Test (MAST).[12] The MAST is a relatively nonthreatening paper-and-pencil questionnaire that has been validated as a reliable diagnostic instrument. The test, which is reproduced in Fig. 1, consists of 24 weighted score questions about alcoholic behavior. A score of 5 or more would place the subject in the "alcoholic" category, and a score of 4 would be suggestive of alcoholism. This test has proved to be highly reliable in detecting alcoholics in the general hospital setting[13,14] and could easily be utilized in a primary-care office practice as a part of routine health maintenance.

6. RATIONALE FOR PREVENTION

The hard data regarding the effectiveness of secondary prevention of substance abuse in reducing morbidity and mortality and in saving money are sparse and incomplete—leaving this a fertile area for research. However, since most of the morbidity and mortality is associated with the direct toxic effects of the substances on the body or with the alterations in behavior by the substances, it follows that any plan that would prevent the abuse of substances primarily or intercede in the disorder prior to the occurrence of complications would markedly reduce morbidity and mortality. A review of 12 studies of the efficacy of alcoholism treatment in reducing medical care utilization, sick days, and accident benefits paid revealed that alcoholism treatment is clearly cost-effective.[15] This is supported by the study of Reiff,[16] which examined cost-effectiveness of alcoholism treatment for a health maintenance organization (HMO). This study unequivocally demonstrated that alcoholism treatment easily pays its own way and, in fact, saves money for the HMO. Similar data supporting the cost-effectiveness of alcoholism treatment are provided by Paredes.[17]

Points			Yes	No
	0.	Do you enjoy a drink now and then?	____	____
(2)	1.	Do you feel you are a normal drinker? (By normal, we mean you drink less than or as much as other people.) (Score 2 points for a negative answer.)	____	____
(2)	2.	Have you ever awakened the morning after some drinking the night before and found that you could not remember a part of the evening?	____	____
(1)	3.	Does your wife, husband, a parent, or other relative ever worry or complain about your drinking?	____	____
(2)	4.	Can you stop drinking without a struggle after one or two drinks? (Score 2 points for a negative answer.)	____	____
(1)	5.	Do you ever feel guilty about your drinking?	____	____
(2)	6.	Do friends or relatives think you are a normal drinker? (Score 2 points for a negative answer.)	____	____
(2)	7.	Are you able to stop drinking when you want to? (Score 2 points for a negative answer.)	____	____
(5)	8.	Have you ever attended a meeting of Alcoholics Anonymous (AA)?	____	____
(1)	9.	Have you gotten into physical fights when drinking?	____	____
(2)	10.	Has your drinking ever created problems between you and your wife, husband, a parent, or other near relative?	____	____
(2)	11.	Has your wife, husband, a parent, or other near relative ever gone to anyone for help about your drinking?	____	____
(2)	12.	Have you ever lost friends because of your drinking?	____	____
(2)	13.	Have you ever gotten into trouble at work because of drinking?	____	____
(2)	14.	Have you ever lost a job because of drinking?	____	____
(2)	15.	Have you ever neglected your obligations, your family, or your work for two or more days in a row because you were drinking?	____	____
(1)	16.	Do you drink before noon fairly often?	____	____
(2)	17.	Have you ever been told you have liver trouble? Cirrhosis?	____	____
(2)	18.	After heavy drinking have you ever had delirium tremens (DTs) or severe shaking, or heard voices or seen things that weren't really there?	____	____
(5)	19.	Have you ever gone to anyone for help about your drinking?	____	____
(5)	20.	Have you ever been in a hospital because of drinking?	____	____
(2)	21.	Have you ever been a patient in a psychiatric hospital or on a psychiatric ward of a general hospital, where drinking was a part of the problem that resulted in hospitalization?	____	____
(2)	22.	Have you ever been to a psychiatric or mental health clinic or gone to any doctor, social worker, or clergyman for help with any emotional problem, where drinking was part of the problem?	____	____
(2)	23.	Have you ever been arrested for drunken driving, driving while intoxicated, or driving under the influence of alcoholic beverages?	____	____
(2)	24.	Have you ever been arrested, or taken into custody even for a few hours, because of other drunken behavior?	____	____

Scoring

5 points or more, high probability of alcoholism; 4 points, suggestive of alcoholism; 3 points or less, low probability of alcoholism.

Figure 1. Michigan Alcoholism Screening Test (MAST). (Source: Selzer.[12])

There are currently many programs that attempt to prevent substance abuse primarily. The majority of these programs are aimed toward children and adolescents in the school systems. This young population at risk has been identified, and the goal is to educate them about the adverse effects of alcoholism and drug abuse with the hope of preventing these diseases in the upcoming generations. This plan must include education and some way of combating the peer and parental pressures to abuse substances. These primary prevention programs are attaining some success and should be of benefit to future generations; however, the problem of substance abuse is a monumental one today. Can we effectively intervene in the early stages of substance abuse disorders and prevent the secondary complications of substance abuse? This is a two-step process which involves, first, the identification of the victims of substance abuse before the complications occur and, second, successful and cost-effective treatment of substance abuse disorders. Both of these are possible—at least in the case of alcoholism, the most prevalent of the substance abuse disorders.

There are a number of tactics currently in effect at various levels that allow secondary intervention in substance abuse disorders. Many state and local governments have alcohol safety action programs, which identify alcoholic automobile drivers and legally force them into treatment via the judicial system. These have been coupled in some states with driving checkpoints, which attempt to identify drunk drivers before accidents occur. Many employers have instituted employee assistance programs, which identify alcoholic and drug-dependent employees and force them into treatment. Employees who sucessfully complete treatment are generally allowed to return to their jobs after treatment. This has been found to be a cost-effective plan for employers—it is cheaper to identify and successfully treat experienced employees and return them to their jobs than to hire and train new employees. Companies have found that for each dollar invested in an employee through its employee assistance program, there is a return of between $2 and $20. Reduced absenteeism alone often results in a savings of approximately $1000 per employee treated. Substance abuse treatment programs associated with employee assistance programs have resulted in recovery rates of between 50% and 90%. Unfortunately, only about 12% of American companies have such a program.

Some companies have instituted preemployment drug/alcohol screening tests, and many of these companies repeat these tests periodically during employment in order to detect employee substance abuse. There are significant limitations to some chemical screening tests, which must be taken into consideration before implementing and acting on the results of these tests. These programs, along with similar school programs, have been very successful in reaching many victims of substance abuse and sending them into treatment before the major complications of the illnesses occur. However, the health care profession has been less responsible and less effective at identifying and treating patients with alcohol and drug dependency early in the illness. Since alcoholics and other substance abusers are such frequent users of health care services, the physician's office and the hospital should be primary locations for high-yield identification of these patients.

Ideally, alcoholics should be identified and treated prior to their developing any of the complications of alcoholism mentioned earlier. If this is done, there unequivocally should be a tremendous cost savings. The investment for the screening tests is minimal, and the cost of alcoholism in this country is more than 60 billion dollars per year in medical costs, disability costs, loss from missed time at work, and so forth. The efficacy of physician prevention and intervention has not been clearly demonstrated because it has not been implemented on a large scale. It is clear, however, that other forms of secondary prevention have been successful in reducing morbidity and mortality from alcoholism. Two good examples of this are apparent. There has been a clear reduction in mortality associated with alcohol-related motor vehicle accidents in states that have instituted drunk driver detection and intervention programs. Another example of the value of secondary prevention in substance abuse is the success of the various employee assistance programs in large companies in the United States. These programs clearly have been successful in reducing lost corporate revenues associated with substance-abusing employees. In addition, they have saved federal and state monies by rehabilitating alcoholic employees rather than placing them on the unemployment rolls. Presumably, physician intervention in the early stages of alcoholism would be equally or more effective in reducing morbidity, mortality, and financial losses. Applying the data from the employee assistance program experience to the total cost for substance abuse in this country, there would be an annual savings of at least 30 billion dollars. More important, approximately 100,000 lives would be saved.

The complications of applying prevention strategies should be insignificant compared to the potential gains. The tests for detection of substance abuse may be somewhat threatening to the patient, but a good physician–atient relationship should be able to tolerate any anxiety produced in the patient. Positive tests should result in more patients being sent into treatment programs of various types. Fortunately, false positive tests are rare.

7. SUBSTANCE ABUSE INTERVENTION: DETOXIFICATION AND REHABILITATION

Patients who are alcohol dependent (i.e., physically dependent) are at significant risk for serious complications during the withdrawal period (5–10 days after discontinuation of the alcohol). For safety this should be accomplished in a hospital setting. Detoxification from alcohol on an outpatient basis is less than optimal because it requires that the alcoholic take a benzodiazepine drug in a decremental dosing fashion over a period of 5–10 days. It is difficult, if not impossible, to be certain how much benzodiazepine the patient will need for the first few days to prevent serious withdrawal consequences, i.e., delirium, seizures, or death. Even if this could be determined with ease, the process would then be dependent on the alcoholic patient's being responsible for correctly taking the prescribed doses of medication on a regular schedule, changing the dose as prescribed every 2–3 days, and not drinking any alcohol during this period, since the combination of alcohol and a benzodiazepine may be lethal. The alcoholic, almost by definition, cannot be responsible for these expectations. In addition, the alcoholic often has many medical complications of his alcoholism which must be treated during the early part of alcoholism treatment/rehabilitation. The initial treatment of addiction to other drugs besides alcohol is also a critical period, although the detoxification from narcotics, cocaine, and amphetamines is generally not as dangerous as the detoxification from alcohol and the sedative/hypnotic agents.

After the initial detoxification process a decision must be made about the appropriateness of further rehabilitation. This may be done on an outpatient or inpatient basis, depending on the specific details of the patient's illness. Certainly, outpatient treatment is less expensive than inpatient treatment; however, many patients do not have the reliability to attend outpatient treatment. The biggest hurdle that must be crossed in the initial phase of alcoholism treatment is the patient's denial of his illness. This denial is virtually always present and often prevents the patient from continuing in treatment or complying with the various aspects of treatment. It is true that the aspect of alcoholism treatment that seems to have the greatest success rate is that of support groups such as Alcoholics Anonymous (AA). It seems that it would be cheap and easy just to refer alcoholic patients to this organization for treatment. Although this is true, it is very difficult to convince a patient to become involved with AA without some type of assistance. Patients who are willing to go for the first time typically do not continue to attend regularly. Overcoming the patient's denial and involving him/her in a support group is one of the primary responsibilities of a formal treatment program—either outpatient or inpatient.

The model inpatient treatment program typically lasts approximately 28 days and consists of a detoxification period of 5–7 days. During this period the treatment team begins to work with the patient on some of the problems that have resulted from his/her substance abuse. Typically cognitive ability is somewhat impaired during the first stage of treatment, and the patient is limited in what he/she can process during this time. During the second stage of treatment the patient is able to look more carefully at his/her life and the role that substance abuse has played in the various disturbances in physiological, psychological, occupational, and social functioning. He/she accepts the fact that he/she is a substance abuser. In the final stage of the inpatient program the patient begins plans for survival outside the hospital without alcohol and drugs. This would include such things as support groups (i.e., Alcoholics Anonymous and Narcotics Anonymous), family support and/or therapy, halfway houses, and Antabuse.

8. SUMMARY

It is clear that alcohol and drug abuse disorders are pervasive in our society and, in general, are becoming more prevalent. They are associated with and cause a great deal of morbidity and mortality because of the adverse effects of alcohol and drugs on individual functioning and relationships. This results in a tremendous financial loss. A number of programs for secondary prevention are now in place, including school identification and prevention programs, employee assistance programs, and state alcohol safety action programs. Since substance abusers are frequent users of the health care system, it is reasonable that the physician's office and the hospital would be high-yield locations for the identification and intervention of substance abuse. Apparently, little known to physicians and nurse practioners is that there are a number of screening tests for the identification of substance abusers—especially alcoholics—which can be applied in the primary-care setting at a minimal expense. Since treatment of substance abuse has been demonstrated to be cost-effective, early identification, intervention, and treatment of substance abusers by primary-care health care professionals should improve quality of life, reduce mortality

and morbidity, and save at least 30 billion dollars in annual health care costs in the United States.

REFERENCES

1. Schuckit, M. A., Goodwin, D. A., and Winokur, G.: A study of alcoholism in half siblings. *Am. J. Psychiatry* **128**:1132–1136, 1972.
2. Goodwin, D. A., Schulsinger, F., Moller, N., *et al.*: Drinking problems in adopted and nonadopted sons of alcoholics. *Arch. Gen. Psychiatry* **31**:164–169, 1974.
3. Alcohol and drug misuse prevention. *Public Health Rep.* **171**(Suppl): 116–120, Sept.–Oct. 1983.
4. National Institute on Drug Abuse: Drug Abuse Warning Network Semi-annual Report Series G, No. 15 DHHS Publication no. (ADM) 85–1393: iv, 1985.
5. Institute of Medicine, Division of Health Promotion and Disease Prevention: *Alcoholism, Alcohol Abuse and Related Problems: Opportunities for Research.* National Academy of Science, Washington, DC, 1980.
6. Caine, D. B., Langston, J. W., Martin, W. R. W., *et al.:* Positron emission tomography after MPTP: Observations relating to the cause of Parkinson's disease. *Nature* **317**:246–248, 1985.
7. West, L. J., Maxwell, D. S., Noble, E. P., *et al.*: Alcoholism, UCLA Conference. *Ann. Intern. Med.* **100**:405–416, 1984.
8. American Psychiatric Association: *Diagnostic and Statistical Manual of Mental Disorders,* (3rd ed.) APA Press, Washington, DC, 1980.
9. Chychula, N. M.: Screening for substance abuse in the primary care setting. *Nurse Practitioner* **9**(7):15–23, July 1984.
10. Whitfield, C. L.: Outpatient management of the alcoholic patient. *Psychiatr. Ann.* **12**(4):447–458, 1982.
11. Ryback, R. S., Eckardt, M. J., and Pantler, C. P.: Biochemical and hematological correlates of alcoholism. *Res. Commun. Clin. Pathol. Pharmacol.* **29**:533–550, 1980.
12. Selzer, M. L.: The Michigan alcoholism screening test: The quest for a new diagnostic instrument. *Am. J. Psychiatry* **127**:1653–1658, 1971.
13. Favazza, A. R., and Pires, J.: The Michigan alcoholism screening test: Application in a general military hospital. *Q. J. Stud. Alcohol* **35**:925–929, 1974.
14. Westermeyer, J., Doheny, S., and Stone, B.: An assessment of hospital care for the alcoholic patient. *Alcoholism* **2**:53–57, 1978.
15. Jones, K. R., and Vischi, T. R.: Impact of alcoholism, drug abuse and mental health treatment on medical care utilization. *Med. Care* **17**:1–82, 1979.
16. Reiff, S.: A cost-effectiveness study of alcoholism treatment in a health maintenance organization. *Substance Abuse* **6**(2):24–28, 1985.
17. Paredes, A.: Cost effectiveness in alcoholism treatment. *Substance Abuse* **6**(2):29–37, 1985.

26

Periodic Health Examination

Julia E. Connelly

1. INTRODUCTION

Periodic health examination is a common and important part of office practice. Its purpose is the detection of asymptomatic illness and the prevention of disease before irreversible pathological changes occur. There are many questions about the content and efficacy of this type of examination.[1] Which conditions are preventable? Which diagnostic tests are useful for screening and case finding? Is this type of prevention cost-effective? Will patients and third parties pay for this type of health care?

Even though controversy is present, physicians must have a strategy for office prevention because patients request checkups and information about preventive health care. The National Ambulatory Medical Care Survey demonstrated that the request for a general health checkup was the most common reason given by patients for an office visit.[2] In order to meet the needs of these patients, the physician must determine what factors motivate the patient to seek health assessment, understand what the patient expects from the examination, and provide individualized recommendations targeted at the detection of preventable asymptomatic conditions.

The purpose of this chapter is to define periodic health examination, present the criteria used to select potentially preventable conditions, discuss the limitations and clinical implications of periodic examinations, and review the historical development of and current recommendations for periodic examinations.

2. DEFINITION OF TERMS

Periodic health examination is defined as "a group of tasks designed either to determine the risk of subsequent disease or to identify disease in its early symptomless state."[3–5] Two approaches to periodic health examinations are used. The first, *screening*, refers to any activity using procedures that classify unselected general populations into two groups: one group with a high probability of having a fatal or disabling condition or an unhealthy lifestyle, and the other group with a low probability of having the condition.[5] Screening may be promoted by the public health department, at health fairs, or by

Julia E. Connelly • Department of Internal Medicine, University of Virginia School of Medicine, Charlottesville, Virginia 22908 local drug stores that promote the detection of colon cancer.[6] No ongoing therapeutic relationship is implied between the two parties involved in screening, and no follow-up of abnormal tests is expected. In general, participants are notified of results and, in turn, request their physician to evaluate abnormal findings. The second approach to periodic health examination is *case finding*. Case finding is the detection of asymptomatic disease using interventions ordered by a physician who has an ongoing relationship with the patient and who will provide follow-up of any abnormality. Case finding incorporates the detection of asymptomatic disease into the routine office visit.

The keystone of periodic health examination is prevention. There are three levels of prevention: primary, secondary, and tertiary (see Fig. 1).[7] Prevention requires an intervention that reduces the probability that a condition will affect a person or that is known to interrupt the progression of the disease. Primary prevention diminishes the probability that a disease will develop in a person. Vaccination for the prevention of rubella is an example of primary prevention. Secondary prevention attempts to detect or impair the progression of a disease while it is asymptomatic. It consists of early diagnosis during the lead time and treatment of disease before irreversible changes occur. Physicians perform secondary screening in their offices when they look for occult stool blood, do Pap smears, or order mammograms in patients asymptomatic for the given disease. Secondary prevention corresponds to case finding. Tertiary prevention attempts to limit progressive disability in

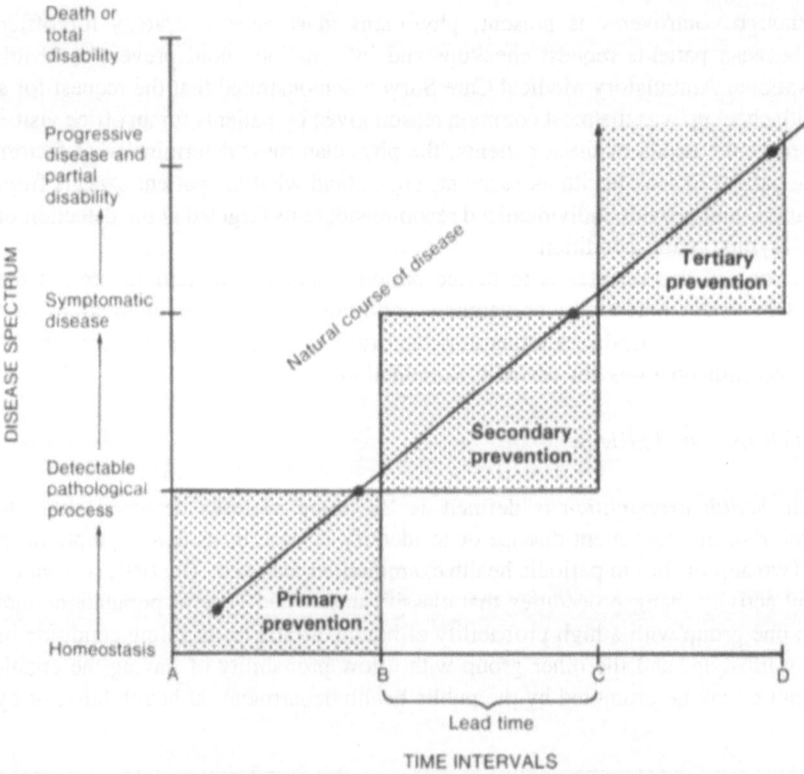

Figure 1. Levels of prevention. (Source: Barker.[7])

individuals with established irreversible disease. An example is the maintenance of strength and mobility in a patient with arthritis by using physical therapy.

3. SELECTION OF PREVENTABLE CONDITIONS

In practical terms not all illness can be prevented. The World Health Organization suggests the following criteria as the most important factors for the selection of conditions that are potentially preventable: (1) the condition must be sufficiently prevalent—common enough to warrant the attempt to detect it, (2) it must have a meaningful impact on an individual's health if not treated, (3) there must be evidence that treatment during the asymptomatic phase improves the untreated outcome of the condition, and (4) the method of detection must be acceptable, affordable, and must have adequate sensitivity and specificity.[8] The primary purpose of laboratory tests used in screening is early detection of asymptomatic disease. Griner and associates defined an acceptable screening test as "one that will be abnormal in almost all individuals with the disease and will provide the physician with confidence that the patient is free of disease when the test is normal."[9] Because it is important to minimize the number of false positive studies that would require further evaluation, the test should be very specific. The chapter on testing discusses further the utility of screening tests, the hazards of their misinterpretation, and the difficulties of screening programs.

4. LIMITATIONS OF PERIODIC HEALTH EXAMINATION

Labeling a patient as having an asymptomatic disease carries potential risks.[10,11] Haynes and associates demonstrated an increase in work absenteeism among asymptomatic patients who were found to have hypertension in a screening program.[12] Such patients may adopt the "sick role" or develop an impaired perception of their own health. Because of the potential adverse reactions to the early detection of disease, treatment during the asymptomatic phase must be known to offer an improvement in clinical outcome greater than treatment in later symptomatic phases. If this is not the case, such detection may increase the patient's burder of suffering. In assessing the benefit of early disease detection, one needs to consider also the possibility of lead time bias and selection bias.[5,7] Lead time bias appears to increase survival because diagnosis and treatment occur before the onset of symptoms. Selection bias may affect survival because patients who request screening may differ from other groups of patients with similar conditions (i.e., they may be more aware of changes in their bodies or more interested in a healthy lifestyle and therefore seek more checkups). Bias in screening programs is also discussed in Chapter 3.

5. CLINICAL IMPLICATIONS OF PERIODIC HEALTH EXAMINATION

Periodic examination is appropriate for all individuals. However, the content of such examinations varies with the patient's age, sex, risk factors, and relationship with the physician. New patients have different screening and prevention requirements than established patients. For example, during the initial visit a thorough history may uncover high-risk conditions, expose the patient's reasons for the examination, and establish a basis for the relationship with the physician. The physical examination may uncover unrecognized problems or define a basis for future comparison. The actual interventions will be determined by specific recommendations based on the patient's age and sex, by the presence of any high-risk conditions, and by the physician's judgment. Whether or not the initial visit should include an electrocardiogram, "routine blood chemistries," urinalysis, or chest x-rays remains controversial. The physician must always use clinical judgment to individualize test ordering. These interventions are not recommended annually in asymptomatic patients who return for periodic follow-up.[5,13–15] It is most important to integrate the periodic health examination with ongoing care. Minimum recommendations for the detection of preventable conditions should not be overlooked for new patients or for those returning for follow-up care.[5,13–15] Although periodic examinations are directed at the detection of asymptomatic disease, patients usually visit physicians with symptoms. After addressing the chief complaint, disease that is asymptomatic and present in other organ systems should be sought. For example, a middle-aged man with chronic obstructive lung disease was found to have colon cancer. Review of his chart revealed that screening for the early detection of colon cancer had not been recommended. It is understandable that the physician's attention should be focused on the treatment of chronic obstructive lung disease, yet such a narrow focus may overlook the detection of preventable conditions. Again, the recommendations are made to detect asymptomatic disease in individuals who may or may not be truly asymptomatic.

Special attention to hidden agendas should be given to patients who request checkups. One study of such patients demonstrated that factors other than screening motivated the majority (76%) to request checkups.[16] Most of these patients were not asymptomatic and often had multiple, covert, nonmedical reasons for the appointment. Reasons that motivated these patients included psychosocial problems, health concerns, bothersome symptoms, administrative issues, the desire to satisfy concerned relatives, and a need for information.

Interest in periodic health examinations is increasing among physicians. One study demonstrated that the majority of internists are doing more to detect cancer than they were 5 years ago, especially for breast, colorectal, and gynecological cancer.[17] In fact, physicians may order more tests than are recommended. Serum cholesterol, blood glucose, hematocrit, urinalysis, Pap smear, and glaucoma testing are often overused.[18] Sometimes patients expect more testing than is currently recommended. Their expectations need to be understood, and educating the patient about current recommendations is a useful substitute for what may be an unnecessary test.

6. HISTORICAL DEVELOPMENT OF PERIODIC HEALTH EXAMINATION

The concept of the periodic health examination is not new. Dobell, an English physician, advocated "periodic health examinations for all" in 1861. The content of such periodic review evolves as understanding of disease states change, as diagnosis of asymptomatic disease improves, and as treatment during the asymptomatic phase is shown to improve morbidity and mortality. To understand current recommendations for periodic examination, it is useful to review the historical development of this concept.[19,20]

In the late 19th century, contagious diseases were the major cause of death. Thus, at school, children were routinely examined for infections, and by the 20th century, this search was extended to general physical impairments.[21] George Gould, an oculist from England, brought the concept of general examinations to the United States. Before the American Medical Association (AMA) he proposed that every American should have a general examination every few years.[22] Physicians affiliated with life insurance companies were the first to actually carry out a program of periodic examinations. Dr. E. L. Fisk established the Life Extension Program of the Metropolitan Life Insurance Company in 1914. Policy holders were offered free examinations, but by 1921 only 2.5% had been examined.[23] During the same years the National Association for the Study and Prevention of Tuberculosis supported the value of the annual examination.[24] The popularity of such examinations increased as a result of World War I, when the rejection rate of supposedly healthy young men from the army was alarmingly high. By 1920 the AMA adopted the slogan "Have a Health Examination on Your Birthday."[25] The support for annual examinations continued as Americans began to own automobiles, and some suggested, "Let your doctor overhaul you once a year."[26]

During the 1930s insurance companies, public services, the military, industrial organizations, and the general population became more interested in the annual health examination. During World War II the rejection rate for the military was again high, and emphasis was placed on screening the general population. In the postwar years, mass screening was possible due to advances in technology. Syphilis and tuberculosis screening centers were established. In 1950 the President's Commission on the Health Needs of the Nation recommended multiphasic screening—"everything for everyone."[27] Multiphasic screening became popular and provided screening for multiple problems at one screening site. It was an attempt to centralize records and decrease screening costs. Opposition arose from many sectors. Individuals were upset because there was no contact with the physician. The therapeutic effects of the relationship between the patient and the physician were eliminated. Physicians were also upset because positive tests were common, and they were obligated to follow up tests they had not ordered and advise individuals they often did not know. Government costs for such programs increased, as did dissatisfaction within the general population. In 1953 Breslow suggested that multiphasic screening be incorporated into the routine office visit to increase case finding. The physician ordered screening tests during the regular office visit and provided follow-up of abnormal tests. This approach pleased both patients and physicians. It was comprehensive, allowed centralized record keeping, and saved time.

Annual examinations for the general population continued throughout the 1960s. Multiphasic screening was suggested for all individuals without regard to age or sex. Executive examinations were popular, and many unsuspected problems were discovered. However, scientific investigations were not available to show that uncovering such maladies actually decreased morbidity and mortality. In the early 1970s results from an 11-year controlled, prospective study demonstrated a decrease in morbidity and mortality for men 45–54 years old who had undergone comprehensive examination annually.[28] In 1975, Frame and Carlson selected 36 diseases and analyzed the feasibility of screening for each one. The criteria for selection were broad, ranging from the effect on quality and length of life to the availability of diagnostic tests. The final proposal recommended screening on the basis of age and sex.[29] In 1977, Breslow and Somers proposed their "Lifetime Health-Monitoring Program." They emphasized the utilization of cost-effective and health-effective preventive interventions.[30] In 1979, the Canadian Task Force on the Periodic Health Examination published recommendations for a "lifetime plan of preventive medicine."[5] Seventy-eight potentially preventable conditions were studied, and recommendations were made by an international group of consultants who considered "the effectiveness of the ensuing treatment or preventive measure, the burden of suffering caused by the condition, and the characteristics of the early detections procedure to be used to find the condition." The Canadian Task Force recommended that the routine annual checkups be replaced by a selective approach determined by the patient's age and sex.[5] In 1980, the American Cancer Society proposed recommendations for the cancer-related examination. These were also based on the patient's age and sex.[31]

7. RECOMMENDATIONS FOR PERIODIC HEALTH EXAMINATION

7.1. Recommendations of the 1970s

During the 1970s four sets of recommendations were made by Frame and Carlson (1975), Breslow and Somers (1977), the Canadian Task Force on the Periodic Health Examination (1979), and the American Cancer Society on the "cancer-related checkup" (1980).[5,29–31] Although the recomendations vary, each group proposed a change to periodic rather than annual examinations, and each advocated a targeted approach aimed at detection of a potentially preventable condition depending on the age and sex of the individual.

7.2. Recommendations of the 1980s

The Medical Practice Committee of the American College of Physicians and the Council of Scientific Affairs of the American Medical Association summarized the four sets of recommendations just mentioned. Neither group offered to select or weigh the importance of the interventions that should be included in periodic health examinations. Each concluded that (1) periodic examinations are important, (2) the optimal frequency and the interventions need to be determined by the age and sex of the patient, (3) the recommendations represent minimum interventions, which should be modified by the patient's relationship with the physician, by the characteristics of the diagnostic tests, and by the prevalence of disease in the population being treated, (4) physicians need to be more skillful at fostering healthy lifestyles, and (5) the recommendations will be updated as necessary.[15]

Figures 2–4 offer a compilation of the four sets of recommendations. These forms can be included in each patient's chart in order to (1) remind the physician about the knowledge base needed when performing periodic health examinations, (2) record the periodic interventions in a centralized place to minimize time spent searching for previuosly ordered tests, and (3) demonstrate to patients what is actually important to look for and when. Copies of these recommendations may be useful to patients, both to inform them and also to remind them when the next periodic evaluation is due.

The recommendations address (1) preventable conditions in the general population, (2) preventive counseling, (3) immunizations, and (4) problems that occur in individuals at high risk.

7.3. Specific Recommendations

7.3.1. Recommendations for the Cancer-Related Checkup (see Chapter 16)

7.3.1a. The Early Detection of Cancer of the Cervix. A Pap smear is recommended yearly between age 16 and 35 years, every 3 years in women between 36 and 60, and every 5 years thereafter.[32] These recent recommendations were presented as an update to the Canadian Task Force. Yearly examinations were recommended because a risk factor for cervical cancer is multiple sexual partners, and many women in the general population have multiple partners.

7.3.1b. The Early Detection of Cancer of the Breast. It is recommended that breast self-examination be taught and reinforced every time a cancer-related checkup is performed.[33–35] Physical examination by the physician is recommended every 3 years from age 20 to 40 and yearly thereafter.[33] Mammography is recommended once between 35 and 40 years and annually between 50 and 60. The Breast Cancer Detection Demonstration Project revealed that mammograms alone significantly increase the detection of asymptomatic cancer in women between 40 and 60.[34–36] However, there has not been a study that demonstrates a decrease in morbidity and mortality when asymptomatic breast cancer detected between 40 and 50 years is treated. The American College of Physicians does not recommend mammography for the early detection of breast cancer in this age group.[33] The Health Insurance Plan of Greater New York demonstrated in a large clinical trial that screening mammography reduced breast cancer deaths in women over 50.[37]

7.3.1c. The Early Detection of Colon Cancer. Stool blood detection is recommended every year after the age of 40. Two samples of three consecutive stools should be tested using a test for occult blood. The stools should be tested within 4 days because the false-negative rate approaches 30% after 6 days. To reduce false-negative tests further, the patient should not take vitamin C 3 days prior to testing.[38] Aspirin and nonsteroidal antiinflammatory drugs can cause false positive results.[38]

Controversy exists about the use of sigmoidoscopy. Rigid sigmoidoscopy was not recommended by the Canadian Task Force because of the risk of perforation, the cost, and the discomfort to the patient.[5] The American Cancer Society did recommend the test.[31] The 35-cm flexible sigmoidoscope is now available and affordable for the physician's office. When it is used by a trained physician, patient discomfort and the risk of perforation are diminished. The American Cancer Society now recommends two flexible sigmoidoscopic studies near the age of 50, followed by repeated examinations every 3–5 years.[39]

7.3.2. Non-Cancer-Related Recommendations

Hypothyroidism is a relatively common condition, affecting approximately 1% of the general population and a much higher proportion of older women.[40] Screening for thyroid

Date

Age	16	17	18	19	20	21	22	23	24	25	26	27	28	29	30	31	32	33	34	35	36	37	38	39
Blood pressure	•			•			•			•			•			•			•			•		
Weight*																								
Pap smear	•	•	•	•	•	•	•	•	•	•	•	•	•	•	•	•	•	•	•	•			•	
Breast exam					•			•			•			•			•			•			•	
Mammogram																				(•)				
Oral exam	•	•	•	•	•	•	•	•	•	•	•	•	•	•	•	•	•	•	•	•	•	•	•	•
Breast self-exam*																								
ETOH abuse*																								
Smoking*																								
Seat belts*																								
Sexual/marital problems*																								

Child abuse/neglect*																								
Poliomyelitis	•																							
Tetanus	•									•									•					
Rubella	•																							
High-risk problems:																								
Cancer of skin*																								
Cancer of breast	•	•	•	•	•	•	•	•	•	•	•	•	•	•	•	•	•	•	•	•	•	•	•	•
Cancer of colon*																								
Cancer of cervix	•	•	•	•	•	•	•	•	•	•	•	•	•	•	•	•	•	•	•	•	•	•	•	•
Gonorrhea	•	•	•	•	•	•	•	•	•	•	•	•	•	•	•	•	•	•	•	•	•	•	•	•
Syphilis	•	•	•	•	•	•	•	•	•	•	•	•	•	•	•	•	•	•	•	•	•	•	•	•
Tuberculosis	•	•	•	•	•	•	•	•	•	•	•	•	•	•	•	•	•	•	•	•	•	•	•	•
Iron deficiency*																								
Malnutrition*																								
Hyperlipidemia*																								
Unwanted 2nd pregnancy*																								
Hepatitis B vaccine*																								
Influenza vaccine	•	•	•	•	•	•	•	•	•	•	•	•	•	•	•	•	•	•	•	•	•	•	•	•
Pneumovax	•																							

Figure 2. Periodic health examination record, ages 16–39. *, No specific interval recommended.

Date																				
Age	40	41	42	43	44	45	46	47	48	49	50	51	52	53	54	55	56	57	58	59
Blood pressure	•	•	•	•	•	•	•	•	•	•	•	•	•	•	•	•	•	•	•	•
Weight*																				
Pap smear	•			•						•			•			•			•	
Stool blood	•	•	•	•	•	•	•	•	•	•	•	•	•	•	•	•	•	•	•	
Sigmoidoscopy											•	•								
Breast exam	•	•	•	•	•	•	•	•	•	•	•	•	•	•	•	•	•	•	•	•
Mammogram	(•	•	•	•	•	•	•	•	•	•)	•	•	•	•	•	•	•	•	•	•
Thyroid exam						•		•		•		•		•		•		•		•
Oral exam*	•	•	•	•	•	•	•	•	•	•	•	•	•	•	•	•	•	•	•	•
Hearing*																				
Breast self-exam																				
Menopause*																				
Retirement distress*																				

Smoking*																				
Seat belts*																				
Sexual/marital problems*																				
Child abuse/neglect*																				
Tetanus	•																			
High-risk problems:																				
Cancer of bladder*																				
Cancer of skin*																				
Cancer of cervix	•	•	•	•	•	•	•	•	•	•	•	•	•	•	•	•	•	•	•	•
Gonorrhea	•	•	•	•	•	•	•	•	•	•	•	•	•	•	•	•	•	•	•	•
Syphilis	•	•	•	•	•	•	•	•	•	•	•	•	•	•	•	•	•	•	•	•
Tuberculosis	•	•	•	•	•	•	•	•	•	•	•	•	•	•	•	•	•	•	•	•
Glaucoma*																				
Hyperlipidemia*																				
Iron deficiency*																				
Malnutrition*																				
Hepatitis B vaccine*																				
Influenza vaccine	•	•	•	•	•	•	•	•	•	•	•	•	•	•	•	•	•	•	•	•
Pneumovax*																				

Figure 3. Periodic health examination record, ages 40–59. *, No specific interval recommended.

Date																										
Age	60	61	62	63	64	65	66	67	68	69	70	71	72	73	74	75	76	77	78	79	80	81	82	83	84	85
Blood pressure	•	•	•	•	•	•	•	•	•	•	•	•	•	•	•	•	•	•	•	•	•	•	•	•	•	•
Weight*																										
Malnutrition	•			•			•			•			•			•			•			•			•	
Progressive changes w/aging	•			•			•			•			•			•			•			•			•	
Pap smear	•					•					•					•					•					•
Breast exam	•	•	•	•	•	•	•	•	•	•	•	•	•	•	•	•	•	•	•	•	•	•	•	•	•	•
Stool blood	•	•	•	•	•	•	•	•	•	•	•	•	•	•	•	•	•	•	•	•	•	•	•	•	•	•
Sigmoidoscopy	•					•					•					•					•					•
Thyroid exam	•			•			•			•			•			•			•			•			•	
Oral disease	•	•	•	•	•	•	•	•	•	•	•	•	•	•	•	•	•	•	•	•	•	•	•	•	•	•
Hearing*																										

Glaucoma*																										
Breast self-exam*																										
ETOH abuse*																										
Smoking*																										
Seat belts*																										
Retirement distress*																										
Influenza vaccine	•	•	•	•	•	•	•	•	•	•	•	•	•	•	•	•	•	•	•	•	•	•	•	•	•	•
Pneumovax	•										•										•					
Tetanus	•																									
High-risk problems:																										
Cancer of bladder*																										
Cancer of cervix*																										
Cancer of endometrium: Sx*																										
Cancer of prostate*																										
Cancer of skin*																										
Tuberculosis	•	•	•	•	•	•	•	•	•	•	•	•	•	•	•	•	•	•	•	•	•	•	•	•	•	•

Figure 4. Periodic health examination record, ages 60–85. *, No specific interval recommended.

disease should rely on history and physical examination. Laboratory tests such as thyroid-stimulating hormone tests are not recommended for asymptomatic patients. The yield would be low, and the treatment of asymptomatic hypothyroidism must be individualized.

Oral examination for dental caries and periodontal disease is recommended yearly, with referral to a dentist as needed. In older patients and patients with tobacco- and alcohol-associated risks, regular inspection and palpation of the oral cavity for incipient oral cancer are necessary.

Attention to problems with hearing is recommended during any appointment. Adults who do not respond to normally spoken conversation or fail to hear sounds during their daily life should be referred for complete hearing evaluation.

Malnutrition is a common problem among the elderly population. Persons living alone are at greater risk. Careful dietary history is important. Home visits offer a unique opportunity to detect probable cases of malnutrition.

Glaucoma is more common in patients over the age of 60. Visualization of the optic disc for cupping and evaluation of the cup-to-disc ratio is probably the most accurate method to detect increased intraocular pressure in the general office.[5] The tonometer lacks sensitivity and specificity. Referral to an ophthalmologist every 2–3 years after the age of 60 may improve the early detection.

7.4. Preventive Counseling

This category includes detection of drug, tobacco, and alcohol abuse; child abuse; marital discord; sexual dysfunction; problems during life changes such as menopause and retirement; and the use of seat belts. During specific life changes stresses may increase and maladjustment may occur. These change should be discussed in advance.

7.5. Immunization

Immunizations are an integral part of every periodic health examination. This important subject is discussed comprehensively in separate chapters on adult immunization (Chapter 4) and advice to travelers (Chapter 20).

REFERENCES

1. Spitzer, W. O., and Brown, B.: Unanswered questions about the periodic health examination. *Ann. Intern. Med.* **83:**257–263, 1975.
2. Cypress, B. K.: *The National Ambulatory Medical Care Survey: 1981 Summary.* U S Department of Health and Human Services, National Center for Health Statistics, Hyattsville, MD, 1981.
3. Delbanco, T. L., and Noble, J.: The periodic health examination revisited. *Ann. Intern. Med.* **83:**271–273, 1975.
4. Delbanco, T. L., and Taylor, W. C.: The periodic health examination 1980. *Ann. Intern. Med.* **92:**251–252, 1980.
5. Spitzer, W. O.: Chairman: Report of the Task Force on the Periodic Health Examination. *Can. Med. Assoc. J.* **121:**1193–1254, 1979.
6. Berwick, M. D.: Screening in health fairs. *JAMA* **254:**1492–1498, 1985.
7. Barker, R.: Preventive care in ambulatory practice, in Barker, L. R., Burton, J. R., and Zieve, P. D. (eds.): *Principles of Ambulatory Medicine.* Williams & Wilkins, Baltimore, 1982, p. 16.

8. Wilson, J. M. G., and Junger, G.: *Principles and Practice of Screening for Disease*. World Health Organization, Geneva, 1968.
9. Griner, P. F., Mayewski, R. J., Mushlin, A. I., and Greenland, P.: Selection and interpretation of diagnostic tests and procedures. *Ann. Intern. Med.* **94**(4, part 2):553–600, 1981.
10. Fienleib, M., and Zelen, M.: Some pitfalls in the evaluation of screening programs. *Arch. Environ, Health* **19**:412–415, 1965.
11. Sackett, D. L.: Screening for the early detection of disease: To what purpose? *Bull. NY Acad. Med.* **51**:39–52, 1975.
12. Haynes, R. B., Sackett, D. L., Taylor, D. W., *et al.*: Increased absenteeism from work after detection and labelling of hypertensive patients. *N. Engl. J. Med.* **299**:741–744, 1978.
13. American College of Physicians' Medical Practice Committee: Periodic health examinations: A guide for designing individualized preventive health care in the asymptomatic patient. *Ann. Intern. Med.* **95**:729–732, 1981.
14. Fletcher, S. W., and Spitzer, W. O.: Approach of the Canadian Task Force to the periodic health examination. *Ann. Intern. Med.* **92**:253–254, 1980.
15. Jones, R. (Council of Scientific Affairs): Medical evaluation of healthy persons. *JAMA* **95**:729–732, 1981.
16. Connelly, J. E., and Mushlin, A. I.: The reasons patients request a "check-up": Implications for office practice. *J. Gen. Med.* **1**:163–165, 1986.
17. American Cancer Society survey of physicians' attitudes and practices in early cancer detection. *CA* **4**:197–213, 1985.
18. Woo, B., Woo, B., Cook, E. F., *et al.*: Screening Procedures in the asymptomatic adult. *JAMA* **254**:1480–1484, 1985.
19. Reiser, S. J.: Emergence of the concept of screening for disease. *Millbank Mem. Fund Q.* **56**:403–425, 1978.
20. Charap, M. H.: The periodic health examination: Genesis of a myth. *Ann. Intern. Med.* **95**:733–735, 1981.
21. Physical examination of school children. *Boston Med. Surg. J.* **152**:587, 1905.
22. Gould, G. M.: A system of personal biologic examinations: The condition of adequate medical and scientific condult of life. *JAMA* **35**:134–137, 1900.
23. Edie, E. B.: Health examinations past and present and their practice in Pennsylvania. *Am. J. Public Health* **15**:602–606, 1925.
24. Croft, B. P.: Benefit of physical examinations. *Boston Med. Surg. J.* **174**:814–815, 1916.
25. Tobey, J. A.: The health examination movement. *National Health* **5**:610–611, 1923.
26. Emerson, H.: The protection of health through periodic medical examinations. *J. Michigan Med. Soc.* **21**:399–403, 1922.
27. President's Commission on the Health Needs of the Nation: *Building America's Health, A Report to the President*, Vol. 1. US Government Printing Office, Washington, DC, 1978.
28. Dales, L. G., Friedman, G. D., and Collen, M. F.: Evaluating periodic multiphasic health checkups: A controlled trial. Kaiser Foundation Research Institue and Permanente Medical Group. *J. Chronic Dis.* **132**:385–404, 1979.
29. Frame, P. S., and Carlson, S. J.: A critical review of periodic health screening using specific screening criteria. *J. Fam. Pract.* **75**(2):29–36, 123–129, 189–194, 1975.
30. Breslow, L., and Somers, A. R.: The lifetime health-monitoring program. A practice approach to preventive medicine. *N. Engl. J. Med.* **206**:601–608, 1977.
31. American Cancer Society report on the cancer-related health check-up. *CA* **30**:194–240, 1980.
32. Fletcher, S.: The peridic health examination and internal medicine. *Ann. Intern. Med.* **101**:866–868, 1984.
33. Health and Policy Committee, American College of Physicians: The use of diagnostic tests for screening and evaluating breast lesions. *Ann. Intern. Med.* **103**:143–146, 1985.
34. Baker, L. H.: Breast Cancer Detection Demonstration Project: Five-year summary report. *CA* **32**:194–226, 1982.
35. Shapiro, S.: Evidence on screening for breast cancer from a randomized trial. *Cancer* **39**(suppl):2772–2782, 1977.
36. American Cancer Society statement on mammography, 1982. *CA* **32**:226–230, 1982.
37. Shapiro, S.: Screening for early detection of cancer and heart disease. *Bull, NY Acad. Med.* **51**:80–95, 1975.

38. Gnauck, R., Macrae, F. A., and Fleisher, M.: How to perform the fecal occult blood test. *CA* **34:**134–147, 1984.
39. Crespi, M., Weissman, G., Gilbertsen, V. A., *et al.:* The role of proctosigmoidoscopy in screening for colorectal neoplasia. *CA* **34:**158–166, 1984.
40. Tunbridge, W. M. G., Everd, D. C., Hall, R., *et al.:* The spectrum of thyroid disease in a community: The Whickhams survey. *Clin. Endocrinol.* **7:**481–493, 1977.

Index